Contributors

MARK S. ATKINS, Children's Seashore House, and University of Pennsylvania School of Medicine, Philadelphia, Pennsylvania 19104

SUSAN E. BARKER, Department of Psychology, Louisiana State University, Baton Rouge, Louisiana 70803-5501

JUDITH V. BECKER, Department of Psychiatry, University of Arizona College of Medicine, Tucson, Arizona 85724

KIM BROWN, Children's Seashore House, and University of Pennsylvania School of Medicine, Philadelphia, Pennsylvania 19104

JAMES E. BRYAN, Department of Medical Psychology, Oregon Health Sciences University, Portland, Oregon 97201-3098

PAUL M. CINCIRIPINI, Department of Psychiatry and Behavioral Sciences, University of Texas Medical Branch, Galveston, Texas 77550

KARLA J. DOEPKE, Department of Psychiatry and Behavioral Sciences, Emory University College of Medicine, Grady Memorial Hospital, Atlanta, Georgia 30335

MINA K. DULCAN, Department of Child Psychiatry, Children's Memorial Hospital, Division of Child and Adolescent Psychiatry, Northwestern University School of Medicine, Chicago, Illinois 60614

MORRIS EAGLE, The Ontario Institute for Studies in Education, Toronto, Ontario M5S 1V6, Canada

JENNIFER L. EDENS, Department of Psychology, West Virginia University, Morgantown, West Virginia 26506

JOSHUA EHRLICH, Department of Psychiatry, University of Michigan, Ann Arbor, Michigan 48104

PAUL M. G. EMMELKAMP, Department of Clinical Psychology, Academic Hospital, 9713 EZ Groningen, The Netherlands

HAROLD M. ERICKSON, JR., Department of Psychiatry, University of Kansas Medical Center, Kansas City, Kansas 66160

v

CYRIL M. FRANKS, Graduate School of Applied and Professional Psychology, Rutgers University, The State University of New Jersey, Piscataway, New Jersey 08855

GERALD GOLDSTEIN, Highland Drive VA Hospital, Pittsburgh, Pennsylvania 15206

DONALD W. GOODWIN, Department of Psychiatry, University of Kansas Medical Center, Kansas City, Kansas 66160

ALAN M. GROSS, Department of Psychology, University of Mississippi, University, Mississippi 38677

MEG S. KAPLAN, New York State Psychiatric Institute, College of Physicians and Surgeons, Columbia University, New York, New York 10032

NADINE J. KASLOW, Department of Psychiatry and Behavioral Sciences, Emory University School of Medicine, Grady Memorial Hospital, Atlanta, Georgia 30335

DEBORAH A. KEOGH, Department of Psychology, University of Notre Dame, Notre Dame, Indiana 46556

LYNN KERN KOEGEL, Autism Research Center, Graduate School of Education, University of California, Santa Barbara, California 93106

ROBERT L. KOEGEL, Autism Research Center, Graduate School of Education, University of California, Santa Barbara, California 93106

KEVIN T. LARKIN, Department of Psychology, West Virginia University, Morgantown, West Virginia 26506

INGRID N. LECKLITER, Department of Medical Psychology, Oregon Health Sciences University, Portland, Oregon 97201

HOWARD D. LERNER, Department of Psychiatry, University of Michigan, Ann Arbor, Michigan 48104

JOSEPH D. MATARAZZO, Department of Medical Psychology, Oregon Health Sciences University, Portland, Oregon 97201

F. DUDLEY McGLYNN, Department of Psychology, Auburn University, Auburn, Alabama 36849-5214

PATRICK W. McGUFFIN, Hahnemann University, Philadelphia, Pennsylvania 19102-1192

PARAS MEHTA, Department of Psychology, University of Houston, Houston, Texas 77204-5341

CYNTHIA L. MILLER, Department of Psychology, University of Notre Dame, Notre Dame, Indiana 46556

J. SCOTT MIZES, Department of Psychiatry, MetroHealth Medical Center, Case Western Reserve University School of Medicine, Cleveland, Ohio 44109

RANDALL L. MORRISON, Response Analysis Corporation, Princeton, New Jersey 08542

MARY F. O'CALLAGHAN, Department of Psychology, University of Notre Dame, Notre Dame, Indiana 46556

KEVIN JOHN O'CONNOR, California School of Professional Psychology, Fresno, California 93721

TIMOTHY J. O'FARRELL, Department of Psychiatry, Harvard Medical School, Boston, Massachusetts 02115, and Veterans Affairs Medical Center, Brockton and West Roxbury, Massachusetts 02401

GARY R. RACUSIN, Connecticut Mental Health Center, Yale University, New Haven, Connecticut 06516

MARK D. RAPPORT, Department of Psychology, University of Hawaii, Honolulu, Hawaii 96822

LYNN P. REHM, Department of Psychology, University of Houston, Houston, Texas 77204-5341

CYD C. STRAUSS, Center for Children and Families, Gainesville, Florida 32606

MARTA C. VALDEZ-MENCHACA, Autism Research Center, Graduate School of Education, University of California, Santa Barbara, California 93106

PATRICIA VAN OPPEN, Department of Psychiatry, Valeriuskliniek, 1075 BG Amsterdam, The Netherlands

STACI VERON-GUIDRY, Department of Psychology, Louisiana State University, Baton Rouge, Louisiana 70803-5501

THOMAS L. WHITMAN, Department of Psychology, University of Notre Dame, Notre Dame, Indiana 46556

ARTHUR N. WIENS, Department of Medical Psychology, Oregon Health Sciences University, Portland, Oregon 97201-3098

MARK C. WILDE, Department of Physical Medicine and Rehabilitation, Baylor College of Medicine, and The Institute for Rehabilitation and Research, Houston, Texas 77030

MARK A. WILLIAMS, Department of Psychology, University of Mississippi, University, Mississippi 38677

DONALD A. WILLIAMSON, Department of Psychology, Louisiana State University, Baton Rouge, Louisiana 70803-5501

DAVID WOLITZKY, The Ontario Institute for Studies in Education, Toronto, Ontario M5S 1V6, Canada

ELIZABETH WOLLHEIM, California School of Professional Psychology, Fresno, California 93721

Preface

Although senior undergraduate psychology students and first year master's- and doctoral-level students frequently take courses in advanced abnormal psychology, it has been almost two decades since a book by this title has appeared. Professors teaching this course have had a wide variety of texts to select from that touch on various aspects of psychopathology, but none has been as comprehensive for the student as the present volume. Not only are basic concepts and models included, but there are specific sections dealing with childhood and adolescent disorders, adult and geriatric disorders, child treatment, and adult treatment. We believe the professor and advanced student alike will benefit from having all the requisite material under one cover.

Our book contains 26 chapters presented in five parts, each part preceded by an editors' introduction. The chapters reflect updates in the classification of disorders (i.e., DSM-IV). In Part I (Basic Concepts and Models), the chapters include diagnosis and classification, assessment strategies, research methods, the psychoanalytic model, the behavioral model, and the biological model. Parts II (Childhood and Adolescent Disorders) and III (Adult and Older Adult Disorders), each containing seven chapters, represent the bulk of the book. To ensure cross-chapter consistency, each of these chapters on psychopathology follows an identical format, with the following basic sections: description of the disorder, epidemiology, clinical picture (with case description), course and prognosis, familial and genetic patterns, and diagnostic considerations. Parts IV and V—on Child Treatment and Adult Treatment, respectively—each contain three chapters that deal with the major modes of therapy: dynamic psychotherapy, behavior therapy, and pharmacological interventions. Thus, the student will gain an understanding not only of childhood and adult psychopathology, but of the existing strategies for remediation of such psychopathology as well.

Many individuals have contributed to the fruition of our efforts here. First, we thank our eminent contributors, who took time out from their busy schedules to partake in this project. We thank Burt G. Bolton, as well, for his technical expertise with respect to the manuscript. Finally, but hardly least, we again thank our friend and editor at Plenum, Eliot Werner, who appreciated the timeliness of our project.

VINCENT B. VAN HASSELT
MICHEL HERSEN

Fort Lauderdale, Florida

Contents

Part II. Childhood and Adolescent Disorders

Part III. Adult and Older Adult Disorders

Part IV. Child Treatment

Part V. Adult Treatment

I

Basic Concepts and Models: Introductory Comments

Over time the discipline of abnormal psychology has become more complex, particularly as it adduces data from its sister disciplines, such as epidemiology, genetics, sociology, anthropology, and biology. Adding to such complexity is the status of theory in this area. The absence of theoretical unity is especially striking, given the distinct, and, at times, contradictory expositions from those of psychoanalytic, behavioral, and biological persuasions. But in spite of such complexity and contradiction, there are some very basic data that the student of abnormal psychology must learn, and these are concerned with diagnosis and classification, assessment strategies, and research methods. Moreover, the student should be familiar with the three basic models of abnormal behavior: psychoanalytic, behavioral, and biological. Part I of this book, therefore, is devoted to an outline of these basic issues and models.

Ingrid Leckliter and Joseph D. Matarazzo, in Chapter 1, consider the various paradigms of psychopathology leading to the *Diagnostic and Statistical Manual of Mental Disorders*, or DSM, and its most recent revisions, DSM-III-R and DSM-IV. They point out that the advent of both specific criteria for categories and structured interviewing techniques have contributed to improvements in diagnostic reliability. In turn, greater diagnostic specificity has resulted in improvements in therapeutic technology. In Chapter 2, which is on assessment strategies, Arthur N. Weins and James E. Bryan examine the referrals for psychological assessment, intellectual and behavioral evaluation and report different kinds of assessment strategies used and ways of obtaining information from family members and other collaterals. As in the previous chapter, the value of structured interviewing is underscored. In Chapter 3, F. Dudley McGlynn outlines the research methods carried out to study the numerous aspects of psychopathology. In addition to considering science and explanation in psychopathology and validity in research on psychopathology, McGlynn describes in detail research on etiology and on intervention.

Howard D. Lerner and Joshua Ehrlich, in Chapter 4, introduce the reader to psychoanalytic theory, and trace historically its developments, since Freud, into

1

the various "overlapping models of the mind." Three primary models are presented: modern structural theory, self psychology, and object relations theory. The authors document how each of the models has its unique focus on personality, development, psychopathology, and therapy. The behavioral model of psychopathology in articulated by Cyril M. Franks in Chapter 5. Examined from its somewhat simplistic beginnings to its much more highly sophisticated present, the underpinnings of the approach are identified. Most important in this chapter is Frank's debunking of the popular albeit erroneous notions still held about behavior therapy. In Chapter 6, the last one in this section, Mark C. Wilde and Paul Cinciripini look at the biological model of psychopathology. In so doing, they describe the genetic model, biochemical determinants, gross brain anatomy and psychopathology, and neuroendocrine functions, disease, and stress. The exciting developments in this intriguing area, in part a function of improved scientific technology, are highlighted throughout this chapter.

Diagnosis and Classification

INGRID N. LECKLITER AND JOSEPH D. MATARAZZO

INTRODUCTION

Almost one third of all individuals who are 18 years or older and live in the United States have experienced, at some time in their lives, an alcohol-abuse, substance-abuse, or mental disorder. In any 1-month period, three of 20 adults living in the United States experience these disorders. When alcohol or substance abuse is excluded from these statistics, the lifetime prevalence for mental disorders is 23%; the 1-month prevalence is 13%. These statistics are reported in the recent National Institute of Mental Health (NIMH) Epidemiologic Catchment Area (ECA) survey, which is the largest, population-based survey of the incidence of mental and substance-abuse disorders among individuals 18 years and older who live in the United States (Regier et al., 1990). Some readers may find these statistics even more striking when they consider that the disorders reflected in this survey are severe conditions, such as schizophrenia, organic brain disorders, depression, and incapacitating anxiety. The statistics exclude millions of Americans who experience disorders of psychological or psychophysiological function, such as depersonalization disorders, disorders of impulse control (e.g., pathological gambling), chronic pain, Type A behavior, sexual disorders, and those individuals who experience dysfunction associated with life crises (e.g., death of a loved one, divorce, or sexual assault). These statistics do not reflect the incidence of mental disorders in childhood and adolescence. Nor does their summary here reflect the wide variability of incidence across factors such as geographic region, socioeconomic status, gender, or ethnicity.

INGRID N. LECKLITER AND JOSEPH D. MATARAZZO • Department of Medical Psychology, Oregon Health Sciences University, Portland, Oregon 97201.

Advanced Abnormal Psychology, edited by Vincent B. Van Hasselt and Michel Hersen. Plenum Press, New York, 1994.

INGRID N.
LECKLITER and
JOSEPH D.
MATARAZZO

Nevertheless, the NIMH ECA survey is important for several reasons. From a practical or applied perspective, relatively dependable statistics are important to developing public policy and to allocating limited public and private resources for human services. From a scientific perspective, when compared with earlier studies, the NIMH ECA survey reflects significant advances in the epidemiology of mental and substance-abuse disorders. Of utmost relevance to this chapter is the advance made because trained interviewers used a standard, highly structured interview instrument [the Diagnostic Interview Schedule (DIS)] to identify disorders. Prior to the NIMH ECA survey, prevalence data varied quite a bit among different studies because different subsamples of the population were examined (e.g., only hospitalized individuals) and different classification schemes were used to define and identify disorders.

The current classification schemes are important because they aim to minimize the problems and inconsistencies found with the idiosyncratic ways disorders were defined and identified among earlier epidemiological investigations. These schemes attempt to describe patterns of internal and external behaviors in ways that reflect the "truth" (i.e., are valid) and in ways that are dependable across clinicians (i.e., are reliable). As suggested above, classification schemes are practical from the point of view of policymakers. They are also practical from the perspectives of researchers who study human behavior, practitioners who offer treatment for disordered behavior, and individuals who experience behavioral problems. Classification schemes provide a basic terminology that facilitates communication and retrieval of information among researchers and other professionals. Classification schemes also guide the development of theories or models of human behavior. These models organize and focus efforts at determining the causes of disordered behavior, predicting future behavior, and developing treatments. The classification and diagnosis of disorders also guide treatment and prognostic decisions. Finally, the economic ramifications of classification are apparent in light of the fact that a diagnosis is required before health insurance companies will reimburse individuals who receive services for mental illness and disordered behavior.

This introductory chapter provides the reader an overview of the history, progress, and issues associated with the diagnosis of behavioral and mental disorders. Three basic premises form its foundation. The first premise reflects the fact that human psychopathology is multidetermined and consequently is understood from a variety of conceptual models or "paradigms." The classification schemes or categories suggested by these paradigms are not proven, tangible entities. Instead, these schemes remain conceptual prototypes that have utility in their ability to further the scientific and clinical understanding of how humans function mentally, emotionally, and behaviorally (Klerman, 1986).

The second premise reflects a phenomenon that is common to scientific endeavors, namely, improvements in measurement technologies often precede changes in conceptual paradigms and scientific advancement. Similarly, advances in the field of mental health and psychopathology have resulted from improvements in our ability to reliably identify conditions or components of conditions that deviate from normal. Further advances toward understanding the etiology and the treatment of these conditions are tied to progress in their reliable identification and objective characterization.

The third premise is that the reliability and validity of diagnostic classification may be evaluated by three standards: strict psychometrics, clinical utility, or progress in the field. When each of these three standards is considered in light of the first two premises described above, it becomes apparent that the diagnosis and classification of human psychopathology are tenable.

PARADIGMS OF PSYCHOPATHOLOGY

Currently in the United States there is no single, dominant model of human psychopathology. The existing models can be conceptualized as broadly falling into two camps, based on a fundamental assumption concerning the nature of psychopathology. One camp postulates that psychopathologies are discrete, categorical entities that are either present or absent, with mutually exclusive boundaries. For example, in medicine, although both affect the lungs, pneumonia and lung cancers are mutually exclusive conditions. That is, their classification boundaries do not overlap because of their different etiologies.

The second camp postulates that psychopathologies represent a continuum of symptoms that all individuals have to one quantifiable degree or another. For example, all individuals have experienced shyness; yet, only some have experienced it so intensely that they are unable to leave their homes for months at a time. In this quantitative model, psychopathologies need not be mutually exclusive, and the boundaries of disorders may overlap.

Current paradigms of psychopathology can also be distinguished by their perspectives on the presumed etiology of mental and emotional disorders. Some paradigms do not have underlying assumptions about etiology. The *multivariate statistical approach* is a good example. This paradigm is not based on presumptions about etiology, but instead attempts to categorize and understand psychopathologies by determining clusters of interrelated behaviors via statistical methods. The paradigm advanced by the neo-Kraepelinian movement, considered the vanguard of the American Psychiatric Association's *Diagnostic and Statistical Manual of Mental Disorders*, and its subsequent revisions (DSM-III, DSM-III-R, and DSM-IV, respectively), represents the primary assumption of a *biological basis* to psychopathology. The *genetic paradigm* represents a classic example of such a presumed biological etiology of psychopathologies. Yet, empirical evidence also exists that *environmental factors* are associated with the occurrence of psychopathology. The *social learning paradigm* exemplifies this view of etiology. Despite the seeming exclusiveness of these paradigms, much of the current literature when taken as a whole reveals that multiple factors contribute to the etiology of psychopathology. In recognition of this multiplicity, the task forces that developed the DSM-III, DSM-III-R, and DSM-IV attempted to avoid paradigmatic biases and aimed to develop a "nondoctrinaire, empirically based" diagnostic manual (Million, 1986). The DSM-III-R represents the current scheme used in the United States for classifying and diagnosing conditions of disordered behaviors, emotions, and/or mental status. DSM-IV, which should be available in May, 1994, further revises DSM-III-R and is compatible with the tenth revision of the International Classification of Diseases (ICD-10), developed by the World Health Organization. Consequently, international and U.S. classification schemes will be quite similar. A brief review of the history of psychiatric and psychological diagnosis follows to provide a basis for understanding the current status of this manual.

INGRID N.
LECKLITER and
JOSEPH D.
MATARAZZO

The word diagnosis is derived from the Greek preposition *dia* (apart) and *gnosis* (to perceive or to know). Thus, knowing the nature of a condition requires being able to separate it from other conditions. Evidence exists that as early as 2600 B.C. attempts were made to differentiate patterns of disordered behavior. The patterns identified at that early era were most consistent with patterns that today are called Major Depressive Episode: Melancholic Type, and Conversion Disorder. Although global classifications of disordered behavior have been evident throughout subsequent eras, the advent of the mental health sciences is a relatively new phenomenon that dates to the early part of this century.

During the early 1940s to mid-1970s, diagnosis and classification were initially of minor concern to mental health experts in this country. Throughout this period, psychoanalytic therapy was generally considered the primary treatment method for *all* conditions. Accordingly, diagnostic distinctions were deemed academic since in practice, psychoanalytic therapy was the treatment of choice and different interventions were generally unavailable (Klerman, 1986). Additionally, manuals that were then in existence for the classification of mental disorders were found incomplete and insufficient to diagnose the array of psychological difficulties, such as psychosomatic disorders seen by military mental health professionals who practiced during the World War II era (Millon, 1986).

The classification and diagnosis of mental health disorders were also de-emphasized during this era because empirical evidence demonstrated little agreement among professionals who diagnosed the same individual. Based on this evidence, the logical argument could be made that diagnostic classification was an unreliable exercise. Perhaps diagnoses were unreliable because the categories were not real conditions but were idiosyncratic constructs shaped by the diagnosticians' own experiential and cultural biases. However, as will be discussed below, it was equally possible that diagnostic unreliability stemmed from the varying and unsystematic methods used to arrive at diagnoses (Matarazzo, 1983).

Further, during the 1960s and 1970s, forces within the school of Humanistic Psychology argued against the classification of mental disorders. This argument was based on the contention that diagnostic classification was an instrument of social control, reflecting the status quo as established by the dominant class. Moreover, it was argued that such systems of classification failed to accept and promote diversity among human beings as desirable, if not at least acceptable (Gergen, 1991).

In the mid-1970s, three factors overrode these arguments against classification and led to a resurgence of interest in the classification and diagnosis of mental health disorders (Klerman, 1986). One of these was the advent of psychometric assessments of personality, behavior, and symptoms, such as with personality inventories (e.g., the Minnesota Multiphasic Personality Inventory) or rating scales (e.g., the Beck Depression Inventory). The concurrent development of high-speed computers facilitated the analysis of large sets of data gathered from multiple sources and methods. Advances in the treatment of mental health disorders with psychopharmacologic and other modalities also contributed to the resurgence of interest in diagnosis and classification. Unlike in earlier decades when professionals had only one choice of treatment for all conditions (psychoanalytic therapy), in the mid-1970s professionals began to recognize the utility of matching diagnostic conditions with treatment modalities (e.g., behavior therapy for treating phobias and tricyclic medication for treating depression).

DSM-III: Its Predecessors and Revisions

DSM-III is truly unique for several reasons (Klerman, 1986; Millon, 1986). When published in 1980, it was the first official system of nomenclature field-tested for reliability by its intended audience in its intended arena of use. It describes "specific and uniform rules of definition" for inclusion and exclusion within a diagnostic category (Millon, 1986, p. 52). Previous psychiatric diagnostic schemes did not provide specific criteria and allowed each clinician to idiosyncratically define the boundaries of diagnostic conditions. This allowance contributed markedly to unreliable diagnoses between clinicians described earlier in this chapter. The authors of the DSM-III also recognized the multiplicity of etiological factors that might result in the presence of a mental disorder and thus attempted to avoid promulgating specific etiological assumptions regarding the conditions described. Theoretical doctrine and bias (i.e., psychoanalytic) is quite evident, however, in earlier DSMs.

The DSM-III (1980) and its 1987 and 1993 revisions also are unique because they code mental disorders (Axis I) and provide additional axes to code broader aspects of peoples' lives, including personality or developmental disorders (Axis II), general medical conditions (Axis III), type and severity of psychosocial or environmental stressors (Axis IV), and highest level of adaptive functioning in the last year (Axis V). In parallel with the nondoctrinaire stance taken by DSM-III's authors, this reconceptualization of the diagnostic process also recognizes the multiplicity of factors that impact the individual's presentation and thus, the diagnostic picture.

Future revisions of the DSM will rely on accumulating empirical evidence to further refine diagnostic criteria. These criteria will likely use multiple methods of assessment such as schemes that quantify symptoms, and procedures that identify or quantify biological markers (among disorders where such markers are recognized). In addition, dimensions such as psychosocial situations (people behave differently in different settings) and interpersonal style may be incorporated into future revisions (Millon, 1986). Ultimately, the ideal goal is to produce a manual that associates diagnostic conditions with empirically validated treatment approaches.

"Project Flower," named after Chairman Mao's declaration to "Let all flowers bloom," was an apparently frustrating attempt to produce just such a document. As described by Millon (1986), an invitation was extended from the DSM-III Task Force to a broad array of professionals of different theoretical orientations to "systematize their knowledge and technology in a manner relevant to diagnosis" (p. 58). The results were decidedly disappointing and were described as follows:

> Most members thought it best that Project Flower be allowed simply to wilt; one primary reviewer was more blatantly sarcastic, recommending that it "be sprayed with a potent herbicide" . . . The Task Force simply could not put its stamp of approval on such pretensions to therapeutic infallibility (p. 58).

Fortunately, as will be described later in the chapter, much greater optimism exists today for the eventual completion of just such a project that will be based on empirical demonstrations of specific treatment efficacy for different diagnostic conditions.

Definition of Mental Disorders

As clearly stated in the DSM-III-R, "no definition adequately specifies precise boundaries for the concept 'mental disorder'" (p. xxii). However, several significant factors are usually considered in attempts to grapple with defining this dynamic, multifaceted concept. One factor is that the *individual* must experience a painful symptom *or* impairment in one or more important areas of functioning (e.g., employment, interpersonal relationships) before a mental disorder can be diagnosed. An additional factor has to do with the recognition that while social values are intertwined with contemporary definitions of what is and what is not beyond the range of normal, mental disorders are manifested dysfunctions within the person and are not dysfunctions associated with conflicts between the individual and societal systems. Thus, for example, the DSM-III eliminated homosexuality as a mental illness unless the individual explicitly stated a desire for heterosexual relationships and that the homosexual orientation was unwanted and a persistent source of distress. In this instance, the diagnosis of "Ego-dystonic Homosexuality" would be considered. However, the diagnosis would be inappropriate among individuals who had no desire for heterosexual relationships and were early in the process of adjusting to transitory distress or discomfort associated with their recently discovered or disclosed sexual preference. The DSM-III-R went even further in response to the complex web of social values and empirical data surrounding homosexual behavior and totally eliminated the label of homosexuality. Instead, the diagnosis of "Sexual Disorder Not Otherwise Specified" is reserved for those individuals with persistent and marked distress about their sexual orientation. DSM-IV has elaborated further on societal systems and psychopathology by introducing an Appendix of syndromes that are unique to only a few of the world's societies (e.g., amok).

In summary, although attempts to identify and distinguish patterns of human suffering and mental disorder are quite ancient, attempts to define these patterns in a more reliable and standardized manner are relatively recent. The current diagnostic system that is used in the United States is unique in that it has operationalized the inclusionary and exclusionary criteria used to define the presence of a mental disorder and in that it has sustained working trials in its intended arena of use. The DSM-III and DSM-III-R reflect attempts to be sensitive to the multiplicity of factors that contribute to the manifestation of a mental disorder in the individual and also to the complexity of social values that contribute to the definition of mental disorders. Although one of the ideal goals of the DSM-III task force, namely pairing treatment with diagnostic conditions, was not realized, current research suggests more optimism that this goal will be realized in the near future.

APPRAISAL OF THE CURRENT SCHEME FOR THE CLASSIFICATION OF MENTAL DISORDERS

What are the qualities of a good classification and diagnostic system? Most experts agree that a good classification system must possess the following qualities: (a) the features of the disorder must be clearly described and defined, preferably in a fashion that is based on observable information gathered from multiple methods of assessment; (b) the features of the disorder should cluster together and covary across situations; (c) disorders should be reliably identified (i.e., two clinicians should arrive at the same diagnosis for the same case) and should be relatively stable over time; (d) the different disorders should be distinguishable from each other and should represent valid constructs as demonstrated by disparate etiologies, differential response to various treatment modalities, and/ or distinct courses; and (e) the classification system should be sufficiently complete so as to describe all mental disorders in the most parsimonious fashion.

In actuality however, several of these qualities receive most of the attention. These are the qualities of reliability and validity of diagnosis. Before each of these qualities is addressed in turn, however, it will be helpful for the reader to remember one of the underlying premises of this chapter. Specifically, the categories suggested by the DSM-III and its revisions are useful conceptual prototypes rather than proven, tangible entities. In light of this premise, and the nature of progress in science, the categories as they are currently conceptualized probably do not represent final classifications. Accordingly, "literal identification . . ." of a mental disorder ". . : with its currently accepted signs and symptoms . . ." is overly simplistic (Meehl, 1986, p. 222).

By illustration, a parallel can be drawn with the development of biological classification. In this system, classification is based on orderly principles that define categories in a hierarchical manner (i.e., kingdom, phylum, class, order, family, genus, species). Species represent the most specific categorical level, while genus and family represent broader classifications. This hierarchical arrangement was recognized intuitively even before specific labels were proposed. Nevertheless, acceptable definitions of categories hinged on the development of a general theory of biology, namely, the theory of evolution, and on more recent advances in molecular biology. In light of the current state of the art and science of psychopathology, which lacks a unified general theory, it is clear that the diagnostic categories represented in the DSM-III and DSM-III-R are not yet sufficiently specific to fall at the species level (Blashfield, 1984).

The work of Cloninger, Bohman, and Sigvardsson (1981) provides an excellent example of the fact that current diagnostic categories are relatively more global, rather than specific classifications of mental disorders. These investigators identified two distinct subgroups of alcoholics who differed primarily in terms of biological risk factors. One group of individuals, labeled "milieu-limited," were the offspring of parents with patterns of mild alcohol abuse and minimal criminality. The second group of individuals, labeled "male-limited," were the offspring of relationships between a normal woman and a man who had both severe alcohol abuse and severe criminality. Environmental risk factors such as being adopted away at a late age or being raised by adoptive parents of lower socioeconomic strata, interacted to produce different outcomes among these two groups. Men among the milieu-limited group who experienced environmental risk were two times more likely to develop alcoholism than men who did not experience these environmental risk factors. In contrast, when compared with men who did not have the same biological risk, men among the male-limited group were nine times more likely to develop alcoholism, regardless of their exposure to environmental risks. Thus, although both groups fit within the more general category of alcoholism, the two subgroups likely reflect different etiological processes with differing prognoses, and likely require disparate treatment strategies. By analogy, using the model of biological classification, the diagnosis of alcoholism would be inaccurately placed at the species level, and probably more accurately placed at the level of genus. Continuing with the analogy, substance addictions in general might fit the more superordinate level of classification, namely, family.

Systems that classify mental disorders have yet to develop concepts analogous to the biological classificatory concepts of kingdom, phylum, class, order, family, genus, and species (Blashfield, 1984). As was true in biology, the development and refinement of hierarchical organizing concepts in the field of psychopathology are tied with progress toward the development of a unified paradigm of psychopathology and more generally of human behavior. Until such unified paradigms are manifest, the appraisal of current diagnostic schemes from the perspective of fine-grained, psychometric analyses of reliability and validity will produce inexact results. Metaphorically, such analyses are reminiscent of attempts to use a fine-toothed comb to groom the muddied and matted fur of a golden retriever just back from a romp in the marshes. This coarse chore would be more effectively accomplished with a wider-toothed comb. The following sections survey the current state of diagnosing mental disorders from the fine-grained perspectives of psychometric properties, such as reliability and validity, as well as from the wider-grained perspectives of progress in the field.

How Reliable Is Psychiatric Diagnosis across Clinicians?

As mentioned previously in this chapter, pre-1950 criticisms against the diagnosis of mental disorders pointed to the poor-to-mediocre levels of diagnostic agreement between clinicians who examined the same individual. Experts argued that diagnoses were unreliable classifications because rather than reflecting true, tangible entities, they reflected the current or idiosyncratic world views of the individuals who made them. A related argument that was offered less often, but was equally plausible, was that diagnoses were unreliable because the processes of making them were unstandardized and varied across clinicians. Thus clinicians, guided by their differing world views and theoretical orientations, might gather certain types of information concerning the individual but neglect to gather (or fail to give credence to) other types of information. As a consequence, the resulting diagnostic judgments would be inconsistent across clinicians (i.e., unreliable).

Contemporary re-analyses of Sigmund Freud's case histories provide a prime example of how prevailing world views may influence the clinician's selective attention to and conceptualization of data gathered about an individual (Lewis, 1981; Masson, 1984). For example, Dora was an 18-year-old woman who entered treatment with Freud due to depression. While in treatment, she disclosed that her father's colleague, Mr. K, had been harrassing her sexually since she was 14 years old. She had complained to her father but he did not believe her. Subsequently, she turned to her mother and Mrs. K (Dora's close friend) for support. They too were aloof to her concerns. Eventually, Dora discovered that Mrs. K and her father were romantically involved and reasoned that the adults rejected her concerns in order to avoid a confrontation with Mr. K. Understandably, Dora was angered and distressed by her circumstances and the unsupportive attitude of those who were closest to her.

As would most good scientist-clinicians, Freud interviewed collateral sources to determine whether Dora's allegations were true. Although these interviews confirmed her story, Freud did not focus treatment on Dora's legitimate feelings of betrayal and anger. Nor did he help her find ways to cope with what must have been an untenable interpersonal situation. Rather, consistent with the social norms of that era, Freud tacitly colluded with the other adults in Dora's life and denied the reality of her concerns. He interpreted them as fantasized constructions of her own repressed sexuality. This intervention is markedly different from how a clinician would address Dora's concerns today. Yet, this example presents a stark illustration of how cognitive perspectives established by the culture's predominant world view and the clinician's theoretical orientation can direct the conceptualization and classification of an individual's emotional distress. For in fact, at one time, Freud formulated the "seduction hypothesis" based on the stories of other women he treated who, like Dora, disclosed similar experiences. Later he repudiated this hypothesis and developed his theory of sexual repression. Masson (1984) suggested that this repudiation stemmed from Freud's desire for professional acceptance. His nineteenth century, Victorian era, Viennese colleagues had dismissed the earlier hypothesis that associated patients' impaired mental health and their earlier sexual victimization or abuse.

Many experts now recognize that scientific endeavors, such as the work of Freud, are influenced by scientists' world views and their location in time and place (Bevan, 1991). Methods of observation and data collection are similarly influenced. For example, historically in psychology and psychiatry, the interview was the observational method of choice, particularly in light of the absence of biological markers for mental disorders. Yet, in the late 1940s through the 1960s, clinicians with seemingly similar professional training and allegiance to the same diagnostic classification system demonstrated limited interclinician reliability based on diagnostic interviews of the same individual. This unreliability likely stemmed from several factors: (a) clinicians elicited different data based on different interviews, (b) clinicians differentially attended to and weighted data based on their own idiosyncratic clinical biases, and (c) clinicians differed in how they chose to operationalize diagnostic categories.

The advent in the 1970s, of structured diagnostic interviews combined with explicit operational definitions of diagnostic categories minimized these three factors and significantly enhanced the reliability of diagnosis. For example, studies conducted before the 1970s revealed average interclinician agreement (i.e., reliability) across diagnostic categories that ranged from kappa coefficients (which control for chance agreements between clinicians) of 0.33 to 0.77. Among these studies, the median kappa coefficient was 0.53. However, with the advent of structured diagnostic interviews and more specific operational criteria used in DSM-III, these reliabilities improved to kappas that ranged from 0.36 to 0.93. Among these later studies, the median kappa coefficient was between 0.73 and 0.79 (Matarazzo, 1983). Accordingly, Matarazzo concluded that the reliability coefficients for psychiatric diagnoses formulated from data obtained by standardized interviews and operational definitions of diagnostic categories "are at levels which traditionally have characterized the best psychological tests from the psychometric standpoint" (p. 115).

Although ample evidence exists that diagnostic reliability is enhanced by the use of structured interviews *and* operational definitions of diagnostic categories, the DSM-III and DSM-III-R provide the latter but not the former. Accordingly,

INGRID N.
LECKLITER and
JOSEPH D.
MATARAZZO

interclinician reliabilities using only these operational definitions are somewhat lower (kappa coefficients in the 0.70s among adults and in the 0.50s among children) than in the investigations previously cited that used both operational definitions and diagnostic interviews. Inasmuch as current diagnostic categories are still evolving conceptual prototypes, it is probably wise that the diagnostic criteria actually used in practice (i.e., DSM-III and DSM-III-R) are made more flexible than criteria from interview schedules. This flexibility recognizes that although reliability is desirable, it does not necessarily mirror utility or the correctness of the diagnostic scheme. In other words, high reliability does not guarantee validity. Until the utility and correctness of diagnostic schemes are determined, it appears wise to retain some element of flexibility in how diagnoses are made.

What evidence exists that the diagnosis of mental disorders is useful? Several sources provide evidence for the validity of diagnosis: (a) evidence related to statistically established clusters of behaviors that form a diagnostic condition, (b) evidence related to the etiology of mental disorders, and (c) evidence related to the treatment of specific disorders with specific interventions. Evidence from these three sources has accumulated subsequent to improved technologies of measurement and statistical analysis. Each of these sources for the validity of diagnosis is considered below with illustrations taken from the examples of paradigms of psychopathology introduced earlier in the chapter.

STATISTICALLY ESTABLISHED BEHAVIORAL CLUSTERS AND THE MULTIVARIATE PARADIGM

Multivariate statistical analyses are relatively new to the study of psychopathology and classification, dating back to the mid- to late 1950s. Basically, multivariate statistics use mathematical procedures to analyze intercorrelated data matrices in an effort to derive clusters of similar or related behaviors and symptoms. Multivariate statistical procedures are too complex and numerous to review here. The interested reader is referred to Grove and Andreasen (1986) and Quay (1986) for introductory articles about these procedures as they relate to differential diagnosis.

Behavioral clusters suggested by multivariate procedures may be used to develop new classification schemes or to mathematically validate existing schemes. The present chapter focuses on the latter mathematical validation of current diagnostic classifications. Quay (1986) provided an example of this focus when he compared the major DSM-III diagnostic categories of mental disorders evident in childhood with the results of multivariate statistical studies. He reviewed 61 multivariate studies that described various patterns of childhood disorders and summarized the disorders along eight dimensions: Undersocialized aggressive conduct disorder, socialized aggressive conduct disorder, attention deficit disorder, anxiety-withdrawal-dysphoria, unresponsive schizoid-disorder, social ineptness, psychotic disorder, and motor overactivity. Although there were "many more DSM-III disorders than there [were] empirically derived dimensions" (Quay, 1986, p. 18), clear counterparts were established between several disorders and dimensions. Specifically, the following DSM-III disorders had good association with empirically derived dimensions: attention deficit disorder with and without motor overactivity, undersocialized and socialized aggressive conduct disorders, anxiety disorder, and schizoid disorder. However, Quay added that clinically accepted disorders such as pervasive developmental disorder and the subtypes of anxiety disorders (e.g., separation anxiety disorder) await further empirical validation.

Literature regarding the empirical validation of adult mental disorders based on multivariate statistics has yet to be reviewed as comprehensively as Quay's summary of the child literature. The reader though, is referred to Andreasen and Grove (1982) and Cloninger, Bohman, and Sigvardsson (1981) for examples of multivariate empirical validations of depression and alcoholism, respectively.

In summary, multivariate statistical procedures provide a relatively new and sophisticated way to validate current diagnostic categories without making assumptions as to etiology. Evidence is available from literature on both child and adult disorders that certain diagnostic classifications are indeed valid constructs.

THE ETIOLOGY OF MENTAL DISORDERS: EXAMPLES FROM GENETIC AND SOCIAL LEARNING PARADIGMS

Although mathematical validation of mental disorders is heuristically useful, the models do not provide the external validation gained from understanding the etiology of mental disorders. The following examples illustrate how investigations into etiology can provide additional validation and information necessary to refine diagnostic groups. Alcohol dependence/abuse and conduct/antisocial personality disorders are offered as examples of two diagnostic groups. These disorders were selected for two reasons: (a) early research that did not distinguish between the two groups resulted in some erroneous conclusions about etiology, and (b) the etiology of these disorders has been investigated from genetic and social learning paradigms. These paradigms were selected for the following reasons: (a) they illustrate how advances in technologies of measurement and data analysis precede advances in paradigm development, and (b) often they are seen as representing opposite poles of the nature–nurture spectrum. In fact, these paradigms are not necessarily mutually exclusive, and their integration one day into a single paradigm will likely facilitate our ultimate understanding of the etiology of mental disorders.

Alcoholism: An Example from the Genetic Paradigm. Genetic bases have been implicated in the differential rates of alcoholism across ethnic groups (Reed, 1985). For example, by using genetic techniques developed in the 1970s, Harada et al. (1982) reported that 44% of the general population of Japan possesses a gene that causes unpleasant biochemical changes associated with alcohol ingestion. These unpleasant changes generally protect the individual against heavy drinking. However, this protective form of the gene is notably infrequent among Japanese individuals who are alcoholic. The relatively recent demonstration of such variations in behavior associated with alternate gene forms at the same chromosomal locus (i.e., allelic variations), has become possible only since the recent advent of genetic markers and linkage studies.

Investigations of twins and the adopted-away offspring of adults who abuse alcohol also provide fairly convincing evidence for the heritability of alcoholism. As described earlier in the chapter, Cloninger et al. (1981) identified two subtypes of alcoholism with differing genetic risks. However, these researchers also documented that environmental factors contributed to whether individuals with differ-

INGRID N.
LECKLITER and
JOSEPH D.
MATARAZZO

ent genetic risks developed alcoholism. Additionally, Heath et al. (1989) studied female identical (monozygotic) and fraternal (dizygotic) twin pairs and demonstrated that marital status buffered the genetic effects of alcohol use among women. Specifically, unmarried women, of both zygosity groups, were at greater risk for heavy alcohol use than were their married cohorts. Obviously these data suggest that genetic studies of behavior and mental disorders must consider both biological and environmental influences. Accordingly, such investigations are quite complex.

Plomin and Rende (1991) reviewed three reasons for this complexity. Behavior is an observable, measurable characteristic or "phenotype," in genetic terminology. This phenotype is more complicated to study than the dichotomous phenotypes of Gregor Mendel's peas (e.g., smooth versus wrinkled) because it is usually quantified on a continuous rather than dichotomous scale, such as smooth or wrinkled. Further, behavior is substantially influenced by the environment and also by many genes, each of which contributes small effects. As a consequence of these factors, investigations into the underlying genetic etiology of mental disorders is extremely complicated. Diagnostic classifications are based on the phenotypic resemblance of patterns or clusters of behaviors (such as in the multivariate approach described above). While these diagnoses may appear similar in phenotype, they may in fact be different disorders in which differing etiological processes affect the same final pathway. Thus, as exemplified in the work of Cloninger and colleagues reviewed above, and the work of Patterson and colleagues reviewed below, the phenotypes for alcoholism and for conduct/antisocial disorders actually may be caused by different genotypes or genotype–environment interactions.

Conduct Disorder and Antisocial Behavior: An Example from the Social Learning Paradigm. Alcoholism occurs frequently among individuals who exhibit persistent patterns of conduct/antisocial behavior (e.g., criminal activity, "conning" others for personal profit or pleasure, reckless disregard for one's own or other's personal safety). Early studies of alcoholics led to the hypothesis that both disorders resulted from the same underlying bioenvironmental processes. However, later investigations demonstrated that alcoholism among individuals with antisocial behaviors is different from alcoholism among individuals for whom alcoholism is the sole diagnosis. Specifically, individuals with the primary diagnosis of alcoholism generally do not demonstrate antisocial behaviors prior to the development of alcoholism. On the other hand, alcohol abuse is just one of the many antisocial behaviors exhibited by individuals with antisocial disorders (Vaillant, 1983).

The research efforts of Gerald Patterson and his colleagues at the Oregon Social Learning Center have contributed to a better understanding of the etiology of antisocial behavior patterns. As in the field of genetics, improved measurement and data analysis technologies facilitated the development of the social learning paradigm, particularly in relation to antisocial behavior patterns. Specifically, Patterson and colleagues developed observational methods that allowed for sequential, interactional, microanalysis and prediction of children's future social behavior (reaction) from adults' antecedent behavior (action) (Patterson, 1982). These fine-grained analyses resulted in a model that has accounted for almost 40% of the variance in children's antisocial behavior patterns among two studied cohorts (Patterson, 1986). This model implicates a direct causal link between inept parental discipline and child antisocial behavior. Explosive discipline, unenforced threats, scolding, and nagging are among some of the adult behaviors that were observed to comprise inept parental discipline. However, child coercion (e.g., when the child's counterattack caused a family member to withdraw), also helped determine inept parental discipline.

Continued research into antisocial behavior has resulted in a developmental model that further implicates inept parenting and a variety of contextual variables (e.g., family stress, such as unemployment or violence) as the first step in a sequence of relatively predictable steps. This pattern is followed by the second step of child conduct problems leading to academic failure, peer rejection, and depression. The third step involves the identification of the academically and socially inept older child or adolescent with a deviant peer group, which facilitates further training of antisocial and delinquent behaviors (Patterson, DeBaryshe, & Ramsey, 1989). Eventually, this model may help identify subtypes of individuals with early patterns of antisocial behaviors who go on to develop adolescent delinquency (about 50% of antisocial children) and eventually become full-blown adult offenders (about 75% of adolescent delinquents). Such etiological subtyping of the relatively more global diagnostic categories of conduct/antisocial disorders will have implications for prognostic and treatment decision making. Eventually, prevention studies that target three factors, namely, effective child behavior management by parents, social skills training for parents and children, and academic remediation for children should help demonstrate the external validity of this model.

The Treatment of Mental Disorders: Example from Unipolar Depression and Attention Deficit Hyperactivity Disorder

As implied in former sections of this chapter, the validity of diagnoses can be established by identifying and matching specific treatments to specific diagnostic conditions. For example, although pharmacotherapy and cognitive-behavioral-interpersonal interventions generally are seen as stemming from different paradigms of psychopathology, each has been evaluated as a treatment strategy for both unipolar depression and attention deficit hyperactivity disorders (ADHD). Hollon, Shelton, and Loosen (1991) reviewed the literature on the efficacy of cognitive therapy versus pharmacotherapy (usually with tricyclics) for the treatment of unipolar depression. They suggested that both approaches, more or less, are equally effective for the treatment of acute depressive episodes. However, individuals who received cognitive therapy during the acute depressive episode (either combined with or in isolation from pharmacotherapy) were less likely to *relapse* after treatment was terminated (21% relapsed in the combined approach and 23% relapsed in the cognitive therapy only approach). Seventy-eight percent of the individuals who received only pharmacotherapy relapsed. Thus, they concluded that specific and successful methods are available for treating individuals with unipolar depression. Nevertheless, Hollon et al. (1991) recommended further research to control for heterogeneity among individuals diagnosed with unipolar depression because some individuals were nonresponsive to pharmacotherapy.

Whalen and Henker (1991) similarly reviewed the literature on various treatment strategies for children with ADHD. They too remarked on the heterogeneity of individuals included within the ADHD diagnostic category and suggested that treatment strategies need to be specified for different child characteristics, such as

INGRID N.
LECKLITER and
JOSEPH D.
MATARAZZO

age or developmental level. For example, they reported that behavioral therapies are more effective when used with younger children than with adolescents. Nevertheless, they reviewed findings that suggested that stimulant pharmacotherapy and behavior therapy (e.g., contingency management) are effective treatments for ADHD.

In summary, current research and practice suggest that different treatment modalities have disparate levels of effectiveness with distinct mental disorders. This evidence provides further validation for the existence of different diagnostic categories. Nevertheless, current diagnostic classes still reflect a great deal of heterogeneity among persons within any given class, and further research is required in order to define the optimal treatment for an individual.

SUMMARY

Specific examples have been used to address broad issues in this chapter on diagnosis and classification. The three broad issues of focus are:

1. Current diagnostic classifications are conceptual prototypes that continue to evolve concurrent with the field's evolution of a paradigm of psychopathology. As in the field of biology, the advent of a unifying model or paradigm in psychopathology will allow for greater specificity in the classification of mental disorders. Current diagnostic categories are still at relatively superordinate classification levels, and researchers and clinicians recognize that heterogeneity exists among individuals who meet current criteria for a particular diagnosis. Contemporary research into the subtypes of alcohol abuse and dependency is an example of this.

2. Improvements in technologies of measurement and data analysis enhance diagnostic reliability and paradigm development. Structured diagnostic interviews and operational criteria, the latter of which are exemplified by the DSM-III, DSM-III-R, and DSM-IV, help to reduce idiosyncratic diagnostic biases associated with variability in the subjectively developed world views of clinicians and researchers. Additionally, technological improvements, as illustrated by gene mapping or microanalysis of interactional social behaviors, increase our understanding of the etiology of disorders. Etiology is an important but still too little understood variable that will promote more reliable and valid identification of mental disorders. Multiple environmental and individual factors need to be considered in order to better understand the causes of mental disorders.

3. Greater precision in diagnostic classification and recognition of the multiplicity of factors that contribute to the occurrence of mental disorders has resulted in the advancement of treatment technologies. Treatments specific to different mental disorders are now being investigated for their relative efficacy. Examples of treatment–diagnostic pairings that have demonstrated efficacy for unipolar depression and ADHD were provided. Research in these arenas is more promising than a decade ago when each clinician's own theoretical orientation appeared to be the primary factor that determined treatment modality.

In light of these issues, history and progress are the critical standard by which to judge the utility of diagnosis and classification of mental disorders. Although the identification of discrete human psychopathologies may date back at least as far as Greco-Roman times, the scientific study of mental disorders is relatively new, dating back only to the turn of the century. Diagnosis and classification are in even greater infancy, with promising empirical research having been started only three decades ago. In these three decades, the field has articulated strategies to deal with the biasing influences of individual clinicians' and researchers' views of mental disorders. Further, the field has witnessed significant scientific advances in measurement and data analysis technologies that have and will continue to facilitate greater understanding of the etiology and treatment of mental disorders. In light of this progress, it is an exciting time to enter and explore the field of psychopathology.

REFERENCES

American Psychiatric Association (1980). *Diagnostic and statistical manual of mental disorders*, 3rd Edition. Washington, DC: Author.

American Psychiatric Association (1987). *Diagnostic and statistical manual of mental disorders*, 3rd Edition, Revised. Washington, DC: Author.

American Psychiatric Association (1993). *DSM-IV draft criteria*. Washington, DC: Author.

Andreasen, N. C., & Grove, W. M. (1982). The classification of depression: A comparison of traditional and mathematically derived approaches. *American Journal of Psychiatry, 139*, 45–52.

Bevan, W. (1991). Contemporary psychology: A tour inside the onion. *American Psychologist, 46*, 475–483.

Blashfield, R. K. (1984). *The classification of psychopathology: Neo-Kraepelinian and quantitative approaches.* New York: Plenum Press.

Cloninger, C. R., Bohman, M., & Sigvardsson, S. (1981). Inheritance of alcohol abuse: Cross-fostering analysis of adopted men. *Archives of General Psychiatry, 38*, 861–868.

Gergen, K. J. (1991). *The saturated self: Dilemmas of identity in contemporary life.* New York: Basic Books.

Grove, W. M., & Andreasen, N. C. (1986). Multivariate statistical analysis in psychopathology. In T. Millon & G. L. Klerman (Eds.), *Contemporary directions in psychopathology: Toward the DSM-IV* (pp. 347–362). New York: Guilford Press.

Harada, S., Agarwal, D. P., Goedde, H. W., Tagaki, S., Ishikawa, B. (1982). Possible protective role against alcoholism for aldehyde dehydrogenase isozyme deficiency in Japan. *Lancet, 2*, 827.

Heath, A. C., Jardine, R., & Martin, N. G. (1989). Interactive effects of genotype and social environment on alcohol consumption in female twins. *Journal of Studies in Alcoholism, 50*, 38–48.

Hollon, S. D., Shelton, R. C., & Loosen, P. T. (1991). Cognitive therapy and pharmacotherapy for depression. *Journal of Consulting and Clinical Psychology, 59*, 88–99.

Klerman, G. L. (1986). Historical perspectives on contemporary schools of psychopathology. In T. Millon & G. L. Klerman (Eds.), *Contemporary directions in psychopathology: Toward the DSM-IV* (pp. 3–18). New York: Guilford Press.

Lewis, H. B. (1981). *Freud and modern psychology.* New York: Plenum Press.

Masson, J. M. (1984). *The assault on truth.* New York: Farrar, Straus, & Giroux.

Matarazzo, J. D. (1983). The reliability of psychiatric and psychological diagnosis. *Clinical Psychology Review, 3*, 103–145.

Meehl, P. E. (1986). Diagnostic taxa as open concepts: Metatheoretical and statistical questions about reliability and construct validity in the grand strategy of nosological revision. In T. Millon & G. L. Klerman (Eds.), *Contemporary directions in psychopathology: Toward the DSM-IV* (pp. 215–231). New York: Guilford Press.

Millon, T. (1986). On the past and future of the DSM-III: Personal recollections and projections. In T. Millon & G. L. Klerman (Eds.), *Contemporary directions in psychopathology: Toward the DSM-IV* (pp. 29–70). New York: Guilford Press.

Patterson, G. R. (1982). *A social learning approach: Coercive family process* (Vol. 3). Eugene, OR: Castalia Publishing Co.

Patterson, G. (1986). Performance models for antisocial boys. *American Psychologist, 41*, 432–444.

INGRID N.
LECKLITER and
JOSEPH D.
MATARAZZO

Patterson, G., DeBaryshe, B. D., & Ramsey, E. (1989). A developmental perspective on antisocial behavior. *American Psychologist, 44,* 329–335.

Plomin, R., & Rende, R. (1991). Human behavioral genetics. *Annual Review of Psychology, 42,* 161–190.

Quay, H. C. (1986). Classification. In H. C. Quay & J. S. Werry (Eds.), *Psychopathological disorders of childhood* (3rd ed.) (pp. 1–34). New York: John Wiley & Sons.

Reed, T. E. (1985). Ethnic differences in alcohol use, abuse, and sensitivity: A review with genetic interpretation. *Social Biology, 32,* 195–209.

Regier, D. A., Farmer, M. E., Rae, D. S., Locke, B. Z., Keith, S. J., Judd, L. L., et al. (1990). Comorbidity of mental disorders with alcohol and other drug abuse. *Journal of the American Medical Association, 264,* 2511–2518.

Vaillant, G. E. (1983). *The natural history of alcoholism.* Cambridge: Harvard University Press.

Whalen, C. K., & Henker, B. (1991). Therapies for hyperactive children: Comparisons, combinations, and compromises. *Journal of Consulting and Clinical Psychology, 59,* 126–137.

2

Assessment Strategies

Arthur N. Wiens and James E. Bryan

Introduction

It is likely that all of the authors who prepared chapters for this volume in advanced abnormal psychology, and all of its readers, will, upon reflection, realize that they have assumed some definition of normality and abnormality in human behavior. For example, some may have assumed that normality equates with "health" and that behavior is assumed to be within normal limits when no manifest psychopathology is evident. Others may have in mind an "ideal" of optimal functioning. Still others, including many psychologists, may think of normality in terms of "average" levels of functioning and consider both very low and very high scores on various assessment procedures as deviant. This approach to describing abnormality is based on the mathematical principle of the bell-shaped curve and describes variability of behavior within the context of the total group, and not within the context of one individual. We will leave it to other chapter authors to elucidate this definitional issue of normality and abnormality. We did want to call the reader's attention to the fact that there may be few absolute definitions of abnormality and few clear-cut boundaries between normal and abnormal.

We also want to remind the reader that "abnormal" behavior, or diagnosable mental disorder, is widespread in our society. The field of psychiatric epidemiology is the study of the pattern of occurrence of mental disorders and deals with the distribution, incidence, prevalence, and duration of psychiatric illness with respect to the physical, biological, and social environment in which people live. A recent definitive study of psychiatric epidemiology has been conducted and is being analyzed by Darrel Regier and his associates at the Division of Biometry and

Arthur N. Wiens and James E. Bryan • Department of Medical Psychology, Oregon Health Sciences University, Portland, Oregon 97201-3098.

Advanced Abnormal Psychology, edited by Vincent B. Van Hasselt and Michel Hersen. Plenum Press, New York, 1994.

ARTHUR N.
WIENS and
JAMES E. BRYAN

Epidemiology of the National Institute of Mental Health. One objective of their study is to provide the most accurate estimates of the incidence of alcohol, drug abuse, and other mental disorders in the United States.

The five sites for their studies were: New Haven, Connecticut; St. Louis, Missouri; Baltimore, Maryland; Durham, North Carolina; and Los Angeles, California. In each site, adults aged 18 years and over were selected from rural, suburban, and urban neighborhoods; the total sample size was 18,571. The NIMH Diagnostic Interview Schedule (DIS), discussed later in this chapter, was used as the case-identification instrument. A 1-month time frame of prevalence rates allowed an assessment of current illness and minimized recall problems. The authors concluded that 15.4% of the population 18 years of age and over fulfilled criteria for at least one alcohol, drug abuse, or other mental disorder during the period 1 month before interview. The prevalence rates of DIS disorders varied from 12.9% in St. Louis to 19.8% in Baltimore. Higher prevalence rates of most mental disorders were found among younger people (<45 years), with the exception of severe cognitive impairments. Men had higher rates of substance abuse and antisocial personality, whereas women had higher rates of affective, anxiety, and somatization disorders.

Rates for any DIS disorder covered an increase from 15.4% for a 1-month prevalence, to 19.1% for a 6-month period, and to 32.2% for a lifetime prevalence (Regier, Boyd, Burke, Rae, Myers, Kramer, Robins, George, Karno, & Locke, 1988).

The point that we want to make in these introductory comments is that the purview of abnormal psychology is very broad and that it encompasses many different people at various stages in their lives.

Referrals for Psychological Assessment

To give the reader of this chapter a further look at how assessment in abnormal psychology is practiced, we will review aspects of our own clinical practice in a medical psychology clinic that is located in a health sciences university that includes many different outpatient clinics, two hospitals, and several psychiatric inpatient wards. The clinic is also the setting for a residency training program in medical psychology.

Faculty clinicians and residents in medical psychology respond to referral requests for assessment of patients on the psychiatric inpatient wards, on various inpatient medical wards, and from many of the fifty, or so, outpatient clinics; and to requests for assessment that are self-initiated by persons from the community.

Consultation requests for inpatient psychiatry services provide a good example of the multiplicity of assessment approaches that may be used in acute-care situations. Within our own clinic we have found that such consultation requests most often involve difficult diagnostic questions, where clarification of diagnosis and related cognitive and/or emotional symptoms can have significant bearing upon treatment and discharge placement decisions.

While this has been a long-established role of psychologists in hospitals, relatively little has been written about the effectiveness of assessment data in improving diagnosis and treatment. Recently, Zacker (1989) used a quasi-experimental approach to examine the impact of psychological assessment on diagnostic outcome in a series of 70 hospital referrals in a community mental health center. He found high concordance between the diagnoses of those based on psychological assessment and those made by the referring clinicians. Concordance improved after the assessment findings were reported; while the rate of agreement was 71% at the time of admission between the psychologist and attending clinician, it improved to 94% at discharge (using four broad diagnostic categories). Assessment findings contributed to change of diagnosis in a significant number of these cases. As the psychologists' conclusions were accepted in almost every instance, specialized assessment information was clearly highly valued.

Such referrals to our clinic typically involve cases where information about cognitive performance, intellectual level, and personality style help the hospital team conceptualize diagnosis and treatment approach. In a series of 30 recent consultation requests over a 4-month period, we found that 83% asked for assistance with diagnosis. The others involved cases where diagnosis was already clearly established (e.g., mental retardation and at least moderate-stage dementia), and assistance was requested with behavior management and help in identifying sources of recent increases in agitation and disruptive behavior.

Cognitive and neuropsychological assessment was employed in 63% of these referrals, involving differential diagnostic questions such as schizophrenia vs. drug-induced encephalopathy; presence of mental retardation and/or schizophrenia; early-onset dementia vs. schizophrenia; dementia secondary to HIV and/or substance abuse; and degree of depression.

Personality measures, both objective (e.g., MMPI, SCL-90-R) and projective (e.g., Rorschach, Thematic Apperception Test, Incomplete Sentences), were used in 73% of the referrals, which included questions of: major depression and/or presence of personality disorder; schizophrenia vs. major depression with psychotic features; personality disorder and/or posttraumatic stress disorder.

Many cases also involved both types of measures, for several purposes. Personality measures were routinely employed in inpatient neuropsychological evaluations, for example, to determine both the types of symptomatology that the patients were reporting (e.g., were these consistent with neurological and/or psychotic dysfunction?), and the extent of their emotional distress. Cognitive and intellectual measures were similarly employed in schizophrenia-related assessment. In these cases, WAIS-R performance was qualitatively analyzed (e.g., assessing looseness of association or unusual linguistic errors on the open-ended verbal subtests). Visual–perceptual and organizational functioning was also assessed as required in the copy reproduction and recall trials of the Rey-Osterreith Complex Figure Test. Diagnostic conclusions in most cases thus involved a combination of quantitative and qualitative assessment.

Communication with the referring clinician before, during, and following the evaluation is emphasized routinely, and has further enhanced the value of formal test findings. At the outset, review of medical records and briefing with the clinician helps determine the selection of tests and analysis of results in regard to pertinent questions. Follow-up reporting to both the clinician and the patient helps coordinate test results with treatment and discharge planning and enhances collegial and collaborative relationships (Zacker, 1989).

Many different assessment/referral questions are presented by patients from medical wards or from other clinics in our health care center. Familiar diagnostic issues about depression, bipolar affective disorders, anxiety, panic attacks, and so on, are often presented. We also see many patients who are concurrently evaluated by psychologists and physicians because of the awareness that both

ARTHUR N.
WIENS and
JAMES E. BRYAN

psychological and physical factors are intertwined in the symptoms and distress the patient experiences, e.g., patients presenting with fibromyalgia, chronic fatigue syndrome, chronic pain. Patients are also seen for evaluation of stress reactions and stress management or temper outbursts and anger management. Many patients experience a decrement in cognitive abilities: Complaints about memory impairment are often received and are assessed. The cognitive sequelae of head injury are evaluated and the progressive dementia that may accompany HIV/AIDS is often monitored by referral for serial psychological evaluation.

Other groups of patients that we see in our clinic are those who have been exposed to industrial or other toxins and fear that they may have suffered central nervous system damage. Still other patients feel that their psychological or physical impairments are so severe that they are disabled from any gainful employment; both patients and governmental agencies may request psychological assessment to help evaluate such claims.

There are also referral requests that arise out of new and innovative health care procedures, and the psychologist may be called upon to devise assessment procedures and protocols to address questions that may be entirely new. The scientist-professional education and training background of the psychologist is often invaluable to devise innovative assessment techniques and establishing the protocols that will allow systematic evaluation of the reliability and validity of the new techniques, and even the validity of the new health care interventions that are being used. Some of the new interventions include organ transplantations that involve the psychological assessment of a patient's capacity to withstand the rigors of the procedures, as well as the patient's ability to comply with the medical management regimens that follow. Another important question has to do with the quality of a patient's life after a particular medical intervention; this will be described further in a later section of this chapter. As the reader of this chapter has no doubt already surmised, we view assessment in abnormal psychology to be very wide-ranging. The successful practitioner in this area needs to be broadly and intensively educated and trained.

PRACTICE DATA MANAGEMENT

An important assessment strategy in abnormal psychology or, in any other aspect of psychological practice, is to establish the reliability and validity of the psychologist-assessor. To this end the successful psychologist will establish those practice data management procedures that will allow a detailed description of patients seen, verification of diagnosis or other assessment conclusions, and ultimately the determination of those patient groups that a given psychologist can successfully diagnose and treat. Practice in psychology is becoming increasingly specialized, and specific expertise in an area of practice will have to be demonstrated in the future.

In our own clinic we have developed a clinic management program or clinic appointment activity report that allows us to see how many of the patient appointments that were scheduled were kept, not kept, or canceled. We can describe the age and sex distribution of our patients, the procedures that were completed with them, and the diagnoses assigned to them. We can examine the data for all of our clinicians combined or for a given clinician; for example, each of the residents in our program can have a printout report of the patients that he or she has seen. This activity report has administrative, professional, and educational uses. It allows each resident to track and have a record of the assessment procedures done and the diagnoses of the patients seen. This also creates the possibility of assigning certain kinds of patients to remedy deficits in training. The reports create documentation that the resident can later use when asked to verify the nature and extent of training experiences.

To illustrate again the variety of assessment demands in abnormal psychology, we can note that over a 3-month period our residents saw about an equal number of males (49.2%) and females (50.8%). Approximately 10% of the patient appointments involved children and adolescents under 21 years of age, and 8.6% of the appointments involved patients 65 years of age or older. About 17% of the appointments involved psychiatric inpatients and about 16% involved inpatients from various medical wards. Many of those seen were outpatients referred either from other clinics or from the community. For administrative purposes, we also note that only about 10% of our patients were nonsponsored (i.e., the majority of our patients were covered by commercial insurance carriers or other health care contracts).

Approximately one-half of our clinic patient appointments were for treatment procedures, e.g., couples' therapy, individual therapy, tension-pain therapy, or brief visits. The assessment procedures that were completed included:

- Parenting Evaluation and Report
- Consultation Interviews
- Intellectual Evaluations
- Intellectual-Personality Evaluations
- Neuropsychological Evaluations (complete)
- Neuropsychological Evaluations (partial)
- Personality Evaluations
- Psychophysiologic Evaluations
- Behavioral Evaluation and Report
- Intellectual and Developmental Evaluation and Report

Intellectual and Behavioral Evaluation and Report. The most common procedure done in our clinic for the time period reviewed here was the Neuropsychological Evaluation (partial). In addition to a Clinical Interview and a Psychological/Social History Questionnaire, the modal psychological test battery in this evaluation includes the Wechsler Adult Intelligence Scale—Revised, the Wide Range Achievement Test—Revised-2, the California Verbal Learning Test, The Rey-Osterreith Complex Figure Test, Trail Making Test—Parts A & B from the Halstead-Reitan Neuropsychology Test Battery, the Hopkins Symptom Check List (SCL-90-R), and often the Minnesota Multiphasic Personality Inventory.

It is also useful to note the diagnoses assigned to the patients seen to illustrate the range of referral questions that can be inferred from these diagnoses. The assigned diagnoses in this period were as follows:

- presenile dementia, uncomplicated
- senile dementia with delirium
- alcoholic psychoses
- amnesic syndrome
- dementia in conditions classified elsewhere
- other specified organic brain syndromes (chronic)

- paranoid type schizophrenia
- schizo-affective type schizophrenia
- unspecified schizophrenia
- major depressive disorder, single episode
- major depressive disorder, recurrent episode
- bipolar affective disorder, unspecified
- paranoid states
- anxiety state, unspecified
- panic disorder
- neurotic depression
- somatization disorder
- affective personality disorder, unspecified
- schizoid personality disorder, unspecified
- schizotypal personality
- histrionic personality disorder
- dependent personality disorder
- antisocial personality disorder
- borderline personality
- other personality disorders
- alcohol dependence syndrome
- other and unspecified alcohol dependence
- barbiturate and similar sedative/hypnotic dependence
- cannabis abuse
- other, mixed, or unspecified drug abuse
- tics
- tension headache
- brief depressive reaction
- prolonged depressive reaction
- specific academic or work inhibition
- adjustment reaction with anxious mood
- adjustment reaction with mixed emotional features
- other adjustment reaction with emotion disturbance
- adjustment reaction, emotion and conduct disturbance
- adjustment reaction with physical symptoms
- unspecified adjustment reaction
- frontal lobe syndrome
- organic personality syndrome
- postconcussion syndrome
- other brain damage, nonpsychotic mental disorders
- unspecified brain damage, non-psychotic mental disorders
- socialized conduct disorder
- overanxious disorder
- unspecified delay in development
- psychic factors associated with diseases classified elsewhere
- mental retardation: mild, severe, profound
- other specified mental retardation
- migraine headache

From the list of diagnoses found for these patients it seems clear that many different assessment strategies would have to be used in assessing them.

ASSESSMENT STRATEGIES

Interviewing

THE CLINICAL INTERVIEW

The topics to be covered in an initial clinical interview are relatively consistent from one clinician to the next. The general objective is to carefully obtain a history that can be the foundation for the diagnosis and treatment of the patient's disorder. More specific objectives of the clinical interview are to understand the individual patient's personality characteristics, including both strengths and weaknesses; to obtain insight into the nature of their relationships with those closest to them, both past and present; and to obtain a reasonably comprehensive picture of the patient's development from the formative years to the present.

In preparing a written record of a clinical interview, most clinicians begin by presenting *identifying information*, such as the patient's name, age, marital status, sex, occupation, race, place of residence and circumstances of living, history of prior clinical contacts, and referral and information sources. The *chief complaint*, or the problem for which the patient seeks professional help, is usually reviewed next and is stated in the patient's own words or in the words of the person supplying this information. The intensity and duration of the presenting problem is noted, specifically the length of time each symptom has existed and whether there have been changes in quality and quantity from a previous state. It is also useful to include a description of the patient's appearance and behavior. In reviewing a *present illness* or presenting problem, the clinician looks for the earliest and most disabling behavior or symptoms and for any precipitating factors leading to the chief complaint. Often the precipitating or stress factors associated with onset of symptoms may be subtle and require the clinician to draw on knowledge of behavior and psychopathology to help with inquiry regarding relevant life change events. The clinician should also report on how the patient's problems have affected his or her life activities. It is important to review *past health history* for both physical and psychological problems—for example, physical illnesses that might be affecting the patient's emotional state. Prior episodes of emotional and mental disturbances should be described. The clinician also needs to inquire about and report prescribed and nonprescribed medication and alcohol and drug use. Possible organic mental syndromes must be noted. *Personal and social history* usually includes information about the patient's parents and other family members and any history of psychological or physical problems. The account of the patient's own childhood and developmental experiences may be detailed. Educational and occupational history are noted as well as social, marital, military, legal, and other experiences. The personal history should provide a comprehensive portrait of the patient independent of his or her illness (Siassi, 1984). The mental status examination is also included in the initial clinical interview but will be reviewed separately in the next section. The section of the interview on initial impressions or *findings* should include deductions made by the clinician from all sources available to this point about the patient's past history, description of the present problems, and results of the clinician's examination as determined from the mental status examination, results of psychological testing, contributions of family members and significant others, and so on. Finally, *recommendations* are presented about what kind of treatment the patient should receive for what problems and target symptoms.

MENTAL STATUS EXAMINATION

The mental status examination is reviewed under the following headings: general appearance and behavior; mood, feelings, and affect; perception; speech and thought; sensorium and cognition; judgment; insight; and reliability.

An example of a mental status examination report that was printed from responses recorded in a structured interview (Harrell, 1984) is presented below:

Ms. Doe was generally cooperative with the interviewer although her specific interactions were defensive. Level of consciousness during the interview was unimpaired. She was not under the influence of alcohol or drugs. Ms. Doe was oriented to time, place, person, and situation. No apparent deficits were evidenced in attention and concentration. Comprehension of simple commands was unimpaired. There *was* evidence of impairment in short-term memory. No indications of amnesia were present. Current intellectual level appeared to be average and fund of information was below average. Current intellectual functioning appears to be consistent with that evidenced prior to onset of the present condition. Abstract thinking appeared intact. No impairment was evidenced in simple computational skills. There was no evidence of specific neurological impairment. Examination of perceptual processes did not reveal any illusions, hallucinations, or other perceptual dysfunctions. No unusual aspects of thought content were noted. There was no evidence of phobias. The predominant mood during the evaluation was moderate anger, which was consistent with thought content. Secondary moods included mild depression. Generally, affective reactions were appropriate to status or complaints. Appropriate variability in affective reactions was observed. There was no evidence of significant cyclic mood changes. There was no indication that Ms. Doe is currently at risk for suicide. Current risk of danger to others appears to be low. No current self-destructive behavior patterns were identified. Level of impulse control was estimated to be limited and judgment generally appeared to be below average. Level of insight was characterized by some awareness of problems with some denial.

COMMUNICATION BETWEEN DOCTOR AND PATIENT

Although a treatise on the importance of the doctor–patient relationship is beyond the scope of this chapter, it is necessary to point out that a clinical interview, or mental status examination, cannot be conducted with validity unless reasonable rapport is established and the doctor and patient are listening to each other.

In a study of more than 1000 encounters between internists and patients, Beckman and Frankel (1984) have reported that most people are interrupted by their physicians within the first 18 seconds of beginning to explain what is wrong with them. This practice often prevents people from completing the purpose of their visit.

Typically, people go to their physicians with about three concerns, and the most troubling complaint is not always presented first. No relationship was found between the order of presentation and the importance of the complaint. This finding challenges the prevailing hypothesis that the first complaint is the most important. Once interrupted early in the encounter, patients rarely return to any additional concerns. The researchers found no differences between male and female doctors in the tendency to interrupt and control the interview. They also found that an encounter averages about 15 minutes in the United States and about half that in Great Britain.

The doctor–patient encounter can be made more useful if patients think beforehand about what they want to say and get out of the visit and take more control of the interview. It appears that older people are less willing to assert themselves in this manner than younger people, and thus they may be at particular risk for not having their concerns heard. Basically, patients want clinicians who will work with them and who will understand them, and a very important strategy in assessment in abnormal psychology is the establishment of rapport or a working relationship between doctor and patient.

STRUCTURED INTERVIEWS

A major source of unreliability in diagnosis in abnormal psychology is the variability of information about a patient that is available to a given clinician. For example, some clinicians may talk with patients' families and others may not. Similarly, some clinicians may ask questions concerning areas of functioning and symptoms and other clinicians may not.

To deal with such information variance, psychologists and psychiatrists have developed structured clinical interviews that reduce that portion of the unreliability variance based on different interviewing styles and coverage. The structured clinical interview is used routinely in clinical research and increasingly in daily clinical patient examinations. A structured clinical interview essentially outlines a list of target behaviors, symptoms, and events to be covered, and some guidelines or rules for conducting the interview and recording the data. Interview schedules vary in that some offer only general and flexible guidelines and others have strict and detailed rules (i.e., some are semistructured and others are highly structured). With the latter, wording and sequence of questions, recording responses, and rating responses are all specified and defined. The interviewer may be regarded as an interchangeable piece of the assessment machinery. Clinical judgment in eliciting and recording information is minimized and, given the same patient, different interviewers should obtain the same information. The impact of computers in standardized interviewing also appears decisive, in that they allow for efficient retrieval of information. Computers can also be used to apply an algorithm to yield reliable diagnoses from raw data.

DIAGNOSTIC INTERVIEW SCHEDULE (DIS)

The DIS (Robins, Helzer, Croughan, & Ratcliff, 1981) is a fully structured interview schedule designed to enable clinicians to make consistent and accurate DSM-III psychiatric diagnoses. It was designed to be administered by persons not professionally trained in clinical psychiatry or psychology, and all of the questions and the probes to be used are fully explained. It reminds interviewers not to omit critical questions and presents well-tested phrasing for symptoms that are difficult to explain or potentially embarrassing to patients. Questions about symptoms cover both their presence or absence and severity (e.g., taking medication for the symptoms, seeing a professional about the symptom, and having the symptom significantly interfere with one's life). In addition, the interview ascertains whether the symptom was explained entirely by physical illness or injury or as a complication of the use of medication, illicit drugs, or alcohol. The age at which a given diagnostic symptom first appeared is also determined, along with the most recent experience of the symptom. These questions are designed to help determine whether a disorder is current (i.e., the last 2 weeks, the last month, the last 6 months, or the last year). Demographic information, including age, sex, occupation, race, education, marital status, and history of treatment, is also determined.

Current functioning is evaluated by ability within the last 12 months to work or attend school, maintain an active social life, act as head or cohead of a household, and get along without professional care for physical or emotional problems.

Aside from a few open-ended questions at the start of the interview to allow the interviewee the opportunity to voice the chief complaint and to give the interviewer some background for understanding answers to close-ended questions, the interview is completely precoded. Symptoms assessed by the computer are precoded at five levels: (a) negative, the problem has never occurred; (b) present but so minimal as to be of no diagnostic significance; (c) present and meets criteria for severity, but not relevant to the psychiatric diagnosis in question because every occurrence resulted from the direct or side effects of prescribed, over-the-counter, or illicit drugs or alcohol; (d) present and meets criteria for severity but not relevant to the psychiatric diagnosis in question because every occurrence resulted from medical illness or injury; and (e) present, meets criteria for severity, and is relevant to the psychiatric diagnosis under consideration.

The DIS has been translated into different languages, and its use is now underway, or planned, in about 20 different countries. Cross-national comparisons in psychiatric and psychological epidemiology are possible due to the growing number of population surveys in various countries that have used the DIS. Similarly, cross-cultural surveys of anxiety disorders and prevalence, and symptomatic expression and risk factors in alcoholism have been planned.

Computerization of the DIS makes direct patient administration possible either in its entirety (18 sections) or one section at a time. The computer printout lists all DSM-III diagnoses for which the patient meets criteria. It also presents additional information about each diagnosis including the recency of symptoms, duration, and age of onset. In addition, the printout lists for the clinician what other diagnoses must be ruled out before this diagnosis can be assigned according to the DSM-III hierarchy. The diagnostic categories that are surveyed include the following:

- Tobacco Use Disorder
- Somatization Disorder
- Panic Disorder
- Generalized Anxiety Disorder
- Phobic Disorder
- Depression
- Manic Episode
- Schizophrenia
- Anorexia Nervosa
- Bulimia
- Alcohol Abuse and Dependence
- Obsessive Compulsive Disorder
- Drug Abuse
- Conduct Disorder
- Psychosexual Dysfunction
- Antisocial Personality Disorder
- Pathological Gambling

We have been using the Computerized-DIS (Blouin, 1985) in our clinic for some time. As part of our assessment strategy we wanted to include a procedure that clinician/researchers in other settings could follow if they wished to replicate our clinical data. We have been using the DIS routinely in examination of fibromyalgia patients. This is an example of a particular patient population in which we assumed that psychological factors had an important role either as an etiological factor in the development of the illness or as a consequence of suffering from it.

To date, after more than 100 referrals, no patient has yet been unable to complete the DIS. Our patients appear to be willing, and perhaps to welcome the opportunity, to respond to the various questions about their health status and history. Time at the computer screen to complete the DIS has varied from about 45 minutes to more than 2 hours, depending on how many different question branches the patient's responses would yield. With knowledge of the diagnostic presence of one or another DSM-III disorder, it is possible to tailor the patient's treatment program to be more comprehensive by taking psychological factors/ needs into account. First developed to help in making DSM-III diagnoses, the DIS was later modified to assist in making DSM-III-R diagnoses. It will undoubtedly be modified again to assist in making DSM-IV diagnoses (American Psychiatric Association, 1993).

Psychological/Social History Report

Another standardized data collection questionnaire that we use routinely is the Psychological/Social History Report (Rainwater & Coe, 1988). The questions are in a multiple-choice response format that permits computer scoring of the responses with a narrative printout of the results. Question categories include family/developmental experiences, educational experiences, employment experiences, military history, alcohol and drug use history, medical history, marriage history, diet, psychological history, and presenting problems. As with many questionnaires, the patient is asked to respond to many more questions than a face-to-face interviewer might have patience to pursue. Responding to all of the questions prevents overlooking a critical problem area in the patient's life, that might later turn out to be an important assessment omission.

Research has indicated (Young, O'Brien, Gutterman, & Cohen, 1987) that structured interviews increase, by a factor of two to one, the number of clinical observations (e.g., number of problem areas) and the amount of relevant patient information that is recorded. Clinicians using structured interviews tend not to be limited to the presenting symptoms in their diagnostic formulations; their results have higher reliability. Interviewers using structured interviews consider themselves equally as emphatic as when using free-flowing interviews. With practice, they can use structured interviews with increasing efficiency, so that this method requires about the same amount of time as traditional clinical interviews.

AutoSCID II

The AutoSCID II (First, Gibbon, Williams & Spitzer, 1991) is a computer-administered version of the "Structured Clinical Interview for DSM-III-R Personality Questionnaire" (SCID II PQ). It has been designed to assist in the assessment of personality disorders and can be used to collect diagnostically relevant historical data directly from the patient using SCID II PQ questions. The clinician can be prompted by the responses the patient has made to the screening questions to inquire further about evidence for the different personality disorders. It can be used to screen for the presence of adult Axis II disorders, as identified in the DSM-III-R.

This diagnostic approach to personality disorder views personality traits as enduring patterns of perceiving, relating to, and thinking about the environment and oneself, which are exhibited in a wide range of important social and personal contexts. It is only when personality traits are inflexible and maladaptive and cause either significant functional impairment or subjective distress that they constitute personality disorders (DSM-III-R: American Psychiatric Association, 1987). To be rated as present the described characteristic must show evidence of being pathological, persistent, and pervasive. Pathological characteristics must be beyond those experiences that one would expect to see in nearly everyone; for example, social anxiety would have to be clearly extreme. To be diagnosed, a characteristic should have been present over a period of at least 5 years. The characteristic should also be apparent in a variety of contexts, such as at work and at home, or in different relationships.

Computer-Administered Interviews

Computers have long played a significant role in assessment. Much modern test construction has been dependent on the availability of computing resources. As test administration itself became more feasible with the advent of microcomputers, one of the questions raised concerned the comparability of data obtained with traditional paper-and-pencil administration and computerized administration. Lukin, Dowd, Plake, and Kraft (1985) obtained no significant differences between scores on measures of anxiety, depression, and psychological reactance across administration formats. Most important, while producing results comparable to the pencil-and-paper assessment, the computerized administration was preferred to the pencil-and-paper administration by 85% of the subjects.

More recently, Choca and Morris (1992) compared a computerized version of the Halstead Category Test to the standard projector version of the test using neurologically impaired adult patients. Every patient was tested with both versions and the order of administration was alternated. Results indicated that difference in mean number of errors made between the two versions of the test was not significant. The scores obtained with the two versions were seen as similar to what would be expected from a test-retest administration of the same instrument. The authors note that one advantage of the computerized version is that it assures an error-free administration of the test. Secondly, the computer version allows the collection of additional data as the test is administered, such as the reaction time and the number of perseverations when a previous rule is inappropriately used. Finally, it may be eventually possible to show that promptings from the examiner do not make a significant difference in terms of the eventual outcome. If this were the case, the computer version would have the added advantage of requiring a considerably smaller time commitment by the examiner (Choca & Morris, 1992, p. 11–12).

There is evidence (Giannetti, 1987) that automated self-reports have advantages for both clinical practice and research. Patients accept and enjoy responding to online computerized questionnaires and frequently prefer them to clinical interviews or paper-and-pencil questionnaires. Even chronic and disturbed inpatients can answer computer-presented questions without assistance. There are indications that respondents are more likely to report socially undesirable behavior to a computer (e.g., reporting greater alcohol consumption to computers than to interviewers). Self-report and interviewer-collected history data show high agreement. Finally, it may be cost saving to complete interviews by computer rather than by traditional means.

Adams and Heaton (1987) called attention to a further administrative/research role of computers in clinical practice: creating and maintaining an informational database. This database might include information concerning patient demographics, referral sources, historical data, criterion test results (e.g., brain tests), psychological test findings, and clinical outcome. Such information is valuable in documenting the sources of patients, their demographic and base-rate profiles, the relationship of neuropsychological tests to other results, and the impact of testing, or other services, on patient outcome. Such data are of importance in quality assurance and in evaluation research. External reviewers and third-party agencies increasingly request data showing accuracy of diagnosis and relationship to hospital/clinic utilization, more appropriate care, and improved outcome. Practice data are important to have, given the current climate in health services delivery. Once this view is accepted, it follows that the optimal way to gain control of the quality and accuracy of such data is to implement one's own system to generate them.

Information from Family Members and Other Collaterals

The clinical usefulness of psychological test results is determined by its relation to the person's functioning in everyday life. Literature as to the "ecological validity" of psychological assessment consistently compares psychometric test data with other measures of real-world functioning (e.g., Baird, Brown, Adams, & Schatz, 1987). Information obtained from others who live with and know the person is essential to understanding the nature of the condition and predicting its long-term effects. Such information from family members and others closely involved with the person ("collaterals") can serve many purposes.

In diagnosis, other persons can help describe changes in the person's functioning, in terms of deterioration of general social roles (e.g., employment status and quality, domestic responsibilities, recreation and activity level), or global change in personality and emotional style. They can also help specify clinically significant symptoms that may not emerge through psychometric methods or that the individual may not recognize or acknowledge (e.g., the "positive spouse sign" is familiar to interviewers of early-stage dementia patients, when the spouse points out significant deficits that the patient minimizes or fails to mention).

In terms of ongoing behavior management, family members may be able to alert the clinician to specific problematic or at-risk behaviors requiring rapid attention. The degree of discrepancy between family members' and patients' ratings of functioning on the same measure can be informative. Discrepancies may point to the patients' lack of awareness of symptoms, as well as to possible hypervigilance and overinvolvement of the relatives. As a source of outcome data, the same measures can be administered to relatives over time, before and after treatment and at successive intervals afterward. Family members may be able to describe the effectiveness of interventions and provide suggestions to better apply methods to their own situation.

Family rating methods typically address global estimation of adjustment and role function as well as more specific important behaviors and cognitive/emotional symptoms. They represent a systematic means of gaining highly relevant dispositional information about the person, to complement clinical psychometric information or supplement it when complete testing may not be possible. Issues of psychometric reliability and validity are central to their meaningfulness and usefulness. These are commonly in the form of self-administered paper-and-pencil measures as well as structured face-to-face or telephone interviews. Some of the more commonly employed measures will be described here.

These are completed by the collateral member alone, and typically involve scoring level of functioning on a variety of general and specific items. The *Katz Adjustment Scale-Relatives Form* (Hogarty & Katz, 1971) is a measure of quality of life for both patient and relative. It has been used in a wide variety of studies involving health care conditions that compromise everyday functioning. Relatives rate two areas: (1) the person's current level of performance across a wide variety of daily social role functions; and (2) their estimation of how well they feel the person is meeting what they *expect* of them in that capacity. This provides both a measure of level of function as well as of discrepancy from the relative's expectations.

The *Cognitive Behavior Rating Scales* (Williams, 1987) address common sequelae of neurological conditions. The raters indicate their observations of the presence and degree of severity of a range of emotional and behavioral symptoms, neurological signs, and cognitive deficits. These are organized under nine scales entitled Language Deficit, Apraxia, Disorientation, Agitation, Need for Routine, Depression, Higher Cognitive Deficits, Memory Disorder, and Diffuse Dementia.

Briefer and more behaviorally specific rating forms have been developed with particular purposes in mind. An example is the *Patient Competency Rating Form* developed by Prigatano (1986), as part of a comprehensive neuropsychological rehabilitation program. This measure rates observations of the patient's ability to perform a variety of daily living skills, from hygiene to cooking, with the degree of difficulty presented by emotional and cognitive symptoms. The *Disability Rating Scale* (Rappaport, Hall Hopkins, Belleza, & Cope, 1982) is a similar brief measure of self-care, cognitive level, and occupational functioning designed for head-injured patients in clinic and at home.

FAMILY INTERVIEW MEASURES

Other family rating systems are placed in the context of a structured interview. This permits rating of the same sorts of areas noted above, but in a more qualitative and content-oriented format of contact with the family member. The *Vineland Adaptive Rating Scales* (Sparrow, Balla, & Cicchetti, 1984) are among the most widely used in this regard. They allow highly useful information to be obtained about the adaptive functioning of impaired and mentally retarded persons, which cannot be as clearly described by test data, particularly for severely impaired persons. They are scaled by norm group and age equivalent in four broad domains: Communication, Socialization, Motor Skills, and Maladaptive Behavior. This format allows an estimation of general level of function in each area, as well as the drawing of a profile of adaptive strengths and weaknesses in the person's daily living.

Other behaviorally oriented interviews include the *Social Behavior Assessment Schedule* (Platt, Weyman, Hirsch, & Hewett, 1980), designed to assess the extent of dysfunction of schizophrenic patients, and its impact upon persons who live with them. In this format, the family member is asked to rate degree of severity in a variety of behavioral and psychiatric-symptom-related areas, along with the extent to which they find those symptoms distressing to them. This has been applied to other populations, such as the head injured, and used as a measure of subjective burden involved in caregiving for such persons at home (Bryan & Strachan, 1992). *The Burden Interview* (Zarit, Orr, & Zarit, 1985) is a brief, symptom-focused rating system also designed to assess the degree of distress associated with caring for dementia patients.

Observed Interactions

PARENT–CHILD INTERACTION

The opportunity to observe individuals interacting with each other often provides a great deal of information about each of the individuals as well as their relationship. Observed interaction is often of critical importance in evaluating children, whose behavior may in large part be a reflection of the stimulus values and reinforcement behaviors of the parents. Robinson and Eyberg (1981) asserted that direct observation is a critical component of clinical child assessment and described an observational system to do such assessment. They described a study in which they standardized and validated the Dyadic Parent–Child Interaction Coding System (DPICS), a comprehensive observational system for conduct problem children. Both parent and child behaviors are observed and coded. Each parent (i.e., mother and/or father, if available) was observed in two 5-minute interactions with each child in a playroom. There were two types of interaction. In the child-directed interaction, the parent was instructed to allow the child to choose any activity and to play along with him/her. In the parent-directed interaction, the parent was instructed to select an activity and keep the child playing according to the parent's rules.

Interrater reliability was assessed; the mean reliability coefficient for parent behaviors was 0.91 and for child behaviors, 0.92. Validity was investigated by examining differences between normal and conduct problem families. Parents of conduct problem children made more critical statements and direct commands and gave fewer descriptive questions than did parents of normal children. In addition, the conduct problem parents gave a higher percentage of direct commands to their children than did normals. The conduct problem children demonstrated more whining, yelling, and noncompliance than normal children. For example, the average normal child noncomplied 6.1 times, whereas the average conduct problem child noncomplied 14.2 times during 10 minutes of observation. The DPICS correctly classified 94% of families and predicted 61% of the variance in parent report of home behavior problems.

Robinson and Eyberg (1981) suggest that continuous recording contributes to validity and utility by providing a complete account of all behavior, and that it allows data to be collected in less time than typically is required by interval sampling methods. They also note that the structure of the situations permits both the parent and the child to proceed naturally under varying degrees of parental control, thus maximizing the possibility of observing interactional dysfunction in conduct problem families. The authors explicitly acknowledge that characteristics of the parent as well as those of the child contribute to the diagnosis of conduct problem. Finally, they point out that their observational procedure can be used serially to guide the course of treatment and to document treatment change.

The DPICS has been used clinically in different assessment situations. As already noted, it can be used to assess conduct problems between parent and child and to monitor change with treatment intervention. It has also been used in clinical assessment when there are clinical/forensic questions, such as determination of child custody and termination of parental rights. The generation and availability of empirical observation data can be useful in such decision making.

INPATIENT WARD OBSERVATION METHODS

Among the most important sources of information about patients is observation of how they function while in the hospital. In order to sensibly interpret and organize the inpatient observation information, structured rating scales have been developed. These typically place high value upon being brief and convenient, while also seeking to adapt acceptable levels of reliability and validity. The best known of these methods have evolved from inpatient psychiatry. They tend to be structured around diagnostically significant behaviors and related observable symptoms. Clinically, they are used to help diagnose and track changes in patients' mental state and functional status over time. They are also used to help establish the validity of diagnostic systems through research on large groups of patients, making use of the wealth of available information from patients within a controlled setting.

The most common inpatient psychiatric rating methods have been in use for decades, including the *Brief Psychiatric Rating Scale* (BPRS) (Overall & Gorham, 1962), the *Present State Examination* (Wing, Cooper, & Sartorius, 1974), and the *Nurses' Observation Scale for Inpatient Evaluation* (NOSIE) (Honigfeld, Gillis, & Klett, 1966). They enjoy widespread use, with continuing refinement of psychometric and diagnostic discriminatory properties. These typically rate both global level of functioning and specific descriptive subscales.

Recent modifications of the BPRS include development of an 18-item format in which the clinicians rate on a scale of very mild to severe, items described by one or two sentences. The BPRS-18 includes the following six scales: Anxiety-Depression, Lack of Energy, Thought Disturbance, Hostility-Suspiciousness, and "Schizophrenia" (including unusual thought content, hallucinations, blunted affect, and emotional withdrawal). Hafkenscheid (1991) found that the thought disturbance and schizophrenia scales and the global scale showed adequate reliability and discriminatory power. The NOSIE has also been found to be convenient and sensitive to clinical change. Recent studies have reported good reliability and identified six main factors: Social Competence, Social Interest, Personal Neatness, Irritability, Psychoticism, Retardation, and Depression (Dingemans, Bleeker, & Frohn-DeWinter, 1984).

These scales have been adopted in current research on "positive" and "negative" symptoms in diagnostic subtypes of schizophrenia. Positive symptoms involve abnormal and maladaptive functions such as hallucinations, bizarre behavior, and disturbed thought. Negative symptoms relate to the absence or lack of aspects of normal functioning and include poor initiative, social withdrawal, flat affect, and impoverishment of thought and speech. Dingemans (1990) found that both the BPRS and NOSIE contributed to reliable identification of positive symptoms, although negative symptoms were less consistently measured. Greater use of these scales to track patient progress and operationalize diagnostic constructs is expected.

QUALITY OF LIFE ASSESSMENT

Advances in the effectiveness and expense of clinical health procedures have raised pressing questions about how and when they should be applied. The benefits versus costs of medical procedures are the focus of crucial economic and biomedical ethical decision making. The concept of *quality of life* has evolved as the measure of worth to be balanced against the efforts, costs, and risks of intervention methods. The impact on the quality of life of recipients is addressed at many levels, from political/social resource distribution, to measures of the effectiveness of drug, surgical, or psychological treatment, to clinical contact with individual patients involving the ongoing assessment of their progress and response. Quality of life is further used as an outcome measure in individual and epidemiologic studies, and as the basis for establishing standard of care in many areas.

While a crucial construct, quality of life is also broad and vague. It is generally agreed that it can best be conceived as a multidimensional construct, an aggregate of distinguishable and closely related factors affecting response to the disease and/or treatment. Definitions of the construct typically include:

1. Physical aspects, including mobility, pain, and appearance
2. Psychological and emotional aspects, including cognitive/intellectual function, self-esteem, and subjective sense of well-being
3. Social aspects including role functioning, contact versus isolation, and reciprocation in relationships (Siegrist & Junge, 1989)

Shumaker, Anderson, and Czajkowski (1990) have further added productivity and intimate involvement with others as relevant dimensions. Spilker (1990) has proposed a system-based definition that couches the safety, efficiency, and cost of treatment in terms of outcomes of physical status, psychological well-being, social interactions, and economic status. The patient's values, beliefs, and judgments represent moderating factors also affecting outcome.

Given the broad definition and wide range of applications of this construct, its meaning is being established through specific uses and measurement strategies. Shumaker et al. (1990) recommend a hypothesis-testing approach, with emphasis upon the specific areas considered to be relevant to a particular treatment. "Quality of life" seems all-encompassing, while prediction about types of expected effects forces the examiner to consider which dimensions are most relevant to the clinical trial.

Considerable attention has been given to the psychometric foundations of measures of quality of life. Objective, reliable, and standardized measurement is especially important in such a value-laden area. As a result, most measures emphasize the types of specific dimensions mentioned above. Some approaches include all of them within a single instrument, while other authors advocate a battery of individual tests. To be useful and meaningful, such measures must meet standards of reliability and validity (in all forms). Further, they must be sensitive indicators of change, providing information about which dimensions are affected by treatment, in which directions, and at which times.

A variety of approaches have been employed in quality of life assessment. They include scaled observer ratings and triangulation of information from different sources such as family members, co-workers, and physicians (Siegrist & Junge, 1989). The self-report questionnaire format is by far the most common, due to many advantages of data collection, cost-efficiency, and applicability to a range of patients. They are most effective when compared with other indices of physical, psychological, and social functioning, including ratings by physicians and others who know the person well.

Many self-report measures have been developed, the most common of which will be summarized as examples of the types of dimensions addressed and questions utilized. The *General Health Questionnaire* (Goldberg, 1979) is a 60-item scale developed as a screening measure of somatic symptoms, mood and affective states, subjective feelings of distress, and social interactions. The *Symptom Checklist-90-Revised* (Derogatis, 1983) is a similar 90-item rating scale of symptoms primarily in nine psychiatric categories, and yields both separate scale scores and a Global Symptom Index. The *Chronic Illness Problem Inventory* (Kames, Naliboff, Heinrich, & Schag, 1984), permits rating of perceived severity of limitation upon a wide range of areas of daily functioning among persons affected by debilitating illnesses. The *Quality of Life Scale* (Burkhardt, Woods, Schultz, & Tiebarth, 1989) is a brief, 16-item scale that yields a summary satisfaction score regarding broad areas of life. Specific scales have been developed for more circumscribed populations, such as the *Quality of Life Rating Scale* (Walker, Blankenship, Ditty, & Lynch, 1987), a nine-item Likert-scaled measure designed for clients within a head-injury rehabilitation program.

The *Quality of Well-Being Scale*, developed by Kaplan and Anderson (1990), is a functional health measure completed by the clinician. It consists of three scales that focus upon elementary aspects of daily functioning: social role activity, physical activity, and mobility. These provide a description of level of general function, while an extensive list of 25 specific symptoms that can impeded function is also included. Each of the functional levels and symptom is assigned a "preference weight," which then comprises a global quality of well-being score. Preference weighting of this sort has been used as the basis for health care cost-utility analysis, placing relative weighted value upon types of symptom combinations. They are the basis of actuarial systems employing indices such as "quality-adjust life-years," or QALYs.

Psychological Testing

We have saved our discussion of psychological testing as the last topic in our brief and selective overview of psychological assessment activities. This is not because we consider it the least important. Indeed, to the contrary, it is the most important of a psychologist's assessment activities, and we do not consider that any psychological assessment consultation is complete unless, or until, some form of psychological testing has been done and some testing data have been recorded.

STANDARD OF CARE

In our discussion of psychological testing we want to introduce several assessment concepts and strategies that have become the norm in clinical practice. The first issue we want to highlight can be labeled "standard of care." The psychologist is no longer an island of practice unto him/herself. Under our almost universal third-party coverage, insurance companies want to know the quality of care for which they are paying. Similarly, with the rising number of malpractice complaints, both patients and their attorneys want to know what are accepted standards of care and whether the patients' care was at such a level.

Quality of care and patient satisfaction are defined by patient perceptions and expectations, perhaps even more than by standards established by the profession. We have already discussed the importance of doctor–patient communication. Two additional very important components of patient satisfaction are accessibility and availability of services. Our clinic has tried to attend to timely availability to patients and has established and monitored efforts toward this goal.

TIMELINESS

An important assessment strategy is to respond promptly when a request for a psychological consultation is made. Many inpatients are hospitalized for relatively short periods of time and, if psychological consultation findings and/or recommendations are to be included in decision making, the consultation assessment needs to take place within 24 hours. For outpatient consultations, the patient should also be contacted within 24 hours to arrange a mutually convenient appointment time.

QUALITY ASSURANCE

In our health care setting, as in most others where hospital or other health facility accreditation is involved, we must show what efforts we make to monitor, evaluate, and improve clinical services. One aspect of such monitoring and evaluation function is to have established standards of care and then to assess whether we are delivering services according to those standards. Standard of care is clearly involved when we consider what constitutes acceptable psychological testing in response to various consultation referrals.

For example, our clinical faculty has established a standard of care in assessing questions of intellectual ability level in patients. When seeing a patient for such a referral question, the core procedures include use of the Wechsler Adult Intelligence Scale—Revised, The Wide Range Achievement Test—Revised-2, and a review of the patient's educational history with a review of school transcripts when these can be obtained. In our Quality Assurance monitoring we review records to confirm that these core procedures have indeed been completed,

TESTING PROTOCOLS FOR DIFFERENT PATIENT GROUPS

We have no doubt that, in time to come and in the interests of establishing and assuring appropriate standards of care, testing protocols appropriate to various patient groups, and to various referral questions, will be established. Although practicing psychologists have long discussed the uniqueness of each patient, the advantages of flexible testing, and the desirability of tailoring assessment to each individual, such approaches to assessment raise some important questions in our minds. For example, one cannot know what relationship scores from one test have to scores from another test unless the tests have been used consistently and systematically with each other so that through research or extensive experience such relationships can be identified. When different tests are used with each patient, it is not possible to observe or establish patterns of test response within a given patient group.

It is also important to observe standard testing procedures. As pointed out by Faust, Ziskin, and Hiers (1991), when a clinician alters standard instructions or test procedures, then short of research on these changes, one does not know how this impacts upon test scores, or what scores would have been achieved had the standard instructions been used.

When consistent test protocols are not used with particular patient groups, or referral questions, it becomes more difficult to determine effectiveness or accuracy across different assessment cases. One has essentially performed a unique set of procedures with every individual, and must conduct a separate "experiment" for each case seen (Faust, Ziskin, & Hiers, 1991). Overall, an approach that allows different assessment procedures among a given diagnostic category of patients, is likely to result in significant variability across different clinicians, is quite difficult to evaluate scientifically, and seems open to examiner bias.

As an assessment strategy in our clinic, we have developed testing protocols for different patient groups. One of these consists of patients referred from the Rheumatology Clinic with a presumed diagnosis of fibromyalgia. Most fibromyalgia patients require some form of psychological intervention, and all of the patients are seen for psychological evaluation when they are accepted into our treatment program (Bennett, Campbell, Burckhardt, Clark, O'Reilly, & Wiens, 1991). We wanted a psychological test battery that would reproduce assessment procedures used by other clinician/investigators and that could be replicated by other clinicians in turn. We chose the following procedures to constitute our protocol: Clinical Interview, C-DIS, Psychological/Social History Questionnaire, MMPI, Cornell Medical Index Health Questionnaire, the Shipley Institute of Living Scale, and a Quality of Life Inventory. We have been able to describe the psychological characteristics of this patient population to a number of different professional audiences.

In concert with clinicians in our Occupational Health Clinic and the Department of Neurology, we believe that behavioral and neurophysiologic changes may be the earliest, and sometimes the only, indicators of acute or chronic neurotoxicity. That is, we view behavior as a sensitive indicator of central nervous system impairment. The literature has suggested that neurotoxins interfere with at least four distinct aspects of central nervous system functions: memory, visuomotor performance, affect, verbal concept formation. We have proposed measurement of behavior by neuropsychological tests for the objective assessment of early neurologic deficit and for the detection of preclinical nervous system changes resulting from environmental or occupational exposure to neurotoxic agents. The core psychological test protocol that we selected for our neurobehavioral examination is as follows: WAIS-R, MMPI, Halstead-Reitan Neuropsychology Test Battery (15 subtests), Rey Auditory Verbal Learning Test, Rey-Osterreith Complex Figure Test, Cornell Medical Index Health Questionnaire, and a Structured Interview. The interview has a number of foci: previous health history, medications, use of alcohol/drugs, present symptoms and history, general orientation, physical appearance and gait, speech, affect, personality characteristics, and general competence to handle daily activities. We have been able to describe the modal cognitive, personality, and physical complaints of these patients and to differentiate among them those who show no identifiable emotional or cognitive dysfunction, those who show primarily emotional/chacterological concerns and no significant evidence of cognitive impairment, those who have a history of episodes of emotional dysfunction and show evidence of cognitive impairment, and those who have evidence of cognitive impairment as the primary finding. We do not believe that we could have made the observations that we have of this patient group without a standardized testing protocol.

Clinical versus Actuarial Judgment

In this final section we can only introduce discussion of a topic that will preoccupy psychologists increasingly in time to come. In talking about assessment, almost all psychologists would suggest that, in arriving at assessment conclusions the clinician has to "integrate" the assessment data with all of the historical data available. This integrative function is often subsumed under the heading of "clinical judgment." Faust, Ziskin, and Hiers (1991), have challenged us with the following statement:

> Although the need to "integrate all of the data" and the ability to do so are often taken for granted, it is extremely doubtful that clinicians can perform such cognitive operations (p. 279).

Paul Meehl (1954) introduced the issue of clinical versus actuarial judgment to a broad range of social scientists in 1954 and his lucid exposition stimulated a great deal of research on this topic. Dawes, Faust, and Meehl (1989) have more recently reviewed much of this research and have again concluded that research comparing these two approaches shows the actuarial method to be superior. Clinical diagnosticians must be aware of these research findings and face a significant challenge in planning how to incorporate them into clinical practice.

Faust and Ziskin (1988) also addressed the topic of factors limiting clinical judgment. They note, to begin with, that mental health practitioners are limited by the state of their science, in that psychology lacks a formalized, general theory of human behavior that permits accurate prediction. For example they cite the dozens of personality theories and hundreds of approaches to psychotherapy. More specifically, on the point of limitations in clinical judgment, they suggest that clinicians often underutilize information about frequency of occurrence, or base rates. For example, if a suicide indicator occurs in 80% of true cases and 10% of negative cases, and if suicidal intent is present in one per 1000 patients, the one patient is likely to be identified correctly by such a suicide indicator but about 99 will be misidentified. Faust and Ziskin express concern that clinicians often overvalue supportive evidence and undervalue counter-evidence. Clinicians expect to and typically find evidence of abnormality in individuals they examine, even normal persons. Faust and Ziskin also note that clinicians often practice under conditions that do not promote experiential learning; that is, they often receive little or no outcome information or feedback about their judgments. With reference to psychotherapy outcome, it is usually the satisfied patients who may make follow-up contact with the clinician to express their satisfaction. Patients who were unhappy with the clinicians' judgments may simply absent themselves from further contact.

Dawes et al. (1989) make clear that clinical judgment should not be equated with a clinical setting or a clinical practitioner. A clinician in psychiatry, psychol-

ARTHUR N.
WIENS and
JAMES E. BRYAN

ogy, or medicine may use the clinical or actuarial method. The definition of the clinical method is that the decision-maker combines or processes information in his or her head. In the actuarial or statistical method the human judge is eliminated and conclusions rest solely on empirically established relations between data and the condition or event of interest. Dawes et al. go on to say that:

> . . . the actuarial method should not be equated with automated decision rules alone. For example, computers can automate clinical judgments. The computer can be programmed to yield the description "dependency traits," just as the clinical judge would, whenever a certain response appears on a psychological test. To be truly actuarial, interpretations must be both automatic (that is, prespecified or routinized) and based on empirically established relations (1989, p. 243).

Dawes et al. (1989) add that virtually all types of data are amenable to actuarial interpretation. Qualitative observations (e.g., patient appears withdrawn) can be coded quantitatively and incorporated into a predictive equation. Actuarial output statements can be written for virtually any prediction of human interest.

A well-known example of actuarial prediction is the Goldberg Rule in differentiating neurosis from psychosis on the MMPI. (The following research is discussed with an important caveat to the reader: The research was carried out during the years when clinical diagnoses, as noted earlier, were not as reliably made as they are now. It would be of interest to know whether the same findings would result if the research were implemented with present-day clinical diagnostic procedures. Nonetheless, the Goldberg research is of considerable interest.) Goldberg (1965) showed that the most effective rule for distinguishing psychosis from neurosis was quite simple: Add scores from three scales and then subtract scores from two other scales. A cutting score was selected; if the sum falls below 45, the patients is diagnosed neurotic and if above 45 the patient is diagnosed psychotic. The criterion was the patient's discharge diagnosis. The decision rules were then applied to new cases and also compared with clinical judges. In each of seven different settings the Goldberg Rules performed as well as or better than clinical judges. In another study, judges were given training packets and even the outcome of the Goldberg rule for each MMPI, and were free to use the rule when they wished. Judges generally made modest gains in performance, but none could match the rule's accuracy; every judge would have done better by always following the rule. In an interesting elaboration of this research, Goldberg (1970) constructed mathematical models of the judges' decision making. In principle, if a judge weights variables with perfect consistency, the same data will always lead to the same decision and the model will always reproduce the judge's decision. Goldberg found that the judges were not always consistent, and in cases of disagreement the models were more often correct than the very judges on whom they were based.

Dawes et al. (1989) note that the perfect reliability of the models is likely to explain their superior performance in this and related studies. After reviewing a sample of 100 studies that showed the superiority of actuarial decision making in almost every case, Dawes et al. (1989) concluded that the actuarial advantage is general and likely encompasses even judgment tasks not yet studied. They felt that there is no other body of research in psychology in which the findings are coming out as uniformly as they are in the studies of clinical versus actuarial prediction.

In thinking about factors underlying the superiority of actuarial methods, Dawes et al. (1989) note, first of all, that actuarial procedures, unlike the human judge, always lead to the same conclusion for a given data set. Second, the mathematical features of actuarial methods ensure that variables contribute to conclusions based on their actual predictive power and relation to the criterion of interest. Individuals often have difficulty in distinguishing valid and invalid variables and may develop false beliefs in association between variables. Clinicians often do not obtain immediate feedback on the validity of their diagnoses. Self-fulfilling prophecies may come into play as when prediction of an outcome leads to decisions that influence or bias that outcome. The clinician may also be exposed to a limited or skewed sample of humanity and, without exposure to truly representative samples, may not be able to determine relationships among variables. One cannot determine whether a relation exists unless one also knows whether the sign occurs more frequently among those with, versus those without, the condition. As Dawes et al. (1989) point out, if 10% of brain-damaged individuals make a particular response on a psychological test and only 5% of normals, but nine of ten clinic patients are not brain-damaged, most patients who show the feature will not be brain-damaged.

Although surpassing clinical methods, actuarial procedures are also fallible and sometimes can achieve only modest results. They need to be periodically reevaluated, and they need to be established for each new setting. Reevaluation is aided by the fact that actuarial methods are explicit and can be subjected to informed criticism and be made freely available to other members of the scientific community who might wish to replicate or extend research. Clinician-researchers must lament with Dawes et al. (1989) that the investigations on clinical versus statistical judgment have had so little impact on everyday decision making, particularly within its field of origin (clinical psychology). Although of demonstrated value, actuarial interpretation of interviews is still rarely used. As relevant research findings accumulate, actuarial interpretation will be relied on much more heavily in the future. When actuarial methods prove more accurate than clinical judgment, the benefits to individuals and society are apparent. Much would be gained, for example, by increased accuracy in the prediction of violent behavior and parole violation, the diagnosis of disorder, and the identification of effective treatment (Dawes et al., 1989). Even lacking any outcome information, it is possible to construct models of judges' decision making that will likely surpass their clinical judgment accuracy.

SUMMARY

The assessment strategies that we have been discussing can be expected to lead to a diagnosis of a patient's condition. A great deal of thought has gone into thinking about criteria for diagnoses and sources of unreliability in diagnostic formulations. Spitzer, Endicott, and Robins (1975) noted five sources of unreliability and then determined that two of these contributed most heavily to diagnostic unreliability. The first source of unreliability they noted was *subject variance*, which occurs when patients actually have different conditions at different times. Spitzer et al. gave the example of the patient who may show alcohol intoxication on admission to a hospital but develop delirium tremens several days later. A second source of unreliability is *occasion variance*, which occurs when patients are in different stages of the same condition at different times. An example of this would be a patient with a bipolar disorder, who is depressed during one

ARTHUR N.
WIENS and
JAMES E. BRYAN

period of illness and manic during another. A third source is *information variance*, which occurs when clinicians have different sources of information about their patients. Examples here include information from clinicians who talk with patients' families and those who do not, or from interviewers who question patients concerning areas of functioning and symptoms about which other interviewers do not ask. A fourth area of unreliability is *observation variance*, which occurs when clinicians notice different things although presumably observing the same patient behavior. Clinicians may disagree as to whether a patient was tearful, hard to follow, or hallucinating. A fifth source is *criterion variance*, which occurs when clinicians use varying diagnostic criteria (e.g., whether a formal thought disorder is necessary for the diagnosis of schizophrenia or precludes a diagnosis of affective disorder). Spitzer et al. (1975) concluded that the largest source of diagnostic variability by far was criterion variance. Their efforts in the development of DSM-III diagnostic criteria obviously reflected their confidence in this conclusion.

Their research efforts to reduce information variance (the second most important source of unreliability) led to the development of structured clinical interviews that reduce that portion of the unreliability variance based on different interviewing styles and coverage.

We can predict that the unstructured assessment clinical interviews of the past will be replaced in the future by structured interview schedules for routine clinical assessment. This shift is supported by trends toward use of operational criteria for diagnosis, well defined taxonomies, almost exclusive use of structured examinations in research settings, and the growing influence of clinician-researchers. Further, the demand for accountability has also forced a problem-oriented type of record-keeping system in most institutions, with emphasis on branch-logic systems of clinical decision making, and progress notes that reflect resolution of symptom-syndromes and changes in problem status rather than changes in psychodynamics. Finally, the impact of computers appears decisive in that they allow for more efficient retrieval of information than is possible with records of noncomputerized narrative clinical interviews. Computers can also be used to apply an algorithm to yield highly reliable diagnoses from raw data (Siassi, 1984).

The comprehensiveness of the information that can be collected with structured interviews is leading to their use in routine clinical practice. The availability of personal computers is contributing to their increased use in patient self-administration of various structured interviews, including psychosocial history interviews and diagnostic interviews. With assessment strategies that allow patients to contribute data about themselves ever more directly, it should be possible to reduce information variance even more in the future. We have attempted to illustrate both the principles and techniques of assessment strategies in the practice of abnormal psychology through examples and data from our own ongoing clinical work. What we still have to research is how such expanded information bases can be used most validly in assessment/diagnosis and in assisting the persons who come to us for help.

REFERENCES

Adams, K. M., & Heaton, R. K. (1987). Computerized neuropsychological assessment: Issues and applications. In J. N. Butcher (Ed.), *Computerized psychological assessment* (pp. 355–365). New York: Basic Books.

American Psychiatric Association (1987). *Diagnostic and statistical manual of mental disorders*, 3rd Edition, Revised. Washington, DC: Author.

American Psychiatric Association (1993). *DSM-IV draft criteria*. Washington, DC: Author.

Baird, A. D., Brown, G. G., Adams, K., & Schatz, M. W. (1987). Neuropsychological deficits and real-world dysfunction in cerebral revascularization candidates. *Journal of Clinical and Experimental Neuropsychology, 9*, (4), 407–422.

Beckman, H. B., & Frankel, R. M. (1984). The effect of physician behavior on the collection of data. *Annals of Internal Medicine, 101*, 692–696.

Bennett, R. M., Campbell, S., Burckhardt, C., Clark, S., O'Reilly, C., & Wiens, A. N. (1991). A multidisciplinary approach to fibromyalgia management. *The Journal of Musculoskeletal Medicine, 8*, (11), 21–31.

Blouin, A. (1985). *Computerized psychiatric diagnosis: Manual*. Ottawa: Ottawa Civic Hospital.

Bryan, J. E., & Strachan, A. M. (1992). Expressed emotion, coping, and subjective burden in family caregivers of the closed head injured. *Journal of Clinical and Experimental Neuropsychology, 14*, (1), 29.

Burkhardt, C. S., Woods, S. L., Schultz, A. A., & Tiebarth, P. M. (1989). Quality of life in adults with a chronic illness: A psychometric study. *Research in Nursing and Health, 12*, 347–354.

Choca, J., & Morris, J. (1992). Administering the Category Test by computer: Equivalence of results. *The Clinical Neuropsychologist, 6*, (1), 9–15.

Dawes, R. M., Faust, D., & Meehl, P. E. (1989). Clinical versus actuarial judgment. *Science, 243*, 1668–1674.

Derogatis, L. R. (1983). SCL-90-R: Administration, scoring, and procedures manual. Towson, MD: Clinical Psychometric Research.

Dingemans, P. M. (1990). The Brief Psychiatric Rating Scale (BPRS) and the Nurses' Observation Scale for Inpatient Evaluation (NOSIE) in the evaluation of positive and negative symptoms. *Journal of Clinical Psychology, 46*, (2), 168–174.

Dingemans, P. M., Bleeker, J. A. C., & Frohn-DeWinter, M. L. (1984). A cross-cultural study of the reliability and factorial dimensions of the Nurses' Observation Scale for Inpatient Evaluations (NOSIE). *Journal of Clinical Psychology, 40*, (1), 169–172.

Faust, D., & Ziskin, J. (1988). The expert witness in psychology and psychiatry. *Science, 241*, 31–35.

Fast, D., Ziskin, J., & Hiers, J. B. (1991). *Brain Damage Claims: Coping with Neuropsychological Evidence*, Volume I. Los Angeles: Law and Psychology Press.

First, M. B., Gibbon, M., Williams, J. B. W., & Spitzer, R. L. (1991). *AutoSCID II for Personality Disorders*. Toronto: Multi-Health Systems, Inc. & American Psychiatric Association.

Giannetti, R. A. (1987). The GOLPH psychosocial history: Response-contingent data acquisition and reporting. In J. N. Butcher (Ed.), *Computerized psychological assessment* (pp. 124–144). New York: Basic Books.

Goldberg, D. (1979). *Manual of the general health questionnaire*. Windsor, England: NFER Publishing.

Goldberg, L. R. (Ed.). (1965). Diagnosticians vs. diagnostic signs. The diagnosis of psychosis vs. neurosis from the MMPI. *Psychological Monographs, 79*(9).

Goldberg, L. R. (1970). Man versus model of man: A rationale plus some evidence, for a method of improving on clinical inferences. *Psychological Bulletin, 73*, 422–432.

Hafkenscheid, A. (1991). Psychometric evaluation of a standardized and expanded Brief Psychiatric Rating Scale. *Acta Psychiatrica Scandinavica, 84*, (3), 294–300.

Harrell, T. H. (1984). *Intake evaluation checklist: Clinician version*. Indialantaic, FL: Psychologistics, Inc.

Hogarty, G. E., & Katz, M. M. (1971). Norms of adjustment and social behavior. *Archives of General Psychiatry, 25*, 470–480.

Honigfeld, G., Gillis, R., & Klett, J. (1966). NOSIE-30: A treatment-sensitive ward behavior scale. *Psychological Reports, 19*, 180–182.

Kames, L. D., Naliboff, B. D., Heinrich, R. L., & Schag, C. C. (1984). The chronic illness problem inventory: Problem-oriented psychosocial assessment of patients with chronic illness. *International Journal of Psychology Medicine, 14*, 65–75.

Kaplan, R. M., & Anderson, J. P. (1990). The general health policy model: An integrated approach. In B. Spilker (Ed.), *Quality of Life Assessments in Clinical Trials* (pp. 131–149). New York: Raven Press, Ltd.

Lukin, M. E., Dowd, E. T., Plake, B. S., & Kraft, R. G. (1985). Comparing computerized versus traditional psychological assessment. *Computers in Human Behavior, 1*, 49–58.

Meehl, P. E. (1954). *Clinical versus statistical prediction: A theoretical analysis and a review of the evidence*. Minneapolis: University of Minnesota Press.

Overall, J. E., & Gorham, D. (1962). Brief psychiatric rating scale. *Psychological Reports, 10*, 799–812.

Platt, S., Weyman, A., Hirsch, S., & Hewett, S. (1980). The Social Behavior Assessment Schedule (SBAS):

Rationale, contents, scoring, and reliability of a new interview schedule. *Social Psychiatry, 15,* 43–55.

Prigatano, G. (1986). *Neuropsychological Rehabilitation.* Baltimore: Johns Hopkins Press.

Rainwater, G. D., & Coe, D. S. (1988). *Psychological/Social History Report: Manual.* Melbourne, FL: Psychometric Software, Inc.

Rappaport, M., Hall, K. M., Hopkins, K., Belleza, T., & Cope, D. N. (1982). Disability Rating Scale for severe head trauma: Coma to community. *Archives of Physical Medicine and Rehabilitation, 63,* 118–123.

Regier, D. A., Boyd, J. H., Burke, J. D., Rae, D. S., Myers, J. K., Kramer, M., et al. (1988). One-month prevalence of mental disorders in the United States. *Archives of General Psychiatry, 45,* 977–986.

Robins, L. N., Helzer, J. E., Croughan, J., & Ratcliff, K. (1981). National Institute of Mental Health Diagnostic Interview Schedule. *Archives of General Psychiatry, 38,* 381–389.

Robinson, E. A., & Eyberg, S. M. (1981). The Dyadic Parent–Child Interaction Coding System: Standardization and validation. *Journal of Consulting and Clinical Psychology, 49,* 245–250.

Shumaker, S., Anderson, R. T., & Czajkowski, S. M. (1990). Psychological tests and scales. In B. Spilker (Ed.), *Quality of Life Assessments in Clinical Trials* (pp. 95–113). New York: Raven Press, Ltd.

Siassi, I. (1984). Psychiatric interview and mental status examination. In G. Goldstein & M. Hersen (Eds.), *Handbook of psychological assessment* (pp. 259–275). Elmsford, NY: Pergamon Press.

Siegrist, J., & Junge, A. (1989). Conceptual and methodological problems in research on the quality of life in clinical medicine. *Social Sciences Medicine, 29,* (3), 463–468.

Sparrow, S. S., Balla, D. A., & Cicchetti, D. (1984). *Vineland Adaptive Behavior Scales.* Circle Pines, MN: American Guidance Service, Inc.

Spilker, B. (1990). Introduction. In B. Spilker (Ed.), *Quality of Life Assessments in Clinical Trials* (pp. 3–9). New York: Raven Press, Ltd.

Spitzer, R. G., Endicott, J., & Robins, E. (1975). Clinical criteria for diagnosis and DSM-III. *American Journal of Psychiatry, 132,* 1187–1192.

Walker, D. E., Blankenship, V., Ditty, J. A., & Lynch, K. P. (1987). Prediction of recovery for closed-head-injured adults: an evaluation of the MMPI, the Adaptive Behavior Scale, and a "Quality of Life" Rating Scale. *Journal of Clinical Psychology, 43,* 699–707.

Williams, J. M. (1987). *Cognitive Behavior Rating Scales: Manual.* Odessa, FL: Psychological Assessment Resources, Inc.

Wing, J., Cooper, J., & Sartorius, N. (1974). *The Measurement and Classification of Psychiatric Symptoms.* Cambridge: Cambridge University Press.

Young, G., O'Brien, J. D., Gutterman, E. M., & Cohen, P. (1987). Structured diagnostic interviews for children and adolescents. *Journal of the American Academy of Child and Adolescent Psychiatry, 26,* 611–620

Zacker, J. (1989). It only takes one psychologist to demonstrate the impact of psychological assessment. *Journal of Personality Assessment, 53,* (1), 173–179.

Zarit, S. H., Orr, N. K., & Zarit, J. M. (1985). *The hidden victims of Alzheimer's disease: Families under stress.* New York: New York University Press.

3

Research Methods in Psychopathology

F. DUDLEY MCGLYNN

INTRODUCTION

Psychology began as a taxonomy of experience: as a classification system for mental events such as sensations, images, and feelings. When mental taxonomy failed, it was replaced by alternative schema for organizing the new science (i.e., the classical psychological "schools" of functionalism, behaviorism, Gestalt psychology, and psychoanalysis). When none of the classical schools was able to win the day, psychology became fragmented into clusters of specialized methods and narrow research problems (e.g., general and special theories about learning, perception, and emotion). As a consequence, general psychology incorporates an astonishingly diverse array of research methods and problems (Staats, 1991).

The history of abnormal psychology is much the same as that of general psychology. Biological, psychodynamic, behavioral, cognitive, and developmental approaches, each with its own unique research methods and theories, have been relatively prominent at one time or another, but none has won the day. As a consequence, modern psychopathology is a confusing array of general and special theories that oftentimes are manifestly incompatible, and of research methods that mirror disparate scientific assumptions. It is possible to articulate commonalities among the various research approaches only by focusing on the fundamentals of the scientific method.

F. DUDLEY MCGLYNN • Department of Psychology, Auburn University, Auburn, Alabama 36849-5214.

Advanced Abnormal Psychology, edited by Vincent B. Van Hasselt and Michel Hersen. Plenum Press, New York, 1994.

F. DUDLEY
McGLYNN

A branch of philosophy known as epistemology is concerned with the origins of knowledge; epistemology asks how do we know something. The fundamental character of modern science was shaped by two schools of epistemology in ancient Greece. An epistemic position known as rationalism held, in general, that knowledge can be ascertained through reason (e.g., through deductive logic). An epistemic position known as empiricism held, in general, that knowledge can be ascertained through observation. Science is a compromise; reason and observation are linked together so as to produce rationo-empirical statements about natural phenomena. They are called rationo-empirical statements because they contain terms with rational (conceptual) implications and terms with empirical (observable) implications.

The business of the scientific psychopathologist is to link reason and observation so as to make rationo-empirical statements about those behaviors that are said to manifest or to reflect psychopathology. In general, the statements made by scientific psychopathologists have to do with description, explanation, prediction, and control of those behaviors.

Description and explanation are at opposite ends of a continuum of rationo-empirical statements. Descriptions are statements that portray psychopathological behaviors and the events or conditions that are observed to precede, accompany, or follow them regularly. Scientific descriptions have a predominantly empirical character; they are "if–then" statements about observed states of affairs. Scientific explanations are empirical, "if–then" statements also but they are something more; they carry the rational implication that the presence of the "if" term is somehow necessary to the presence of the "then" term.

From the perspective of the philosophy of science, "explanation" is a concept that can take on a variety of meanings; what it means to explain something varies from one scientific context to another. Two approaches to explanation are prominent in psychopathology. For researchers working within the biological perspective, an explanation is an "if–then" statement in which the "if" term is stated with a vocabulary that is more molecular or more "basic" than is the behavioral vocabulary of the "then" term. For example, when an "if" term from anatomy (such as microorganismic infection of the brain) precedes a "then" term about behavior (such as disorganized speech and locomotion), an explanation of the behavior has been achieved. For psychopathology researchers working within the behavioral perspective, on the other hand, an explanation is an "if–then" statement in which the "if" term describes the procedures or conditions that are necessary and sufficient to produce or control the behavior in the "then" term. For example, explanatory terms, such as positive reinforcement, negative reinforcement, and punishment, refer to means of controlling rates of a behavior via controlling its consequences.

Notwithstanding the popularity of biological and behavioral explanations in psychopathology, other approaches to explanation clearly are possible. From the perspective of information theory (Attneave, 1959), for one example, an explanation of a phenomenon is a statement that reduces uncertainty: a statement that provides information about the phenomenon above and beyond the information contained in its description. The concept of explanation as uncertainty reduction is of considerable potential value in psychopathology because it focuses attention on the risks of some explanations. When a given array of behaviors is explained with a term such as "personality disorder" or "schizophrenia," does that explanation tell us anything we didn't already know?

Arguments over the propriety of alternative approaches to explanation clearly are possible. The biological scientist can argue that the behavioral scientist's explanations are merely descriptive. The behavioral scientist can argue that the biological scientist's explanations are narrow and naively reductionistic. The information theorist can challenge any other theorist to show that he or she is doing something more than restating the same information with a different vocabulary.

Validity in Research on Psychopathology

Concern over scientific validity cuts across all varieties of the rationo-empirical method. Four types of research validity are customarily distinguished: internal validity, external validity, theoretical validity, and statistical validity (Cook & Campbell, 1979).

INTERNAL VALIDITY

The dimension of internal validity refers to the degree to which changes in the phenomena under study are known to be related to the research variable(s) of interest, not to other factors. Internal validity is conceptualized as a dimension because different research strategies yield different degrees of internal validity. Simple case studies (below), for example, are low on the dimension of internal validity because they do nothing to rule out unknown influences on the phenomena of interest in the case. Well-executed experiments (below), on the other hand, can be high on the dimension of internal validity because procedural and/or statistical controls over unknown influences on the phenomena of interest are brought to bear. Other research strategies, e.g., quasi experiments (below), typically fall in-between simple case studies and experiments along the dimension of internal validity.

EXTERNAL VALIDITY

External validity refers to the degree to which the rationo-empirical statements produced by research are accurate when they are applied in contexts other than the research contexts used to produce them. Again, external validity is a dimension because different research strategies afford different degrees of external validity. Simple case studies are low on the dimension of external validity because they provide no information at all about other contexts in which the statements yielded by the case might be applicable. True experiments tend to be low on the dimension of external validity also because the procedures used to maximize internal validity tend to produce artificiality with respect to events in the real world. Well-executed quasi experiments can be high on the dimension of external validity because they typically are conducted in real-world settings.

THEORETICAL VALIDITY

Theoretical validity refers to the degree to which the procedures used in research represent satisfactorily the events that one or more theories purport to explain. In some models of science, a theory is used to derive a hypothesis or prediction about what will happen in an experiment or other empirical undertaking. The empirical work is then conducted, and the theory is retained, discarded, or modified in light of the results. This rationo-empirical approach can succeed only when the rational requirements of the theory are captured faithfully by the empirical features and products of the research. For example, a general theory maintains that the behaviors of sociopathic humans reflect subtle neurologic peculiarities. Gorenstein and Newman (1980) tested hypotheses derived from that theory by experimenting with rats whose brains they had purposefully damaged. The question of theoretical validity centers on the degree to which the empirical connections between experimental lesions and behaviors among rats represent faithfully the rational (theoretical) connections between neurologic peculiarities and sociopathic conduct among humans.

STATISTICAL VALIDITY

According to the discipline of mathematical statistics, proper inference from observations made on research samples (e.g., 30 schizophrenic subjects vs. 30 normal subjects) to observations that might be made on sampled populations (e.g., schizophrenics vs. normals at large) requires that the numbers used in statistical analyses be produced in certain ways and have certain properties. For example, the numbers should be obtained from random independent samples of target populations, they should be normally distributed, and they should be based on number-assignment (measurement) operations such that the sizes of differences between the phenomena designated by different pairs of adjacent numbers are the same. According to the traditional account, a given research product is statistically valid to the extent that such desiderata have been met. However, it is known empirically that some statistics are viable even when one or more of the aforementioned desiderata are not met. A statistic is said to be "robust" when the conclusions it produces are not influenced unduly by numbers that violate the theoretical assumptions of mathematical statistics. In practice, statistical errors are rife within the published literature in psychology. In principle, a given research product is statistically valid when the numbers used in statistical analyses meet the various desiderata for those analyses or when the statistics used are robust.

RELATIONSHIPS AMONG TYPES OF VALIDITY

Internal validity is important fundamentally; internal validity permits us to make statements about what leads to what. Statistical validity is likewise important fundamentally (in paradigms that make use of inferential statistics); statistical validity is the basis of accurate inference from observed samples to observable populations. External validity is not important fundamentally; it becomes important when the purpose of research is to make statements that are applicable directly to one or more real-world contexts (e.g., clinics, hospitals). Theoretical validity is not important fundamentally either; it becomes important when the purpose of research is to make statements about the value of one or more theories.

Some writers have argued that the various forms of validity must be achieved simultaneously. Bernstein and Paul (1971), for example, argued that behavior therapy analogue research (discussed later) is not worthwhile unless it is valid theoretically, internally, and externally. Actually, however, the various types of research validity rarely are achieved simultaneously in a single research project. Rather, they are achieved to varying degrees depending upon the specific methods and exact purposes of the given research effort. In turn, overall validity in a scientific arena derives from the cumulation of findings produced by heterogeneous research methods that complement one another along the various validity dimensions. This theme will be repeated herein from time to time.

RESEARCH ON ETIOLOGY

Psychopathology research takes place in many different arenas, for example those of etiology (the study of causes), epidemiology (the study of population prevalence), classification, intervention, and prevention. In each arena research methods that are basically the same are adapted to serve special purposes. The arenas of etiology and intervention are used here to organize the narrative. Within the section on etiological research, activities are subdivided into four general methods: case studies, correlational studies, quasi experiments, and experiments. Each method occupies a legitimate place in the scientific quest and, as noted earlier, the various methods can and should play complementary roles.

The Case Study Method

The case study method has played an influential role in the history of psychopathology. Case studies reported in the middle of the nineteenth century initiated interest in an apparent constellation of behavioral phenomena that would later be called schizophrenia (Bleuler, 1911). A case study of the Genain quadruplets (Rosenthal, 1963) stirred subsequent interest in a genetic contribution to the phenomena of schizophrenia. The cases of Little Hans (Freud, 1909) and of Anna O. (Breuer & Freud, 1895) influenced the formulation of psychoanalytic theory and the "talking cure" for psychoneuroses.

An etiologic case study is a narrative that describes a patient's symptoms, and the circumstances that brought the symptoms about, usually as interpreted from some systematic theoretical perspective (e.g., psychoanalysis, conditioning theory, genetics). From within the scientific context of discovery, the case study method has considerable merit. It is, perhaps, the only method that portrays the ontogeny of psychopathology with all its subtlety and complexity. As such it is an important component of the overall scientific effort. From within the scientific context of confirmation, however, the case study method is sorely lacking, save for certain types of intervention case studies (discussed elsewhere). Among other shortcomings, case studies are without the observational conditions that are necessary to make trustworthy statements about what leads to what, and case studies are open to major biases introduced by the reporter's theoretical perspective. Notable of the latter problem is the ease with which behavioral theorists (Wolpe & Rachman, 1960) challenged the putative evidence for a psychodynamic etiology in Freud's (1909) case of Little Hans.

Correlational Research

Most etiological research in psychopathology is nonexperimental research, often called "correlational research." In nonexperimental research, measures are

F. DUDLEY
McGLYNN

taken of historical and/or biological and/or psychological variables, then mathematical relationships among those measures are described. In univariate correlational research, one etiologic variable and one measure of psychopathology are of interest. In multivariate correlational research, many etiologic and psychopathologic variables are studied simultaneously. There are numerous statistical variations in "correlational" research, and some of these variations are very sophisticated mathematically. In general, however, correlational research belongs in the scientific context of discovery. Correlational research produces statements about relationships between variables, but the statements need confirmation and clarification by other methods. Only some subsets of correlational methodology are overviewed here and only a few examples are provided. Examples appear throughout the text; the narrative here should assist in understanding methodological terminology in those examples.

EX POST FACTO COMPARISONS

In true experiments (below) the phenomena of interest are created by what the experimenter does. In nonexperimental research the phenomena of interest are brought to the investigator by the subject; they have been created already. Most *ex post facto* comparison research seeks to discover how the phenomena of interest were created, by discovering one or more potentially causal differences between persons who manifest the phenomena and persons who do not. Even though psychopathology researchers from all theoretical perspectives make use of *ex post facto* comparisons, they are particularly common in the biological literature.

Widespread use of the method of *ex post facto* comparison occurs in the study of genetic influences on psychopathology. In family history studies, the incidences of psychopathologies among the blood relatives of affected persons (probands) are compared with the incidences of the same and related psychopathologies among the blood relatives of unaffected persons. Higher incidences among the relatives of affected probands suggest genetic influence. For example, the incidence of panic disorder among the first-degree relatives of panic-disordered probands is 17 to 20.5%, whereas the incidence of panic disorder among the first-degree relatives of normal and other controls is 1.8 to 4.2% (FIDIA Research Foundation, 1992). In twin studies, the co-incidences of psychopathologies among genetically identical (monozygotic) twins are compared with those among fraternal (dizygotic) twins. Higher co-incidence among identical than among fraternal twins suggests genetic influence. For example, the co-incidence of panic disorder among identical twins is 22 to 31%, while the co-incidence of panic disorder among fraternal twins is 0% (FIDIA Research Foundation, 1992). In adoption studies, the incidences of psychopathologies among the adopted-away children of affected versus control mothers are studied. Because the children are adopted at a very early age, maternal influences based on learning and similar factors are eliminated; hence higher incidences of psychopathology among the children of affected mothers than those of control mothers point to genetic influence. In some adoption studies the influence of the adoptive parents/family is studied along with the mother's genetic influence. For example, Tienari, Lahti, Sorri, Naarala, Moring, Wahlberg, and Wynne (1987) were able to show that incidence of schizophrenia spectrum disorders among adoptees was influenced both by the birth mother's psychiatric status and by the level of disorganization (stress) within the adoptive family.

Other noteworthy exemplars of *ex post facto* research from within the biological perspective are studies of the neuropathology and neuroradiology of schizophrenia. Bogerts, Meertz, and Schonfeldt-Bausch (1985) compared postmortem brain specimens from 13 schizophrenics and control subjects and found relatively less volume in the basal ganglia and limbic system among those with the schizophrenia diagnosis. DeLisi, Dauphinais, and Gershon (1988) compared magnetic resonance imaging (MRI) data from 24 schizophrenics and control subjects and found that the schizophrenics had relatively less total area of hippocampus, parahippocampal gyrus, and amygdala. Magnetic resonance imaging provides pictures of the living brain. Imaging of brain structures, such as the hypothalamus, is potentially informative because schizophrenics suffer from disordered emotion, and the hypothalamus and related structures in the limbic system (phylogenetically old brain) participate in emotional expression.

Ex post facto comparisons sometimes involve more than one comparison variable. When a researcher is interested in several factors that might act in combination to produce differences between clinical groups or subgroups and others, a multivariate (see below) technique known as discriminant analysis can be used. In discriminant analysis, values for groups of variables are used to form a composite score, called the discriminant function, that discriminates between the comparison groups as much as is possible, and that quantifies the importance of each predictor variable to the optimal discrimination. Discriminant analysis is similar to a multiple regression procedure (below) in which the criterion variable is categorical (i.e., each research subject is assigned to one category or another). It allows researchers to evaluate the separate and combined effects of etiologic factors that lead to membership in different diagnostic/nondiagnostic categories. For example, Fraser, King, Thomas, and Kendall (1986) formed a discriminant function composed of language variables (fluency, complexity, and accuracy) to distinguish between schizophrenics, mood disordered patients, and normal controls.

Valid *ex post facto* comparisons have rarely, if ever, produced clearcut differences. Furthermore, even if very large differences were produced any causal implication would be weak necessarily. *Ex post facto* comparisons are low on the dimension of internal validity; numerous unknown factors can be confounded with the variables under study. *Ex post facto* comparisons also fail to reveal the directions or temporal flow of causal relationships among the phenomena of interest. For example, a diagnosis of schizophrenia might mean that subjects have been taking neuroleptic medication, and the medication might contribute to an observed neurologic difference between schizophrenics and others.

Beyond the inherent shortcomings of *ex post facto* comparisons, many are weakened unnecessarily by the use of diagnostic categories to form comparison groups. A group of diagnosed schizophrenics probably will include some individuals whose symptomatic behaviors do not overlap. A comparison group of non-schizophrenics probably will include individuals whose behaviors overlap with some of the behaviors seen among the schizophrenics. Hence, it is unclear what behaviors are being explained by results of comparisons across diagnostic categories. *Ex post facto* comparisons across diagnostic categories can be improved somewhat by using relatively homogeneous research diagnoses such as the presence of "negative symptoms" (Crow, 1985); however, some ambiguity remains. Persons (1986) argued that comparisons should be made across relatively discrete behavioral categories such as the presence or absence of thought disorder. This is an eminently reasonable argument because the recommended comparison focuses more attention on the behavior of subjects, and less attention on the behavior of diagnosticians.

SIMPLE CORRELATION AND SIMPLE REGRESSION

Simple correlation research makes use of only two variables. For example, mothers and their children might be asked to rate on a scale of 1 to 7 the degree to which they are frightened by each of N objects or events such as dogs, spiders, dental visits, violent weather. A coefficient of correlation can then be calculated to quantify the extent to which the mothers and their children provided similar/dissimilar fear-intensity ratings for the various objects and events. A coefficient of +1.00 would indicate that the fear ratings among the children are exactly the same as those of their mothers. A coefficient of −1.00 would indicate that the fear ratings supplied by the children are totally opposite those provided by their mothers. A coefficient of 0.00 would indicate that no relationship exists between the fear ratings of children and those of their mothers. The mathematical model of simple correlation assumes only that the two variables are somehow mutually dependent. Therefore, causal statements are not possible. A large positive correlation between the fears of mothers and their children might prompt research to determine the extent to which maternal fears influence childhood fears, the extent to which childhood fears influence maternal fears, and the extent to which fears of mothers and their children are shaped by other factors that mothers and their children have in common.

Simple regression research likewise makes use of only two variables; values for a predictor variable are given and are used to predict values for a criterion variable. Unlike the mathematical model of correlation, the mathematical model of regression assumes that values for the criterion variable are in some way dependent upon values for the predictor variable. Hence, research narratives say that one variable "predicts" or "explains" the other. At the level of calculation, however, simple regression is the same as simple correlation. Hence, the words prediction and explanation have no important causal implication.

MULTIPLE CORRELATION AND MULTIPLE REGRESSION

Classical descriptions of the experimental method state that the effects of one (independent) variable on another (dependent) variable are studied while effects on the dependent variable from all other potential sources of influence are ruled out. In brief, the classical method isolates and studies one variable at a time. Contemporary methodology is quite different. Owing to advances in mathematical statistics over the past three decades, multivariate techniques exist that allow for the study of many variables at a time. Most frequently, multivariate techniques are associated with nonexperimental research. However, mathematically equivalent multivariate methods are available for analyzing complex data sets from actual experiments.

The multivariate techniques of multiple correlation and multiple regression are used to describe the strongest linear covariations that exist between groups of two or more variables on one side of an equation and one variable on the other side of the equation. The mathematical models are simple extensions of the two-variable models just described. In general, multiple correlation and regression are used to form the "best" (i.e., the most highly correlated or most predictive) composites from among the groups of two or more variables, and to describe linear relationships between those composites and the single variable on the other side of the equation. For example, McNeal and Berryman (1989) examined some possible origins of dental phobia (odontophobia) by studying the "best" predictors of self-report scores for dental fear among self-report scores for other fears. Self-reported dental fear scores were used as the criterion variable for a multiple regression procedure in which the composite predictor variable was potentially made up of scores for fear of pain, of being closed in, of mutilation, and of social encounters. Scores for fear of pain and for fear of being closed in were included in the best prediction of self-reported fear of dentistry among males. Scores for fear of mutilation also had to be included to achieve the best prediction of fear of dentistry among females. Scores for fear of social encounters were not useful in predicting self-reported dental fear scores among subjects of either gender.

OTHER "CORRELATIONAL METHODS"

There are several special-purpose mathematical approaches to understanding relationships among multiple nonexperimental measures. One of these, discriminant analysis, was discussed above. Another is termed canonical correlation. As noted, multiple correlation and multiple regression extend their simple models by identifying groups of two or more variables on one side of an equation that yield the "best" correlation or regression with respect to a single variable on the other side of the equation. The method of canonical correlation extends the simple models still further by finding the strongest association or best possible predictions that exist among composites or groups of variables on both sides of the equation (Marascuilo & Levin, 1983).

Another special-purpose approach is termed loglinear analysis. Multiple regression is not robust when the measures that are used violate the assumptions of mathematical statistics (above). At the same time, much multivariate research in psychopathology makes use of categorical assignments that constitute measurement violations (e.g., diagnosis, gender, assignment to one research cohort vs. another). Loglinear analysis is a method for describing multivariate relations among large numbers of categorical variables (Marascuilo & Busk, 1987).

Another set of correlational techniques is termed factor analysis. Researchers in psychopathology often deal with numerous variables (e.g., scores on tests or test items about personality or psychopathology, measures of the symptoms of anxiety, depression, or schizophrenia). Factor analysis is a group of procedures with which a set of variables can be reduced in number to form a smaller set of intercorrelated variables called latent variables or factors. In general, factor analysis serves to simplify research by reducing the numbers of variables, but often there is an implication that the smaller set of latent variables or factors helps explain the larger set of variables. Confirmatory factor analysis and exploratory factor analysis bear different relationships to theory. In confirmatory factor analysis one or more a priori theories guide the factor analytic work by specifying the factors that are theoretically expected. The factor analytic procedure then confirms or fails to confirm the theoretical expectation(s). In exploratory factor analysis (Harmon, 1967) the factor analytic work proceeds without theoretical guidance as to the factors expected. For example, Johnson, Mayberry, and McGlynn (1990) used exploratory factor analysis to reduce responses to a 60-item dental fear question-naire down to four latent (provisionally explanatory) variables: fear of pain, of being closed in, of negative social evaluation, and of loss of control.

Another multivariate technique that has recently become popular is referred to as structural equation modeling, causal modeling, or covariance structure analysis. Structural modeling is a rationo-empirical method that is used to test one or more theories about causal mechanisms that might account for patterns of correlation in nonexperimental data. In structural modeling the data take the form of factor analytically derived latent variables or factors. The hypotheses are theo-retically derived statements about how the latent variables should be related to one another and to the measured variables. The mathematical treatment boils down to a regression analysis (above) using factor scores (e.g., Bentler, 1985). Given particular outcomes of the regression, each theoretical model of causal mechanisms under-lying the correlations is or is not rejected. For example, Hammen, Burge, and Stansbury (1990) showed that a factor derived from measures of psychopathology and dysfunction among the children of depressed mothers was explained by a model composed of two other reciprocally interacting factors derived from mea-sures of maternal functioning and of child characteristics.

COMMENT

There are methods for multivariate analysis of nonexperimental data other than those overviewed here (e.g., cluster analysis, multidimensional scaling). There also are many nuances involved in applications of the approaches just overviewed. Advances in statistics, the availability of computer software packages, and the widespread availability of personal computers, have made correlational research attractive. Perhaps correlational research is too attractive. Very frequently the numbers used in nonexperimental research are of dubious or demonstrably weak empirical meaning. Certainly the scientific product of multivariate research, even research using the most sophisticated of methods, can be no better than is the empirical quality of the numbers that are analyzed. Considerable caution should be used when encountering words such as explanation, prediction, and cause as they are used in the context of multivariate analysis of nonexperimental measures, because the data are fundamentally correlational in nature. Also, considerable attention should be paid to the measurement operations by which the numbers for multivariate "correlational" research are acquired.

Quasi-Experimental Research

The generic feature of "correlational research" is that the investigator has no actual control over the phenomena being studied or over any of the variables that might influence the phenomena being studied. The identifying feature of experi-mental research (below) is that, in principle at least, the investigator has control over all of the variables that might be influential, while he or she manipulates some of them. There is a general experimental strategy that falls between correlational and experimental research on the dimension of experimental control/manipulation. The term quasi-experimental research denotes (typically naturalistic) research in which some potentially influential variables are controlled and others are not, and one or more variables are manipulated (Cook & Campbell, 1979).

There are several quasi-experimental designs that, in various ways, accommodate for influential variables that cannot be controlled. In general, a causal nexus between two variables is argued when one variable precedes the other in time, when a credible scientific theory of the relationship between the two variables exists, and when other explanations of the relationship have been ruled out. Some quasi-experimental work is discussed briefly later in the narrative about intervention research. Research on cognitive behavior among schizophrenics is used here to illustrate the general quasi-experimental approach.

Most authorities agree that schizophrenia is fundamentally a syndrome of disordered thinking. Therefore, a considerable amount of quasi-experimental research has attempted to pinpoint or describe the nature of the cognitive disorder. The research is quasi-experimental because subjects are neither selected nor assigned to experimental conditions randomly. Rather, experimental and comparison groups are made up of schizophrenic and normal subjects who are locally available. Contemporary work begins with some theory of how information-processing behaviors among schizophrenics differ from information-processing behaviors among normals. The theory is then used to design an information-processing task on which schizophrenics and normals should perform differently if the theory is correct. Finally, the task performances of schizophrenics and normals are compared in order to retain, modify, or discard the theory. Saccuzzo, Hirt, and Spencer (1974), for example, theorized that schizophrenics are slower than normals in terms of the speed with which visual images are stored in short-term memory. Therefore, they had schizophrenic and normal subjects perform a task in which, after various time intervals, they were to identify targets that had been imbedded in a complex visual display. When the durations of opportunities to store the display in short-term memory were limited, by exposing subjects to a competing visual stimulus, normals performed better than did schizophrenics. Thus, the theory of relatively slow processing among schizophrenics was retained.

The term quasi-experimental research is somewhat unfortunate because it implies that the research is not quite experimental, or not quite good enough. In fact, very few experimenters succeed in controlling all of the variables that might influence the phenomenon of interest. Hence, differences between quasi-experimental and experimental projects are differences of degree. The strength of quasi-experimental, as opposed to experimental, design logic is that it prompts researchers to identify the uncontrolled variables so as to be aware of their implications for interpreting the data that are acquired. For example, Campbell and Stanley (1966) listed eight possible sources of unwanted influence that can compromise the internal validity of an experiment, and four common threats to external validity.

Experimental Models

The paradigm of the experiment begins with the reproduction of some phenomena of interest under carefully controlled conditions of observation. The effects of one or more independent (manipulated) variables on the phenomena are then studied while other potential sources of variance in the phenomena are taken into account in one way or another. Two recent examples of this sort of work are attempts to develop animal models of anxiety disorders via aversive conditioning procedures (Mineka, 1987), and attempts to produce delusions, compulsions, and dissociation via hypnotic induction (Hilgard, 1977; Kihlstrom, 1979).

The common element of true experiments in psychopathology is that the phenomena of interest are produced by something the experimenter does to the subject; they are not brought to the laboratory by the subject then studied by the experimenter. In principle, an ability to produce and control psychopathological phenomena would be a powerful demonstration that the phenomena are understood. (Indeed, as noted earlier, prediction and control amount to explanation from the vantage point of those who espouse a behavioral position.) However, there are noteworthy problems with the classical experiment as it is used currently in the context of psychopathology research.

Ethical considerations preclude attempts to reproduce bona fide psychopathology in humans. The experimental psychopathologist must, therefore, be content with animal models or with subclinical human analogues. In the case of animal models the fact of phyletic discontinuity imposes inherent limits on the accuracy of statements made about humans. Similar problems arise with subclinical human models; because the human experimental psychopathologist is explicitly prohibited from producing the exact clinical phenomenon of interest, there is always room to question the adequacy of experimental approximations.

A related problem is that the reproduction of any phenomenon in an experiment requires considerable knowledge, or at least agreement, about the nature of the phenomenon that is being reproduced. The state of our knowledge about the events of psychopathology augurs against ready or routine agreement about when those events have and have not been reproduced satisfactorily. Finally, experiments often have an artificial character. As noted earlier, the procedures that are necessary to create controlled conditions of observation often have the collateral effect of weakening the external validity of the statements produced by the experiment.

Notwithstanding criticisms such as those above, true experimental modeling of psychopathology is a potentially valuable undertaking. This would be especially true if the psychopathologists could shift fundamentally the focus of their experimental work. Most criticisms of experimental psychopathology boil down to allegations of suspect external validity with respect to events in clinical settings. The traditional response to this state of affairs has been to attempt to improve the external validity of experiments by matching experimental events to clinical events in various ways (Abramson & Seligman, 1977). An alternative response is to articulate experimental purposes that circumvent the problem of suspect external validity. One way to do this is to explicitly place experimental psychopathology in the context of scientific discovery, not of scientific confirmation. Having done so, the statements derived from particular experiments are not judged in terms of external validity; rather, they are judged in terms of the degree to which they serve to direct methodologically different confirmatory research that has the property of external validity, e.g., quasi-experimental research with clinical patients in clinical settings. Another way to circumvent the problem of suspect external validity in true experimentation is to orient the work explicitly toward theoretical hypothesis testing. Research that tests a theory is judged not in terms of external validity but, rather, in terms of theoretical validity. A given theory can be tested with experiments that have the property of theoretical validity and with quasi experiments that have the property of external validity. In this way experiments, theories, quasi experiments, and other methods can be interlaced so as to produce rationo-empirical statements that are based on controlled and externally valid research without attempting to meet the ill-conceived requirement that experimental control and external validity be achieved at the same time.

RESEARCH ON INTERVENTION

The remainder of this chapter is about research on psychological intervention into psychopathology. Various approaches to research are discussed: simple case studies; intrasubject replication experiments; behavior therapy outcome experiments; behavior therapy analogue experiments; psychotherapy process and outcome research, and meta-analytic methods.

The Case Study Method

The case study has always been a basic and important aspect of research on intervention into psychopathology. Over the course of the past century, intervention case studies have evolved from being little more than stories to being legitimate pieces of science. In the contemporary case study considerable detail is provided about the measures used to quantify the patient's problem, about the interventions that were used, and about the measurable changes that were wrought, usually in both the short and long term. While the case study is a legitimate and important part of therapeutic science, its limitations should be clearly understood.

Simple (assessment-intervention-repeat assessment) case studies lack internal validity because numerous unknown factors can coincide with intervention and influence the measurements that are targeted by the intervention. Examples of such factors are cycles in the targeted problem(s), extra-therapeutic influences on the targeted problem, effects of repeated evaluations on measures of the targeted problem, and the like. Simple case studies lack external validity also because no data are provided about the effects of the intervention when it is provided by other persons, when it is provided to other persons, etc. As with the etiologic case study, therefore, proper scientific use of the simple intervention case study occurs in the scientific context of discovery; case studies suggest clinical and theoretical possibilities that must be confirmed by more rigorous methods before they are accepted.

Intrasubject Replication Experiments

Intrasubject replication methodology (sometimes called single-subject methodology) is a general approach to psychological science (Skinner, 1953; Johnston & Pennypacker, 1980). It takes, as a point of departure, the argument that most behavioral research methods are designed to make statements about populations or population samples, not statements about the individuals whom the populations or samples comprise. It is offered as a corrective methodology that affords scientific statements about the behavior of individuals.

Intrasubject replication methodology is well suited to the intervention case study arena (e.g., Hersen & Barlow, 1976). In general, intrasubject replication research seeks to demonstrate repeated changes in behavior that are coterminous with repeated changes in the subject's environment (or changes in some other variable, such as the initiation of treatment). Repeated changes in behavior immediately after repeated environmental changes are used to support the argument that the environmental change produced the behavioral change (i.e., the behavioral change was not produced by some unknown and temporally confounded factor). In an intrasubject reversal experiment about positive reinforcement, for example, the rate of a behavior is recorded during an unconstrained baseline period, during a subsequent period when the behavior leads to reward, during a third period when the behavior is again unconstrained, and during a fourth period when the behavior once again leads to reward. Demonstrations of relatively lower rates of behavior during the first and third (baseline) periods than during the second and fourth (reward) periods support the argument that the contingent reward served to increase rates of the behavior (i.e., that the behavior was under the control of positive reinforcement). In an intrasubject multiple baselines experiment about positive reinforcement, for another example, the rates of three or so behaviors are recorded during an unconstrained baseline period. During a second period, two of the behaviors are still unconstrained but the third behavior leads to reward. During a third period, one of the behaviors remains unconstrained, while the second and third behavior both lead to reward. Finally, there is a period when all three behaviors lead to reward. A demonstration that the rate of each behavior changes only during the period(s) when it is rewarded is used to support the argument that reward produced the change.

The common feature of intrasubject replication experiments is that close correspondence between recorded events in behavior and manipulated events in the environment is used to argue that the behavioral events were produced by the environmental changes. Unwanted influence from temporally contiguous and unknown confounds, such as natural cycles in the target behavior, is controlled by requiring that records of the behavior reveal a stable rate before contingencies or other experimental variables are introduced or withdrawn.

Each of the intrasubject replication strategies has strengths and weaknesses. The intrasubject reversal design, for example, can be used only when the effects of treatment are transient; permanent or long-lasting treatment effects would preclude a return to baseline and forestall opportunity to demonstrate repeated effects of treatment. Intrasubject multiple baselines experiments can be used to evaluate permanent or long-lasting interventions, but they require that the three or so target behaviors be relatively independent. If the behaviors vary together, then successful intervention with one will influence the other two also, and will preclude opportunity to demonstrate the orderly sequence of environment/behavior correspondences that the logic of the design requires.

Behavior Therapy Outcome Research

Behavior therapy often takes the form of using fairly well defined intervention procedures or sets of procedural "packages" to influence relatively well defined problematic behaviors. For example, procedures such as systematic desensitization (Wolpe, 1990) and guided exposure (Marks, 1981) are used with patients who present with anxiety disorders such as simple, social, and agoraphobia. Therefore, research in behavior therapy generally involves comparing behavioral changes among a group of treated patients with behavioral changes among groups of patients who receive competing treatments.

In the most simple behavior therapy outcome experiment one group of patients is assessed and treated while, simultaneously, another is assessed but not treated. Differential change in simultaneously assessed target behaviors (dependent variables) between the two patient groups is construed as reflecting the influence of the experimental treatment (independent variable). Given that various methodological desiderata have been met (i.e., the experimental treatment is a faithful representation of clinical treatment or of a theory about clinical treatment; the experimental measures are ecologically valid indices of adaptively significant behavior), the simple treatment vs. no-treatment experiment can, with narrow external validity, demonstrate the effectiveness of a behavior therapy. This is so because data from the untreated patients allow for control over potential confounds, such as cycles in the target behavior and effects on the target behavior from repeated assessments during the experiment.

For all approaches to treatment, the validity of treatment vs. no-treatment comparisons is extended by incorporating quasi-experimental design logic into research protocols. As noted earlier, quasi-experimental designs are useful when researchers know that experimental controls are necessarily incomplete (Cook & Campbell, 1979). An exemplar quasi-experimental strategy that can reduce unwanted influences in therapy outcome studies is called the interrupted time series design.

In the simplest experiment, the intervention target is measured twice, once before and once after treatment. In an interrupted time series experiment, the intervention target is measured repeatedly and at regular intervals before, during, and after a period of treatment. The data from multiple measures of the target allow the researcher to portray what would be expected to happen in the absence of treatment, and to identify treatment effects as departures from that expectation. For example, Harlow, Anglin, and Douglas (1984) measured chronic heroin addicts' heroin use, marijuana use, and employment status several times before and after the addicts entered a methadone maintenance program. (Methadone is an alternative drug that mimics the effects of heroin but is less dangerous.) Time series analyses of the multiple, repeated measures showed that entry into the program was associated with decreased heroin use, with increased use of marijuana, and with improved employment status.

Sometimes patients improve simply because they are "in treatment." When treatment vs. no-treatment comparisons are used, any nonspecific effects from "being in treatment" are added inadvertently to the effects of the behavior therapy itself and can lead researchers to overstate the power of the therapy. Hence, research strategies have evolved that separate nonspecific from specific effects. A historically prominent strategy is use of the psychological placebo (Thorne, 1950) in which one (control) group of patients is "in treatment" but they receive an experimental regimen that theoretically should not influence the target behavior. In principle, the behaviorally inert psychological placebo controls for the effects of "being in treatment" by providing patients with attention, time, etc. equivalent to that experienced by patients receiving the behavior therapy of interest (e.g., Paul, 1966). In practice, however, there have been significant problems associated both with designing "treatments" that are consensually described as inert, and with demonstrating the equivalence of nonspecific influences within therapeutic and inert placebo regimens (Kazdin & Wilcoxon, 1976). A more contemporary strategy is, simply, to compare the effects of two or more behavioral treatments, while simultaneously monitoring a group of temporarily untreated patients (e.g., patients on a waiting list for treatment). Presumably, all of the treated patients are influenced nonspecifically by being "in treatment", hence, different outcomes across treatment vs. no-treatment comparisons are construed as reflecting differences in specific therapy effects.

Behavior therapy outcome experiments have been used not only to evaluate the effects of competing treatment packages, but also to evaluate the effects of combined therapeutic tactics. For example, the effects of behavioral and cognitive treatments, alone and in combination, on panic disorder with agoraphobia have been described experimentally (e.g., Kleiner, Marshall, & Spevack, 1987) as have the separate and combined effects of behavioral and pharmacological approaches to treating simple phobia (Marshall & Segal, 1986). When researchers wish to study therapy effects on several or many measures of outcome, multivariate statistics of the type described earlier are available, e.g., multivariate analysis of variance.

Behavior Therapy Analogue Research

Owing to ethical constraints on dealings with patients, and to practical limitations associated with research in clinical settings, behavior therapy outcome experiments are often weak on the dimension of internal validity. Therefore, room exists for research that takes place in settings other than clinics, and that uses subjects other than patients. The term "analogue research" is used to refer to such efforts, even though virtually all experimental events are analogues of their naturalistic referents in one way or another. Some analogue research uses actual laboratory settings and animal subjects. For example, Delprato (1973) used aversively conditioned rats to evaluate the effects of an experimental version of systematic desensitization (Wolpe, 1990) and of various procedural components. Most behavior therapy analogue research, however, has made use of nonclinical human subjects: persons who are not patients but who are recruited for research via media solicitations or in some other way.

The potential benefit of behavior therapy analogue research is enhanced internal validity relative to clinical investigations. This is so because analogue researchers have relatively more control over the experimental events to which their subjects are exposed. For example, subjects can more readily be given a theoretically inert treatment; interventions can be tape recorded so that identical treatments(s) are provided for subjects. The inherent weakness of behavior therapy analogue research is in external validity. This is so by definition; interventions, subjects, and intervention targets are approximations of treatments, patients, and behavioral phenomena in the clinic.

Much controversy has surrounded the value of behavior therapy analogue research. In some degree the controversy has rested on the widespread misconception that the statements produced by therapy analogue research must be high on the dimension of external validity (Bernstein & Paul, 1971). Most of the controversy has been unnecessary. The proper role of behavior therapy analogue research within the overall research enterprise parallels that of experimental modeling of psychopathology (discussed earlier). Valuable behavior therapy analogue research will be high on the dimensions of internal validity and theoretical validity. External validity can then be emphasized in experimental and quasi-experimental behavior therapy outcome research with actual clinic patients. Optimally, internally valid analogue research and externally valid clinical outcome research will play complementary roles in developing scientific theories of behavior therapy effects.

Psychotherapy Research

Unlike research in behavior therapy, research in psychotherapy does not begin with well defined treatment packages. Sometimes the activities of psychotherapy are regularized by providing research therapists with treatment manuals similar to those used in behavior therapy research. However, even the authors of such manuals lament their incompleteness in the psychotherapy context; questions remain about what goes on during psychotherapy. Similarly, psychotherapy research ordinarily does not deal with discrete and readily identifiable target behaviors. Rather, dependent variables take the forms of patient and clinician ratings of improvement, changes in scores on psychometric measures of self-esteem, or of psychopathology, etc. In general, therefore, psychotherapy research is much more complex than is behavior therapy research and, notwithstanding substantial methodological improvement during the past decade, the dividend from psychotherapy investigations has not been comparable to that from work in the behavioral arena. Only a few major themes can be touched on here.

PSYCHOTHERAPY PROCESS RESEARCH

"Psychotherapy process" research seeks to discover which events or other aspects of psychotherapy sessions are important, and how those events affect patients within and outside the therapy context. "Psychotherapy outcome" research seeks to determine how much benefit is achieved. Recently, psychotherapy process and correlated outcomes have been studied simultaneously (Greenberg, 1986).

Psychotherapy process research seeks to identify the important events in psychotherapy, then to describe the flow of those events as patients and therapists interact (Mahrer & Nadler, 1986). Some researchers have defined as important those psychotherapeutic events that presumably are related to improvement on treatment-outcome criteria (Orlinsky & Howard, 1978). Others have defined as important those psychotherapeutic events that demonstrably are related to reductions in the patient's problems or to positive evaluations of therapy sessions by patients and/or therapists (e.g., Stiles, 1980). Still others have defined as important those events that comport well with some theory of psychotherapeutic practice (see the discussion of "task analysis" below) or with some theory about the psychological determinants of the patient's problems. In the latter case, for example, if excessive self-criticism is construed theoretically as a determinant of patients' problems, then events that signal a lessening of self-criticism are defined as important (e.g., Rice & Greenberg, 1984).

The great bulk of research on the flow of important events in psychotherapy has used a "frequency approach" (Russell & Trull, 1986) to describing patient and therapist language as recorded and transcribed from psychotherapy sessions. The frequency approach begins by developing language categories and coding strategies (Russell & Stiles, 1979). Content category systems, for example, classify words or phrases by their denotative, connotative, referential, or metaphorical meanings (e.g., death, mother, sexual anxiety, unconscious dependence). Given a language category system and a coding strategy, the frequency approach continues by recording the frequencies with which therapists and/or patients exhibit the coded language variables during and across psychotherapy sessions.

At best, the frequency approach provides tallies of the frequencies with which various classes of verbalizations occur during psychotherapy sessions. Importantly, it tells us nothing about how the patient's language influences the therapist's language or vice versa; that is, it tells us nothing about the patterning or sequencing of patient and therapist verbalizations. This is very problematic because knowledge of moment-to-moment reciprocal influences between patients and therapists lies at the very core of understanding psychotherapy process.

Some psychotherapy process researchers have attempted to redress weaknesses in the frequency approach by using a rationo-empirical method known as task analysis (Greenberg, 1986). The analytical unit in task analysis is a "change event" that incorporates the verbalizations of both patients and therapists and that serves, therefore, to identify interactions between the two. Task analysis begins with identifying some recurring change event to study (e.g., resolution of a conflict). Next the researcher uses an accepted theory of change (e.g., of conflict resolution) to generate theoretically perfect examples of change performances (e.g., performances that show movement from self-criticism to self-acceptance). And then the researcher undertakes intensive study of the actual change performances of individual patients and therapists (e.g., conflict resolution performances) and, having done so, revises the theoretical example so as to fit the performances actually observed. The newly described theoretical performance is then used to guide further study of actual performances, further revisions of theoretical performances, etc. Using the task analysis approach, Greenberg (1984) was able to show that patients who resolved an intrapsychic conflict and patients who did not (as judged by patient and therapist report) differed in terms of change events such as alterations in voice quality and in depth of experiencing.

Other psychotherapy process researchers have attempted to redress weaknesses in the frequency approach by using sequential analysis methods (Sackett, 1979) to describe serial dependencies between patient and therapist language categories. In general, sequential analysis in psychotherapy process research begins with the development of a language category system such as that described above. Simultaneous time-series descriptions (language category sequences) of the language of the patient and of the therapist, as their interaction unfolds through time, are then examined for serial dependencies that exist between the two time-series variables. For example, a serial dependency between the language of a therapist and the language of a patient would be said to exist if changes in the patient's voice quality occurred a disproportionately high number of times immediately following a specific category of therapist behavior, e.g., interpretation.

Time-series descriptions of psychotherapy process are limited in several ways. For example, the coding systems for patient and therapist behaviors necessarily have a preliminary character; time-series work seeks to elucidate psychotherapy process, but something must be known already about the psychotherapy process to derive the codes for time-series description. Second, time-series description ordinarily is restricted to dependencies between events on one time series variable and the immediately preceding events on the other. Hence, temporally delayed influence is missed, and the flow through time of psychotherapeutic transactions is chopped into bits and pieces. In principle, a method known as lagged sequential analysis can be used to identify dependencies between events on one time series and events on another that are further back in time than the immediately preceding one, e.g., a patient's response to something the therapist said 10 minutes before. Lagged sequential analysis, however, does not solve the problem of describing multi-element sequences (i.e., the "flow" of psychotherapy) (Russell & Trull, 1986).

Some recent research has combined the methods of task analysis and sequential analysis to study the flow of events in psychotherapy. The combined tactic reduces problems associated with the use of preliminary or arbitrary language categories to form category sequences (time-series variables). Wiseman and Rise (1989), for example, derived change-event categories from task-analytic iterations based on a theory of how the therapist's voice quality influences the patient's voice quality and the depth of the patient's emotional experiencing during client-centered therapy. They than performed sequential analyses using categories of the therapist's voice quality to form one time-series variable, and categories of the patient's voice quality and of the patient's depth of experiencing to form two other time-series variables. Some serial dependencies were detected, e.g., the therapist's voice quality influenced both the patient's voice quality and, for some categories, the patient's depth of experiencing.

COMPARATIVE PSYCHOTHERAPY OUTCOME RESEARCH

In general, comparative psychotherapy outcome research pits psychotherapies against one another in order to decide which therapies are best. The work proceeds by assessing patients' problems, randomly assigning patients to different treatments, conducting somewhat standardized versions of the different treatments, and re-assessing patients' problems, so as to allow for comparisons of therapeutic efficacy. In principle, comparative psychotherapy outcome research is straightforward and has much to recommend it as a means of choosing psychotherapeutic approaches. This is particularly true given recent advances in methodology (e.g., concern over the representativeness of research psychotherapies, the availability of treatment manuals that regularize research psychotherapies, interest in the validity of outcome measures). Comparative psychotherapy outcome research also provides opportunities to study psychotherapy process (above) and to develop theory in the psychotherapy arena. In practice, however, there are significant reasons to question the value of comparative psychotherapy outcome research (Kazdin, 1986). Individual research projects are expensive and time consuming, and there are several hundred approaches to psychotherapy that might be candidates for comparative evaluation. The effects of various therapies on measures of outcome often are too small to permit statistical tests based on reasonable numbers of patients to reveal actual differences between them (Kazdin & Bass, 1989). The number of potential confounds across the compared treatments is very large, sufficiently large to raise questions about the degree to which random assignment of reasonable numbers of patients controls for all of them (Hsu, 1989).

Meta-Analysis

For reasons such as those just mentioned, individual psychotherapy outcome experiments rarely if every suffice to determine how well a particular intervention works, or which intervention is better than another. Rather, knowledge about the

F. DUDLEY
McGLYNN

comparative effects of an intervention emerges slowly through the cumulation of information from multiple comparative outcome trials involving different therapists, different patients, different settings, different outcome measures, different outcomes, etc. The term meta-analysis refers to a set of statistical methods through which heterogeneous information from diverse empirical sources can be standardized and pooled for comparative purposes. In the psychotherapy outcome arena, meta-analysis is sometimes used to compare the magnitudes of therapeutic benefits, termed the effect sizes, that are associated with different therapy approaches (Smith, Glass & Miller, 1980). The value of statements based on meta-analytic psychotherapy outcome research has always been controversial, and the popularity of meta-analysis seems to be diminishing. Among the significant problems of meta-analysis in psychotherapy is the variable, and often questionable, quality of the individual research reports that contribute to calculated effect sizes.

SUMMARY

The focus of this chapter was on research methods: on their strengths, on their weaknesses, and on the kinds of statements they do and do not produce legitimately. The methods described were chosen from among many that are used because they are fundamental and/or of contemporary interest. Many contemporary research techniques were not included because of the methodological focus, and because they are discussed elsewhere in the text.

The theme of the chapter is that the business of science is to make statements, and that case studies, nonexperimental research, quasi-experimental research, and experimental research afford different kinds of statements. The statements afforded by each set of methods occupy a legitimate place in psychopathology. It is incumbent upon scientists to recognize areas of legitimacy, and to appreciate the role of methodological complementarity in building the body of knowledge.

The future of psychopathology research presents both opportunities and challenges. There have been significant advances in statistical treatment of research data. Major advances in biological research and in psychological research hold out the possibility of providing improved data for advanced statistical treatment. For example, the influence of single genes on psychopathology can be studied by tracing genetic markers, called restriction fragment length polymorphisms, through families. That technology, coupled with modern conceptions of polygenetic transmission, and with modern statistics, should render obsolete the twin studies, and family studies so popular until now. At the same time, progress is hindered by conceptual allegiance to prescientific diagnostic categories, and by methodological allegiance to procedures that were designed to make statements about samples and populations, not statements about individuals. It will be of some interest to find out if our conceptualizations of psychopathology research problems keep pace with our mathematical and technological skills.

REFERENCES

Abramson, L. Y., & Seligman, M. E. P. (1977). Modeling psychopathology in the laboratory: History and rationale. In J. P. Maser & M. E. P. Seligman (Eds.), *Psychopathology: Experimental models* (pp. 1–26). San Francisco: W. H. Freeman.

Attneave, F. (1959). *Applications of information theory to psychology: A summary of basic concepts, methods, and results*. New York: Holt, Rinehart and Winston.

Bentler, P. (1985). *Theory and implementation of EQS: A structural equation program*. Los Angeles: BMDP Statistical Software.

Bernstein, D. A., & Paul, G. L. (1971). Some comments on therapy analogue research with small animal "phobias." *Journal of Behavior Therapy & Experimental Psychiatry, 2*, 225–237.

Bleuler, E. (1911). *Dementia praecox oder gruppe der schizophrenien*. Aschaffenburger Handbuch der Psychiatrie, Leipzig und Wien.

Bogerts, B., Meertz, E., & Schonfeldt-Bausch, R. (1985). Basal ganglia and limbic system pathology in schizophrenia. *Archives of General Psychiatry, 42*, 784–791.

Breuer, J., & Freud, S. (1895). *Studien uber hysterie*. Vienna: Franz Deuticke.

Campbell, D. T., & Stanley, J. C. (1966). *Experimental and quasi-experimental designs for research*. Chicago: Rand McNally.

Cook, T. D., & Campbell, D. T. (1979). *Quasi-experimentation: Design and analysis issues for field settings*. Chicago: Rand McNally.

Crow, T. J. (1985). The two syndrome concept: Origins and current status. *Schizophrenia Bulletin, 11*, 471–486.

DeLisi, L. E., Dauphinais, I. D., & Gershon, E. S. (1988). Perinatal complications and reduced size of brain limbic structures in familial schizophrenia. *Schizophrenia Bulletin, 14*, 185–191.

Delprato, D. J. (1973). An animal analogue to systematic desensitization and elimination of avoidance. *Behaviour Research and Therapy, 11*, 49–55.

FIDIA Research Foundation. (1992). *Neuroscience Facts, 3*, 1–4.

Fraser, W. I., King, K. M., Thomas, P., & Kendall, R. C. (1986). The diagnosis of schizophrenia by language analysis. *British Journal of Psychiatry, 148*, 275–278.

Freud, S. (1909). Analysis of a phobia in a five-year-old-boy. In *Collected works of Sigmund Freud* (Vol. 10). London: Hogarth, 1956.

Gorenstein, E. E., & Newman, J. P. (1980). Disinhibitory psychopathology: A new perspective and a model for research. *Psychological Review, 87*, 301–315.

Greenberg, L. (1984). A task analysis of intrapersonal conflict resolution. In L. Rice & L. Greenberg (Eds.), *Patterns of change: Intensive analysis of psychotherapy process* (pp. 67–123). New York: Guilford Press.

Greenberg, L. (1986). Change process research. *Journal of Consulting and Clinical Psychology, 54*, 4–9.

Hammen, C., Burge, D., & Stansbury, K. (1990). Relationship of mother and child variables to child outcomes in a high-risk sample: A causal modeling analysis. *Developmental Psychology, 26*, 24–30.

Harlow, L. L., Anglin, M., & Douglas, D. (1984). Time series design to evaluate effectiveness of methadone maintenance. *Journal of Drug Education, 14*, 53–72.

Harmon, H. H. (1967). *Modern Factor Analysis* (2nd Ed.). Chicago: University of Chicago Press.

Hersen, M., & Barlow, D. H. (1976). *Single-case experimental designs: Strategies for studying behavior change*. New York: Pergamon Press.

Hilgard, E. H. (1977). *Divided consciousness: Multiple controls in human thought and action*. New York: Wiley-Interscience.

Hsu, L. M. (1989). Random sampling, randomization, and equivalence of contrasted groups in psychotherapy outcome research. *Journal of Consulting and Clinical Psychology, 57*, 131–137.

Johnson, B., Mayberry, W. E., & McGlynn, F. D. (1990). Exploratory factor analysis of a sixty-item questionnaire concerned with fear of dentistry. *Journal of Behavior Therapy & Experimental Psychiatry, 21*, 199–203.

Johnston, J. M., & Pennypacker, H. (1980). *Strategies and tactics of human behavioral research*. Hillsdale: Lawrence Erlbaum Associates.

Kazdin, A. E. (1986). Comparative outcome studies of psychotherapy: Methodological issues and strategies. *Journal of Consulting and Clinical Psychology, 54*, 95–105.

Kazdin, A. E., & Bass, D. (1989). Power to detect differences between alternative treatments in comparative psychotherapy outcome research. *Journal of Consulting and Clinical Psychology, 57*, 138–147.

Kazdin, A. E., & Wilcoxon, L. A. (1976). Systematic desensitization and nonspecific treatment effects: A methodological evaluation. *Psychological Bulletin, 83*, 729–758.

Kihlstrom, J. F. (1979). Hypnosis and psychopathology: Retrospect and prospect. *Journal of Abnormal Psychology, 88*, 459–473.

Kleiner, L., Marshall, W. L., & Spevack, M. (1987). Training in problem solving and exposure treatment for agoraphobics with panic attacks. *Journal of Anxiety Disorders, 1*, 219–238.

Mahrer, A. R., & Nadler, W. P. (1986). Good moments in psychotherapy: A preliminary review, a list, and some promising research avenues. *Journal of Consulting and Clinical Psychology, 54*, 10–15.

Marascuilo, L. A., & Busk, P. L. (1987). Loglinear models: A way to study main effects and interactions for multidimensional contingency tables with categorical data. *Journal of Counseling Psychology, 34*, 433–455.

Marascuilo, L. A., & Levin, J. R. (1983). *Multivariate statistics in the social sciences*. Monterey: Brooks/Cole.

Marks, I. M. (1981). *Cure and care of neurosis: Theory and practice of behavioral psychotherapy*. New York: Wiley.

Marshall, W. L., & Segal, Z. (1986). Phobias and anxiety. In M. Hersen (Ed.). *Pharmacological and behavioral treatment: An integrative approach* (pp. 260–288). New York: Wiley.

McNeal, D. W., & Berryman, M. L. (1989). Components of dental fear in adults? *Behaviour Research and Therapy, 27*, 233–236.

Mineka, S. (1987). A primate model of phobic fears. In H. Eysenck, & I. Martin (Eds.). *Theoretical foundations of behavior therapy* (pp. 81–111). New York: Plenum.

Orlinsky, D. E., & Howard, K. I. (1978). The relation of process to outcome in psychotherapy. In S. L. Garfield, & A. E. Bergin (Eds.), *Handbook of psychotherapy and behavior change* (pp. 283–329). New York: Wiley.

Paul, G. L. (1966). *Insight vs. desensitization in psychotherapy*. Stanford, Calif: Stanford University Press.

Persons, J. (1986). The advantages of studying psychological phenomena rather than psychiatric diagnoses. *American Psychologist, 41*, 1252–1260.

Rice, L. N., & Greenberg, L. S. (1984). The new research paradigm. In L. N. Rice, & L. S. Greenberg (Eds.), *Patterns of change: Intensive analysis of psychotherapy process* (pp. 7–25), New York: Guilford Press.

Rosenthal, D. (Ed.). (1963). *The Genain Quadruplets*. New York: Basic Books.

Russell, R. L., & Stiles, W. B. (1979). Categories for classifying language in psychotherapy. *Psychological Bulletin, 86*, 404–419.

Russell, R. L., & Trull, T. J. (1986). Sequential analysis of language variables in psychotherapy process research. *Journal of Consulting and Clinical Psychology, 54*, 16–21.

Saccuzzo, D. P., Hirt, M., & Spencer, T. J. (1974). Backward masking as a measure of attention in schizophrenia. *Journal of Abnormal Psychology, 83*, 512–522.

Sackett, G. P. (1979). The lag sequential analysis of contingency and cyclicity in behavioral interaction. In J. D. Osofsky (Ed.), *Handbook of infant development* (pp. 623–649). New York: John Wiley and Sons.

Skinner, B. F. (1953). *Science and human behavior*. New York: MacMillan.

Smith, M. L., Glass, G. V., & Miller, T. I. (1980). *The benefits of psychotherapy*. Baltimore, MD: Johns Hopkins University Press.

Staats, A. W. (1991). Unified positivism and unification psychology: Fad or new field? *American Psychologist, 46*, 899–912.

Stiles, W. B. (1980). Measurement of the impact of psychotherapy sessions. *Journal of Consulting and Clinical Psychology, 48*, 176–185.

Thorne, F. C. (1950). Rules of evidence in the evaluation of the effect of psychotherapy. *Journal of Clinical Psychology, 8*, 38–41.

Tienari, P., Lahti, I., Sorri, A., Naarala, M., Moring, J., Wahlberg, K.-E., & Wynne, L. C. (1987). The Finnish adoptive family study of schizophrenia. *Journal of Psychiatric Research, 21*, 437–445.

Wiseman, H., & Rice, L. H. (1989). Sequential analysis of therapist-client interaction during change events: A task focused approach. *Journal of Consulting and Clinical Psychology, 57*, 281–286.

Wolpe, J. (1990). *The practice of behavior therapy* (4th ed.). New York: Pergamon.

Wolpe, J., & Rachman, S. J. (1960). Psychoanalytic "evidence," a critique based on Freud's case of Little Hans. *Journal of Nervous and Mental Disease, 131*, 135–147.

4

Psychoanalytic Model

Howard D. Lerner and Joshua Ehrlich

Introduction

Sigmund Freud, through his discoveries about the inner workings of the mind, offered people a revolutionary way in which to view themselves. His discoveries suggested that mental life was vastly more complex than psychologists and philosophers had previously believed. As an important example, psychologists before Freud believed that mental functioning was conscious. Freud's revolutionary method of studying the mind, which he called psychoanalysis, indicated that what is mental includes far more than what is merely conscious or accessible to consciousness. His illumination of unconscious thought processes dramatically expanded the depth, range, and scope of psychology and altered our understanding of human nature. The enduring impact of the founder of psychoanalysis upon the field is truly striking. Though psychoanalytic thought and method have evolved enormously since Freud, 50 years after his death Freud and psychoanalysis are still considered synonymous in people's minds.

Psychoanalysis is a term that has two related meanings. First, it is a theory of personality. As we will see, psychoanalysis, in fact, has evolved since Freud into different though overlapping theories of human development: the working of the human mind, and psychopathology. Second, psychoanalysis is a procedure: a method of studying mental functioning and a form of psychotherapy. In the discussion that follows, we will offer some insights into the psychoanalytic approach to psychotherapy.

The impact of psychoanalysis on popular thought in the past century has been immense. It has influenced theories and values in regard to childrearing, education, sexuality, human relations, and numerous other domains of human experi-

Howard D. Lerner and Joshua Ehrlich • Department of Psychiatry, University of Michigan, Ann Arbor, Michigan 48104.

Advanced Abnormal Psychology, edited by Vincent B. Van Hasselt and Michel Hersen. Plenum Press, New York, 1994.

HOWARD D.
LERNER and
JOSHUA
EHRLICH

ence. Terms, such as *identity, identification, defense,* and the *unconscious,* which originated with Freud, are now part of everyday language. Anyone interested in the mind must have some knowledge of psychoanalysis and its contribution to our understanding of mental processes.

Interestingly, Freud's original theories applied exclusively to psychopathology, to the symptoms of mental illness. Freud demonstrated convincingly that unconscious mental processes, wishes, fantasies, emotions, and memories determine the nature and type of symptoms. He showed that ideas and feelings of which the patient was unaware contributed significantly to psychopathology. For the first time, the study and treatment of psychopathology became part of psychology. This revolutionary understanding of psychopathology was only a beginning. Freud extrapolated from the processes and experiences involved in psychopathology to illuminate those responsible for mental health. As his theories developed, it became increasingly apparent that the same conflictual wishes, ideas, fantasies, and memories that underlie psychopathology also determine what is normal.

THE THREE PSYCHOLOGIES OF PSYCHOANALYSIS

In approaching psychopathology from the perspective of psychoanalytic theory it is crucial to understand that psychoanalysis does not offer a single, coherent theoretical system. Psychoanalysis does not represent the monolithic, uniform theory it is purported to be. To begin, Freud, through the course of his writings, advanced evolving, often divergent, conceptualizations of the human mind to account for new observed clinical phenomena. The transformation from one set of formulations to another did not indicate that one necessarily superseded the other. Freud assumed that a given set of clinical phenomena might be best understood by using one frame of reference whereas another set of data demanded a different set of concepts for its understanding.

Of even greater importance than the numerous and complex shifts in Freud's own theorizing, psychoanalysis since Freud has undergone enormous revisions and transformations that have altered many fundamental aspects of Freud's ideas. Profound shifts in the psychoanalytic understanding of female sexuality, of infant and child development, and of severe psychopathology are crucial examples of the altered psychoanalytic landscape.

As psychoanalytic theory has evolved, divergences in the understanding of early development, psychopathology, treatment, and more fundamentally, the nature of the human mind have led to the development of different theoretical approaches or models within psychoanalysis. Within contemporary psychoanalytic thought, three conceptual approaches—modern structural theory, self psychology, and object relations theory—are most influential. Each theory or model offers a coherent account of early development and psychopathology and, emanating from these, of how treatment should proceed.

BASIC ASSUMPTIONS OF THE THREE PSYCHOANALYTIC MODELS

These three models, which we will explore at length below, are neither mutually exclusive nor exhaustive. Each offers a coherent model that can stand alone but also overlaps in many subtle and less subtle ways with each other model. Several areas of convergence appear most important. First, a continuum concept underlies all psychoanalytic approaches to psychopathology. It is widely thought that all mental disorders lie on a continuum, with psychosis and neurosis or mental health at opposite ends. Psychopathology can be thought of as a unitary process based on a concept of homeostasis, with disorders ranked according to their degree of deviation from a baseline. The continuum concept stresses the similarities and differences among all disorders. The model further implies that any individual can move along the continuum, depending on life circumstances and crises.

The continuum concept points to the importance of human development from birth onwards, and leads to a second area of substantial agreement between theories: early childhood development is crucial to later functioning and adults reenact early childhood experience and fantasy in their adult lives. The influence of early parent–child interaction is thought to be crucial for later development.

Third, all psychoanalytic models appreciate the profound significance of unconscious mental processes—unconscious thinking, memories, feelings, and fantasies—on determining behavior and personal meaning. With the assumption and belief in unconscious mental processes, psychoanalytic theorists place less emphasis on overt behavior and focus a sharper lens on underlying structures and meanings.

A fourth area of convergence involves the approach to treatment. All psychoanalytic theorists advocate an intensive, more long-term form of psychotherapy that involves the use of free association, a neutral or objective stance on the part of the therapist, and the reenactment of childhood experience, fantasy, and conflict in relationship to the analyst. The notion of the repetition of the past in the present in relationship to the analyst is termed, "transference." The working through and understanding of the transference is viewed by theorists as the critical therapeutic task within all three psychoanalytic psychologies.

A fifth area of significant convergence among theorists revolves around the significance of theory and clinical data. Since the formative days of psychoanalysis, its theory has been intimately connected with clinical observations and with the techniques of the psychoanalytic method. New clinical findings have been reflected in theoretical changes, and theoretical reformulations have, in turn, affected clinical observation. Throughout the remainder of the chapter, Table 1 (The

TABLE 1. The Three Psychoanalytic Models

	Classical	Object-relations	Self
Contributors	Freud Brenner Arlow	Freud Klein Winnicott Kernberg Adler	Kohut
Core focus	Conflict	Relationships	Self
Key concept	Compromise formation	Object representation	Self-object
Development	Psychosexual stages	Separation individuation	Transmuting internalizations
Psychopathology	Neurosis	Borderline psychosis	Narcissism
Treatment method	Interpretation	Analyst-as-new-object	Empathy

Three Psychoanalytic Models) will serve as a reference point for comparing each model in terms of major contributions, focus, key concepts, developmental theory, psychopathology, and treatment method.

MODERN STRUCTURAL THEORY

History

Freud offered models of the mind that gradually evolved—from the topographical (unconscious and conscious) to the structural (ego, superego, and id). Modern structural theory, an enormously complex, rich theoretical system, represents a refinement and elaboration of Freud's original structural theory. Structural theory, above all, is a conflict theory. From the perspective of structural theory, all psychic phenomena, including psychopathology, are manifestations of conflict. Recognizing and effecting shifts in conflicts are the main tasks of treatment. Some psychoanalysts believe that psychoanalytic theory *is* above all a conflict theory, and some question whether nonconflict models (such as self psychology) are psychoanalytic at all. Many structural theorists integrate self psychology and other conceptual frameworks into their theoretical understanding and their clinical work.

As Boesky (1991) suggests, tracing the evolution of models of conflict within psychoanalytic theory is a monumental task, essentially equivalent to tracing the history of psychoanalytic thought itself. In broadest strokes, Freud first proposed a model involving conflict between the conscious and unconscious (the topographical model). The structural model, which posited conflict between the three agencies of the mind—ego, superego, and id—represented a more complex, refined approach to psychic functioning. Arlow (1991) summarized this model succinctly:

> The ego is the final arbiter over the conflicting claims of derivative expressions of the instinctual drives, collectively designated as the id, and moral imperatives and ideal aspirations collectively designated as the superego. In its role as mediator, the ego integrates the realistic concerns of the individual for survival, adaptation, and inner harmony (p. 4).

Boesky (1991) details how, in the last 50 years, psychoanalysis has gradually elaborated Freud's structural model, although the tripartite structure of superego, ego, and id remains its cornerstones.

The Compromise Formation and the Components of Psychic Conflict

As structural theory has evolved, the concept of *compromise formation* has moved to the fore, becoming the central theoretical construct in the explication of psychic functioning, including psychopathology. The most prominent proponent of modern structural theory, Charles Brenner, a New York-based psychoanalyst, has offered the most influential contributions to the understanding of compromise formation. Brenner's *The Mind in Conflict* (1982) has become the most important single contribution to modern structural theory.

According to structural theory, the mind is constantly in a state of dynamic tension. Derivatives of basic drives (aggressive and/or sexual) constantly seek gratification. The term "drive derivative" is used because drives are thought to be biological; the term "derivative" indicates the psychological representation of the biological drives. The ego functions to oppose these drive derivatives sufficiently to ward off experiences of unpleasure (anxiety and/or depressive affect). The consequence of this dynamic tension is always a compromise between the competing components of the mind, termed a *compromise formation*. All compromise formations have four components: (1) a drive derivative; (2) anxiety and/or depressive affect; (3) defense; and (4) an aspect of superego functioning. According to Brenner (1982), *all* psychic phenomena—moods, wishes, dreams, fantasies, plans, etc.—represent compromise formations. That is, all psychic phenomena represent compromises between the derivative of an instinctual drive, the accompanying depressive and/or anxious affect, defense, and an aspect of superego functioning. All manifestations of psychopathology represent compromise formations, too, according to modern structural theory. Below, we will illuminate each component of the compromise formation, explore how the compromise formation works, then explore pathological compromise formations.

DRIVE DERIVATIVE

Within structural theory, instinctual drives are viewed as the force that propels the mind into action and motivates human behavior. Structural theorists posit two fundamental drives: sexual and aggressive. As our discussion of self psychology will suggest, the notion of primary instinctual drives is controversial. The controversy over drives extends well beyond the scope of this discussion. In exploring structural theory, it is essential to understand that instinctual drives are viewed as primary motivators of human behavior, that they are evident from early on in psychic development, and that manifestations or representation of these drives (drive derivatives) play an integral role in all psychic conflict.

ANXIETY AND/OR DEPRESSIVE AFFECT

The second component of the compromise function is anxiety and/or depressive affect. According to Brenner (1982), affects (what we commonly call emotions) are complex psychic phenomena that contain sensations of pleasure or unpleasure (or a combination of the two), plus ideas. Structural theory posits an intrinsic tension in all people's lives: between the wish for the gratification of instinctual drives and the feelings of unpleasure that such drives often arouse. The unpleasure can take the form of a fear of a future occurrence (anxiety) or a repetition of a previously experienced catastrophe (depression). The fundamental tension between drive and unpleasure stood as the centerpiece of Freud's conflict theory.

"CALAMITIES OF CHILDHOOD"

Why do instinctual drives often arouse unpleasure and thus produce intrapsychic conflict? The answer, according to structural theory, is rooted in what are termed the "calamities of childhood"—imagined dangers that all children attempt to cope with in play and fantasy. As noted, all affects contain sensations and ideas. The ideas bound up with all sensations of unpleasure can be traced to the "calamities of childhood." These are: object loss (the loss of a parent), loss of love, castration, and superego condemnation. The "calamities of childhood" represent normative developmental experiences for the child that involve intense feelings of unpleasure (anxiety and/or depressive affect). When a psychoanalyst describes a "calamity of childhood," he or she is describing a fantasied experience, a purely intrapsychic event, though these may become entangled with events in reality (e.g., castration fears may be heightened by having surgery as a child; fear of loss of a parent's love may be exacerbated by a parent's withdrawal from a child). It is essential to have some understanding of the "calamities of childhood" because they provide the crucial link between childhood experience and fantasy and adult psychic functioning, including psychopathology.

DEVELOPMENT

Structural theorists have focused most attention on what they term *oedipal development* during childhood and the ongoing impact of the psychic "calamities" from that period of development on all ensuing development. Neurotic (as opposed to more severe) difficulties are usually associated with oedipal-level conflicts. According to Brenner (1982), oedipal development occurs approximately between the years 2½ and 5. While psychological development is enormously complex during this time, a brief summary will suffice here. In normal development, the oedipal triangle takes place when the daughter is attached to the father (an attachment that includes aggressive, competitive wishes directed toward the mother and sexual wishes directed toward the father) and fears that the mother will punish her for this attachment. The opposite situation occurs for the boy through his attachment to the mother and his fears of his father's retaliation. A principal "calamity" during oedipal development involves the fear of or fantasied experience of castration (or bodily harm). This is often evident in the child's play, dreams, and fantasies. Other calamitous worries—fears of losing the parents' love or of losing the parents altogether—also bound in the fantasy-filled mind of the young child, grappling with the intensity of his or her own aggressive and sexual wishes and the complex world that surrounds him or her. Fantasies, wishes—and also fears—from the oedipal period of development *persist* in psychic life from childhood onward. Often, these contribute significantly to adolescent and adult psychological difficulties, as we will describe below.

We are now ready to look at the emergence of the compromise formation. According to structural theory, drive derivatives, pressing for gratification, often arouse anxiety or depressive affect (which is intrinsically bound up with one or more of the calamities of childhood). When this occurs, the ego, which seeks not only to facilitate gratification of drives but also to reduce anxiety or depressive affect, opposes the expression of the drive by implementing a defense. The dynamic tension between drive derivative and defense forms the centerpiece of the compromise formation. The compromise formation, according to Brenner (1982), functions to allow the greatest degree of satisfaction of drive derivatives without the arousal of too much anxiety and/or depressive affect. Brenner suggests that the ego functions as a mediator of satisfaction unless the drive derivatives arouse unpleasure; then, the ego functions appear as defense.

DEFENSES

According to Brenner (1982), defenses, the third component of the compromise formation, are aspects of mental functioning that can be defined only in terms of their function or consequence: the reduction of anxiety or depressive affect aroused by a drive derivative. Certain defenses—repression, denial, sublimation—have become well known within the popular culture. The final component of the compromise formation, an aspect of superego functioning, involves the moral component to each compromise formation. The superego contribution to compromise formation often involves the experience of guilt.

An example of a compromise formation from everyday life might be helpful here. A college student, a young man, has a crush on his teacher, a female professor in her forties. His frankly sexual wishes toward her (a sexual drive derivative) arouse anxiety because they are associated with forbidden incestuous wishes from his childhood (thus, the childhood calamity associated with his anxiety is the fear of castration; the superego component involves his feelings of guilt). He therefore implements a defense, denial, against these sexual wishes. If one were to ask him about sexual wishes toward his professor, he would answer in all honesty that he does not harbor such wishes because, in fact, they never enter his consciousness. He is, however, able to entertain with pleasure the fantasy of kissing the teacher, just once, at the end of the schoolyear. He also has a sexual dream about her two times in which she appears in disguised form. His sexual wishes, in other words, achieve *a degree* of satisfaction. To return to the compromise formation, this young man achieves a compromise between the gratification of the drive derivative (the sexual wish toward the professor) and the unpleasure associated with the drive derivative (anxiety, which is tied to fears of castration). This whole process is unconscious, though the young man may, at moments, be aware of feeling slightly anxious in this teacher's classroom without knowing why.

Pathological Compromise Formations and the Structural Approach to Neurosis

Not all compromise formations work. That is, they might not achieve a reasonable balance between the expression of the drive and the need to maintain unpleasure within tolerable limits. Brenner (1982) suggests that a compromise formation is pathological when a combination of any of the following conditions exists: too much restriction of gratification of drive derivatives; too much anxiety or depressive affect; too much inhibition of one's capacity to exert mastery in the world; too great a tendency to injure or destroy oneself; or too great a conflict with those around one. In the instance of the young man above, for example, the student's anxiety about his sexual wishes might become so intense that he withdraws from the class the woman professor teaches. Or, because of his guilt about his sexual wishes, he might begin failing the class in an unconscious effort at atonement. In such instances, we would suggest that the compromise formations—catalyzed by his sexual wishes toward his professor—are pathological.

As suggested, structural theorists since Freud have focused most attention on neurotic difficulties, which, they believe, are rooted predominantly in oedipal development. The possible roots of neurotic conflict within childhood are complex and multiply determined and as varied as the individuals who have them. We have talked briefly about oedipal-level conflict. In discussing the emergence of conflict in childhood, the structural theorists tend to place less emphasis on external circumstances—for instance, unempathic parenting—than on the powerful impact of instinctual drives and unconscious fantasy. In this, they differ profoundly from the self psychologists. Structural theorists stress that normative developmen-

HOWARD D.
LERNER and
JOSHUA
EHRLICH

tal experiences are often internalized in profoundly distorted ways because of the intensity of the child's wishes, the impact of defensive efforts, and the level of the child's cognitive functioning (Tyson, 1991).

As a common example, a 5-year-old boy, angrily competing with his father, often projects his hostile, destructive wishes onto his father in an effort to disown them. In his own mind, then, his *father* is the angry one even when, in reality, the father may be a benign, nonhostile presence in the boy's life. The boy might internalize an image of himself in violent conflict with a destructive man, bent on harming him. This, in fact, is often the critical feature in the development of castration anxiety: The child projects his or her own aggressive wishes onto the parent and then fears retaliation. The intensity of the child's own instinctual drives, the primitive nature of his or her defenses (projecting wishes) and his or her limited cognitive capacities combine to create a monster in the child's mind. Selma Fraiberg (1959), in her book *The Magic Years*, poignantly describes how preschoolers, through magical thinking, develop fears and phobias in response to everyday occurrences. What is crucial is that these childhood experiences often reverberate throughout life. The boy's unconscious fear about a man's retaliation may reemerge when he competes with other boys on the ballfield (which he unconsciously associates with competing against his father) or, later, attempts to consummate a sexual relationship with a woman (which he unconsciously associates with the forbidden sexual wish for the mother).

While structural theorists emphasize the power of wishes, primitive thinking, and unconscious fantasy, they do not deny that childhood events in reality can profoundly affect children. They stress, however, that the child does not internalize events *as they are* but filters them through the lens of his or her own wishes and fears. As a fairly common example, a single mother might sleep in a bed with her son following a divorce and, because she is lonely, might place him in the role of the man of the household, despite his age. Such an experience often makes boys acutely anxious because they fantasize that they have, in fact, won the oedipal competition. They then live in dread of the father's retaliation. Such boys, anxious in childhood, will potentially develop significant inhibitions in the sexual realm and in self-assertion. What is crucial here is that the meaning of the life event, according to the structural theorist, can only be understood in the context of the child's fantasy life.

CLINICAL EXAMPLE OF NEUROSIS

As a more in-depth example of the structural view of neurotic-level functioning, let us look at M.T., a 32-year-old graduate student at a major university.

> M.T. struggled intensely with worries about his competence in many domains of his life: in work, in athletics, and, most painfully, in terms of his sexual functioning and attractiveness to women. Although he was successful as a student (he was close to completing his doctorate), managed his day-to-day life with relative ease, and had engaged in two, generally positive, long-term relationships with women, he still worried about his adequacy and competence and suffered from chronic, mild depressive symptoms and, at times, from painful feelings of anxiety.
>
> In reflecting on his intimate relationships with women, M.T. related that he had longstanding fears that "something bad" might happen. Further explora-

tion suggested that these fears were associated with fiercely critical and aggressive thoughts that welled up inside him when he engaged in close heterosexual relationships. He worked hard to suppress these thoughts, but was unable to do so. A gentle man, who, in fact, had never been violent in reality, M.T. took a harsh view of himself as a "jerk" and "insensitive" because he harbored such thoughts.

Constantly worried that he might hurt others' feelings, M.T. tended to assume a passive stance in his relationships. He let women take the lead, both in the bedroom and other domains, and worked, sometimes desperately, to inhibit any overt expression of anger. In school and on the ballfield (he played intramural soccer), he functioned adequately, but he tended to inhibit himself because he worried about asserting himself fully, which felt like an aggressive act. Thus, he failed to come close to achieving his potential.

Historically, M.T.'s neurotic difficulties appeared bound up to a great extent in his trouble negotiating the triadic relationship with his mother and father. As a boy, M.T. had aligned himself closely with his mother, who, he described, served as his "confidante." His father tended to be angry and, at times, explosive; he frightened M.T. and angered M.T.'s mother. While M.T. had admired certain qualities of his father—his outgoing style and competitive drive—he had feared aligning himself with him for fear of losing his alliance with his mother. M.T. described how furious he had been at his father for demanding so much attention from family members and also for denigrating him. Afraid of how angry he felt, however, he tended to retreat from confrontation with his father and to seek a safe haven in his mother's arms. Unconsciously, it appeared, he felt profoundly guilty for what he experienced as having a closer relationship with his mother than his father did.

As an adult, in an unconscious defensive maneuver, M.T. shifted back and forth between these two primary identifications. At moments, he identified with his father and his father's competitive, self-assertive strivings. Then, anxious about his emerging aggressive wishes and fears of alienating the woman, he shifted to an identification of what he experienced as the woman's "softer features." From this position, he suffered less anxiety about his aggressive wishes, but also found himself unable to assert himself fully—sexual or otherwise. He felt inhibited, according to his own description, and out of touch with his masculinity.

In returning to the notion of compromise formation, we see how, in typical neurotic ways, M.T.'s compromise formations were what Brenner would term pathological. He suffered from feelings of anxiety and depression, which appeared tied to his inability to adequately modulate his aggression wishes. His guilt (emanating from the superego component of his compromise formations) led him to inhibit himself, so that he failed to perform with the mastery and pleasure expected were he less conflicted.

The Structural Approach to Severe Psychopathology

Where the psychopathologists have placed most emphasis on an explication of narcissistic disorders, and object relations theorists, at least recently, on borderline disorders, structural theorists, as the above discussion should suggest, have focused most attention on neurotic disorders. The structural theory of intrapsychic conflict involving drive and defense offers a powerful model for illuminating such common neurotic difficulties as inhibitions of sexual and aggressive wishes and

HOWARD D.
LERNER and
JOSHUA
EHRLICH

excessive guilt. Critics, such as Kohut, argue, however, that structural theory is less adequate in explaining more severe psychopathology.

In contrast to the self psychologists and object relations theorists who tend to stress *deficits* in psychic structure as underlying severe psychopathology (i.e., the self psychologists speak of an "impoverished" or inadequate self structure), structural theorists tend to stress the role of *conflict* in the etiology of severe psychopathology. Structural theorists generally believe that conflicts from all developmental levels contribute to more severe disorders. And, as one would expect, all symptoms represent pathological compromise formations.

As an example of this approach, we will turn briefly to a segment of a psychoanalysis of a woman with borderline tendencies, conducted by a psychoanalyst whose predominant approach is structural (Willick, 1991). The patient, a woman in her late twenties, was often depressed, chronically anxious, had no friends, showed significant impairments in her parenting, and was locked into a miserable marriage in which she functioned as an "obedient slave." In the analysis, typical of borderline patients, she quickly developed an intense transference to the analyst, which involved painful fears of separation and the troubling experience of not being able to remember the analyst during her separation from him over the weekends. In contrast to the object relations theorist, who might view her inability to recall the analyst as originating in a developmental deficit involving a lack of object constancy or evocative memory, Willick viewed her difficulty as emanating from a *conflict*. As he interpreted to the patient, she failed to remember him because were she to allow herself to picture him, she would feel a more terrible longing that she could not be with him. In other words, according to the analyst, the "not remembering" was a symptom of conflict: It represented a defensive effort by the patient to fend off intensely painful feelings about her separation from the analyst. In a similar fashion, structural theorists tend to view the borderline's subjective experience of "emptiness" or inner "deadness" as manifestations of psychic conflict, as opposed to a symptom of deficient psychic structure.

As biological psychiatry has come to dominate the contemporary understanding of severe psychopathology, especially psychotic disorders and major depressive disorders, structural theorists have sought to integrate biological approaches with their understanding of conflict and its ubiquitous role in psychic life. While structural theorists recognize that constitutional impairments often contribute to such severe disorders as schizophrenia, they continue to focus on the manifestations of conflict in understanding the patient's psychic life. Willick (1990) summarized this approach succinctly: "No matter what organic impairments are present in the psychoses, they still manifest themselves through the patient's mind . . ." (p. 1078).

The Structural Approach to Treatment

The structural approach to psychoanalytic treatment follows directly from the conceptual model of the compromise formation. In the most basic terms, the analyst, through interpreting the patient's defenses, seeks to facilitate the emergence of different transferences in relation to the analyst. These transferences are understood in terms of compromise formations: They contain derivatives of instinctual drives (now directed toward the analyst), defenses, affects, and a superego component.

The analyst's central task is to help the patient gradually understand how he or she constructs the world according to childhood experience and fantasy: how, for example, a person inhibits himself or herself because of unconscious fears of retribution for sexual thoughts, or how a person behaves in self-destructive ways because of guilt due to aggressive wishes. Where Freud in his early writing and Freudian theorists focused on making the unconscious conscious (the "cathartic method"), modern structural theorists have a more complex, ambitious task. They seek to help the patient understand *all* aspects of his or her mental functioning, beginning with an understanding, through gradual, painstaking analysis, of how the patient seeks to fend off feelings of unpleasure through a variety of defensive maneuvers.

This should not be viewed as a dry, intellectual approach, involving one person offering didactic seminars to a compliant patient. The analyst's persistent interpretation of defenses facilitates the emergence of intense affects and a painful confrontation for the patient with his or her own primitive wishes and fantasies. Interpretation generally is seen to be useful only when conflicts have emerged, usually with emotional intensity, in the transference. At the same time, the structural theorist does emphasize *insight*. Where the self psychologist and object relations theorists tends to stress the role of the therapeutic relationship itself in therapeutic change, the structural theorist tends to focus on the mutative role of *interpretation*. Interpretations, properly timed, in the context of the transference, can produce shifts in the dynamic tension of the compromise formation, according to structural theory. A patient, for instance, might come to allow himself or herself more gratification of drive derivatives with less guilt and inhibition, or might come to assert himself or herself more actively without precipitating conflict with others.

As an example, let us return briefly to our young college student, sitting, mildly anxious, in the class of the woman professor. Let us imagine one aspect of a psychoanalytic treatment with him. Gradually, through the analyst's consistent interpretation of his denial about his sexual wishes toward the professor (and, perhaps, other older women), he comes to understand that he, indeed, harbors such wishes and that they make him intensely uncomfortable. Over time, he comes to understand, perhaps through a persistent, anxiety-provoking fantasy that his male analyst will attack him for having sexual thoughts, that his anxiety resides in castration fears. As he comes to understand his fear of his analyst, he might come to see that this fear, unfounded, is rooted in childhood fantasy, tied to his parents, that his sexual wishes for his mother would elicit his father's wrath. As he gains this insight, he becomes more comfortable with his sexual fantasies. He finds that he is freer to enjoy sex and that he worries less that something is somehow wrong with him for his sexual desires.

SELF PSYCHOLOGY

History

Self psychology, the newest of the three conceptual frameworks we are exploring, offers an approach to human development—and to psychopathology and its treatment—that diverges sharply from the theory of drives and conflict, rooted in Freudian theory, that continues to be the dominant psychoanalytic approach. Its emergence as an important contemporary psychoanalytic approach can be attributed to the contributions of Heinz Kohut, a Chicago-based psychoanalyst. Kohut's central contributions—*The Analysis of the Self* (1971) and *The Restoration of the Self* (1977)—stand as the cornerstones of self psychology. Kohut's work has been elaborated on and expanded by his followers. However, it still stands as the definitive conceptualization of the self psychological approach.

Wallerstein (1983) suggests that Kohut's most important theoretical contribution was to bring to the fore the central role of narcissism in psychological functioning. Narcissism, a complex concept of a long, varied history within psychoanalysis, has been defined in various ways by psychoanalysts and has also come to assume important meanings within the popular culture. Here, we will use the functional definition offered by Stolorow (1975): the "structural cohesiveness, temporal stability and positive affective coloring of the self-representation." In simpler terms it means a consistent, relatively realistic sense of self through time and across situations. Adler (1989) has suggested that Kohut's contributions on narcissistic disorders shifted the term narcissistic from being a pejorative term meaning *entitled* to a concept that spoke to an individual's sense of incompleteness and poor self-worth.

Kohut believed that classical psychoanalytic formulations, which focused on biological drives and conflict, offered little toward an understanding of the role that narcissism plays in both healthy and pathological development. He offered a comprehensive developmental theory that explored the vicissitudes of narcissistic development in early childhood and the maintenance of narcissism throughout the life cycle. Kohut and his followers have emphasized the role that the caregiver's empathy toward the young child plays in the development of the child's—and subsequent adult's—healthy sense of self. While empathy was not a topic new to psychoanalysis, Kohut's careful explication of this important concept catalyzed significant interest in it within psychoanalysis, both as it pertained to early development (the caregiver's empathy toward the child) and also to the treatment situation (the analyst's empathy toward the patient).

Kohut's conceptual framework is termed self psychology because he places the development of the self at the center of his theory. The "core of the personality," according to Kohut and Wolf (1978), the self is "an independent centre of initiative, an independent recipient of impressions." In contrast to structural theory, which views instinctual drives (e.g., aggressive, sexual) as the primary motivator behind all human behavior, self psychology is based on the motivational primacy of self-experience. The individual is concerned with maintaining a vital, complete, nonfragmented sense of self (Stolorow, 1983). From the perspective of the self psychologist, manifestations of infantile instinctual drives (e.g., destructive rage, sexual "fixations") are not primary but emerge when the self has been threatened in some way. As an important example, the structural theorist tends to view aggression as an instinctual given, while the self psychologist tends to view the emergence of aggression as secondary to narcissistic trauma or injury. Structural theorists have criticized self psychologists for failing to appreciate what they believe is the formative role of inborn sexual and aggressive drives in early development and in the development of psychopathology.

Development

In the self psychologist's theory of development, the caregiver's capacity to respond empathically to the child's psychological needs is central. Kohut terms the caregiver of the infant and child a *selfobject* because the developing child, who has not yet established a firm sense of self, experiences the parenting figure as part of the self (in an effort to facilitate understanding of this complex notion, Kohut and Wolf (1978) suggest that the infant and developing child expect to control the selfobject in a manner similar to an adult's expectation of controlling his or her own body or mind).

According to Kohut and Wolf (1978), the child has two overriding emotional needs in relation to the caregiver. First, the child needs the selfobject to "confirm the child's innate sense of vigour, greatness and perfection" (p. 414). This is termed the *mirroring* selfobject. It refers to the child's need for caregivers who can appreciate and affirm his or her special qualities and respond with pleasure to his or her initiatives. Second, the child needs a selfobject "to whom the child can look up and with whom he can merge as an image of calmness, infallibility and omnipotence" (p. 414). This is termed the *idealizing* selfobject. In day-to-day terms, this refers to the child's need for a calm, capable parent whose sense of himself or herself in the world is secure and who can provide the child with a sense of stability and self-confidence with which the child can identify.

In ordinary circumstances, the parents are able to provide the child sufficiently with the selfobject functions described above, so that the child develops a healthy self. The caregivers' calm and self-confidence and also their pleasure and affirmation of the child is gradually internalized by the child as he or she develops so that he or she can maintain, at least much of the time, a sense of self-confidence, enthusiasm, and positive feeling, despite life's inevitable frustrations and disappointments. If an individual has developed a firmly established self, according to Kohut and Wolf (1978), he or she can tolerate wide swings of self-esteem and cope with the dejection of failure and the pleasure of success, experiences that often lead to acute psychological distress in those with more precariously established selves.

The gradual processes through which the child internalizes the parental function of helping the child maintain narcissistic equilibrium are termed *transmuting internalizations* by the self psychologist. These occur when the child's sense of calm and omnipotence is disturbed by minor and inevitable failures in the caregiver's response. For example, a parent does not understand why an infant is crying and thus is unable temporarily to soothe him or her, or, at a particular moment, a parent fails to pay attention to a child who is urgently seeking affirmation. In response to these ordinary empathic failures, the child attempts to maintain a sense of narcissistic perfection by establishing grandiose or exhibitionistic images of the self or by attributing narcissistic perfection to the parenting figure. Gradually, however, the child relinquishes archaic images of his or her own and the caregiver's narcissistic perfection. In doing so, he or she slowly acquires increments of inner psychological structure. To put it in other terms, repeated, tolerable disappointments in the caregiver lead the child over time to develop the capacity for self-soothing and the modulation of tension, and to an increasing capacity to regulate his or her own self-esteem.

Disorders of the Self

In contrast to ordinary, circumscribed lapses in empathy that contribute to the internalization of parental functions and, gradually, the development of a healthy self, serious, persistent failures in parental empathy lead to narcissistic traumas and, potentially, severe psychopathology, according to self psychologists. Kohut and Wolf (1978) stress that single traumatic incidents are rarely critical in the development of disorders of the self. Instead, ongoing failures of the caregivers to provide the child with adequate mirroring and idealizing selfobjects are critical. These failures potentially lead to weakened or defective self, the core of psychopathology in narcissistic patients. As examples of the sorts of ongoing failures in empathy that the self psychologists describe, one might consider a father, chronically angry, struggling with feelings of inadequacy, who constantly derides his son, a toddler, for not being more competent, every time the boy tries something new (e.g., putting on a shirt, drawing). Or, one might envision the experience of a 1-year-old daughter of a chronically anxious, overburdened mother who cannot sit still for more than a few moments at a time. When the child wishes to be held at vulnerable moments, she is put down again after a few seconds because the mother is too preoccupied to respond for a longer period of time. In essence, the parents' own self pathology prohibits them from attending to the child's needs for mirroring and idealizing selfobjects.

When adequate selfobject functions are lacking, the child develops an inadequate sense of self. He or she fails to develop the internal structures that allow him or her to regulate his or her own narcissistic equilibrium. Instead, the child (and, later, the adult) retains an archaic grandiosity and the wish to continue the fusion with an omnipotent selfobject in order to maintain an archaic sense of self as a defense against painful states of anxiety and depression (Blatt & Lerner, 1991). Often, the self-perceptions of these patients are fragmented and discontinuous. Often they seek in others a replacement for the psychological structures that they lack (an urgent search for affirmation, for instance, and mirroring).

In the gravest instances of what self psychologists term *disturbances of the self*, the individual develops a chronic psychosis. This occurs, according to Kohut and Wolf (1978), when the self is noncohesive, lacking in even the most basic capacities for self-esteem regulation. Psychotic disorders are the outcome of inherent biological tendencies, of a childhood lacking in even minimally effective mirroring, or of a combination of both biological and environmental factors. On the continuum of primary disorders of the self, borderline states represent the second most severe disturbance. Borderline states, according to Kohut and Wolf (1978), emanate from the permanent break-up or enfeeblement of the self. In contrast to the more blatant manifestations of psychotic disorders, borderline disorders are more muted due to overlay of complex defense mechanisms. From the self psychological perspective, borderline states are rooted in part in the caregivers' chronic inability to understand the developing child's need to establish autonomy. The psychological view of borderline disorders has been criticized by many theorists for failing to take heed of the central role of overwhelming aggressive impulses in the formation of the disorder (e.g., Adler, 1989).

Many disorders of the self, resulting from unempathic caregiving during infancy and childhood, are less severe than the psychotic and borderline disorders noted above. Kohut and Wolf (1978) offer a subtyping of self disorders, though they caution that these groupings do not do justice to the complexity of any one individual's clinical presentation. These classifications are useful because they tie particular problems in child development to their later behavioral and experiential manifestations. The *understimulated self* arises in the face of insufficient stimulation from caregivers in childhood. Individuals with an understimulated self experience themselves as boring; they are apathetic and lack vitality. They seek excitement in an effort to ward off feelings of deadness and depression. An understimulated toddler might engage in headbanging, a school-age child in compulsive masturbation, an adolescent in daredevil activities, and an adult in a range of perverse sexual and addictive behaviors. The *overstimulated self* results from unempathic overstimulation during childhood, especially excessive response to the child's grandiose-exhibitionistic strivings. Flooded by unrealistic fantasies of greatness, which produce acute anxiety, individuals with an overstimulated self urgently seek to avoid situations in which they might be the center of attention and often suffer severe inhibitions. The *overburdened self* arises when a child has not had a calm, soothing selfobject with whom he or she can merge and thus has not internalized a self-soothing function. The individual with an overburdened self is unable to regulate his or her own emotions, and is thus subject to traumatic levels of anxiety. A *fragmented self* develops in individuals whose caregivers were unable to offer integrating responses. States of fragmentation, which often arise in response to an experienced lack of empathy in others, vary in degree. More severe manifestations include profound anxiety and hypochondriacal worry.

The Understimulated Self: A Clinical Example

R.D., a 14-year-old high school freshman, was referred for treatment by his school guidance counselor and the local police. Recently, both the parents and the police began to accumulate evidence that R.D. was responsible for stealing over $23,000 from relatives and neighbors through a series of break-ins. He also was suspected of dealing and using drugs. Interestingly, these allegations were always difficult to prove conclusively and, despite an early history of head banging, erratic school performance, and large deposits into his bank account, R.D.'s behavior only recently had come to the attention of his parents. R.D.'s history reveals that he was adopted at 6 weeks of age. His mother recalls that he had severe diaper rash and never smiled. Indeed, upon meeting R.D., the therapist was struck by how sad, depressed, and apathetic he appeared. The little that he did have to say was that he felt that he had no problems, was doing fine in school, and really had no interest in anything. It became increasingly apparent that R.D.'s late night break-ins, operation of a gambling ring, and use of drugs were a desperate attempt to create excitement in order to ward off the subjective experience of deadness. Despite good social skills, he preferred to be alone, and every step along the way he would recklessly sabotage his own achievements and skills. For example, he used his lucrative baseball card collection as a front for stolen money. Once this was uncovered, he seemed to lose any interest that he had in collecting baseball cards.

Self psychologists have focused most attention on individuals with disorders in the narcissistic realm. Such individuals have severe difficulties in the maintenance of self-esteem. In the interpersonal realm, these narcissistic patients are extremely sensitive to what they experience as disappointments, failures, and slights. Kohut and Wolf (1978), again with cautions about oversimplification, offer a typology of narcissistic personality types. The *mirror-hungry personality* urgently seeks affirmation from others. Chronically seeking to counteract painful feelings of worthlessness, these individuals persistently display themselves in an effort to induce selfobjects to admire them and thus bolster their self-esteem. *Ideal-hungry personalities* constantly search for relationships with others whom they can admire for their intelligence, wealth, beauty, or other attributes. Usually, this new self-object relationship cannot fill the individual's sense of deficiency, and, disappointed, he or she sets out once again to find a special someone in whose glory he or she can bask. *Alter ego personalities* seek relationships with selfobjects who, by conforming to the self's values, appearance, and opinions, affirms the existence of the self. *Merger-hungry personalities* control others in relationships in an effort to find in others the structure they need for their own fragmented selves. *Contact-shunning personalities* avoid others because their need for others is so great. They fear rejection and, on a deeper level, fear that their self will be lost in the yearned-for fusion with the selfobject.

Throughout life, individuals with narcissistic disorders unconsciously and, generally, without success seek to repair longstanding deficits in their selves through their current relationships. Extraordinarily vulnerable to rejections and disappointments and, in essence, seeking the improbable in their relationships (that these current relationships can somehow repair the damage done by unempathic selfobjects during childhood), these individuals often have short-lived or shallow, extremely frustrating relationships. Absorption in their own desperate psychological needs, too, contributes to their interpersonal difficulties because they are unable much of the time to focus empathically on others' needs. The outward qualities that characterize many individuals with narcissistic disorders—self-absorption, aloofness, arrogance, grandiosity, ragefulness—often make it difficult for others, including clinicians, to maintain empathy with them and to recall that these personality characteristics, in fact, represent an effort to contend with feelings of worthlessness, depression, and incompleteness.

Mirror-hungry Personality: A Clinical Example
A.E., a 23-year-old graduate student, was initially referred for treatment because of anorexia nervosa. She was painfully thin, like a waif. She reported secluding herself in her dorm room only to emerge at dinner time to parade herself through the dining room "to be seen by everyone" as she took a small salad and again retreated to her room. She became even more secluded as her friends pleaded with her to eat. Her history revealed that her father died suddenly when she was 10 years old, and that she had an overly close, enmeshed relationship with her mother, in which A.E. actually mothered the mother. She reported that as a little girl she would frequently come home from school, eager to tell her mother about her excellent grades or success in basketball. But the mother, rather than listening with pride, habitually steered the conversation from A.E. to herself, and frequently began to talk about either her own needs at the moment or her previous successes, which overshadowed those of her young daughter. What emerged in her treatment was A.E.'s self-righteous demands for exclusive attention, praise, and reassurance. This was surprising in the sense that she presented herself as being painfully shy and inhibited and, in her own words, "always putting other people's needs ahead of my own." Because of A.E.'s experience that her own needs would not be echoed with understanding empathy, she felt deep shame, which, in turn, led her to suppress all of her needs—including the need to eat—which she manifested in her eating disorder, depression, and hopeless withdrawal. Her "parading" through the dining room in the dorm was an angrily expressed exhibitionistic demand that the "wrongs" that had been done to her be set right.

The Self Psychology Approach to Treatment

As to treatment, the self psychologist focuses on the emergence of *selfobject transference* within the treatment situation. This occurs when the patient revives, in relation to the analyst, a childhood need for either mirroring or idealizing, a need that had been insufficiently responded to by the original caregivers. In the mirroring transference, the patient seeks from the analyst the acceptance and confirmation that he or she failed to receive earlier in life. In the idealizing transference, the patient seeks merger with the analyst as an idealized source of strength and calmness. Kohut and Wolf (1978) stress the need for the analyst to maintain a calm, empathic stance in the face of the narcissistic patient's often rageful and incessant demands. The analyst must neither exhort, attempt to educate, or blame the patient for his often unreasonable behavior:

> But if he can show to the patient who demands praise that, despite the availability of average external responses he must continue to "fish for compliments" because the hopeless need of the unmirrored child in him remains unassuaged, and if he can show to the raging patient the helplessness and hopelessness that lie behind his rages, can show him that indeed his rage is the direct consequence of the fact that he cannot assert his demands effectively, then the old needs will slowly begin to make their appearance more openly as the patient becomes more empathic with himself (p. 423).

As the patient's old needs gradually reemerge in the treatment situation, the analyst can help the patient understand how unfulfilled needs from childhood continue to dominate his or her current life. Most importantly, the analyst assumes a new selfobject function for the patient. By offering the patient a mirroring and idealizing selfobject—and analyzing his or her empathic failures and their effect on the patient—the analyst facilitates the process of internalization of parental functions that had been incomplete in the patient's childhood.

OBJECT RELATIONS THEORY

History

The history of psychoanalysis has been punctuated by theoretical debates, but no debate has been as wide-ranging and has had such profound implications as that involving object relations theory. Object relations theorists address questions of the relationship between what is psychologically "internal" and what is "external," as well as how significant early formative relationships become internalized and affect our subsequent experience of ourselves and other people. What aspects of our early relationships determine those we choose as lovers, spouses, or friends? What is the dynamic nature of our internal object world? How does it evolve and what are the implications for treatment? What is biologically innate in the psychology of the person and what is modulated by direct environmental experience? What is the nature of motivation? Is it the pressure of instinctual wishes or the seeking of relationships with other people?

Interest in the study of object relations evolved as Freud's interest extended beyond basic biological predispositions to include the cultural and family context and their influence on psychological development. His interest in the superego, defined as the internalization of cultural prohibitions and values, led him to a fuller appreciation of the family as a mediating force in the transmission of cultural values. Freud focused increasing attention on the role of parents in shaping psychological development. Development came to be viewed as a consequence of

HOWARD D.
LERNER and
JOSHUA
EHRLICH

the care-giving patterns of significant people in the child's early environment. Later, knowledge gained from psychoanalytic work with children and the observation of normal and disrupted development of infants and children contributed further to the psychoanalytic appreciation and understanding of early developmental phases, their role in normal personality development, and the occurrence of psychopathology throughout the life cycle.

Object Representation

Our sense of who we are in relation to others begins in infancy and evolves throughout the life cycle. A key concept in object relations theory is that of *object representation*. Broadly defined, according to Blatt and Lerner (1991), object representation refers to conscious and unconscious mental schemata—including cognitive, affective and experiential components—of significant interpersonal encounters. Beginning as vague, diffuse, variable experiences of pleasure and unpleasure, schemas gradually develop into differentiated, consistent, relatively realistic representations of the self and the world of other people. Earliest forms of representation are based on those action sequences and behaviors associated with the gratification of basic needs; later forms are based on specific perceptual and functional features of the self in relationship to care-giving agents; and higher forms are more symbolic and conceptual. There is a constant and reciprocal interaction between past and present interpersonal relations and the development of representations. Schemas evolve both developmentally and in psychoanalytic treatment from the internalization of interpersonal relationships. New levels of object and self-representation provide a revised internal organization for subsequent interpersonal relationships.

Object relations theory is not a unitary theory but rather a way of thinking and a movement within psychoanalysis representing the convergence of two sources of information—the clinical observations of patients in psychoanalysis and psychotherapy and systematic observations of infants in relation to their mothers. The most influential developmental studies in the United States on object relations have been those of Margaret Mahler and her colleagues, summarized in the book, *The Psychological Birth of the Human Infant* (1975). Other investigators, such as Bowlby (1969, 1973), convincingly demonstrated the importance of early mother–infant bonding and attachment in establishing a sense of self and others. The cognitive studies of Jean Piaget have had a profound impact on object relations theory in general and the development of object representation in particular. These seminal psychoanalytic observations have been integrated by Kernberg (1975, 1976) in his theoretical approach to psychopathology. The mental processes he observed in patients with borderline personality organizations (patients located in the middle of the psychopathology continuum between neurosis and psychosis) have striking parallels to the behavior of children in certain phases of development.

Development

Based on the study of severely disturbed infants, Mahler and her colleagues conducted a 10-year observational study of normal children and their mothers. These children entered the study in their first few months of life. Psychoanalytically trained researchers observed them, both alone and in interaction with their mothers, through their third year. Their remarkable series of detailed and empathic observations were then used to delineate what Mahler called "the psychological birth of the human infant."

According to these investigators, the infant, through the first 2 months of life, remains in a psychological shell. As the child develops a dawning awareness of self and others, the child and mother begin to form two poles of a dyadic unity of symbiosis (2–6 months). Slowly differentiating from the mother, the infant enters the separation–individuation phase and its specific subphases: differentiation, practicing, and rapprochement. The child becomes increasingly aware of the mother as a separate agent during the differentiation or "hatching" subphase (6–10 months). With increased motor and cognitive skills, the child, during the practicing subphase (10–16 months) appears to be intoxicated, in a "love affair with the world." Taken with his or her own sense of power, the child easily "darts away" from the mother as if she were not needed. Yet, with increased growth there is an awareness of separateness and helplessness which ushers in the subphase of rapprochement (16–24 months). The child is then observed to move back and forth, separating and returning, willful yet dependent. As what is termed the "rapprochement crisis" resolves, the child begins to display a confidence in the mother's continued loving presence despite her occasional absences. The ability to retain an image or representation of the mother as a caring, gratifying presence but also frustrating is called emotional object constancy (24–36 months). With this, the child develops an increasingly stable and more complex sense of individuality, along with an increasingly stable sense of significant others.

Borderline Personality

Extensive clinical and research studies of the borderline personality over the past 25 years have played a significant role in the development of object relations theory. Developmentally, borderline disorders display conflicts and issues that appear consistent with the rapprochement subphase. Kernberg, in two major books, *Borderline Conditions and Pathological Narcissism* (1975) and *Object Relations Theory and Clinical Psycho-Analysis* (1976), advanced the most thorough psychoanalytic understanding of people who had what he termed borderline personality organization. He described these patients as having certain symptoms, personality characteristics, and developmental features in common. For over 50 years the term "borderline" referred to patients who were thought to have features of both neurosis and psychosis and who seemed to shift back and forth between the two. Kernberg argued instead that these patients had a remarkably specific and stable form of psychopathology. In terms of symptoms, these patients are impulsive, intensely angry, prone to addictions, promiscuity, and reckless, self-defeating behaviors; prone to intense, often short-lived but intense chaotic relationships; and chronically plagued with diffuse anxiety.

Glen Close's portrayal of Alex in the movie *Fatal Attraction*, offers an excellent example and caricature of the borderline individual. Unlike more neurotic individuals, Alex was unable to maintain relationships with others by expressing warmth, concern, and dedication. It is extremely difficult for such individuals to maintain empathy and understanding in a relationship once conflicts arise. Yet, paradoxically, they are unable to separate or take perspective. As a result, the relationships of borderline individuals are often chaotic and embellished with either idealization or aggression. As with Alex, manipulation often replaces empathy as a way of

HOWARD D.
LERNER and
JOSHUA
EHRLICH

relating to others. These individuals tend to overreact to external stimuli, often aggressively and self-destructively. Underneath the often contradictory, misleading, and vexing clinical picture of the borderline patient, according to Kernberg, are specific and relatively stable forms of coping, specific defensive operations, and highly pathological and "split" internalized self and object representations. The chaotic symptom picture coupled with relatively stable underlying structural features results in these patients being "stable in their instability." The poor coping skills of borderline individuals are termed "ego weakness," which consists of difficulty modulating anxiety, regulating the intensity of emotions, a lack of impulse control, and poor social judgment.

According to Kernberg, a characteristic feature of the borderline individual is intense aggression. Because of either a constitutional predisposition to aggression, excessive frustration during development, and/or trauma such as sexual, physical, and emotional abuse, these individuals tend to split off internalized good self and object representations from bad self and object representations. Further, they tend to project excessively bad (aggressive) self and object representations onto other people. The combination of splitting and projection leads to an incapacity to integrate good and bad self- and object-representations during the rapprochement subphase of development.

The category of borderline personality organization from a psychoanalytic perspective is a broad one and includes individuals thought to be schizoid (excessively withdrawn), paranoid (extremely suspicious and distrustful), and antisocial or psychopathic personalities. These disorders are thought to exhibit similar underlying, internal object relations, ego weakness, and what is termed primitive defensive operations, such as splitting, excessive projection or projective identification, idealization, and devaluation. It should also be stated that these symptoms often exist alongside some very admirable skills and talents. Again, Glen Close's portrayal of Alex in *Fatal Attraction* illustrates the paradox of how outstanding intellectual and work functions can coexist with other more primitive features of the personality.

CLINICAL EXAMPLES OF BORDERLINE PERSONALITY

The impulsivity of many borderline individuals resembles that of toddlers. Without fully considering consequences, they may swiftly move toward what seems gratifying at the moment, forgetting what's frustrating.

> R.G., a 19-year-old female college student, was told to learn a more efficient laboratory procedure by her physics instructor. Her professor valued her and was trying to help, but R.G. could not experience the help while simultaneously tolerating the frustration of accepting criticism and needing to learn something new. She forgot that she was an honor student with a history of success in laboratory sciences. She impulsively dropped the class, drank excessively, and sought out friends for comfort and to complain to. A week later, feeling lonely, bored, and anxious about what she did, she returned to the professor in an attempt to get back into the class. Her life away from the lab now became frustrating and the class once again "looked good."

Patients such as R.G. often turn to drugs, alcohol, or sexuality in a frantic attempt to soothe pain and gratify needs. When the drugs or sexual relationships cause frustration and the lowering of self-esteem, they will impulsively leave them, only to return. This is similar to what observers of infants have noted about the "rapprochement" child's movement away from and back to the mother. This movement also extends to treatment. Often these patients seek treatment to escape feelings of loneliness and emptiness. While initially feeling safe and less alone, once they find therapy frustrating, they seemingly forget its good aspects and leave treatment just as quickly as they entered it.

The sudden shifting of self and object representations also causes difficulty in relationships. Borderline individuals often experience new relationships as "all good" and gratifying and are prone to form intense infatuations that can be extremely exciting. The boundary-blurring of the all-good self and other experience, reminiscent of the symbiotic stage, can swiftly turn to the experience of an all-bad self-other experience because there is a lack of object constancy, that is, an inability to remember the presence of the good object or to recall good memories in the face of frustration. Alex's sudden shift in mood and experience around any separation from her lover illustrates the consequence of a lack of object constancy on the object relations of a borderline patient.

When borderline individuals feel unloved in a relationship, they desperately attempt to change their feelings, less by coping than by manipulating others. They believe they could feel good if only the other "could make it happen." When ungratified or frustrated, they tend to throw tantrums, threaten, and even make suicide attempts. As can be seen in the case of Alex, the suicide attempt is often prompted by separation and is less an attempt to kill oneself than to manipulatively force the return of the all-good object and to punish the all-bad object. These individuals are unable to recognize that the person whom they experience as ignoring them or not loving them at one moment is the same person they felt loved by at a previous moment.

The intense anger of borderline individuals also derives from splits in the internal representation of self in relationship to others. The intense sadism seen in Alex—exemplified by her blowing up her lover's car, kidnapping his daughter, and boiling the daughter's pet rabbit—all demonstrate what is termed in the literature "borderline rage."

Identity disturbance, characteristic of borderline personality organization, stems from an absence of object constancy and internal splitting along all-good and all-bad dimensions. Many individuals actually describe themselves as having a "good self" and a "bad self."

> R.B., a 20-year-old student, had a history of academic success and did very well in school as long as she was in a structured situation in which her assignments were clear and her professors supportive. On weekends, however, she experienced feelings of loss of identity and desperately sought contact and soothing through alcohol abuse, dangerous relationships, and compulsive exercising.

In the absence of object constancy, such individuals are unable to maintain a sense of well-being if relationships are temporarily frustrating. They are unable to recall that life is generally satisfying and that people care about them when they are feeling deprived or alone. With a supportive person, they may feel exhilarated. The extremes of all-good and all-bad self–other experiences make the borderline individual prone to constantly shifting moods.

The all-bad self–other state can often precipitate extremes of stimulating, self-damaging acts.

> One 19-year-old student felt so enraged at her boyfriend, whom she experienced as ignoring her, that she repeatedly leaped off the top of her bunk bed, hurling herself against the wall and onto the floor. She binged and drank wildly and then attempted to force herself to throw up. In an attempt to focus herself and gain control, she painstakingly removed all of the "fuzz" from a peach pit.

Adler (1985), among others, has suggested that the early history of borderline patients includes parents who were unable to competently empathize, soothe, and confirm, so that the child did not have the opportunity to learn or internalize this function. As a result, borderlines do not have the capacity to empathize with themselves, to self-soothe, and to regulate the intensity of their own feelings. Masterson and Rinsley (1975) have described a classic pattern that is thought to take place during the rapprochement subphase in borderline families. During this subphase, in which it is critically important for the child to both separate from and return to the mother and for the mother to be a steady, empathic beacon, the mothers of borderline patients need to cling to their children to meet their own frustrated dependency needs. The mothers offer excessive approval, support, and love for clinging behavior. They are threatened by separation and become "attacking, critical, hostile, angry, withdrawing supplies and approval in the face of assertiveness or other efforts toward separation-individuation" (p. 169). This behavior not only reinforces the child's all-good and all-bad split object representations but also leads the child to feel abandoned for behaving maturely and to constantly seek overly enmeshed, clinging relationships.

PSYCHOTIC PERSONALITY ORGANIZATION

As with borderline personality organization, patients with psychotic personality organization are unable to maintain a stable integration of self and object representations. This seriously undermines their capacity to realistically appraise themselves and other people over time and in different situations. Similar to the borderline patient, patients with a psychotic-level personality organization employ a range of "primitive" defenses—such as splitting and projective identification—which further undermine their coping skills. The reason for utilizing these defensive operations, however, are different in borderline and psychotic patients. According to Kernberg (1975), splitting and other defenses protect the borderline patient from intolerable feelings of ambivalence and the overwhelming rage that interferes with all significant relationships. In contrast, the psychotic individual utilizes these defenses in an effort to avoid the experience of disintegration or merger. Merger refers to the internal fusion or blurring of self- and object-representations. The regressive experience of merger manifests in a total and frightening loss of reality testing: in delusions, hallucinations, and confusion between self and other.

Object relations theory has illuminated how and when people develop a sense of reality as well as how they lose and regain it. The ability to adapt to the world and experience daily events requires a capacity to distinguish between self and other, and yet to remain in relationship to the other. To maintain a stable experiential world, there must be a differentiation of self from other. Without contrast, that is to say, separateness, there would be fusion and symbiotic oneness—an inability to develop a self in relationship to another. Without the sense of differentiation and contrast, these individuals develop self–other boundary confusion or psychosis.

As the self-image dissolves, becomes swallowed up by the image of the other, the psychotic person can literally feel the self disappearing into the other. This loss of self is catastrophic and is experienced in terms of ceasing to exist, a disintegration. Consequently, while psychotic patients seek fusion, they also fear and avoid it. Burnham and her colleagues (1969) characterized this tendency among psychotic patients as the "need–fear dilemma."

> One 18-year-old psychotic boy in the throes of the "need–fear dilemma" was brought to the emergency room by his mother. With one hand he grasped the mother's hand like an infant while with the other he attempted to hit her.

> The dorm room of an 18-year-old freshman was described as a "virtual altar" to his mother, with her pictures and letters arranged in an almost religious fashion. He complained of feeling "lost, isolated, listless, distant from others, and unable to concentrate." As his disjointed speech, hallucinations, and withdrawal gradually increased at school, he began to behave in increasingly bizarre ways, which culminated with him attacking his mother with a knife. His delusional beliefs, visual hallucinations, and concrete thinking represented desperate attempts to maintain a boundary or distinction between self and other.

The Object Relations Approach to Treatment

Object relations theory has not drastically changed psychoanalysis as much as it has subtly influenced its focus. This influence comes from the evolving therapeutic framework of object relations and with its insight about interpersonal and internal development, which has helped provide better therapeutic maps for explorations of borderline and psychotic conditions. Object relations theory has also focused on aspects of the therapist–patient interaction that have not been focused upon from other psychoanalytic perspectives.

Object relations theory focuses upon the internalization of significant interpersonal relationships that initially resulted in the child's understanding of reality and his or her construction of the representational world of self, of others, and their interactions. It is thought that these cognitive–affective structures, constructed around important interpersonal relationships, generalize and provide structures for understanding other dimensions of reality. If the representational world and the sense of reality are established through the internalization of significant interpersonal interactions, then these concepts have relevance for understanding and directing significant directions of the psychotherapeutic process. Presently, formulations about therapeutic action—that is, what is therapeutic in psychoanalysis—increasingly emphasize the therapeutic relationship as a significant interpersonal interaction in which the treatment relationship is the mediator for the patient's development of increasing levels of organization. It is thought if the internalization of object relations results in the formation of psychological structures during normal development, then the internalization of significant interactions between the patient and the therapist plays an important role in the therapeutic process. The therapist becomes available as a new object by eliminating, step by step, the interpersonal distortions (transference) that interfere with the establishment of new object relationships. It is the internalization of new and relatively undistorted relations with the therapist that leads to therapeutic change.

The formulations and clinical examples presented in this chapter suggest that there are different types of distortions in the representational world in various forms and levels of psychopathology. These differences are expressed in the therapeutic process in terms of the nature of the therapeutic relationship, that is, the transference. Given an adequate psychotherapeutic environment—the "holding environment"—reminiscent of the early mother–infant relationship, treatment interventions are aimed at promoting differentiation and integration. They facilitate the patient's evolving awareness of self as having a coherent identity and they assist in the development of a fuller and deeper appreciation of others.

SUMMARY

Psychoanalysis, from its inception, has been concerned with the theory and treatment of psychopathology. Psychoanalysis has evolved since Freud into different, although overlapping models of the mind. Three major psychoanalytic models of psychopathology have been presented: modern structural theory, self psychology, and object relations theory. Each model specifies a unique perspective on personality, development, psychopathology, and treatment. In practice, however, all psychoanalysts address issues of conflict, of narcissism, including self-esteem, and of interpersonal relationships. What makes these models or perspectives on psychopathology specifically psychoanalytic in nature includes a continuum concept of psychopathology, the significance of early childhood development for later functioning, the profound significance of unconscious mental processes, and the utilization of more intensive, long-term treatment with a focus on the psychotherapeutic relationship. Psychoanalytic theories have always been intimately connected with clinical observation. We have presented what is most current in psychoanalytic perspectives on psychopathology and have illuminated theoretical concepts with clinical illustrations.

REFERENCES

Adler, G. (1985). *Borderline psychopathology and its treatment*. New York: Jason Aronson.

Adler, G. (1989). Uses and limitations of Kohut's self psychology in the treatment of borderline patients. *Journal of the American Psychoanalytic Association, 37*, 761–785.

Arlow, J. A. (1991). Conflict, trauma, and deficit. In S. Dowling (Ed.), *Conflict and compromise: Therapeutic implications* (pp. 3–14). Madison, CT: International Universities Press.

Blatt, S. J., & Lerner, H. (1991). Psychodynamic perspectives on personality theory. In M. Hersen, A. E. Kazdin, & A. S. Bellack (Eds.), *The clinical psychology handbook—second edition* (pp. 147–169). New York: Pergamon Press.

Boesky, D. (1991). Conflict, compromise, and structural theory. In S. Dowling (Ed.), *Conflict and compromise: Therapeutic implications* (pp. 15–30). Madison, CT: International Universities Press.

Bowlby, J. (1969). *Attachment and loss, Vol. 1: Attachment*. New York: Basic Books.

Bowlby, J. (1973). *Attachment and loss, Vol. 2: Separation: Anxiety and anger*. New York: Basic Books.

Brenner, C. (1982). *The mind in conflict*. New York: International Universities Press.

Burnham, D., Gladstone, A., & Gibson, R. (1969). *Schizophrenia and the need-fear dilemma*. New York: International Universities Press.

Fraiberg, S. (1959). *The magic years*. New York: Norton.

Kernberg, O. (1975). *Borderline conditions and pathological narcissism*. New York: Jason Aronson.

Kernberg, O. (1976). *Object relations theory and clinical psycho-analysis*. New York: Jason Aronson.

Kohut, H. (1971). *The analysis of the self*. New York: International Universities Press.

Kohut, H. (1977). *The restoration of the self*. New York: International Universities Press.

Kohut, H., & Wolf, E. S. (1978). The disorders of the self and their treatment: An outline. *International Journal of Psycho-Analysis, 59*, 413–425.

Mahler, M., Pine, F., & Bergman, A. (1975). *The psychological birth of the human infant*. New York: Basic Books.

Masterson, J., & Rinsley, D. (1975). The borderline syndrome, the role of the mother in the genesis and psychic structure of the borderline personality. *International Journal of Psycho-Analysis, 56*, 163–177.

Stolorow, R. (1975). Toward a functional definition of narcissism. *International Journal of Psycho-Analysis, 56*, 179–185.

Stolorow, R. (1983). Self-psychology–a structural psychology In J. D. Lichtenberg, & S. Kaplan (Eds.), *Reflections on self psychology* (pp. 287–296). Hillsdale, N.J.: Lawrence Erlbaum Associates.

Tyson, R. L. (1991). Psychological conflict in childhood. In S. Dowling (Ed.), *Conflict and compromise: Therapeutic implications* (pp. 31–48). Madison, CT: International Universities Press.

Wallerstein, R. S. (1983). Self psychology and "classical" psychoanalytic psychology—the nature of their relationship: A review and overview. In J. D. Lichtenberg & S. Kaplan (Eds.), *Reflections on self psychology* (pp. 313–337). Hillsdale, N.J.: Lawrence Erlbaum Associates.

Willick, M. D. (1990). Psychoanalytic concepts of the etiology of severe mental illness. *Journal of the American Psychoanalytic Association, 38*, 1049–1081.

Willick, M. D. (1991). Working with conflict and deficit in borderline and narcissistic patients. In S. Dowling (Ed.), *Conflict and compromise: Therapeutic implications* (pp. 77–94). Madison, CT: International Universities Press.

5

Behavioral Model

Cyril M. Franks

Introduction

Virtually all students have heard about behavior therapy and most have opinions concerning what it is, what it has to offer, its strengths, and its weaknesses. In teaching introductory behavior therapy, it has been my custom to begin with a questionnaire, which students retake at the start of the final class. At the last meeting, we discuss changes in student perspectives that have been brought about as a result of my teaching endeavors. The responses never cease to intrigue and inform me. Even more important, this dialogue usually leads to changes in both format and content the next time the course is offered, a two-way process that characterizes much of what goes on in behavior therapy today.

To determine your initial perceptions of behavior therapy, turn to Appendix 1 *before reading any further*. The remainder of this chapter will be concerned with such matters as origins, nature, conceptual uniqueness, basic strategies, current status, and unresolved issues in behavior therapy. Having read the chapter carefully, refer back to Appendix 1 to see how, if at all, your impressions have changed. In so doing, keep in mind that one chapter can provide little more than a brief introduction to what is a complex field of inquiry requiring much study. Were this a full-length course rather than a single chapter, formal lectures would be supplemented by a film, case presentations, demonstrations of specific techniques, and possibly a visit to a psychiatric facility. Unfortunately, little of this can be integrated into a single chapter. Based on the premise that many how-to manuals are available for those who wish to learn what behavior therapists actually do, I have chosen to focus on principles and issues rather than procedures. I hope it will become readily

CYRIL M. FRANKS • Graduate School of Applied and Professional Psychology, Rutgers University, The State University of New Jersey, Piscataway, New Jersey 08855.

Advanced Abnormal Psychology, edited by Vincent B. Van Hasselt and Michel Hersen. Plenum Press, New York, 1994.

apparent by the conclusion of this chapter that behavior therapy is unique among all intervention systems in that is rests upon data and scientific inquiry.

FOUNDATIONS OF BEHAVIOR THERAPY

Behavior therapy, a term used here interchangeably with behavior modification, has a long past but a short history. Reinforcement and punishment have been used intuitively long before understanding of principles emerged. For example, two thousand years ago the Roman scholar, Pliny the Elder, graphically described the creation of an aversion to alcohol by putting putrid spiders in the bottom of the drinker's glass. And in the nineteenth century, Maconochie, a well-meaning naval officer in charge of a British penal colony in Australia, developed a token economy system in which each prisoner was awarded points for successful performance of selected tasks and social behaviors. Unfortunately, despite apparent success, the "powers that be" disapproved of his innovative methods and the project was abandoned.

Until the middle of the last century, psychology was a armchair discipline housed in university departments of philosophy. It was not until psychology matured sufficiently to abandon philosophical speculation in favor of hard evidence that the ground became ready for behavior therapy to germinate. And it was not until the 1950s that this actually occurred, fertilized by the burgeoning influences of Pavlovian classical conditioning, Watson's neobehaviorism, Thorndike's laws of learning, and Skinner's operant conditioning—names and principles that can readily be found in most texts of experimental psychology and learning theory.

Behavior therapy is now entering its fourth decade. The first decade (the late 1950s and early 1960s) was a pioneering era of ideology and polemics in which behavior therapists strove to present a united front against what they perceived as the common psychodynamic "foe." During those turbulent times, and despite much resistance from the established therapeutic milieu, behavior therapy began to establish itself as a potentially respectable method of treatment. As the second decade unfolded, the emphasis switched to construction rather than defense. Competitive missionary zeal was abandoned in favor of a search for new clinical horizons. In the late fifties, experimentally validated techniques were rare and relatively straightforward (e.g., social or material reinforcers for strengthening desirable behaviors and punishment for the elimination of undesirable activities such as alcohol abuse). As the limited utility of these procedures became apparent, behavior therapy became more sophisticated and more far-reaching.

Behavior therapists began to emphasize overall lifestyle in addition to the presenting problem. For example, while a direct assault was made upon excessive drinking by the use of aversion conditioning, behavioral procedures were also being developed for dealing with the myriad of specific problems that interfered with the alcoholic's everyday life. These spanned the individual's entire lifestyle—sexual difficulties, problems at work, and whatever else ongoing behavioral assessment revealed. This was the era of biofeedback, psychopharmacological behavior therapy, behavioral community psychology, and the extension of behavior therapy into the worlds of administration and government. Traditional stimulus–response learning theory was expanded to develop new concepts, methodologies, and ways of viewing data unheard of less than a decade previously. In the third and fourth decades, where we are at present, this trend continues. More sophisticated methods of treatment, improved methodology, and more effective outcome evaluation procedures are being developed; and, as we shall see shortly, the "cognitive revolution" is invading behavior therapy as it is most areas of psychology.

Some Regional Origins of Behavior Therapy

Great Britain

In the British Isles, behavior therapy arose out of attempts to develop realistic alternatives to the then prevailing psychodynamic mode of intervention— procedures that, by and large, were time consuming, ineffective, expensive, and suitable only for a small segment of those in need. Hans Eysenck and his associates at the University of London Institute of Psychiatry (Maudsley Hospital) had an ambitious and bold plan to map out human personality in terms of a small number of operationally defined dimensions and their hypothesized underlying physiological determinants. These findings were then to be applied to the development of theory-based intervention strategies in which efficiency could be experimentally confirmed first in the laboratory and then in the clinic. As a result, data and systematic inquiry took precedence over ideology, a perspective that remains true of behavior therapy to this day even if Eysenck's aspirations have been only partially realized.

Many psychological models were considered and discarded, and it was only stimulus–response learning theory (in particular, Pavlovian classical conditioning) that seemed at that time to offer promise for the development of predictions that were both relevant and testable. And so it was that the term "behavior therapy" was coined at the Maudsley Hospital circa 1958 to describe these innovations.

South Africa

Meanwhile, in South Africa, Joseph Wolpe, a physician who had become disenchanted with psychodynamic therapy for reasons similar to those stated above, developed what came to be known as psychotherapy by reciprocal inhibition and the technique of systematic desensitization. Full descriptions of this procedure can be found in most manuals of behavior therapy. It is particularly successful for the elimination of the pervasive anxiety that certain individuals experience in such situations as entering crowded stores, flying, driving over bridges, or public speaking. By exposure to a series of gradually increased anxiety-providing situations coupled with some relaxation-producing images, first in the imagination and then in the real-life situation, the hitherto anxious individual becomes innured to situations that would ordinarily cause great distress.

Prior to the advent of desensitization, conditioning techniques were viewed as simplistic procedures suitable primarily for working with animals or children with mental retardation. In sharp contrast, systematic desensitization was shown to be effective with highly sophisticated adults for whom, other than medication, psychodynamically based traditional psychotherapy was the only alternative. Wolpe's "talk-therapy" set the stage for a new era. The fact that his laborious procedure has been modified many times as the result of subsequent study and the fact that his original theoretical explanation is open to question in no way detract from the significance of this accomplishment.

Two other South African pioneers who have achieved world prominence, at first in the United Kingdom and then in the United States and Canada, are Stanley Rachman and Arnold Lazarus, respectively. It should be noted, however, that, while still broadly behavioral (as contrasted with behaviorist), Lazarus no longer calls himself a behavior therapist. By his own affirmation, he practices "multimodal therapy," a procedure described in most manuals of behaviorally related techniques.

Curiously enough (or perhaps not so curious in view of the increasing commonality of thinking among scientists), about the same time that Eysenck coined the term "behavior therapy" in the United Kingdom, Lazarus independently used this same term to describe psychological treatment based upon conditioning and learning theory.

United States

If behavior therapy in the United Kingdom was based initially on classical conditioning, the same cannot be said about the United States. At more or less the same time that Pavlov was studying classical conditioning, B. F. Skinner at Harvard and Thorndike at Columbia were investigating instrumental or operant conditioning, as it came to be called. Classical conditioning is based on Aristotelian association by contiguity. For example, dogs salivate naturally to food; if the food is preceded by some simple stimulus such as a bell, an association between the two will eventually be made and the dog will salivate to the bell alone. In sharp contrast, operant conditioning involves increasing or decreasing a behavior by the use of either positive or negative rewards or through punishment.

The term "operant conditioning" is used to make the point that the behavior operates on the environment. Perhaps because of the pioneering belief in the United States that the environment is there to be conquered and that there are few or no limits to human capacities for so doing, the emphasis was and is on operant or environmental influences rather than constitutional determinants. Thus, this new form of conditioning is quite different from the earlier Pavlovian model. Operant conditioning carries with it the implication that people act on the world and change it, and, in turn, are themselves changed by the consequences of their actions.

By giving meaningful rewards to hospitalized schizophrenics, Ogden Lindsley, a graduate student of Skinner's, trained these patients to perform simple but meaningful tasks. In 1953, Lindsley and his associates independently coined the term "behavior therapy" to describe this new procedure. Later, "applied behavior analysis" became the term of choice to refer to the application of operant conditioning principles to psychological problems and, from this time onwards, the growth of operant-based behavior therapy in the United States and throughout the world was remarkable. Operant principles were applied to the treatment of children's behavior problems, and Theodore Ayllon developed the first comprehensive token economy for psychiatric residents within a state hospital, to name but two of these many developments. In this latter respect, it might be noted that Ayllon, like most early behavior therapists, had to contend with much resistance from the far more numerous traditionally oriented staff members within his institution.

THE EXPANDING HORIZONS OF BEHAVIOR THERAPY

The roots of behavior therapy can be traced back to diverse schools of thought and philosophical systems, to contrasting methodologies, to different countries, and to numerous pioneers. There is no one leader, guru, or "party-line" in behavior therapy. Primarily, what the numerous behavior therapy societies that have sprung up throughout the world have in common is a behavioral science methodology and an allegiance to some form of stimulus–response learning theory. As of 1992, some 30 regularly published behavioral journals, mostly in English, were available. National, international, and world congresses in behavior therapy form part of a well-developed network. Themes covered extend from children to geriatrics, from practical case management to esoteric theoretical interests, from working with the individual to large-scale problems of business and government, from specific stimulus–response units within a school- or hospital-based token economy to field-oriented programs involving complex interactions, and much more.

Early behavior therapy was simplistic. Because the technology for more complex application had not as yet emerged, the emphasis was on one-to-one stimulus–response relationships of a highly specific nature. In addition, largely as a negative reaction to pervasive psychodynamic influences, early behavior therapy was anti-cognitive and anti-mentalistic. Now that behavior therapy, in common with psychology at large, is "going cognitive," this defensive stance is no longer necessary.

Most encouraging, whereas the strongest critics of behavior therapy used to be its opponents, informed criticism now likewise comes from within its group of advocates. Having reached the point where it is no longer necessary to convince outsiders and doubters of its merits, behavior therapists are sufficiently secure to engage in self-evaluation. Numerous articles and several books extol the advantages of examining behavior therapy failures. Behavior therapists are also learning how to function in an interdisciplinary milieu without either losing their identity or becoming confrontational.

CHARACTERISTICS OF CONTEMPORARY BEHAVIOR THERAPY

Well over a decade ago, Kazdin (1978) listed what he considered to be the salient characteristics of behavior therapy. These included: a focus on current rather than historical determinants of behavior; an emphasis on overt change as the main criterion by which treatment is to be evaluated; specification of treatment in objective terms so as to make replication possible; a reliance on basic research in psychology for the generation of testable clinical hypotheses and specific therapeutic techniques; and finally, specificity with respect to definition, accountability, treatment, and measurement.

While these criteria still apply, behavior therapists have broadened their horizons to take into account related disciplines. Another major development is that behavior therapists now view stimuli and responses as reciprocally interacting rather than discrete events. Further, while still more or less embedded in stimulus–response learning theory and the methodology of behavioral science, this methodology itself is now open to question. Behavior therapists are willing to consider the possibility that under different circumstances, other methodologies may also be of value.

But for most behavior therapists what remains unchanged is the emphasis on data and the avoidance of unwarranted speculation. Behavior therapy remains theory-based yet empirical, emphasizing doing as well as talking. Multidimensional methods are preferred, together with a focus on professional accountability, client responsibility, and a problem-solving milieu characterized by mutually informed interactions. Unlike many of their predecessors, contemporary behavior therapists emphasize empathy, therapeutic warmth, listening, and talking with patients—but always keep in mind that presenting problems are rarely the same as those that lie just below the surface. (These, of course, are ideals, which are not always attained. Behavior therapists are only human and, no matter how hard they try, not all behavior therapists invariably manage to practice what they preach.)

Nowhere is the emphasis on behavior therapy as an approach rather than a series of techniques more clear than in the manner in which the Association for Advancement of Behavior Therapy (AABT), the largest professional behavioral organization in the United States and perhaps in the world, had changed its name. It was originally known as the Association for Advancement of the Behavior Therapies. In 1967, two unknown graduate students—later to become leaders in the field—drew attention to the fact that the various techniques of behavior therapy all shared a common approach and that the use of the plural "therapies" was quite incorrect. From then on, the organization became "singular" in more senses than one and the name was officially changed to the Association for Advancement of Behavior Therapy.

DEFINING BEHAVIOR THERAPY

Current definitions of behavior therapy reflect the above developments. But it was not always so. Early definitions were both limited and vague. For example, Eysenck (1959) defined behavior therapy in terms of something vaguely called "modern learning theory" and left it at that. Since that time, definitions of behavior have evolved and proliferated. Most definitions fall into one of two classes: doctrinal and epistemological. Doctrinal definitions attempt to link behavior therapy to specific doctrines, theories, laws, or principle of learning. Epistemological definitions are more inclined to characterize behavior therapy in terms of what behavior therapists do. Doctrinal definitions tend to be exclusive, rejecting whatever does not lie between narrowly defined borders as not being therapy at all. On the other hand, epistemological definitions can be so accommodating that virtually any procedure can be classified as behavior therapy. The more flexible and comprehensive the definition, the greater the potential for overlap with non-behavioral systems. But when a definition is so broad that it excludes virtually nothing, it loses its discriminatory properties.

It may be that a definition that is acceptable to the majority of behavior therapists is not possible at this time and that all that can be done is to adopt a descriptive definition in terms of unifying characteristics. For example, Erwin (1978) feels that it is sufficient to define behavior therapy as "a nonbiological form of therapy that developed largely out of learning theory research and that is normally applied directly, incrementally, and experimentally in the treatment of specific maladaptive patterns" (p. 44).

In an ambitious attempt to cover all fronts, in 1975 AABT endorsed the following still generally accepted definition:

> Behavior therapy involves primarily the application of principles derived from research and experimental and social psychology for the alleviation of human suffering and the enhancement of human functioning. Behavior therapy emphasizes a systematic evaluation of the effectiveness of these applications. Behavior therapy involves environmental change and social interaction rather than the direct alteration of bodily processes by biological procedures. The aim is primarily educational. The techniques facilitate improved self-control. In the conduct of behavior therapy, a contractual agreement is usually negotiated in which mutually agreeable goals and processes are specified. Responsible practitioners using behavioral approaches are guided by generally accepted ethical principles (Franks & Wilson, 1975, p. 1).

THEORETICAL FOUNDATIONS OF BEHAVIOR THERAPY

There are at least three approaches to treatment: the rational, in which theories are used to generate testable predictions leading to the development of empirically validated treatments; the empirical, in which theory is secondary to empirical validation (what works); the notional, an intuitive, sometimes anti-intellectual way of thinking about therapy, which, regrettably, is characteristic of many nonbehavioral clinical psychologists to this day. For these individuals, neither theory-based rationality nor validated empiricism is of much significance; it is only what feels good between client and therapist in the here and now that matters.

Contemporary behavior therapists try to take the positive aspects of all three strategies into account. Ideally, intervention procedures should be theory based. If this is not possible for the time being, at the very least they should be empirically validated for the population concerned. At the same time, that spark of creativity, the notional, needs to be given free rein but only as a first step along the road to empirical evaluation and eventual theoretical confirmation. It is this dynamic interplay that characterizes contemporary behavior therapy.

It is convenient to think of four or possibly five major streams within behavior therapy [see Fishman & Franks (1992) for a more extended discussion of these issues]. As noted, applied behavior analysis is the term used to describe the application of principles derived from operant conditioning to a wide range of clinical and social problems. Applied behavior analysts are usually radical behaviorists whose basic assumption is that behavior is exclusively a function of its consequences. There is no intervening variable, mentalistic inferences are disavowed, and the emphasis is on single-case designs in which a subject serves as his or her own control. The techniques consist primarily but not exclusively of reinforcement, stimulus control, punishment, and numerous extinction strategies.

The second approach, the neobehavioristic mediational S-R model involves primarily classical conditioning as exemplified in the work of Pavlov, Mowrer,

Spence, Wolpe, and Hull, among others. Intervening variables are acceptable and hypothetical, publicly unobservable processes, such as the imaginal representation of anxiety-eliciting stimuli in systematic desensitization are in order.

Together with cognitive behavior therapy, the third approach, Bandura's social learning theory, exemplifies much of mainstream contemporary behavior therapy. In its most advanced form (e.g., Bandura, 1982), social learning theory is interactional, interdisciplinary, and multimodal. If radical behaviorists tend to ignore or deemphasize the role of cognition, and cognitive therapists tend to minimize the importance of performance, social learning theorists stress both cognition and performance. Classical conditioning focuses on external events and association by contiguity. Operant conditioning also focuses on the environment but in terms of reinforcement contingencies. Cognitive and behavioral changes become interdependent and social learning theory takes into account both situations. Self-efficacy theory and modeling are used to develop bridging mechanisms. Self-efficacy refers to the expectations of personal effectiveness that play a vital role in successful coping behavior; modeling refers to the premise that learning acquired through direct experience can also be acquired vicariously through observation.

The fourth approach, of such significance that it warrants a section of its own in this chapter, pertains to the "cognitive revolution" that permeates psychology at large as well as behavior therapy. Whether cognitive behavior therapy is qualitatively different from behavior therapy or merely one facet of behavior therapy is a matter to which I shall return shortly. Finally, there is Staat's social behaviorism, now updated as paradigmatic behaviorism (Eifert & Evans, 1990), the culmination of an ambitious and sustained attempt over the years to integrate conditioning theory with traditional concepts in personality theory, clinical psychology, and social psychology.

BEHAVIOR THERAPY AND ASSESSMENT

Unlike traditional psychotherapy, in which overt activities are viewed primarily as signs of "something" going on beneath the surface, behavior therapy is a more direct problem-solving approach for the here and now in which assessment and intervention continuously interact. By and large, behavior therapists avoid using psychodynamically based procedures such as the Rorschach and Thematic Apperception Test. Psychometric measures such as standardized intelligence tests are more acceptable. When behavior therapists do use traditional diagnostic categories, they are employed primarily to satisfy the classification requirements of hospitals and insurance agencies. For several years, this process was facilitated by use of various forms of the American Psychiatric Association's Diagnostic and Statistical Manual of Mental Disorders (DSM), a periodically updated manual based largely on explicit psychodynamic theory. In 1980, the DSM began to include overt behaviors as isolated diagnostic criteria, which were never conceptualized in terms of any systematic behavioral framework. This fragmented use in isolation of a few behavioral measures does not constitute behavioral assessment. It is the manner in which a procedure is used as well as the method that makes it behavioral. For example, the interview, a commonly deployed assessment method in most forms of psychotherapy, is hardly unique to behavioral assessment. But unlike its psychodynamic counterpart, the behavioral interview concentrates on definable and measurable events operating in the present. Behavioral assessment is geared toward gathering specific information, regarding specific problems. The emphasis is on both presenting concerns and issues that emerge tangentially as the interview develops. The past is incorporated only to the extent that it serves to maintain the present.

Behavioral assessment can include any or all of the following procedures, to name but a few: interview, self-recalling, systematic observation, self-report inventories and check lists, rating scales by the subject and/or by others, naturalistic observation, and a variety of physiological measures. Behavioral assessment is an integral component of behavior therapy. For further details, readers are referred to the many journals and books that deal exclusively with these matters.

Some Behavioral Strategies and Techniques

It is impossible to make more than passing reference to the literally hundreds of behavioral procedures in current use. Most have adequate empirical validation, some are theory-generated, and virtually all are periodically reevaluated in the light of incoming assessment data. *Reinforcement* in some form is probably the most widely utilized behavioral procedure among professionals and lay persons alike. The concept of reinforcement is not the sole prerogative of behavior therapists. What behavior therapists have done is to specify the principles of reinforcement so that they can be applied systematically and reliably to bring about desired changes. Reinforcement refers to the strengthening of behavior to increase the probability of the desired response being performed. The individual is reinforced for engaging in the desired activity, the reinforcement is contingent upon performance, and it always involves an increase in frequency of the desired behavior. If the consequence is presented whenever the behavior is performed, this is known as *positive reinforcement* and the consequence is termed a positive reinforcer. When a consequence, usually unpleasant, is removed or avoided following performance of the desired behavior, this is known as *negative reinforcement*.

Both positive and negative reinforcement are very different from punishment, a rarely used procedure in which the frequency of occurrence of an undesired response is decreased by the presentation of an aversive stimulus whenever the undesirable behavior occurs. Reinforcers can take many forms: material rewards, praise, social interaction, or other intangibles, or tokens to be exchanged for some reward mutually agreed on at a later date. In the token economy, the reinforcers are part of a systematized program for modifying the daily life of entire groups such as the residents of psychiatric wards, prison inmates, or a classroom of children in a public school setting.

All behavior is maintained by reinforcement. If the reinforcer is no longer available, the individual stops engaging in the behavior. This process is known as *extinction*. Many strategies have been developed for bringing about extinction. Reinforcements can be delivered in a real-life situation (*in vivo*) or through the imagination, a procedure known as covert conditioning. Studies show that appropriately paired and monitored stimuli, pleasant or unpleasant, can serve as effective behavior change agents even when they occur only in the imagination.

When working with literate adults, *systematic desensitization* is probably the most extensively used behavioral procedure. Beginning in the imagination and then extending into real life, it generally involves three steps. *First*, the patient is taught a response that is incompatible with anxiety. People rarely feel anxious and relaxed at the same time and muscular relaxation is used to counter anxiety. Training in deep muscle relaxation involves the graduated relaxing of various muscle groups in the body on a programmed basis. Once relaxation training and the delineation with the patient of an individualized hierarchy of anxiety-provoking situations are completed, desensitization to the events associated with specific anxieties can begin. Small, successive steps are used to train the relaxed patient to feel at ease in situations that used to cause anxiety. This process can be facilitated by associating the anxiety-provoking stimulus with some pleasant imagined scene. Finally, the patient it exposed to gradually increasing real-life encounters with the anxiety-provoking situation. This is called *in vivo* desensitization. For example, the client with a fear of flying progresses through a series of increasingly long and arduous imaginary flights to real-life journeys either with or without the therapist present. Public speaking and not easily avoided social encounters are common anxiety-provoking situations that can be treated in a similar fashion.

In *flooding*, the patient is exposed either in imagination or real life to a highly aversive situation for a period long enough for discomfort to reach a maximum and then decline. This traumatic experience should be employed only after careful behavioral assessment to assess both the need for this drastic treatment and the emotional stability of the patient. In *modeling*, the observer watches either a live model or a video reenactment. Modeling can be used to teach new behavior, to motivate more effective performance of existing behavior, to reduce anxiety associated with the performance of this behavior, or to discourage unwanted behavior. People can benefit from the experiences of others and modeling uses a variety of strategies to maximize these benefits.

Interpersonal skill deficits sometimes contribute to performance inadequacies. To correct such deficiencies, numerous remediation packages are now available, depending on the needs of the situation. For example, in *social skills training*, interpersonal competencies may be developed by direct observation or by participant role playing and feedback. Assertive behavior, the ability to function assertively but not aggressively in interpersonal situations, is a related skill that is amenable to behavioral training.

The *behavioral contract* is another frequently employed procedure. Client and therapist work out a mutually acceptable contractual agreement in which specified positive consequences follow successful completion by the client of an agreed sequence of events. If the subject fails to honor the commitment, then less desirable consequences become effective.

Last but far from least, there is cognitive behavior therapy, probably the most prominent development of the present decade. All behavioral procedures involve cognition. It does not seem possible for a human being to carry out any activity without some form of cognition. In cognitive behavior therapy, the emphasis is on strategies for modifying the faulty cognitions that (so it is argued), maintain the disorder. Most behavior therapists now classify themselves as either cognitive behavior therapists or social learning theorists.

In cognitive restructuring therapies, clients are taught to modify distorted or otherwise erroneous thoughts that maintain the problem behaviors and to replace them with more adaptive cognitions. Cognitive restructuring therapies are particularly helpful when the problems are maintained by excessive maladaptive thoughts. In *thought stopping*, the client is trained to disrupt the disturbing thought whenever it surfaces by some such procedure as a loudly shouted "stop" accompanied by a moderately painful flick of a rubber band worn around the wrist. A pleasant thought is then immediately substituted for the unpleasant one. In Rational-Emotive Therapy, a technique developed by Ellis more than 25 years ago, *cognitive restructuring* is used to change the irrational thoughts that cause anxiety, depression, guilt, or anger.

THE FLEXIBILITY OF BEHAVIOR THERAPY

Behavior therapy is now secure enough to tolerate a variety of viewpoints. As already noted, there is no one authority figure or essential set of procedures that all behavior therapists must follow. Within certain behavioral constraints, divergence is tolerated and even encouraged. For example, most behavior therapists stress specific situational determinants rather than any enduring personality structure. Other behavior therapists—such as Eysenck who, it will be recalled, was one of the originators of the term behavior therapy—strongly defend the notion of empirically validated, physiologically based dimensions of personality, which are present regardless of the situations in which they occur. Then there are those who emphasize environmental determinants of behavior to the virtual exclusion of anything else and there are those for whom physiological variables, biological determinants, and genetic endowment are highly relevant to an individual's behavioral repertoire. For a small but growing minority, the guiding framework is that of theoretical radical behaviorism with its complete rejection of any intervening variable between stimulus and response. Denying the existence of mental states as useful postulates, radical behaviorists tend to be nonmediational and antimentalistic, and never inferential. In sharp contrast, the majority of behavior therapists are behavioral rather than behavioristic, identifying only with the generally accepted methodology of behavioral science. It is possible to be a methodological behavior therapist and countenance such notions as free will, self-control, cognition, and awareness—none of which is acceptable to the radical behaviorist for the reasons stated above.

For some behavior therapists, a stimulus–response conditioning foundation is sufficient. Others believe that it is desirable to broaden behavior therapy to include principles drawn from social psychology, physiology, and sociology. Readers interested in additional information on these topics are referred to the many excellent texts that are readily available. In particular, the reader is urged to consult Fishman, Rotgers, and Franks (1988) and Erwin (1978). The latter is one of the very few volumes of substance to deal exclusively with scientific and conceptual problems within behavior therapy. It is perhaps of significance that Erwin is a philosopher, not a psychologist!

COGNITIVE BEHAVIOR THERAPY

Reacting against the "stigma" of mentalism led early behavior therapists (circa 1958) to ignore cognition and focus exclusively on overt responses. It was also easier to utilize immediate and concrete reinforcers on a one-to-one basis, in that the technology for working with complex stimuli on a group basis did not as yet exist. Two not unrelated events changed this situation. *First*, as behavior therapists became more secure, it became both acceptable and necessary to account in behavioral terms for the indisputable presence of cognitive variables in the lives of all individuals. *Second*, mainstream psychology was itself becoming increasingly cognitive.

The so-called cognitive revolution, spearheaded by such leaders as Michael Mahoney and Aaron Beck, is of major significance in behavior therapy on both the above accounts, so much so that it is sometimes argued that a paradigm shift of momentous significance has occurred. For Kuhn (1970), who first made the term popular, the notion of a paradigm pertains to the integrative model or framework of explicit and implicit assumptions to which a discipline adheres in its conduct, an organizing principle or cognitive map of reality involving both conceptual and sociological determinants. If this sounds complex and vague, this is in part because Kuhn himself is not consistent. To make matters worse, Kuhn confines his discussion of paradigms to the natural sciences, and behavior therapy is not a natural science. In any event, it is debatable whether the notion of a paradigm as a general explanatory model exists in either psychology at large or behavior therapy in particular. A compelling argument can be made for the thesis that behavior therapy is still in a preparadigmatic stage, rather like the natural sciences in the sixteenth and seventeenth centuries, when it was as much as investigators could manage to think of in terms of specific phenomena let alone general principles.

This shaky ground notwithstanding, many behavior therapists herald cognitive behavior therapy as a new approach that can no longer be classified as part of mainstream behavior therapy. Others, myself included, maintain that all behavior therapy employs cognition to a greater or lesser extent and that it is extremely difficult to conceive of any behavioral procedure that does not involve some form of cognition. From this perspective, no paradigm shift has occurred and behavior therapy is able to take cognition in its stride.

Behavior Therapy and Psychoanalysis

With the advent of cognition came a campaign to effect a rapprochement between behavior therapy and psychoanalysis. Many individuals in both camps, again myself included, view this as a retrogressive step. Behavior therapy and psychoanalysis are fundamentally different in virtually every respect. For example, behavior therapists evaluate clinical improvement in terms of overt, measurable changes such as better work performance or enhanced family relationships, whereas psychodynamic clinicians (the words "psychodynamic" and "psychoanalytic" are used interchangeably for the purposes of this discussion) think in terms of more global enrichment in which the primary goal is to bring about insight and personality growth. Viewpoints concerning what constitute acceptable data are also different. For the behavior therapist, data must be measurable and precisely defined. For the psychodynamic clinician, subjective data derived entirely from the clinical situation are valid. For the psychoanalyst, direct intervention is rarely acceptable and objective data are used primarily as springboards for second-order conjectures. These are some of the ground rules of psychoanalysis and it is within these limits that psychoanalysis should be appraised. Principles and rules developed for application within one system do not have to be valid for another. It becomes pointless and sometimes destructive to think in terms of which system is better.

The notion of "stimulus substitution" is a case in point. For the psychoanalyst, the symptom is a reflection of some underlying process within the psyche. For the behavior therapist, who thinks in terms of specific behaviors and procedures for the modification of these behaviors, the notion of a symptom as defined above has no meaning. For the psychoanalyst, removal of a symptom without attending to hypothesized, underlying determinants can lead to the unconscious substitution of a different symptom. This is known in psychoanalytic circles as symptom substitution.

Since the notion of a symptom does not exist within behavior therapy, it becomes meaningless to debate whether symptom substitution does or does not occur. What is appropriate for the behavior therapist to discuss is the fact that new, maladaptive behaviors sometimes occur following the elimination or modification of the target behavior. For example, it is now unknown in the behavioral treatment of enuresis (nocturnal bedwetting) for elimination of the bedwetting to be followed by the eventual emergence of head banging or other attention-seeking behavior. It is then incumbent upon the behavior therapist to create and validate a behavioral program that takes these developments into account. For the psychodynamic clinician, the new behavior problem illustrates the hazards of treating the symptom rather than attending to its meaning in terms of more deep-rooted, unconscious processes.

Similar arguments apply to the phenomenon of "the unconscious," a notion that has meaning only within psychoanalytic theory, and "transference," the positive or negative feelings engendered during various stages of the client–therapist relationship. As far as the psychoanalyst is concerned, transference has antecedents that can be traced back to parent–child relationships within both client and therapist. According to the behavior therapist, the observation that selective changes occur within the patient–therapist relationship is valid but both explanation and management are different. What this amounts to is that at the present stage or development, behavior therapy and psychoanalysis are fundamentally incompatible at both conceptual and clinical levels. Behavior therapists and psychoanalysts alike are best advised to proceed with caution, humility, and a sensitivity to differences rather than to engage in futile quests for superiority or premature integration (Franks, 1984).

Licensing, Ethical, and Legal Concerns

Today, the ethical sensitivities of behavior therapists are shared by most mental health professionals. One area in which behavior therapists led the way was in the development of procedures for the measurement of accountability and consumer satisfaction. But in the process, it became increasingly evident that values and science are not necessarily in accord. Values contribute to the selection of the goal; science is more concerned with evaluation and use. Thus, no matter how rigorous the behavioral program, ethical considerations that may or may not be amenable to scientific conceptualization may have to be taken into account. Whether it is possible to treat values as a set of behavioral variables or whether behavior therapists will have to go outside the world of science in the search for an ethical superstructure remains unresolved.

There are many closely related issues for behavior therapists to consider. For example, when modifying client behavior, which behaviors should be changed and in what sequence? What ethical and legal justifications are to be involved in answering such questions? Are the answers to be found through the application of behavioral principles or through subjective value declarations? I can only raise these matters here. You will have to attempt a resolution that is good for you.

While few legal decisions apply exclusively to behavior therapy, there are some rulings that are particularly relevant to a behavioral setting. For example, in planning a token economy for a psychiatric setting, court rulings affirming the rights of all patients to certain basic amenities have to be taken into account. Part of the problem is that behavior therapists and lawyers deploy different language systems. Law is steeped in mentalistic language. In legal parlance, terms like "free-will," "duress," and "coercion" are commonplace and generally accepted. If these words are anathema to most behavior therapists, we should also be alerted to the fact that behavioral terms such as "control" or "behavior modification" are in the same way offensive to many lawyers.

Although guidelines have been tentatively established by many professional organizations for the protection of patients and research subjects, as yet consensus is less than total. This is true even of the attempts by behavior therapists to develop appropriate procedures for working with specific populations such as families of autistic children, prison groups, or patients in hospital settings. Fortunately, most professionals share similar concerns when it comes to the welfare of their clientele. And behavior therapists, in particular, are giving much thought to these matters. A number of voluntary and state-monitored regulations have been proposed and most are still under review. In the interim, probably the best that behavior therapists can do is to be guided by the policies that prevail in their parent profession—be this social work, psychiatry, clinical psychology, or whatever.

THE RESEARCH–CLINICAL PRACTICE GAP, TRAINING, AND THE RISE OF PROFESSIONALISM WITHIN BEHAVIOR THERAPY

More than any other mental health profession, behavior therapy is predicated upon a close relationship between theory and practice. Unfortunately, there is still a gap between, on the one hand, theory and what clinicians say they do and believe and, on the other hand, what they actually do. Even among behavior therapists, clinical research seems to have surprisingly little influence on clinical practice. One corrective measure is for behavioral training programs to emphasize this close association between research and practice in their supervision. Another is for researchers to think more directly in terms of clinical utility in planning and implementing their projects. At the same time, behavior therapists need to return to their foundations. AABT, it will be recalled, began as an interest group geared toward data-based scientific understanding, rather than the enhancement of a guild mentality. Unfortunately, it is the latter model which sometimes prevails and, it is clinical and professional concerns which assume prominence in behavior therapy today. Books, articles, and workshops on how to start a private practice, how to become state licensed and insurance eligible, and how to avoid law suits seem to rule the day. Hopefully, the recent formation of a Special Interest Group within AABT geared explicitly toward the study and application of theoretical and conceptual interests heralds the beginning of a return to founding principles.

THE IMAGE OF BEHAVIOR THERAPY

There is a regrettable tendency for members of the public and even some professionals to view behavior therapy primarily as a collection of powerful and potentially harmful techniques for the promotion of conformity and control, with little regard for the rights and feelings of others. Behavior therapy is still sometimes equated by the uninformed with psychosurgery, brainwashing, the use of drugs, sensory deprivation, and even torture. These negative images are reinforced by behavior therapy terminology—words such as "control," "punishment," and "aversion conditioning" Even the seemingly innocuous term "modification" can have negative connotations for those who mistakenly equate behavior modification with behavior control. While it may not be feasible at this stage to change the nomenclature of behavior therapy, words such as "control" are best used sparingly and, following due process, aversion techniques used only when unavoidable.

Of equal importance is the need to modify public misconceptions through reeducational programs. To the extent that this is feasible, behavior therapists have to think in terms of public relations and the necessity for keeping patients and those who need to know informed at all stages of the intervention process. For example, behavior therapists in private practice could make available written descriptions of their treatment procedures and policies. As yet, little more than lip service is given to these important matters.

PRESENT STATUS, CURRENT ISSUES, AND A LOOK INTO THE FUTURE

In its early days, behavior therapy was limited primarily to the treatment of a small number of self-contained disorders. As time went by, both techniques and conceptualizations became more sophisticated and more generally applicable. The notions of stimulus and response broadened to include the total environment. As therapeutic interventions became multidimensional and more cognitive, behavior therapy became increasingly applicable to a wider range of disorders and settings.

While these developments bear witness to the vitality of behavior therapy, they also contain within them a potential for fragmentation. Whether behavior therapy will continue to be able to accommodate this diversity is a matter for the future to decide. It could also be that, despite technological advances, we have reached a temporary plateau as far as conceptual innovations are concerned. With the possible exception of the "cognitive revolution," no significant conceptual innovation seems to have occurred within the past three or more decades.

Nevertheless, the events detailed in this chapter are encouraging despite the problems that remain. As noted, behavior therapy is an emerging new science rather akin to physics and medicine in the sixteenth and seventeenth centuries. It is far too early to expect all or even most problems to be resolved, and it is equally premature to think in terms of conceptual integration. What is more certain is that behavior therapy is alive, well, and living in many worlds; further, it is likely to continue in this fashion in one form or another. In the unlikely event that the term behavior therapy should vanish from the face of the earth, this would not necessarily be a total disaster if the goals and aspirations toward which we all strive are brought about. After all, our primary concern as theoreticians is with the advancement of knowledge and our primary concern as professionals is with the alleviation of suffering.

Summary

In this chapter, the history of behavior therapy is traced from its unsophisticated beginnings to its present status, with all that this implies with respect both to accomplishments and to problems yet to be overcome. The point is made that the many streams of behavior therapy's reflect a commonality of approach based on the methodology of the behavioral scientist and some form of learning theory rather than a series of isolated techniques. Of equal significance, rigorous as behavior therapy strives to be, this must never be at the expense of ethical considerations, the welfare of the patient, and the maintenance of ideals. Return now to Appendix 1 and your answers to the questions raised prior to your reading this chapter. Mark in red what your opinions are now that you have read the chapter. In my opinion, all the items listed there should be marked FALSE. What do you think? Whatever your conclusions, if the reading of this chapter makes you think afresh about these matters, it will have served its purpose. If not, at the very least, you will have learned what I think behavior therapy is all about.

Appendix 1

Read each of the following statements and note in pencil in the margin which items you believe are mainly TRUE and which you believe are mainly FALSE. Having read the chapter with care, refer back to this list and reexamine your responses to see how, if at all, your opinions have changed.

1. Contemporary behavior therapy is based exclusively on some form of conditioning and a simple stimulus–response model.
2. Warmth, empathy, and the development of a trusting relationship are of little concern in behavior therapy.
3. Behavior therapy should be used only for the treatment of relatively direct problems, such as public speaking anxiety or fear of riding in elevators.
4. Behavior therapists regard the symptom as the disease, treat the symptom directly, and ignore underlying problems. For behavior therapists, underlying problems are either irrelevant or nonexistent.
5. Psychosurgery (e.g., leucotomy) and ECT (electro-convulsive therapy) are behavioral procedures sometimes used in the practice of behavior therapy.
6. Behavior therapy is directive. The therapist makes the decisions and tells the client what the goals of therapy are to be and how these are to be brought about.
7. Behavior therapy is ill-equipped for dealing with problems relating to feelings.

8. Behavior therapy is not appropriate for changing thought processes.
9. Behavior therapists rely heavily on the use of punishment and aversive stimuli to bring about change.
10. Behavior therapy rests largely on the use of tokens and simple reinforcers to change specific behaviors.
11. Positive reinforcement works best with children, feeble-minded adults, and animals. It is not appropriate for working with the problems of verbally sophisticated adults.
12. Most mental health professionals and carefully selected lay persons can be taught to use most behavior therapy techniques with minimal supervision or training. These procedures are easy to learn and apply. Knowledge of behavioral theory and clinical practice are of little relevance. This is the major advantage of behavior therapy.
13. Behavior therapy techniques are best viewed as useful adjunctive procedures for the treatment of specific problems uncovered during the more meaningful process of psychodynamic therapy.
14. In behavior therapy, verbal interchange between patient and therapist is usually neither relevant to successful treatment outcome nor very important.
15. One big advantage of behavior therapy is that most bad habits can be successfully eradicated in five sessions or less.
16. Behavior therapy is antidemocratic. There is little accountability to patients or other professionals and the therapist "calls the shots" with minimal explanation or discussion.
17. Behavior therapists deal exclusively with the here and now. "Whys," maintaining circumstances, "hows," are never of interest or concern.
18. In behavior therapy, the use of punishment in prisons and psychiatric settings to bring about compliance with rules and regulations is quite acceptable.
19. Behavior therapists focus primarily on environmental contingencies to bring about change. Individual differences, biological and constitutional variables, and genetic and physiological determinants are never considered to be important in behavior therapy.
20. The potency and effectiveness of aversive conditioning procedures have led to widespread use by behavior therapists.
21. Behavior therapy can be useful for the treatment of mild or minor neurotic disorders or bad habits; it is not likely to be helpful in working with psychotic or seriously depressed individuals.
22. Behavior therapy is simplistic. The focus is on presenting problems, thereby overlooking what is really going on. It is not considered important in behavior therapy to talk to the patient in an attempt to uncover unrecognized issues.
23. Personal freedom, freedom of choice, and human dignity are not important in behavior therapy. All that matters is changing undesirable behavior by the use of well-validated conditioning procedures.
24. Behavior therapists oversimplify and thereby miss the richness and complexity of living.
25. In behavior therapy, it is neither essential nor even desirable to secure informed patient consent prior to treatment.

They are, of course, *all* false.

CYRIL M.
FRANKS

References[1]

Bandura, A. (1982). Self-efficacy mechanisms in human agency. *American Psychologist, 37,* 122–147.

Eifert, G. H., & Evans, I. M. (Eds.). (1990). *Unifying behavior therapy: Contributions of paradigmatic behaviorism.* New York: Springer Publishing Company.

Erwin, E. (1978). *Behavior therapy: Scientific, philosophical and moral foundations.* New York: Cambridge University Press.

Eysenck, H. J. (1959). Learning theory and behaviour therapy. *Journal of Mental Science, 105,* 61–75.

Fishman, D. B., & Franks, C. M. (1992). Evolution and differentiation within behavior therapy: A theoretical and epistemological review. In D. K. Freedheim (Ed.), *History of psychotherapy: A century of change* (pp. 159–196). Washington, DC: American Psychological Association.

Fishman, D. B., Rotgers, F., & Franks, C. M. (Eds.). (1988). *Paradigms in behavior therapy: Present and promise.* New York: Springer Publishing Company.

Franks, C. M. (1984). On conceptual and technical integrity in psychoanalysis and behavior therapy: Two fundamentally incompatible systems. In H. Arkowitz & S. B. Messer (Eds.), *Psychoanalytic and behavior therapy: Is integration possible?* (pp. 223–247). New York: Plenum Press.

Franks, C. M., & Wilson, G. T. (1975). *Annual review of behavior therapy: Theory and practice* (Vol. 3). New York: Brunner/Mazel.

Kazdin, A. E. (1978). Behavior therapy: Evolution and expansion. *The Counseling Psychologist, 7,* 34–37.

Kuhn, T. S. (1970). *The struction of scientific revolutions* (2nd. Ed.). Chicago: University of Chicago Press.

---

[1]An ongoing chronicle and evaluation of major developments within behavior therapy is to be found in a series edited and later written by Franks, Wilson, and associates entitled *Annual Review of Behavior Therapy: Theory and Practice,* New York: Brunner/Mazel. The first volume appeared in 1973.

6

Biological Model

Mark C. Wilde and Paul M. Cinciripini

Introduction

Biological models of psychopathology emphasize the relationship between a specific constellation of symptoms and an underlying abnormality in physiologic function. Such disorders may be treated with medication and other approaches that are thought to directly alter the underlying biological abnormality (Andreasen, 1984). Modern biological models of psychopathology may be traced to the work of Emile Kraepelin and other European psychiatrists of the late nineteenth and early twentieth centuries, who developed nosological distinctions between major psychiatric disorders, as had been done with major systematic disorders (Andreasen, 1984). Although Kraepelin focused on the development of a diagnostic nosology (with little emphasis on etiology), he believed that disorders such as schizophrenia were caused by underlying biologic factors (Arieti, 1974). In recent years, biological models of psychopathology have increased in popularity, and research has intensified in biologically oriented therapies. Based on animal models, inference from responses to medication, and advanced research methods using sophisticated laboratory imaging techniques and biochemical assays, several hypothesis have been suggested to explain the possible biological basis of certain mental disorders. The present chapter provides an introduction to the biological basis of psychopathology, and presents the reader with the conceptual basis of contemporary biological models, including: genetic, biochemical, neuroanatomical, and neuroendocrinological.

Mark C. Wilde • Department of Physical Medicine and Rehabilitation, Baylor College of Medicine, and The Institute for Rehabilitation and Research, Houston, Texas 77030.   Paul M. Cinciripini • Department of Psychiatry and Behavioral Sciences, University of Texas Medical Branch, Galveston, Texas 77550.

Advanced Abnormal Psychology, edited by Vincent B. Van Hasselt and Michel Hersen. Plenum Press, New York, 1994.

MARK C. WILDE
and PAUL M.
CINCIRIPINI

THE GENETIC MODEL

Basic Assumptions and Background

The role of environmental versus inborn factors in the development of human traits is a long-standing controversy in psychology, medicine, and philosophy. Historically, dichotomous arguments have developed between those who believed that major traits and behavioral predispositions were solely under the control of environmental contingencies, versus those who believed that they were determined by inborn or inherited factors. Strict environmentalist views are exemplified by the ideas of the seventeenth-century philosopher John Locke, who likened the mind at birth to a blank slate, which is shaped and filled by experience. The view that human behavior is largely determined by innate factors, commonly called *nativism*, a philosophical predecessor to genetic theories, was espoused by Wilhelm Leibnitz. Leibnitz believed that the mind at birth possesses innate ideas or dispositions that actively shape our experience. Today, people rarely talk in the dichotomous nature-nurture terms of these early philosophers. Rather, it is generally recognized that many psychologically relevant traits are composed of both environmental and genetic contributions. The field of behavioral genetics has been in the forefront of recognition and is discussed below.

Genes and Patterns of Inheritance

Genes function to carry the chemical and metabolic information responsible for endowing the organism with the major characteristics and fundamental biological processes that constitute the individual. Genes are composed of strands of deoxyribonucleic acid (DNA), which are organized on 23 pairs of chromosomes found in the nucleus of every cell in the body. Twenty two of these pairs are called autosomes. Each of the 22 pairs of autosomes carries complementary genetic information, with one chromosome inherited from the father and the other from the mother. The twenty-third pair (the sex chromosomes) determines gender and carries other genetic information.

The dynamics of inheritance are understood through several key patterns of genetic transmission. Specifically, there are two important general patterns of inheritance. The first is single gene inheritance by which a disorder or trait is expressed through the action of one gene. There are four basic patterns of single gene inheritance, which follow the laws originally discovered by Gregor Mendel. They are: autosomnal dominant, autosomnal recessive, sex-linked dominant, and sex-linked recessive inheritance.

According to the model of autosomnal dominant transmission, all persons carrying the dominant gene with a recessive gene are affected because the trait's physical expression, called phenotype, requires the presence of only one dominant gene on one chromosome. Because the gene is dominant, only one gene contributed by one parent is required for the disorder to be inherited. As a result, offspring of a union with one affected parent have a 50/50 chance of inheriting the trait and every generation in the family should have at least one affected person. An example of a genetically based disorder of this variety is Huntington's disease, a neurologic disorder characterized by spasmodic involuntary movements, and subsequent declines in cognitive and personality functioning, eventually resulting in dementia.

The expression of autosomnal recessive traits requires that the affected individual possess two genes coding for the same disorder or trait, each of which is inherited from both parents. The trait is said to be recessive because if an individual were to inherit only one gene coding for the disorder paired with a dominant version on the other chromosome, the dominant version of the gene would override or cancel out the disorder's expression. The person who inherits one version of the recessive gene along with a dominant gene on the other chromosome is called a carrier since he or she possesses the recessive gene but does not manifest the trait. If a carrier mates with an individual who does not possess the recessive gene, their offspring have a 50/50 chance of being carriers. However, none of them will inherit the trait or disorder. In the case where one parent is a carrier and the other possesses the recessive trait, two out of four will be carriers while two out of four will inherit the trait. A disease found to follow the autosomnal recessive pattern of inheritance is phenylketonuria (PKU), an inborn error of metabolism in which the amino acid phenylalanine is not properly converted into tyrosine. If this disorder is left untreated, it commonly results in mental retardation.

Sex linkage (or X linkage) refers to inheritance of genes located on the X sex chromosome. Genetically, the female gender is determined by the presence of two X chromosomes, one inherited from each parent. On the other hand, the male gender is determined by the presence of one X and one Y chromosome. In addition to female sex characteristics, the X chromosomes carry other genes not related to gender while (with several rare exceptions) the male Y chromosomes carry only information related to male sex characteristics and play a relatively minor role in the inheritance of diseases. As a rule, X linked traits, when transmitted by the father, will affect his daughters and none of his sons since he contributed a copy of one of his X chromosomes to his daughters but a copy of his Y chromosome only to his sons. If a mother possesses the dominant gene on her X chromosome, her sons and daughters both have a one-in-two chance of inheriting the disorder. Sex-linked recessive traits show a mother-to-son pattern of inheritance since the trait always expresses itself on the X chromosome and cannot be modified or nullified by the effects of a second X chromosome. An example of a disorder with this type of genetic pattern is hemophilia, a blood disease characterized by a failure in the clotting mechanism in the blood.

In a polygenetic inheritance pattern, the trait is determined by the combined action of many genes. The known principles underlying polygenetic inheritance are very complex. It should be noted here that more complex models of inheritance have been hypothesized, which include combinations of single major gene inheritance along with moderating polygenetic contributions (Vandenberg, Singer, & Pauls, 1986).

Research Methods

The focus of behavioral genetic research has been on the separation of environmental and genetic determinants of a behavioral characteristic. Four basic research methods are employed in this endeavor. Twin studies separate genetic and environmental similarity. In twin studies, the rates for a particular trait or characteristic are compared between monozygotic (MZ) and dizygotic (DZ) twin pairs, and sometimes nontwin siblings. Since monozygotic or identical twins originate from the same fertilized egg, they are essentially genetically identical and any variation in traits is presumed to be the result of different experiences. Dizygotic twins originate from two separately fertilized eggs, but gestate in the same intrauterine environment, and may be reared under highly similar conditions. They are assumed to genetically resemble nontwin siblings, but at least theoretically share a common environment. From these methods, it is possible to compute what is called a concordance rate, which is expressed as the correlation between groups of MZ and DZ twins, or nontwin siblings, on a particular trait. These correlations are then compared between twin pairs to derive estimates of the percentage of the variability on the trait that is presumed to be environmentally determined and that which is thought to be the result of shared genes. In an ideal model, when comparing twins on a trait that is presumed to have a genetic basis, one would expect correlations of 1.00 for MZ twins, suggesting that 100% of the variance on the trait is under genetic control. However, a correlation of 0.50 for DZ twins and nontwin siblings would be expected, suggesting that about 50% of the variance is due to inherited genetic factors for both groups. Thus, when MZ and DZ twins are compared, if the resemblance between MZ twins is greater than between DZ twins, it is assumed to be due to the fact that MZ twins are genetically identical and DZ twins share about 50% of the genetic material. Further, since twins theoretically experience similar environmental conditions and intrauterine environments, while nontwin siblings do not, a comparison of DZ twins and nontwin siblings also yields a measure of nonshared environmental influence.

There are some problems with this methodology. *First*, the assumption that twins do indeed share the same environment has been disputed since there may be many intervening factors that make each individual's life different. To control for this confound, some have attempted to compare MZ twins raised in disparate environments with genetically unrelated people. Theoretically, if the trait of interest is genetically based and not environmentally determined, both twins will develop the trait; and if the trait is environmental, the twins should not have the same trait any more than other children raised in distinct environments. Unfortunately, the phenomenon of MZ and DZ twins reared apart is rare and collection of sufficient sample sizes to test various hypothesis has been difficult to obtain (Vanderberg et al., 1986). Nevertheless, twin studies have provided evidence of genetic contributions to personality traits, mood disorders, intelligence, and sociopathy (Plomin & Rende, 1991). However, the degree of genetic contribution has varied with trait and study.

Another method that attempts to separate genetic from environmental influences is the adoption/separation study. In its simplest form, the concordance rates in adopted children with affected parents are compared with those of adoptees of unaffected biologic parents. Another variant of this approach is to compare the concordance rates for a particular disease or trait in the biologic and adoptive parents of unaffected control adoptees. This method is predicated on the assumption that if a trait is genetic, then children should resemble biological relatives more closely than adoptive relatives. These methods provide the opportunity to determine the extent to which the environment influences a trait. For example, in the second design, if children resemble their adoptive more than their biologic parents, then the trait is presumed to be environmental. Adoption studies have provided suggestive evidence of a genetic component for many traits and disorders, including some personality traits, delinquent behavior, and schizophrenia (Bertelsen, 1985; Loehlin, Willerman, & Horn, 1988).

Adoption studies also present some methodological difficulties. *First*, there is the problem of selective placement, in which social forces in adoption procedures cause children to be adopted out to adoptive parents who resemble the biologic parents. *Second*, it is often difficult to gather accurate diagnostic information on biological parents due to the retrospective nature of the design. *Third*, in order to answer questions regarding patterns of inheritance, it is necessary to collect diagnostic data from several generations. Thus, adoption studies, like twin studies, are useful insofar as they can provide suggestive evidence that genetic factors might be important.

The family study method is another means by which genetic influences can be examined. The basic design of all family studies involves comparing illness rates in several generations of the families of affected individuals. These rates are then compared with those from a matched control group of families of unaffected persons or disease rates in the general population. From this, risk estimates are derived. Family studies can be used to demonstrate the degree to which a particular disorder runs in families, through the demonstration of increased prevalence in relatives of affected individuals (Weissman et al., 1986). Moreover, detailed studies of extended families can be performed in order to examine the degree to which family aggregation of a disease follows one of the patterns of inheritance discussed above. In segregation analysis, which is a variant of the family study method, genetic hypotheses are tested by pooling data from pedigrees to compare the observed proportion of affected relatives with that expected according to a given genetic hypothesis using complex mathematical modeling procedures.

Family studies have presented evidence suggesting a familial pattern to a number of psychiatric disorders. For example, investigations have shown that the risk of developing schizophrenia for first degree (close) relatives of affected individuals is approximately 10 to 12 times the risk for the general population and that the distribution of risks suggests both a single and polygenetic inheritance pattern (Bertelsen, 1985). Since aggregation can theoretically result from genetic or shared environmental factors, genes and family environment are confounded in determining the similarity among relatives. Thus, the results from family studies suggesting familial aggregation do not prove a genetic basis for that trait (Vandenberg et al., 1986).

Once a genetic basis for a disease is suspected, more advanced and complex methods can be used to further examine the apparent association. An example of one such technique is linkage analysis. During meiosis, or sex cell division, the pairs of chromosomes from the parent routinely cross over or recombine, exchanging segments and creating new combinations of genetic material. Recombination of segments of chromosomes forms one of the bases of heterogeneity and occurs by some fairly predictable laws. There are many differences between homologous or complementary pairs of chromosomes. They often carry two disparate versions or alleles of many of their matching genes.

During recombination, the closer two gene loci are on the same chromosome, the less often their alleles will be separated as DNA is exchanged between homologous chromosomes. Thus, both characteristics will be inherited together. Conversely, the farther apart two loci are, the more likely they will separate and the less likely their related traits will be inherited together. Linkage analysis uses common traits with a known genetic basis and chromosomal location, such as the gene coding for blood type. From this information, the degree to which the disease under study and the marker trait occur together or separately in large families or cloistered populations is ascertained. Significance is determined by examining the difference in the probability of observing the two traits being inherited together (linked) rather than independently (independent assortment). A statistically significant finding of deviation from the expected independent assortment for alleles at a known locus for complex disorder provides evidence that there is a major genetic contribution to the disorder and that the gene responsible for a disorder falls on a particular chromosome (Vandenberg et al., 1986). Until recently, the known markers were few in number. However, the application of sophisticated molecular biological techniques and recombinant DNA technology has made it possible to increase the known markers (White & Lalouel, 1988).

Linkage analysis has yielded some interesting findings. For example, Gusella et al. (1983) used this technique to localize the gene for Huntington's disease to chromosome four. Recently, this technique has been employed in an attempt to localize the genes responsible for affective and schizophrenic disorders, but with contradictory results (Egeland et al., 1987; Hodgkinson et al., 1987; Sherrington et al., 1988). Weaknesses and limitations of this technique include the use of small sample sizes and the familiar problems of collecting large amounts of reliable diagnostic data in extended families. Further, one of the basic assumptions behind linkage analysis is a single gene mode of inheritance. However, for mental disorders, there appears to be little evidence supporting the role of single gene inheritance. In this paradigm, it is also difficult to ascertain the contribution of genetic mosaicism, or non-Mendalian patterns of inheritance (Gardner, in press). These facts may, in part, explain why research findings in this area have been contradictory (Vandenberg et al., 1986).

A final and most conclusive method of establishing a genetic basis to a trait or disorder is by searching for aberrations in the number, structure, or rearrangement of chromosomes. By employing a karyotype method, the chromosomes can be visualized and examined in a standard fashion to detect aberrations. This method has been carried out with Down's syndrome, a disorder with such distinguishing features as mental retardation, a high prevalence of heart malformations, and unusual facial characteristics that used to be referred to as mongolism. Down's syndrome has been traced to the existence of an extra autosome (nonsex chromosome) 21.

Issues

Several important issues need to be discussed when evaluating findings from genetic research into mental disorders. In the past, diagnostic criteria for mental disorders and the methods used to measure associated traits often have been unreliable or poorly operationalized (Loehlin, Willerman, & Horn, 1988). More recent studies have rigorously operationalized these disorders through the use of specific diagnostic criteria such as those presented in DSM-III-R (American Psychiatric Association, 1987) and various structured diagnostic interview procedures.

In addition to this, the apparent heterogeneity of mental disorders has complicated the interpretation of genetic research findings. The broad diagnostic classification of depression, for example, can possibly be broken down into a number of subtypes with different possible causes (etiologic heterogeneity) and clinical presentations (phenotypic heterogeneity) (Loehlin et al., 1988). The issue of clinical heterogeneity has been addressed by cleaving disorders along boundaries drawn by traditional clinical features such as age of onset (early versus late), treatment response, and distinctive symptom constellations. Presently, there is hope that genetic research models will have heuristic value in examining the differential familial prevalence of possible disorder subtypes and thereby enable researchers to clarify the underlying nature of boundaries between various possible subtypes and between other disorders (Plomin & Rende, 1991; Weissman et al., 1986).

Finally, a key issue is the role of the environment. Although there is suggestive evidence of genetic influences for many traits, these investigations also provide strong support for the contribution of environmental and other nonfamilial factors. Plomin (1989), for example, notes that concordance rates for disorders such as schizophrenia are about 40%, which leaves 60% of the variance unexplained. Genetic studies also suggest that there are greater differences than similarities in siblings raised in the same environment and that the majority of the similarities between siblings seem to be of genetic origin (Plomin, 1989). These results point out the important influence of nonshared environmental events on the developing individual and also suggest that the effect of these unique events may be more important than shared family environment (Plomin, 1986). The implications of these issues are twofold. *First*, genetic studies have not only lent support to the notion that inherited traits make a contribution to psychiatric disorder, but have also implicated the importance of environmental factors. *Second*, these investigations highlight the importance of studying the unique contribution of environmental events on an individual, and their relationship to the individual's development and pathogenesis of the disorder. Thus, future behavioral genetic research may demonstrate that genetic factors are operative in some types of psychopathology, but that environmental factors (unique to the individual) are important determinants of the time of expression, form, and intensity of the disorder.

BIOCHEMICAL DETERMINANTS

Background and Assumptions

The essential tenet of biochemical theories is that various chemical systems in the brain malfunction to produce mental disorders. It is proposed in these theories that there is an underlying abnormality in: (1) the amount of neurotransmitter released, (2) the methods by which excess transmitter is degraded, or (3) the means by which a transmitter alters cell function or communication. The neuron, or nerve cell, is the basic building block of the nervous system. The brain and spinal cord are made up of tightly packed and organized systems of neurons. A neuron sends its message through an action potential, an electrochemical event that travels down the length of the cell. When the potential reaches the end of the axon, it causes the release of neurotransmitter substances into the synaptic cleft or small gap between a sending nerve terminal and the receiving cell.

Once released, the neurotransmitter diffuses down to the next neuron, where it binds with protein-based structures called receptors. Receptors have two functional components. A recognition site is located on the outer surface of the membrane on which the neurotransmitter binds with the receiving neuron. The second component is called a transducer site. When provoked by the binding of a neurotransmitter, the transducer site initiates the physiological response of the neuron. There are two basic mechanisms by which neurotransmitter binding is converted into a physiological response, and receptors usually function by only one of them. One directly effects the cell and thereby alters its ability to fire. Figure 1 schematically illustrates the means by which a neurotransmitter might act directly on the cell to alter its ability to fire. The other process initiates chemical changes in the neuron via chemicals called second messengers, which mediate between the stimulus and the changes necessary for the propagation of an action potential (Worley, Baraban, & Snyder, 1987). Figure 2 illustrates how a second messenger, referred to as cyclic AMP, affects the permeability of the postsynaptic cell.

There are two types of effects that may result from transmitter binding. Excitatory effects increase the likelihood that a cell will fire and inhibitory effects increase the probability that a cell will not fire. The excitatory or inhibitory effects of a nerve cell are determined by the type of transmitter substance. Generally, the effect of one neuron will not be responsible for the inhibition or excitation of a whole series of cells. Rather, it is the effects of many neurons which determine whether or not a cell will fire. Each neurotransmitter will bind with several types of receptors that may be structurally or functionally different. The neurotransmitter acetylcholine, for example, possesses two types of receptors, called muscarinic and nicotinic. Neurotransmitters do not appear to be released in exact doses and, thus, each neuron has built-in regulatory functions by which the action of a neurotransmitter is limited. One of these processes, called reuptake, occurs when the neuron reabsorbs extra neurotransmitter into the cell for destruction or restorage. Another mechanism involves chemicals that break the neurotransmitter down and thus nullify its potency. An example of one such chemical is monoamine oxidase (MAO), which breaks down a group of transmitters called monoamines at the

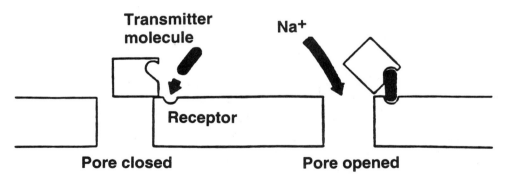

FIGURE 1. A simplified illustration of how a neurotransmitter exerts a direct effect on the postsynaptic cell by altering the permeability of the cell membrane to specific ions. From D. M. Shaw, A. M. P. Kellam, & R. F. Mottram, 1982, *Brain Sciences in Psychiatry* (p. 70), London, UK: Butterworth Scientific Press. Copyright 1982 by Butterworth Scientific Press Ltd. Reprinted by permission.

synaptic cleft. An autoreceptor is located on the sending cell and regulates transmitter release by halting further release when the neurotransmitter binds to it. Figure 3 illustrates the manner in which several of these functions operate.

Chemically, neurotransmitters are complex peptides, amino acids, or neurohormones. A number of presumed or known neurotransmitters have been isolated. For the sake of simplicity, we will refer to only a few that have been widely investigated in the psychiatric literature. They are: norepinephrine, dopamine, serotonin, acetylcholine, and gamma-aminobutyric acid (GABA). The first four are not found in large amounts in the brain, but have been the subject of extensive investigations (Snyder, 1985). GABA, an important inhibitory transmitter, is found in large quantities in the nervous system and has recently become the focus of extensive investigation with respect to anxiety disorders and depression (Lloyd, Morselli, & Bartholini, 1987; Martin, Owen, & Morihsa, 1987).

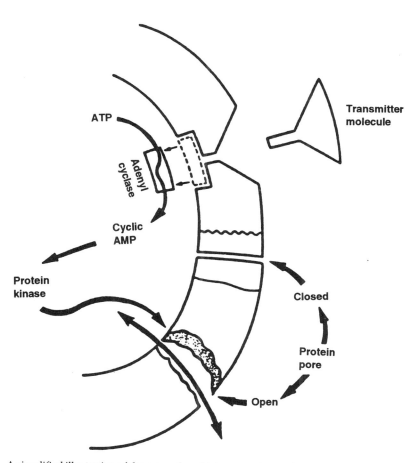

FIGURE 2. A simplified illustration of the means by which a neurotransmitter exerts an indirect effect on membrane permeability through the action of a second messenger called cAMP. From D. M. Shaw, A. M. P. Kellam, & R. F. Mottram, 1982, *Brain Sciences in Psychiatry* (p. 71), London, UK: Butterworth Scientific Press. Copyright 1982 by Butterworth Scientific Press. Reprinted with permission.

MARK C. WILDE
and PAUL M.
CINCIRIPINI

Early biochemical models of psychopathology were based largely on the observation of clinical drug responses. The dopamine hypothesis of schizophrenia, for example, which holds that a fundamental overactivity of central nervous system dopamine is responsible for schizophrenic symptomology, was supported by the observation that medications called phenothiazines appear to be effective in controlling psychotic behaviors (Snyder, Banerjee, Yamamura, & Greenberg, 1974). A similar biochemical theory of depression referred to as the monoamine hypothesis, in its early form, posited that an overactivity of neurons releasing the monoamine neurotransmitter norepinephrine causes mania, while an underactivity leads to depression (Schildkraut, 1965). The monoamine theory of depression initially gained support from drug models based on the observation that depression could be triggered by monoamine antagonists, such as the antihypertensive drug reserpine (Bunney & Davis, 1965). Additional early evidence

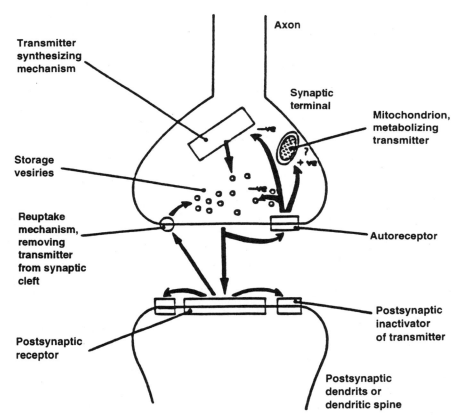

FIGURE 3. A cell synapse and several of the mechanisms controlling the means by which neurotransmitter release is controlled by the neuron. The arrows on the left graphically illustrate how the neurotransmitter is taken back into the cell via reuptake and metabolized by structures within the cell. The middle arrow shows how autoreceptors control the release of neurotransmitter through the binding of extra transmitter substance presynaptically. From D. M. Shaw, A. M. P. Kellam, & R. E. Mottram, 1982, *Brain Sciences in Psychiatry* (p. 73), London, UK: Butterworth Scientific Press. Copyright 1982 by Butterworth Scientific Press, Ltd. Reprinted with permission.

came from examination of the therapeutic effects of antidepressant drugs called tricyclics, which are thought to have their action by blocking the reuptake of norepinephrine into the cell, and monoamine oxidase inhibitors (MAO-I), which essentially block the function of MAO in degrading extra neurotransmitter (norepinephrine). Through these actions, both substances were thought to increase the availability of neurotransmitter and thereby exert their therapeutic effect (Schildkraut, 1965).

Both theories prompted research that sought a presynaptic neurotransmitter abnormality by comparing the concentrations of these neurotransmitters and their metabolites and enzymes in affected and unaffected individuals. Some studies have approached this by measuring such chemicals in the blood, plasma, and cerebral spinal fluid (CSF), while others have utilized postmortem brain samples. These models would predict simple relationships between metabolite, neurotransmitter levels, and disorder. For example, if schizophrenia results from an overactivity of dopamine systems, then levels of dopamine and its metabolites should be higher in unmedicated schizophrenics than in normals. Similarly, the catecholamine hypothesis of depression would predict that levels of norepinephrine and its metabolites should be lower in unmedicated depressives versus normals. Within the depression literature, for example, attempts have been made to compare levels of the major metabolite of norepinephrine called 3-methoxy-4-hydroxy-phenylglycol (MHPG) in the urine and CSF of depressed patients and controls.

Reviews of this literature show that results of these efforts have yielded inconsistent findings (Martin et al., 1987). On the basis of observations that clinically effective antidepressants have effects on the serotonergic system, attempts have also been made to tie serotonin to depression (Eison, 1990). However, comparisons of levels of 5-HIAA, the major metabolite of serotonin, have also yielded inconsistent evidence. Part of the reason why these endeavors have yielded inconsistent results is the possible heterogeneity of these disorders. Some studies claim that subgroups of depressive patients can be differentiated on the basis of urinary, CSF, and plasma levels and that these differences may predict treatment response (Maas, 1975; Westenberg & Verhoeven, 1988). For example, Maas (1975) reviewed the literature on metabolite secretion and treatment response and concluded that two subgroups of depressives, each having a different biochemical abnormality, could be identified. One subgroup was characterized as follows: low levels of secreted MHPG, a favorable response to the antidepressants imipramine and desipramine, improved mood after short-term treatment with an amphetamine, increased MHPG secretion following antidepressant or short-term amphetamine treatment, and poor responses to the antidepressant amitriptyline. A second group showed: normal MHPG secretion, little change or decreasing levels of MHPG in response to antidepressant therapy with imipramine or desipramine, and a positive clinical response to the antidepressant amitriptyline.

Aside from the heterogeneity issue, there are a number of other weaknesses in this methodology. *First*, blood and urine measurements of neurotransmitters and their metabolites are only indirect measures of central neurotransmitter function and can be contaminated by the contributions of transmitter activity outside the central nervous system (Syvalahti, 1987). *Second*, while samples drawn from cerebral spinal fluid provide a more direct measure of CNS metabolites, it is difficult to localize a possible abnormality, since these measurements reflect

MARK C. WILDE
and PAUL M.
CINCIRIPINI

underlying neurotransmitter activity in both the brain and spinal cord (Martin et al., 1987). Finally, while postmortem studies would seem to control for this, one cannot rule out the confound produced by chemical brain changes after death (Martin et al., 1987).

One major weakness of the catecholamine theory is that optimal clinical response to psychotropic medications usually occurs after at least a week of treatment, while the effect of the medication in either blocking dopamine receptors or enhancing norepinephrine function has been shown to occur rapidly upon administration (Prior & Sulser, 1991). This discrepancy, along with the failure to support a presynaptic deficit in metabolite studies, has led researchers to focus on the effects of long-term treatment on the physiology of the postsynaptic receptor. An example of the work done in this area comes from the depression literature. One of the early findings in the attempt to examine the effects of long-term treatment on receptor physiology was that long-term clinically relevant dosages of antidepressants, electroconvulsive therapy (ECT), and sleep deprivation seemed to cause a desensitization (down regulation) of norepinephrine-stimulated syntheses of the second messenger compound cyclic adenosine monophosphate (cAMP) on a specific norepinephrine receptor called the beta receptor. This, in turn, decreased receptor density (Richelson, 1990; Vetulani, Stawarz, Dingell, & Sulser, 1976). These findings led to the proposal that beta norepinephrine receptors are super-sensitive to the effects of this neurotransmitter in depressives, causing a decreased release of neurotransmitter presynaptically via feedback mechanisms on the releasing neuron (i.e., higher availability of the compound in the circulation and decreases in the production and release). This decrease in transmitter synthesis and release would be alleviated by antidepressants that increase the level of available neurotransmitter by inhibiting uptake and degradation, thereby causing a desensitization of the postsynaptic receptors, which, in turn, would cause an increase in further transmitter release (Sulser, 1983). This theory has been an attractive means of explaining the long-term therapeutic effects of antidepressants. However, it has not garnered clear support from clinical research and, as recent reviews point out, it is difficult to tell whether this down regulation is a cause of the depression or an effect of antidepressant therapy (Richelson, 1990).

However, in recent years, increasing attention has been directed to the role of other neurotransmitters and interneurotransmitter interactions that might play a role in psychiatric disorders. The indolamine neurotransmitter serotonin has been hypothesized as an important moderating variable in the cause of affective disease. The importance of serotonin in depression has been supported by research showing that: (1) depressives show abnormalities in the metabolism of tryptophan, an amino acid precursor to serotonin; (2) decreases in serotonin seem to cause depression in recovered depressives; and (3) serotonin receptors are increased or hypersensitive in depression, and that many antidepressants have effects on the serotonin system (Eison, 1990; Meltzer, 1990; Sulser, 1983). With regard to the latter, the now popular antidepressant, Prozac, has been found to be an effective treatment for ameliorating depressive symptoms and is thought to exert its effects by inhibiting the reuptake of serotonin into the presynaptic cell (Baldessarini, 1989; Sommi, Crismon, & Bowden, 1987). Further, recent research has linked serotonin to the down regulation phenomenon of the beta receptors for norepinephrine discussed above. For instance, Brunello, Barbaccia, Chuang, and Costa

(1982) found that if serotonin neurons were destroyed through the use of a chemical lesion, down regulation of the beta norepinephrine receptor did not occur. Current investigations are examining sites at the molecular level in order to find an explanation for these interactions (Prior & Sulser, 1991).

Issues

On the basis of the material just reviewed, several important issues need to be highlighted. *First*, evidence supporting or refuting single transmitter theories is indirect. Data based on drug responses are not sufficient to prove that whatever effect there is in providing symptom relief is directly related to the etiological abnormality of the disorder. The theories described above are based on research that does not separate causal from mediating events, such that one is never certain whether a proposed biochemical abnormality causes the disorder, is a mediating factor reflecting the condition itself, or represents some other aspect in the etiology of the disorder. Therefore, it is not necessarily clear whether medication corrects an underlying biochemical abnormality, or alters some mediating event in the brain that has not been directly observed. Much of the supportive evidence outside of pharmacological models comes from animal studies of receptor physiology and biochemistry or studies of human postmortem brains, or peripheral cells. Future research is needed to ascertain the generalizability of these studies to intact organisms (Martin et al., 1987).

Second, most mental disorders are highly heterogeneous, producing symptoms that traverse a variety of systems. As was the case with genetic studies, this has complicated the interpretation of mixed and sometimes confusing findings. As was the case in the field of behavioral genetics, biochemical psychopathologists have attempted to overcome this obstacle by subtyping syndromes on the basis of symptoms, treatment responses, and their relation to various biochemical markers. However, many of these subtypes have not been observed consistently enough to be entered into the clinical psychiatric nomenclature, and have not garnered enthusiastic support.

Third, single neurotransmitter abnormality theories, such as those discussed, oversimplify the study of a complex phenomenon, namely, a behavioral abnormality. The formation, development, and evolution of biochemical theories have proceeded from simple presynaptic deficit hypotheses to more complex postsynaptic regulatory theories, which have implied interactions with other transmitters (e.g., serotonin). Recent research has favored the more complex of these biochemical interactions as offering a better means to explain contradictory or confounding findings (Prior & Sulser, 1991). It is clear that the study of the biochemical basis of mental disorders has contributed to our knowledge of basic biobehavioral relationships and the therapeutic effects of various neuroleptic drugs. It is also encouraging that research in this area has aimed at increased complexity. Our knowledge of the biochemical basis of mental disorders is, as yet, incomplete. However, future studies may help us learn more about the interaction between affect, behavior, and concomitant changes in neurotransmitter action and their influence on each other. We have assumed a one-way relationship thus far (i.e., biochemical abnormalities lead to changes in affect and behavior). Yet, recent work with obsessive–compulsive disordered patients suggests that changing a patient's behavior may also influence important physiological processes (perhaps underlying the disorder) in the same way as pharmacological intervention does (Baxter et al., 1992).

GROSS BRAIN ANATOMY AND PSYCHOPATHOLOGY

Basic Assumptions and Background

Neuroanatomic models of psychopathology assume that dysfunction or death of comparatively large groups of cell, areas, or structures in the brain causes aberrant behavior. The brain is a complex organ composed of a multitude of cells grouped together into systems and structures. While a detailed discussion of anatomy will not be presented here, it is important to review some of the essential organizational features of the human brain as a reference. Figure 4 illustrates the

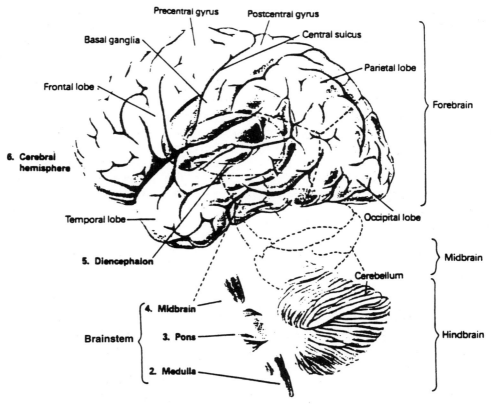

FIGURE 4. The major hierarchical divisions of the human brain. At the highest level are the cerebral hemispheres, which include the frontal, temporal, occipital, and parietal, lobes, along with the important basal ganglia and limbic system. At the next lowest level is the diencephalon, which includes the thalamus and hypothalamus, located subcortically. At the lowest level is the brain stem, including the midbrain, pons, and medulla. From E. R. Kandel & J. H. Schwartz, 1985, *Principles of Neuroscience*, (p. 5), New York: Elsevier Science Publishing Co. Copyright 1985 by Elsevier Science Publishing Inc. Reprinted with permission.

human brain and its hierarchical organization, ranging from the lower centers of the brain stem, pons, and cerebellum to a complex network of structures underlying the cortex, and the cerebral cortex itself. It is the cerebral cortex and underlying structures that will be the focus of later discussions. The cerebral cortex is divided down the midline into the left and right hemispheres. In turn, each hemisphere is divided into four major areas called the frontal, temporal, occipital, and parietal lobes. As shall be demonstrated, some of these divisions may have significance for emotional processes. This section will outline some major findings and theories related to emotional outcome of brain damage, the neuropsychological underpinnings of emotional behavior, and gross anatomical findings in schizophrenia, in an attempt to illustrate current trends.

Exactly how psychological functions are distributed in the brain has been a controversial topic throughout the history of physiological psychology. Historically, two theoretical camps have developed a certain degree of scientific and public popularity. At one extreme were the strict localizationists who believed that distinct psychological functions could be functionally localized to specific areas of the brain. This view is perhaps best exemplified by the work of Franz Joseph Gall, a nineteenth century German physician, who thought that special abilities in one of these areas were reflected in an overdevelopment of that region (Kandel, 1985). Based on this localizationist theory, Gall claimed that special talents, abilities, and traits could be inferred from protrusions of the skull and other physiognomic anomalies. Phrenology, the rather extreme view that psychological characteristics and configurations could be deduced by an examination of these protrusions of the skull, developed from Gall's ideas, and was popularized by his student Spurzheim. While phrenology was very popular outside of the scientific community, it never developed a serious scientific following, and it eventually fell into disrepute. It was not until the work of neurologists such as Broca and Wernicke, who later in the nineteenth century isolated brain areas thought to be critical in language functioning through the study of patients with focal brain lesions, that serious scientific interest in brain localization theory rekindled (Murray, 1983).

An opposing view was presented by the antilocalizationist tradition, which contended that various locations of the brain are not specialized to subserve particular functions. This body of thought is best exemplified by the work of Pierre Flourens, who believed that mental functions are not strictly localized but are instead represented throughout the whole brain (Kandel, 1985). Thus, according to Flourens, any part of the brain was able to mediate all mental abilities.

The ideas of A. R. Luria (1973) represent a more moderate view of brain localization. Luria believed that the brain could be divided into three functional systems composed of a number of specialized cortical zones that work in concert to produce complex behavior. The first unit, which includes the brain stem and structures underlying the cortex and midbrain, is responsible for maintaining arousal and the regulation of attentional processes. The second unit, which consists of the posterior parts of the cortex, including the temporal, parietal, and occipital lobes, is organized into three hierarchical divisions responsible for sensory perception, processing through a single modality, and integration of these modalities. Figure 5 illustrates the areas that roughly correspond to these zones. The primary zones would correspond to primary visual, auditory, and somatosensory areas, while the secondary and tertiary zones roughly correspond to the higher order and/or association cortex. The third unit in Luria's model consists of the frontal lobes and is responsible for maintaining and directing attention, initiating and maintaining goal-directed behavior, and regulating sequential processes (Luria, 1973).

Localization of Emotional Functions in the Brain

Research into the localization of psychological processes in the brain continues today and a great amount of information has been amassed that seems to implicate some systems of interconnected neural structures in various functions. While work into the neural contribution to emotional and personality functions has lagged considerably behind that of cognitive functions, efforts have been made to examine the relationship between various brain areas, emotional processes, and psychopathology.

The limbic system is a loosely defined set of subcortical structures. It is closely connected with many brain areas, including those subserving the endocrine system and frontal lobes, and includes the hippocampus, amygdala, and cingulate gyrus (called the limbic lobe), as well as parts of the thalamus and mammillary bodies (Damasio & Van Hoesen, 1983). It has long been considered an important brain area subserving emotional behavior along with a variety of other functions,

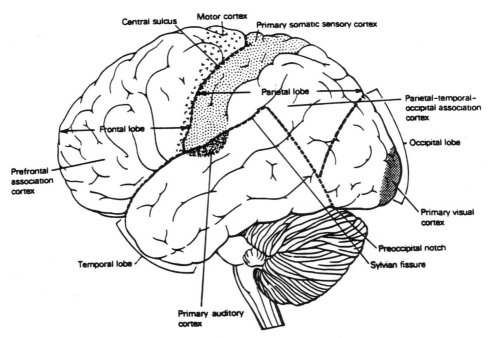

FIGURE 5. The four major cortical divisions (frontal, temporal, occipital, and parietal lobes) and related primary and higher-order processing centers for incoming sensory stimuli in the primary visual, somatic sensory, and auditory cortices, as well as the primary center controlling motor behavior. From E. R. Kandel & J. H. Schwartz, 1985, *Principles of Neuroscience*, (p. 214), New York: Elsevier Science Publishing Co. Copyright 1985 by Elsevier Science Publishing Inc. Reprinted with permission.

including memory, smell, and the regulation of attention. Figure 6 shows the location of the limbic system and other functional brain areas.

The limbic system was first implicated in emotional processes by James Papez (1937), who attempted to map out these subcortical structures and their connections and relate them to emotional functions. More recent work has examined the role of the limbic system in emotion by noting behavioral changes in animals after stimulating various limbic areas, and examining the behavioral responses of animals and man after limbic lesions. While the results of such investigations are not uniform, they seem to reveal a consistent pattern implicating the limbic system in some emotional processes (Heilman, Bowers, & Valenstein, 1985). For example, results of stimulation studies have elicited behavioral changes such as the production of oral automatisms, altering feeding habits, increased anger, flight and fear reactions, increased aggressive behavior, euphoria, and changed pleasure reactions (Macchi, 1989). Of historical importance for lesion studies are the observations of Kluver and Bucy (1937), who demonstrated that bilateral removal of the anterior temporal lobes, which include parts of the limbic system and related structures, caused increased behavior docility and orality in monkeys. Consistent with this finding, experimental lesion studies with animals show an increased threshold of reaction, decreased fear reactions, docility, exaggerated affective reactions, hypersexuality, increased oral and visual exploratory behavior, and hyperactivity (Macchi, 1989). Heilman, Bowers, and Valenstein's (1985) review cited reports of the emotional effects of local brain lesions in humans that have found ragelike reactions, increased sexuality, and increased placidity similar to that described by Kluver and Bucy.

The frontal lobes, which are presumed to be intimately involved in the

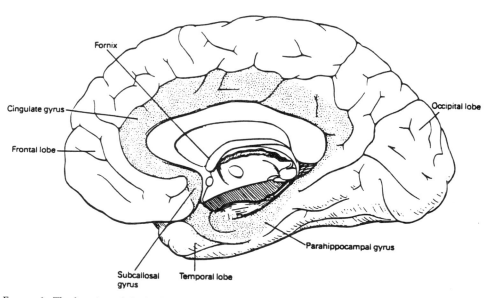

FIGURE 6. The location of the limbic lobe (speckled area) and an underlying deep cortical structure. From E. R. Kandel & J. H. Schwartz, 1985, *Principles of Neuroscience*, (p. 613), New York: Elsevier Science Publishing Inc. Copyright 1985 by Elsevier Science Publishing Inc. Reprinted with permission.

integration and organization of complex information, drive, motivation, self-awareness, and other higher-level abilities, have been the focus of considerable interest in the examination of neuroanatomic factors underlying emotional behavior. A so-called "frontal lobe syndrome" has been observed in patients with lesions affecting this area. It is characterized by prominent personality changes consisting of decreased spontaneity, deficits in goal-directed behavior and planning, outbursts of anger, episodes of euphoria and inappropriate jocularity, hypersexuality, disinhibition of impulses, and poor judgment (Stuss & Benson, 1986). Though many of these symptoms are frequently seen in patients with frontal lobe damage, correlations between specific behavior patterns and frontal lobe damage have been difficult to substantiate (Stuss & Benson, 1986).

Aside from attempting to localize neuroanatomic substrates of emotion in the frontal lobes and limbic system, researchers have also investigated whether or not emotions, or certain aspects of emotional experience, are lateralized in the cerebral hemispheres. The earliest reports that instigated this research were based on observations that emotional changes were seen in patients with left and right hemisphere damage. Briefly, left hemisphere damaged patients, particularly those who possess language deficits, show a "catastrophic" reaction that is characterized by anxiety, agitation, and depressive-like symptoms. Right hemisphere patients, on the other hand, exhibit a marked denial of disabilities and a tendency toward inappropriate humor or jocularity (Gainotti, 1972). While these observations have provided some interesting theorizing on the lateralization of differing emotional states, logical analysis of these syndromes suggests that the left hemisphere catastrophic reaction may be an appropriate response to severely disabling lesions, which frequently disturb language functions. Therefore, they are probably not appropriate analogs of a biologically mediated affective disorder. Right hemisphere emotional syndromes are, however, more clearly inappropriate and may hold keys to differential functioning of the cerebral hemispheres in emotional processes (Gainotti, 1972). This difference has generated a popular theory that emotional behavior is somehow preferentially mediated by the right hemisphere.

Numerous approaches have been used to test the hypothesis that the right hemisphere is intimately involved with emotional experience. Recent reviews in this area find some support for the notion that the comprehension and expression of emotionally related stimuli are preferentially mediated by the right hemisphere (Gainotti, 1989; Heilman, Bowers, & Valenstein, 1985; Strauss, 1983). However, it has not been demonstrated clearly whether the right hemisphere contribution to emotional behavior is related to the recognition of internal emotional experience, the expression of emotional experience, or the understanding of external emotional experience, or whether it is secondary to cognitive factors (Bryden & Ley, 1983; Gainotti, 1989).

There are a number of other factors to consider in the study of the localization of emotional phenomena in the brain. *First*, it is often difficult to generalize and adapt or apply the observed responses in animal research to humans, since it is unknown whether phenomenologically similar responses in the two species represent true analogues of the human emotional experience. *Second*, emotions and emotional experience are difficult to define with sufficient rigor such that they can be measured objectively and discussed consensually. *Third*, it is important to remember that strict theoretical and functional separation cannot be drawn between emotional and cognitive functions. Neuroanatomically, arousal, attention, motivation, memory, hunger, and thirst are cognitive/behavioral states of the organism that are, to some extent, mediated by limbic, frontal, and related brain structures. Changes in these states may play a key role in the "emotional" phenomenon observed in animals and humans after local brain lesions. Further, direct manipulation of the intensity of cognitive variables, through the destruction of underlying brain structures, may provoke emotional change by affecting an organism's ability to understand and organize experience.

Neuropathology of Schizophrenia

Schizophrenia has perhaps received some of the most concentrated attention in the search for associated neuropathological changes. Postmortem studies of schizophrenic brains represented one of the earliest efforts to examine the neuropathological changes in schizophrenia. Suggestive findings in this area are varied and include cellular abnormalities, cortical atrophy, decreased brain weight, abnormal development of glial cells (which is a sign of tissue damage), and the degeneration of myelin within the medial temporal, limbic, and frontal areas (Garza-Trevino, Volkow, Cancro, & Contreras, 1990; Meltzer, 1987; Weinberger, Wagner, & Wyatt, 1983). Neuroradiological techniques have been used to visualize brain structures and compare anatomic variables in normal and patient populations. Pneumoencephalography, for example, is an early technique used to examine the size and shape of ventricles, which are hollow chambers within the brain through which cerebral spinal fluid flows. Recently developed imaging techniques, such as Computerized Tomography (CT) Scanning and Magnetic Resonance Imagery (MRI), developed high-resolution computer-generated visualizations of brain structures. The most consistent finding from use of these techniques has been that schizophrenics show enlarged lateral ventricles and cortical atrophy, which seem to be unrelated to age of disease onset, duration, or medication exposure (Meltzer, 1987; Vita, Sacchetti, Valvossori, & Gazzulio, 1988; Weinberger, Wagner, & Wyatt, 1983).

A more recent imaging technique called Positron Emitting Tomography (PET) allows for the examination of both function and structure of the living brain. By injecting a radioactively labeled compound such as glucose or water into the vascular system, an image can be developed that shows the relative concentrations of these substances throughout different brain areas, presumably reflecting different levels of brain activity in various structures. Some PET studies utilizing glucose have found decreased activity in the frontal and temporal lobes relative to other areas, and increased or decreased basal ganglia activity in schizophrenics relative to normals (Buchsbaum, 1990; Farkas, Wolf, Jaeger, Brodie, Christman, & Fowler, 1984). However, these results have not been consistently replicated and the effects of medication exposure, phenotypic heterogeneity, and disease chronicity remain unclear (Buchsbaum, 1990).

It is interesting to note that a number of investigations utilizing autopsy and brain imaging studies have also found abnormalities in limbic and frontal brain areas in schizophrenics as opposed to normals. However, schizophrenia is a highly heterogeneous disorder, which has complicated the replication of radiological and neuroanatomic findings. A lack of consistency in diagnostic typology and a failure to agree on subtypes has also led to difficulty generalizing results across the studies. Nevertheless, attempts have been made to group patients by neuroradiologic and neuroanatomic findings and their response to treatment. For example, it has been suggested that patients with enlarged ventricles, cortical atrophy, and abnormalities in limbic brain areas also show a range of other characteristics. These include: lower functional premorbid history, prominent negative symptoms (e.g., flattening of affect, social withdrawal, poverty of speech, loss of drive), minor neurological signs and neuropsychological cognitive abnormalities on psychometric scales, and a poorer response to treatment (Weinberger, 1986). It must be noted, however, that findings such as an increased incidence of enlarged ventricles, morphological brain abnormalities, and variations in brain area activity in schizophrenics are nonspecific. They are not pathognomonic of schizophrenia (i.e., they are not found in all schizophrenics), nor do they explain etiology and pathogenesis of the disorder; and they also occur in nonschizophrenic disorders (Garza-Trevino et al., 1990). Consequently, it may be said that some, but certainly not all, cases of schizophrenia are associated with prominent abnormalities in brain structure and function.

NEUROENDOCRINE FUNCTION, DISEASE, AND STRESS

Background and Assumptions

It has long been observed that endocrinological disorders are sometimes associated with mental and psychological symptoms. For example, anxiety, tension, and irritability have been observed in patients presenting with hypothyroidism, while fatigue, indifference, and other depressivelike symptoms have been observed in patients with hypopituitarism (Morely & Krahn, 1987; Wallace & MacCrimmon, 1989).

Neuroendocrine abnormalities have also been associated with major depressive disorder. The hypersecretion of cortisol, a steroid hormone released by the adrenal gland, has been reported to occur more frequently in groups of patients with major depression (Sachar et al., 1980). In fact, cortisol activity has been investigated as a biological marker for this disorder and is thought by some authors to reflect an abnormality in the hypothalamic pituitary axis (HPA) (Sachar et al., 1980). A laboratory clinical procedure called the Dexamethasone Suppression Test (DST) has been developed around this idea. The DST consists of administering a synthetic corticoid hormone called dexamethasone and subsequently monitoring serum cortisol levels at standard times over a 24-hour period. A normal endocrine response to dexamethasone would be to suppress the production of further cortisol because the excess synthetic cortisol should trigger natural feedback mechanisms in the hypothalamic pituitary axis to stop producing cortisol. However, it has been observed that some depressed patients fail to show the expected suppression of cortisol (Sachar et al., 1980). As a result, the DST has been used as a diagnostic test in some centers. However, the usefulness of DST has been questioned. For example, Braddock (1986) argued that there was little support for the notion that a lack of suppression was suggestive of an underlying deficit in endocrine function or neurotransmission. More recent reviews on the topic have suggested much more complex models of the neuroendocrine–cortisol relationships in depression (Charlton & Ferrier, 1989).

Endocrine functions are mediated by chemical messengers called hormones, which are manufactured in the endocrine glands. Hormones contribute to a number of physiological events including lactation, sexual behavior, arousal, growth function, immune function changes, and tissue repair. The hypothalamus, which functions to regulate the internal environment, controls the first steps in hormone release and function. In controlling endocrine function, the hypothalamus releases chemicals known as releasing and inhibiting factors, which travel through a capillary system to the anterior pituitary gland just below the hypothalamus. These factors function to stimulate or inhibit the release of particular tropic hormones that travel to the major endocrine gland (i.e., thyroid, testicles, or adrenals). These tropic hormones, when released, bind with receptors on the endocrine glands and thereby cause the release of hormones, which travel to various target organs where they exert their physiological effects. Like the neurotransmitters, the release of hormones is regulated by a feedback system that prevents excessive production. Through a system of feedback inhibition, receptors at each stage of endocrine release respond to hormones distal to them. The binding of hormones to these receptors then causes a decrease in secretions at higher levels, which ultimately leads to a decrease in releasing factors at the hypothalamic level.

Simple correlations between behavioral symptoms and presumptive, or known, neuroendocrine abnormalities discussed above are but one part of the study of the behavioral aspects of endocrine function. Endocrine behavioral correlates are the focus of study of a field called psychoneuroendocrinology. The fields of study discussed thus far have presumed that some underlying deficit in brain, gene, or neurotransmitter function causes the pathogenesis of a particular mental disorder. Psychoneuroendocrinology, on the other hand, assumes that behavioral and environmental events influence endocrine function, and that the environment can change or effect biological events. Discussions of the endocrinology of stress and disease will be used to illustrate examples of this approach.

Endocrine Function, Stress, and Disease

The relationship between stressful events and hormone function has been widely investigated in animals and humans. The steroid hormone cortisol, which was discussed above, has been extensively studied and is best understood. Cortisol has a number of functions that are important in regulating the stress response, including facilitation of the supply of energy for the body's adaptive defensive reactions through its effects on metabolism. It also facilitates the regulation of immune function and inflammation, allowing the body to adapt to the presence of various potential pathogens (Cox, 1988; Selye, 1982). While a number of hormones other than cortisol have been examined (including the growth hormone, testosterone, and the catecholamines), cortisol will be emphasized here because it has been the focus of considerable scientific study.

Numerous associations have been made between lifestyle factors and the development of disease. While many lifestyle choices (e.g., smoking, ingestion of high cholesterol and caloric foods) have an obvious and direct impact on health, stressful lifestyles have also been associated with disease formation. Selye's (1982) popular theory of general adaptation posits a link between chronic stress exposure, hormone release, and disease processes. According to Selye, exposure to a stressor initiates marshalling of the body's defenses, including hormonal changes involving cortisol, which allow the body to withstand insult from an external

MARK C. WILDE
and PAUL M.
CINCIRIPINI

pathogen. Continued exposure results in a period of adaptation, or resistance, in which the body adapts and attempts to resist the pathogenic forces inherent in continued exposure to stress. The third and final stage in the stress response, called exhaustion, sets in when the body's defenses and adaptive potential have reached their limit. The exhaustion stage, which, according to Selye, is associated with the beginning of a disease process, begins through the degradation of crucial functions or target organ system. Selye's theory implicitly proposes that chronic exposure to stressors results in disease formation through the mediating effects of hormone responses. However, the validity of these assumptions has been questioned. Hormone responses and their relation to disease is complex and related to a number of factors including type of hormone, length of exposure, and coping mechanisms of the individual.

Recent reviews of the literature suggest that increased cortisol release occurs after initial exposure to a number of potentially stressful situations, including the anticipation of surgery, strenuous exercise, examinations, psychological testing, and stressful job tasks (Goldstein & Halbreich, 1987; Rose, 1984). It generally has been found that immediate exposure to a stressor elicits a rapid cortisol response and that this response generally returns to prebaseline levels with continued exposure to the stressor (Rose, 1984). However, unlike cortisol, the catecholamines (also classified as hormones) appear to rise on exposure to a stressor and continue to remain elevated, perhaps as a reflection of increased effort and vigilance required during stressful situations (Goldstein & Halbreich, 1987). Moreover, studies of animals and man have also demonstrated that a number of important moderator variables, such as the type of coping skills, social status, and the individual's personal appraisal of a stressor, are important factors that both define the stressor and regulate the nature of the endocrinological response (Holroyd & Lazarus, 1982; Rose, 1984; Sopolski, 1990).

In an effort to better understand the combined effects of social structure and stress on neuroendocrine response, Sopolski (1990) studied communities of baboons in the wild. His findings highlight important interrelationships between endocrine stress responses, social status, coping behaviors, and disease. Dominant baboons, which generally held a preferred social status in their communities, showed lower levels of cortisol secretion in response to stress than did submissive baboons, which were more frequently in subservient social positions and subject to more social stresses. Sopolski (1990) also found some other interesting relationships. *First*, submissive baboons, in contrast to dominant baboons, failed to normally suppress cortisol in response to dexamethasone administration. *Second*, submissive male baboons appeared to show early indications of disease-prone physiology including lower levels of HDL cholesterol and lower white blood cell counts. *Third*, he found a relationship between lower basal cortisol levels and several personality traits in dominant male baboons. The traits most associated with dominant baboons, which possessed lower cortisol levels, and by implication, less disease-prone physiology were: the ability to differentiate between threatening and neutral stimuli, the propensity to take control of a situation in response to an external threat, and the tendency to displace aggression onto a third party when a fight was lost (Sopolski, 1990).

In humans, exposure to stress and various behavioral variables have been associated with systemic disorders such as cancer, cardiovascular disease, and immunological dysfunction (Cox, 1988). For example, it has been suggested that a patient's cardiovascular response to psychologically challenging situations may influence the action of the catecholamines on the formation of atherosclerotic lesions and promote the development of hypertension through their long-term effects on sympathetic tone and peripheral resistance. Effective behavioral and cognitive coping skills may positively influence these effects (Cinciripini, 1986a,b; Rosenman & Chesney, 1982). What is noteworthy about the links between behavioral factors and cardiovascular disease (and relevant to the study of biological models of psychopathology) is the interaction between behavior, such as poor coping and the effect it has on known psychological mechanisms involved in the etiology of the disease. For cardiovascular disease, numerous links exist. For example, a psychological challenge may precipitate important changes in catecholamine releases, which are directly involved in the development of hypertension or arteriosclerosis process (Cinciripini, 1986a,b). The presence or absence of other behavioral characteristics (e.g., dietary and exercise habits) or constitutional factors (e.g., family history, hyperlipidemia) may influence the extent of the interaction, reducing psychological variables and systemic disease. The closest we have come to this type of modeling in psychopathology is the diathesis-stress formulations of schizophrenia, depression, and other disorders (Dalgleish & Watts, 1990; Gottesman & Shields, 1973). Such notions fall within the realm of behavioral genetics, as discussed earlier. However, they also have relevance to endocrinological models of psychopathology since environmental stressors are considered key elements in both types of formulations.

The diathesis-stress model suggests that a predisposition to develop a disorder (diathesis) combines with specific factors (stress) to trigger the onset of symptoms (Rende & Plomin, 1992). "Stress" refers to specific environmental or cognitive factors, while "diathesis" refers to genetic or constitutional factors. As discussed earlier, the appeal of this model may be related to the fact that a genetic influence has been identified for disorders such as schizophrenia (Plomin & Rende, 1991), bipolar disorder (Tsuang & Faraone, 1990), hyperactivity, autism, and tourretes (Rutter & Pickles, 1991). Yet, the concordance rate for these disorders may be 40% or less (Plomin, Rende, & Rutter, 1991). Thus, factors other than family history must be taken into account to explain variations in the phenotype.

Genetic–environment interactions have been proposed to account for variations in the expression of a broad class of behavioral disorders. For example, it has been suggested that classroom distractions may affect children with a predisposition to attentional problems differently than those without such a predisposition (Kendler & Eaves, 1986; Rende & Plomin, 1992). In the Israeli High Risk Study, the presence of one biological parent with schizophrenia (diathesis) and the experience of environmental stressors during early rearing more accurately predicted both future interpersonal difficulties and the onset of schizophrenic symptoms, as opposed to either factor alone (Hans & Marcus, 1987). Similar observations have also been made between the presence of a positive family history of schizophrenia and being raised in a dysfunctional *adoptive* family (Tienari, Lahti, Sorri, Naarala, Moring, & Wahlberg, 1986).

Recently, Rende and Plomin (1992) underscored the importance of genetic environmental correlations in the development of psychopathology, in addition to the contributions made by genetic–environmental interactions. The correlational model suggests that certain stressful life events may be more frequently encountered by individuals who are high on the genotype of a particular disorder. For example, in the Cambridge Collaborative Depression Study (Bebbington, Brugha, MacCarthy, Potter, Sturt, Wykes, Katz, & Mcguffin, 1988), familial factors were shown to predispose an individual to engage in behaviors that created subsequent stressful life events (e.g., poor relationships, separations, divorce); and these events were associated with the onset of depression. A similar finding has been observed for aggressive delinquent children, who may engage in interpersonally inappropriate behavior, which may result in subsequent stressful circumstances, including trouble with the law, lost friendships, broken marriages, and more intense forms of psychopathology (Rutter, 1991). Such events may be "controlled" by the presence of effective coping behaviors. However, the development of these skills also has been shown to have a strong genetic component (Kendler, Kessler, Heath, Neale, & Eaves, 1991; Plomin, 1989). Thus, certain behaviors may either augment or suppress the development of a disorder by modulating the frequency and intensity of an emotional reaction to stressful life circumstances.

At present, research on genetic–environmental correlations and interactions has suffered from the same difficulties as studies of simple genetic models described earlier in this chapter. Moreover, there have been no attempts to link specific patterns of behavior or the presence of significant stressors to specific biochemical or other physiological changes, which would presumably mediate the expression of the disorder. There is also a need to investigate other factors (e.g., personality, cognitive styles) that may be responsible for a genetic influence on behavior. It should also be possible to show that emerging interpersonal characteristics of patients at risk result in adverse changes in their environment. Future research in this area is needed to support the diathesis-stress model of psychopathology, in a fashion similar to that which has been observed for systemic disorders (e.g., cardiovascular disease).

SUMMARY

An attempt has been made to illustrate the major areas of investigation into biological factors that may underlie psychopathologic disorders. The major areas of exploration include: behavioral genetics, biochemistry, psychopharmacology, neuropathology, neuropsychology, and psychoneuroendocrinology. Exciting trends and core issues have been highlighted and criticisms of existing work have been discussed. Clearly, interest in biological factors has burgeoned in recent years, such that no chapter could do justice to the complexity and breadth of work in the area. While this growth is most evident in psychiatry, a similar trend can be seen in psychology. This is reflected by the growing popularity of neuropsychology and behavioral medicine. However, the increasing enthusiasm for biological models should be tempered by three issues.

First, the review of work on biological theories of mental disorders reveals the complexity of the biological systems involved in regulation of behavior and emotional activity. Efforts at elucidating biochemical or neuropathological factors underlying abnormal behavior have yielded theories that demonstrate an increasing appreciation for the intricacies of brain chemistry, neuroanatomy, cerebral organization, and their interrelationships. However, few definitive causal relationships have been found that demonstrate a one-to-one relationship between a physiological system and clinically abnormal behavior. For example, neurotransmitter regulation theories have garnered strong support for their role in the treatment of mental disorders. However, it is unclear whether their role is causal, correlative, or reflective of some other underlying abnormality. Similarly, neuro-pathological abnormalities found in schizophrenics do not directly point to specific deficits and causes. The findings here are often nonspecific in nature and have not been directly linked to the symptoms of a disorder. Genetic research findings, while suggesting that many mental disorders have inherited components, have neither localized the responsible gene(s), nor identified exactly what is inherited (e.g., metabolic anomalies, structural deficiencies, and/or underlying diathesis). As our knowledge of the contributions of each of the biological systems increases, testable theories can be developed which attempt to integrate these factors into an explanatory network, linking biochemical, genetic, structural, and environmental findings.

Second, an implicit assumption of much of the work carried out on the biology of mental disorders is that there must be an underlying biological abnormality causing these disorders, and that no interaction exists between behavior and biology. Complex human behaviors and their physical substrates are imbedded in social, cultural, personal, and historical contexts. Understanding normal and abnormal behavior may require that all of these factors be taken into account in any explanatory system. Attempts to isolate important variables in understanding human behavior are a necessary reductionistic tool to aid scientific investigation. Yet, to assume that other factors are not important neglects the obvious observations regarding human behavior. A theoretical framework that explains complex behavioral disorders, such as depression, sociopathy, alcoholism, or schizophrenia, solely on the basis of "biochemical imbalance," brain lesions, or metabolic disorders may grossly oversimplify the phenomenon. Without the proper integration of social learning factors, it would be impossible to account for the absence of a disorder in the presence of positive biological findings, or the presence of a disorder where physiological findings are absent. The challenge of integrating both biological and environmental factors into a unitary understanding of human behavior, and separating first-order from second-order causes, will be an important area for scholars in the social and medical sciences.

Third, it became evident in the discussion of psychoneuroendocrinology and diathesis-stress models of psychopathology that biology affects behavior and the environment, and the environment and behavior have important effects on biology. Investigations into the neurobiology of learning and memory, for example, have shown that the formation and storage of new information causes fundamental morphological changes in the neurons and their interconnections, implicating a dynamic process of change within the nervous system (Squire, 1985). Similarly, Rosenzweig (1984) has also demonstrated that animals raised in enriched environments show greater brain weights, changes in synapse size, and number of interconnections in certain brain areas than animals raised in impoverished environments. Research of this type suggests that the relationship among the brain, environment, and behavior is reciprocal and argues against simple models of biochemical or neurological abnormality as the primary cause of behavior disorders. Ignoring the effects of behavioral and environmental factors on brain function reinforces the long discredited notion of mind/body dualism.

With these caveats in mind, it may be emphasized that research on the biological basis of abnormal behavior has made an important contribution toward enhancing our appreciation of the complexity of mental disorders. Investigation of biochemical events, for example, has led to a greater awareness of the intricacies of neurotransmitter function, receptor physiology, and the long-term effects of psychotropic drug use on their function. Further, biologically based studies have been hindered and complicated by the problem of behavioral heterogeneity. Much of the work has served to clarify and illustrate this heterogeneity and provide differentiation between nosological categories.

In closing, it seems prudent to propose that the role of biological influences in mental disorders may be best understood in terms of basic vulnerabilities or strengths of the organism that directly interact and influence the environmental and behavioral factors. These relationships are not unidirectional, as illustrated by the diathesis-stress model. As is the case with systemic diseases, behavioral factors may exert powerful influence on the development of a disorder in the presence of an underlying biologic vulnerability. For example, poor diet, sedentary lifestyle, smoking, and even a Type A behavior pattern may act synergistically with a positive family history of heart disease to increase the patient's risk of developing the disorder. Changing these behavioral factors by quitting smoking, managing stress, etc., reduces the risk of developing the disorder by directly altering the underlying pathophysiology (i.e., lowering the frequency of episodic sympathetic arousal), which may have been related to an underlying genetic vulnerability. Similarly, the etiology of panic disorders may involve a predisposition to react to stressors with an exaggerated cardiovascular response or alarm reaction and an oversensitivity to somatic cues. Learning, manifested through appropriate or inappropriate coping, cognitive appraisal, and social modeling by significant others may determine whether or not these reactions broaden and generalize into unexpected panic attacks and agoraphobic avoidance (Barlow, 1988). From this perspective, it seems conceivable that emotional disorders have multiple pathways leading to their expression. What is clear is that a multifactorial and interactive approach, while difficult to formulate and study empirically, may offer the most comprehensive means of integrating our understanding of biological and social influences.

ACKNOWLEDGMENT.   Support for the writing of this chapter was provided by a grant to the second author from the National Institute of Mental Health (DHHS 5R29DA04520). The authors would like to thank Russell Gardner, M.D. for his helpful comments on earlier drafts of this manuscript.

REFERENCES

American Psychiatric Association (1987). *Diagnostic and statistical manual of mental disorders*, 3rd Edition, Revised. Washington, DC: Author.

Andreasen, N. C. (1984). *The broken brain: The biological revolution in psychiatry*. New York: Harper and Row.

Arieti, S. (1974). *Interpretation of schizophrenia*. New York: Basic Books.

Baldessarini, R. J. (1989). Current status of antidepressants: Clinical pharmacology and therapy. *Journal of Clinical Pharmacology, 50*, 117–126.

Barlow, D. H. (1988). *Anxiety and its disorders: The nature of anxiety and panic*. New York: Guilford Press.

Baxter, L. R., Schwartz, J. M., Bergman, K. S., Szuba, M. P., Guze, B. H., Mazziotta, J. C., Alazraki, A., Selin, C. E., Ferng, H. K., & Munford, P. (1992). Caudate glucose metabolic rate changes with both drug and behavior therapy for obsessive–compulsive disorder. *Archives of General Psychiatry, 49*, 681–689.

Bebbington, P. E., Brugha, T., MacCarthy, B., Potter, J., Sturt, E., Wykes, T., Katz, R., & Mcguffin, P. (1988). The Camberwell Collaborative Depression Study I. Depressed probands: Adversity and the form of depression. *British Journal of Psychiatry, 152*, 754–765.

Bertelsen, A. (1985). Controversies and consistencies in psychiatric genetics. *Acta Psychiatrica Scandinvica, 71*, (Suppl 319), 61–75.

Braddock, M. P. (1986). The dexamethasone suppression test: Fact and artifact. *British Journal of Psychiatry, 148*, 363– 374.

Brunello, N., Barbaccia, M. L., Chuang, D., & Costa, E. (1982). Down-regulation of beta-adrenergic receptors following repeated injections of desmethylimipramine: Permissive role of serotonergic axioms. *Neuropharmacology, 21*, 1145–1149.

Bryden, M. P., & Ley, R. G. (1983). Right hemispheric involvement in the perception and expression of emotion in normal humans. In K. M. Heilman & P. Satz (Eds.), *Neuropsychology of human emotion*, (pp. 6–44). New York: Guilford Press.

Buchsbaum, M. S. (1990). The frontal lobes, basal ganglia, and temporal lobes as sites for schizophrenia. *Schizophrenia Bulletin, 16*, 379–389.

Bunney, W. E., & Davis, J. M. (1965). Norepinephrine in depressive reactions: A review. *Archives of General Psychiatry, 13*, 483–495.

Charlton, B. G., & Ferrier, N. (1989). Hypothalamo-pituitary-adrenal axis abnormalities in depression: A review and a model. *Psychological Medicine, 19*, 331–336.

Cinciripini, P. M. (1986a). Cognitive stress and cardiovascular reactivity I: Relationship to hypertension. *American Heart Journal, 112*, 1044–1050.

Cinciripini, P. M. (1986b). Cognitive stress and cardiovascular reactivity II: Relationship to athero-sclerosis, arrhythmias, and cognitive control. *American Heart Journal, 112*, 1051–1065.

Cox, T. (1988). Psychobiological factors in stress and health. In S. Fisher, & J. Reason (Eds.), *Handbook of life stress, cognition, and health*, (pp. 603–625). New York: John Wiley and Sons.

Dalgleish, T., & Watts, F. N. (1990). Biases of attention and memory in disorders of anxiety and depression. *Clinical Psychology Review, 10*, 589–604.

Damasio, A. R., & Van Hoesen, G. W. (1983). Emotional disturbances associated with focal lesions of the limbic frontal lobe. In K. M. Heilmann & P. Satz (Eds.), *Neuropsychology of human emotion*, (pp. 85–110). New York: Guilford Press.

Egeland, J. A., Gerhard, D. S., Pauls, D. L., Sussex, J. N., Kidd, K. K., Allen, C. R., Hostetter, A. M., & Housman, D. E. (1987). Bipolar affective disorders linked to DNA markers on chromosome 11. *Nature, 325*, 783–787.

Eison, M. S. (1990). Serotonin: A common neurobiologic substrate in anxiety and depression. *Journal of Clinical Psychopharmacology, 10*, 26–30.

Farkas, T., Wolf, A. P., Jaeger, J., Brodie, J. D., Christman, D. R., & Fowler, J. S. (1984). Regional brain glucose metabolism in chronic schizophrenia: A position emission transaxial tomographic study. *Archives of General Psychiatry, 41*, 293–300.

Gardner, R. (in press). Sociobiology and its applications to psychiatry. In H. Kaplan & B. J. Sadock (Eds.) *Comprehensive textbook of psychiatry*. New York: Williams and Wilkins Publishing.

Garza-Trevino, E. S., Volkow, N. D., Cancro, R., & Contreras, S. (1990). Neurobiology of schizophrenia. *Hospital and Community Psychiatry, 41*, 971–980.

Gainotti, G. (1972). Emotional behavior and hemispheric side of the lesion. *Cortex, 9*, 41–55.

Gainotti, G. (1989). Disorders of emotions and affect in patients with unilateral brain damage. In F. Boller & J. Grafman (Eds.), *Handbook of neuropsychology* (Vol. 3, pp. 345–361). New York: Elsevier Science Publishers.

Goldstein, S., & Halbreich, U. (1987). Hormones and stress. In C. B. Nemeroff, & P. T. Loosen (Eds.), *Handbook of Clinical Psychoneuroendocrinology*, pp. 460–469. New York: Guilford Press.

Gottesman, I., & Shields, J. (1973). Genetic theorizing and schizophrenia. *British Journal of Psychiatry, 122*, 15–20.

Gusella, J. F., Wexler, N. S., Conneally, P. M., Naylor, S. L., Anderson, M. A., Tanzi, R. E., Watkins, P. C., Ottina, K., Wallace, M. R., Sakaguchi, A. Y., Young, A. B., Shoulson, I., Bonilla, E., & Martin, J. B. (1983). A polymorphic DNS marker genetically linked to Huntington's disease. *Nature, 306*, 234–238.

Hans, S., & Marcus, J. (1987). A process model for the development of schizophrenia. *Psychiatry, 50*, 361–370.

Heilman, K. M., Bowers, D., & Valenstein, E. (1985). Emotional disorders associated with neurological diseases. In K. M. Heilman & E. Valenstein (Eds.), *Clinical neuropsychology*, (pp. 377–402). New York: Oxford University Press.

Hodgkinson, S., Sherrington, R., Gurling, H., Marchbanks, R., Reeders, S., Mallett, J., McInnis, M., Perturrson, H., & Brynjolfsson, J. (1987). Molecular genetic evidence for heterogeneity in manic depression. *Nature, 325*, 805–806.

Holroyd, K. A., & Lazarus, R. S. (1982). Stress, coping, and somatic adaptation. In L. Goldberger & S. Breznitz (Eds.), *Handbook of stress: Theoretical and clinical aspects* (pp. 21–33). New York: Free Press.

Kandel, E. R. (1985). Brain and behavior. In E. R. Kandel & J. H. Schwartz (Eds.), *Principles of neuroscience* (2nd ed.), (pp. 3–13). New York: Elsevier Press.

Kendler, K. S., & Eaves, L. J. (1986). Models for the joint effect of genotype and environment on liability to psychiatric illness. *American Journal of Psychiatry, 143*, 279–289.

Kendler, K. S., Kessler, R. C., Heath, A. C., Neale, M. C., & Eaves, L. J. (1991). Coping: A genetic epidemiological investigation. *Psychological Medicine, 21*, 337–346.

Kluver, H., & Bucy, P. C. (1937). "Psychic blindness" and other symptoms following bilateral temporal lobectomy in rhesus monkeys. *American Journal of Physiology, 259*, 352–353.

Lloyd, K. G., Morselli, P. L., & Bartholini, G. (1987). GABA and affective disorders. *Medical Biology, 65*, 159–165.

Loehlin, J. C., Willerman, L., & Horn, J. M. (1988). Human behavior genetics. *Annual Review of Psychology, 39*, 101–133.

Luria, A. R. (1973). *The working brain: An introduction to neuropsychology*. New York: Basic Books.

Maas, J. W. (1975). Biogenic amines and depression. *Archives of General Psychiatry, 32*, 1357–1361.

Macchi, G. (1989). Anatomical substrate of emotional reactions. In F. Boller & J. Grafman (Eds.), *Handbook of neuropsychology*, (Vol. 3, pp. 283–303). New York: Elsevier Press.

Martin, M. B., Owen, C. M., & Morihsa, J. M. (1987). An overview of neurotransmitters and neuroreceptors. In R. E. Hales & S. C. Yudofsky (Eds.), *Textbook of neuropsychiatry* (pp. 55–85). Washington, DC: American Psychiatric Press.

Meltzer, H. Y. (1987). Biological studies in schizophrenia. *Schizophrenia Bulletin, 13*, 77–97.

Meltzer, H. Y. (1990). Role of serotonin in depression. *Annals of the New York Academy of Sciences, 600*, 486–497.

Morley, J. E., & Krahn, D. D. (1987). Endocrinology for the psychiatrist. In C. B. Nemeroff & P. T. Loosen, (Eds.). *Handbook of clinical psychoneuroendocrinology* (pp. 3–37). New York: Guilford Press.

Murray, D. J. (1983). *A history of western psychology*. Englewood Cliffs, NJ: Prentice-Hall.

Papez, J. W. (1937). A proposed mechanism of emotion. *Archives of Neurological Psychiatry, 38*, 725–743.

Plomin, R. (1986). *Development, genetics, and psychology*. Hillsdale, NJ: Lawrence Erlbaum Associates.

Plomin, R. (1989). Environment and genes: Determinants of behavior. *American Psychologist, 44*, 105–11.

Plomin, R., & Rende, R. (1991). Human behavioral genetics. *Annual Review of Psychology, 42*, 161–190.

Plomin, R., Rende, R., & Rutter, M. (1991). Quantitative genetics and developmental psychopathology. In D. Cicchetti & S. Toth (Eds.), *Internalizing and externalizing expressions of dysfunction: Rochester Symposium on Developmental Psychopathology*, (pp. 155–202). Hillsdale, NJ: Erlbaum.

Prior, J. C., & Sulser, F. (1991). Evolution of the monoamine hypothesis of depression. In R. Horton & C. Katona (Eds.), *Biological aspects of affective disorders*, (pp. 77–94). New York: Academic Press.

Rainer, J. D. (1985). Genetics and psychiatry. In H. I. Kaplan & B. J. Sadock (Eds.), *Comprehensive textbook of psychiatry*, (pp. 25–42). Baltimore: Williams and Wilkins.

Rende, R., & Plomin, R. (1992). Diathesis-stress models of psychopathology: A quantitative genetic perspective. *Applied & Preventative Psychology, 1*, 177–182.

Richelson, E. (1990). Antidepressants and brain neuro-chemistry. *Mayo Clinic Proceedings, 65*, 1227–1236.

Rose, R. M. (1984). Overview of endocrinology of stress. In G. M. Brown, S. H. Koslow, & S. Reichlin (Eds.), *Neuroendocrinology and psychiatric disorder*, (pp. 95–122). New York: Raven Press.

Rosenman, R. H., & Chesney, M. A. (1982). Stress, type A behavior, and coronary disease. In L. Goldberger & S. Breznitz (Eds.), *Handbook of stress: Theoretical and clinical aspects*, (pp. 547–563). New York: Free Press.

Rosenzweig, M. R. (1984). Experience, memory, and the brain. *American Psychologist, 39*, 356–376.

Rutter, M. (1991). Nature, nurture, and psychopathology: A new look at an old topic. *Development and Psychopathology, 3*, 125–136.

Rutter, M., & Pickles, A. (1991). Person–environment interactions: Concepts, mechanisms, and implications for data analysis. In T. D. Wachs & R. Plomin (Eds.), *Conceptualization and measurement of organism–environment interaction*, (pp. 105–141). Washington, DC: American Psychological Association.

Sachar, E. J., Asnis, G., Swami Nathan, R., Halbreich, U., Tabrizi, M., & Halpern, F. S. (1980). Dextroamphetamine and cortisol in depression: Morning plasma cortisol levels suppressed. *Archives of General Psychiatry, 37*, 755–767.

Schildkraut, J. J. (1965). The catecholamine hypothesis of affective disorder: A review of supporting evidence. *American Journal of Psychiatry, 122*, 509–522.

Selye, H. (1982). History and present status of the stress concept. In L. Goldberger & S. Breznitz (Eds.), *Handbook of stress: Theoretical and clinical aspects*, (pp. 7–17). New York: Free Press.

Sherrington, R., Brynjolfsson, J., Petursson, H., Potter, M., Dudleston, K., Barraclough, B., Wasmuth, J., Dobbs, M., & Gurlin, H. (1988). Localization of a susceptibility locus for schizophrenia on chromosome 5. *Nature, 336*, 164–167.

Snyder, S. H. (1985). Basic science of psychopharmacology. In H. I. Kaplan & B. J. Saddock (Eds.), *Comprehensive textbook of psychiatry*, (pp. 42–156). Baltimore, MD: Williams and Wilkins.

Snyder, S. H., Banerjee, S. P., Yamamura, H. I., & Greenberg, D. (1974). Drugs, neurotransmitters, and schizophrenia. *Science, 184*, 1243–1253.

Sommi, R. W., Crismon, M. L., & Bowden, C. L. (1987). Fluoxetine: A serotonin-specific, second generation antidepressant. *Pharmacotherapy, 7*, 1–14.

Sopolski, R. M. (1990). Stress in the wild. *Scientific American, 262*, 116–123.

Squire, L. R. (1985). *Memory and brain*. New York: Oxford University Press.

Strauss, E. (1983). Perception of emotional words. *Neuropsychologia, 21*, 99–103.

Stuss, D. T., & Benson, D. F. (1986). *The frontal lobes*. New York: Raven Press.

Sulser, F. (1983). Mode of action of antidepressant drugs. *Journal of Clinical Psychiatry, 44*, 14–20.

Syvalahti, E. (1987). Monoaminergic mechanisms in affective disorders. *Medical Biology, 65*, 89–96.

Tienari, P., Lahti, I., Sorri, A., Naarala, M., Moring, J., & Wahlberg, K. (1989). The Finnish Adoptive Family Study of Schizophrenia: Possible joint effects of genetic vulnerability and family environment. *British Journal of Psychiatry, 155*, 29–32.

Tsuang, M. T., & Faraone, S. V. (1990). *The genetics of mood disorders*. Baltimore: Johns Hopkins University Press.

Vandenberg, S. G., Singer, S. M., & Pauls, D. L. (1986). *The heredity of behavior disorders in adults and children*. New York: Plenum Press.

Vetulani, J., Stawarz, R. J., Dingell, J. V., & Sulser, F. (1976). A possible common mechanism of action of antidepressant treatments: Reduction in the sensitivity of noradrenergic cyclic AMP generating system in the rat limbic cortex. *Scandanavica, 78*, 618–621.

Vita, A., Sacchetti, E., Valvassori, G., & Gazzulio, C. L. (1988). Brain morphology in schizophrenia: A two to five year CT scan follow up study. *Acta Psychiatrica Scandanavica, 78*, 618–621.

Wallace, J. E., & MacCrimmon, D. J. (1989). Hyperthyroidism: Cognitive and emotional factors. In G. Holmes (Ed.), *Psychoneuroendocrinology: Brain, behavior, and hormonal interactions* (pp. 323–442). New York: Springer Verlag.

Weissman, M. M., Merikangas, K. R., John, K., Wickramaratne, P., Prussoff, B. A., & Kidd, K. K. (1986). Family-genetic studies of psychiatric disorders. *Archives of General Psychiatry, 43*, 1104–1116.

Westenberg, H. G. M., & Verhoeven, W. M. A. (1988). CSF monoamine metabolites in patients and controls: Support for a bimodal distribution in major affective disorders. *Acta Psychiatrica Scandanavica, 78*, 541–549.

Weinberger, D. R., Wagner, R. L., & Wyatt, R. J. (1983). Neuropathological studies of schizophrenia: A selective review. *Schizophrenia Bulletin, 9*, 193–212.

White, R., & Lalouel, J. (1988). Chromosome mapping with DNA markers. *Scientific American, 258*, 40–50.

Worley, F. F., Baraban, J. M., & Snyder, S. H. (1987). Beyond receptors: Second messenger systems in brain. *Annals of Neurology, 21*, 217–229.

II

Childhood and
Adolescent Disorders:
Introductory Comments

Early writings on child and adolescent psychopathology described the parallels between disorders in these groups and adult populations. Clinical research conducted over the past quarter of a century, however, has revealed the unique and complex developmental characteristics of children and youth that led to disparate manifestations of numerous disorders at early stages of the lifespan. Further, investigative efforts are underscoring the multiple pathways to many of these difficulties. This is reflected by the wide range of symptoms and behavioral disorders observed in children and adolescents within diagnostic categories. Such problems now appear to be a function of the interaction of a variety of psychosocial and biological factors that influence development. The chapters in Part II provide an overview of current findings on each of the major disorders of childhood and adolescence.

In Chapter 7, Cynthia L. Miller, Mary F. O'Callaghan, Deborah Keogh, and Thomas L. Whitman present contemporary approaches to mental retardation. They begin with a discussion of changes in the conceptualization of the disorder over the past 25 years and proceed to the holistic perspective to assessment and treatment (i.e., consideration of behavioral, emotional, and physical functioning, as well as cognitive status) characterizing the field today. Similarly, Lynn K. Koegel, Marta C. Valdez-Menchaca, and Robert L. Koegel examine the role of behavioral, environment, neurological, and physical processes in autism. These authors also describe the three general areas of autism (impaired social interaction, communication deficits, decreased activities and interests), as well as heuristic approaches to evaluation and intervention for each. Strategies and issues pertaining to what is perhaps the most serious and recalcitrant of childhood disorders, attention–deficit hyperactivity disorder, are covered by Mark D. Rapport (Chapter 9). This chapter considers the changes in diagnostic labels for this problem over

141

the years and provides support for the contention that it is a complex and chronic disorder of behavior, the brain, and development.

Mark S. Atkins and Kim Brown (Chapter 10) present an incisive review of conduct disorder, including a description of its various types and its course and prognosis in terms of peer relations, academic functioning, and developmental pathways. These authors emphasize the need to consider the interactive roles of relevant environmental influences (home, school, peer group) and biological and genetic factors. In Chapter 11, Cyd S. Strauss discusses anxiety disorders, which are possibly the most prevalent difficulties in children and adolescents. This chapter includes precise delineations of the symptom patterns comprising the various anxiety disorders as evinced by these age groups. Reliable and valid assessment of these conditions is emphasized.

The distinction between clinical manifestations of child and adult depression is a relatively recent occurrence, with research findings published only since the early 1970s. Nadine Kaslow, Karla J. Doepke, and Gary R. Racusin present an organizational schema that systematically characterizes domains of functioning affected by depressive disorders in children and adolescents. This includes a review of symptoms, and cognitive, affective, interpersonal, family, and adaptive behavior functioning in these individuals. Finally, the eating disorders, anorexia and bulimia nervosa, which have received the most popular attention of all of the disorders in this section, are covered in Chapter 13 by J. Scott Mizes. Here, descriptions of these problems, psychosocial and biological etiologic factors, medical complications, and associated, coexisting disorders (e.g., anxiety, depression, substance abuse) are discussed.

7

Mental Retardation

Cynthia L. Miller, Mary F. O'Callaghan, Deborah A. Keogh, and Thomas L. Whitman

Description of the Disorder

Mental retardation has a long history marked by much change. From its earliest beginnings, society has recognized the presence of individuals who could not meet the demands of everyday life. In Greek writings, mental retardation was mentioned as early as 1500 B.C. Hypocrates wrote in 500 B.C. about skull deformities associated with retardation. Different levels of mental acuity were discussed by the Roman physician Galen. During the Middle Ages, persons with mental retardation were viewed as fools, favored as "innocents of God," persecuted as witches, or considered possessed. In the sixteenth and seventeenth centuries, legal definitions were offered, and in the nineteenth century more sophisticated attempts were made to differentiate mental retardation from mental illness (Scheerenberger, 1987).

During the early twentieth century, a focus on both the environmental and genetic–organic causes of mental retardation, as well as the development of intelligence tests, brought about considerable changes in the way mental retardation was viewed. Workers such as Dugdale and Goddard proposed the term "familial retardation" to describe those individuals who did not have any obvious physical signs of mental retardation, thus recognizing that subgroups of mental retardation existed. The development of intelligence tests provided a measure for assessing subaverage functioning and for distinguishing among different levels of retardation. The terms idiot, imbecile, and moron were introduced to identify those individuals whose test scores fell below 25, 50, and 75 (Scheerenberger, 1987).

Cynthia L. Miller, Mary F. O'Callaghan, Deborah A. Keogh, and Thomas L. Whitman • Department of Psychology, University of Notre Dame, Notre Dame, Indiana 46556.

Advanced Abnormal Psychology, edited by Vincent B. Van Hasselt and Michel Hersen. Plenum Press, New York, 1994.

From approximately 1920 to 1950, a number of workers focused on the variability of functioning in mentally retarded persons of the same mental age. Recognizing the limitations of using intelligence tests as the sole means of classifying the mentally retarded, Porteus developed a test of "planfulness," and Doll proposed what he termed a "measure of social maturity," both of which today would be considered tests of adaptive behavior (Grossman, 1983). This trend toward characterizing mental retardation in terms of both intellectual functioning and adaptive behaviors continued and is reflected in current definitions and classification systems.

In the present chapter, the phenomenon of mental retardation along with its epidemiology will be described. Then, clinical pictures of persons with different levels of mental retardation will be provided along with a discussion of typical courses of development and prognoses associated with this complex disorder. Finally, the diverse causes of mental retardation and issues relating to its assessment will be examined.

Definition and Classification of Mental Retardation

A number of different formal systems for defining and classifying mental retardation have been developed throughout this century. Although these systems have been in general agreement, they differ in the purposes for which they were developed, in the particular aspects of mental retardation that were emphasized, and in the general users for whom they were intended. Several recent definitions will be presented here, including those of the American Association on Mental Retardation (AAMR), the American Psychiatric Association in its *Diagnostic and Statistical Manual of Mental Disorders*, Third Edition, Revised (DSM-III-R) (1987), and the international medical community as part of its International Classification of Diseases-9 (ICD-9). A more encompassing developmental disabilities definition adopted by Congress will also be discussed.

DEFINITIONS

American Association on Mental Retardation. The definition and classification schema proposed by the AAMR is the most widely recognized and utilized system in the United States. The AAMR first published a definition and classification system in 1921. This system has undergone several major revisions since that time. The current AAMR definition of mental retardation (American Association on Mental Retardation, 1992) states that:

> Mental retardation refers to substantial limitations in present functioning. It is characterized by significantly subaverage intellectual functioning, existing concurrently with related limitations in two or more adaptive skill areas. Mental retardation manifests before age 18 (p. 5).

Although this definition seems at first glance somewhat vague, each of the terms in the definition has been further defined. The AAMR classification manual offers the following elaborations of these terms:

> *Limitations in present functioning* is defined as a fundamental difficulty in learning and performing certain daily life skills. The personal capabilities in which there must be a substantial limitation are conceptual, practical, and social intelligence.

Significantly subaverage is defined as approximately an IQ of 70 to 75 or below.

Adaptive skill areas are defined as the effectiveness or degree with which individuals meet the standards of personal independence and social responsibility expected for age and cultural group.

In combination, these terms constitute specific criteria for making a diagnosis of mental retardation. There is, however, some flexibility in making this diagnosis. For example, an IQ of 70, or two standard deviations below the mean on standardized intelligence tests, is given as the cutoff score for mental retardation; however, this limit is intended as a general guideline. It may be extended up through an IQ of 75, depending on the reliability of the intelligence test used. Such flexibility is important in schools or similar settings where it is necessary to formally identify individuals who are in need of special educational services. Although there are standardized tests of adaptive behavior, there is also some flexibility in applying the criterion of adaptive behavior deficits, specifically because of variability in cultural expectations. While mental retardation is a developmental disorder by definition, retardation may occur after the eighteenth birthday as a result of a head injury or other physical trauma, or as the result of central nervous system deterioration. In these cases, however, the condition is formally classified (in the DSM-III-R) as *dementia*, which is an organic mental syndrome characterized by global cognitive impairments.

This most recent revision stresses a multidimensional approach to the classification and diagnosis of mental retardation, with the intent of broadening the conceptualization of mental retardation and avoiding a reliance on IQ for classification. The revision stipulates that a comprehensive diagnosis must include evaluation in four domains. The first domain relates to the core conceptual definition and emphasizes that the cognitive and adaptive deficits are manifested during the developmental period (birth to 18). Within the adaptive skill domain, the following areas of personal competence are articulated: communication, self-care, home living, social skills, community use, self-direction, health and safety, functional academics, leisure, and work. Although deficiencies in at least two of these areas must be present, these deficits may coexist with strengths in other areas of personal competence. This first domain is used to make the formal diagnosis of mental retardation.

After the diagnosis has been made, the individual is evaluated along the other three domains, which encompass psychological/emotional, physical/health, and environmental dimensions. Assessment of the psychological/emotional and physical/health domains involves listing specific disorders that exist in these areas as well as describing the individual's general functioning. Evaluation of the environmental domain consists of providing information about the individual's current living situation, the extent to which that environment facilitates or restricts the individual's life satisfaction, and specification of the optimal environment that would maximize the person's independence, productivity, and community integration. Finally, this proposed system stresses that mental retardation is not always a lifelong condition and that the functioning of individuals with mental retardation can generally be expected to improve with appropriate services.

The Diagnostic and Statistical Manual of Mental Disorders. The DSM-III-R, the most recent revision of the *Diagnostic and Statistical Manual of Mental Disorders*, is intended to provide a common classification system for mental health clinicians and researchers. This system, like the proposed AAMR system, is multidimensional in nature, classifying individuals on the following five axes: Axis I, Clinical Syndromes; Axis II, Developmental Disorders and Personality Disorders; Axis III, Physical Disorders and Conditions; Axis IV, Severity of Psychosocial Functioning; and Axis V, Global Assessment of Functioning. The diagnosis of mental retardation, which falls under Developmental Disorders, is made on Axis II. In addition, a secondary clinical diagnosis may be made on Axis I. The other three axes, which are not necessary for the actual diagnosis, are intended to provide additional information about an individual.

Although the DSM-III-R classification system provides a more comprehensive and detailed assessment than that employed currently by the AAMR system, the actual criteria used in both systems to make a diagnosis of mental retardation are identical: (1) significantly subaverage intellectual functioning, (2) concurrent deficits or impairments in adaptive functioning, and (3) onset before age 18. The DSM-III-R system does differ from that of the AAMR system in that it relies more heavily on clinical judgment in the diagnostic process, especially in assessing the adaptive behavior domain.

Currently the DSM-III-R is undergoing revision. The DSM-IV draft criteria (1993) for mental retardation are similar to the DSM-III-R in that the draft continues to refer to mental retardation in terms of both cognitive and adaptive functioning. However, impairments in the area of adaptive functioning are more specifically defined in the upcoming edition. The DSM-IV draft stipulates that a person must manifest deficits in at least two of the following skill areas of adaptive functioning: communication, self-care, home living, social/interpersonal skills, use of community resources, self-direction, functional academic skills, work, leisure, health, and safety.

International Classification of Diseases. The International Classification of Diseases (ICD) system was developed to provide the international medical community with a standard guide for gathering mortality and morbidity data. The most recent revision of this system, the ICD-9, defines mental retardation as follows:

> . . . a condition of arrested or incomplete development of mind which is especially characterized by subnormality of intelligence. The coding should be made on the individual's current level of functioning without regard to its nature or causation, such as psychosis, cultural deprivation, Down's syndrome, etc. Where there is a specific cognitive handicap—such as in speech—the diagnosis of mental retardation should be based on assessments of cognition outside the area of specific handicap. The assessment of intellectual level should be based on whatever information is available, including clinical evidence, adaptive behavior, and psychometric findings. The IQ levels given are based on a test with a mean of 100 and a standard deviation of 15, such as the Weschler Scales. They are provided only as a guide and should not be applied rigidly. Mental retardation often involves psychiatric disturbances and may develop as a result of some physical disease or injury. In these cases, an additional diagnosis should be recorded to identify any isolated condition, psychiatric or physical (p. 1098).

Additionally, an auxiliary classification of causes, such as injury or poisoning, is included to identify environmental events that lead to mental retardation. The ICD definition differs from the previous two in that it does not use the criterion of adaptive deficits. Moreover, it does not require that onset of mental retardation occur during the developmental period.

Developmental Disabilities. Mental Retardation can also be subsumed under the more general definition of "developmental disabilities." This definition was adopted in 1978 by Congress and included in Section 102(7) of Public Law 95-602, the Developmental Disabilities Assistance and Bill of Rights Act (often referred to as the DD act). It was intended to provide a guideline for identification of individuals who were eligible for government services and funding and not as a clinical criterion. The definition reads as follows:

> The term developmental disability means a severe, chronic disability of a person which (A) is attributable to a mental or physical impairment or a combination of mental and physical impairments; (B) is manifested before the person attains age 22; (C) is likely to continue indefinitely; (D) results in substantial functional limitations in three or more of the following areas of life activity, (i) self-care, (ii) receptive and expressive language, (iii) learning, (iv) mobility, (v) self-direction, (vi) capacity for independent living, and (vii) economic sufficiency; and (E) reflects a person's need for a combination and sequence of special, interdisciplinary, or generic care, treatment, or other services which are of lifelong or extended duration, and individually planned or coordinated.

Developmental disability is sometimes used as a synonym for mental retardation. However, it is important to keep in mind that mental retardation is only one condition among a number of disorders, such as learning disabilities, autism, cerebral palsy, epilepsy, and other neurological impairments, which are collectively labeled developmental disabilities.

CLASSIFICATION

The population of individuals with mental retardation is a very heterogeneous one. Although all individuals with mental retardation have in common low intellectual functioning and deficiencies in adaptive behaviors, there are vast individual differences in the severity of the deficits manifested, the associated physical handicaps and anomalies, the concurrent psychological disorders, and the degree of dependence on environmental supports (Grossman, 1983). For this reason, attempts have also been made to divide mental retardation into more homogeneous subgroups. The three most common subcategorizations of mental retardation have been based on etiology, level of functioning, and educational potential.

Etiological Classification. The American Association of Mental Retardation system divides mental retardation into two distinct subgroups on the basis of general etiology. The first group, which accounts for approximately 25% of the retarded population, is composed of the "clinical types." Individuals in this group have some nervous system pathology, usually fall in the moderate range of intellectual functioning or below, have associated physical handicaps or stigmata, and are usually diagnosed at birth or in early childhood. The second group, which accounts for the majority of cases of mental retardation, consists of individuals who have no apparent neurological damage, have no obvious physical signs of retardation, function in the mild range of mental retardation, and are found in disproportionate numbers in society's lower socioeconomic groups. Typically, diagnosis of this latter group of individuals occurs during the school years

(Grossman, 1983). Although it is possible to distinguish by definition between these two groups, there is no complete professional consensus concerning the utility of this type of dichotomous categorization.

Severity Classifications. Another common method of categorizing mental retardation is by degree of severity of retardation. Both the AAMR and the DSM-III-R systems provide guidelines for distinguishing between four levels of severity. These categorizations, which are made solely on the basis of IQ scores, are as follows:

Mild Mental Retardation   50–55 to approximately 70 IQ
Moderate Mental Retardation   35–40 to 50–55 IQ
Severe Mental Retardation   20–25 to 35–40 IQ
Profound Mental Retardation   below 20 or 25 IQ

A fifth category, unspecified mental retardation, is used when there is reason to suspect mental retardation, but the individual is untestable by standardized IQ tests.

Educational Classifications. Another categorization scheme is the educational classification system. This system, which was developed by schools to determine the need for placement in special educational settings and the potential of a child to benefit from educational instruction, is also IQ-based.

Educable Mentally Retarded (EMR)   50–70 up through 75 IQ
Trainable Mentally Retarded (TMR)   30–50 IQ
Severely Mentally Retarded (SMR)   Below 30 IQ

As can be seen by comparing the educational classification system with a severity classification approach, EMR corresponds roughly to mild retardation, TMR to moderate retardation, and SMR to severe and profound retardation. The EMR child is generally thought to have the potential to learn fundamental academic skills as well as to function independently in the community as an adult. The TMR child is considered capable of learning only rudimentary word and number concepts, and is rarely self-sufficient or independent as an adult. Finally, the SMR child is projected to require almost total care and supervision throughout his/her lifespan (Sinclair & Forness, 1983).

EPIDEMIOLOGY

Epidemiology involves the scientific study of diseases and disorders in populations. Epidemiological research plays an important role in the study of the distribution, causes, treatment, and prevention of mental retardation, and more generally influences the design of public health policies and programs. Epidemiological estimates of mental retardation are dependent upon the method of data collection employed as well as the classification system used. There are two general methods of data collection. The first method involves a random or stratified sampling of a population, in which a representative sample of families is surveyed and asked to identify mentally retarded persons in their household. The second method involves polling social service agencies that serve the mentally retarded. Because the second method is dependent upon people's willingness to seek community services and the service delivery systems' ability to make programs available, the first method usually provides higher and more accurate estimates of mental retardation. The definition and classification system employed also influences epidemiological estimates. For example, 25 years ago, the upper limit for mental retardation was defined by an IQ of 85. Not surprisingly, under this definition, a much larger number of individuals were identified as mentally retarded. Two related measures, incidence and prevalence, are typically used to describe epidemiological findings.

INCIDENCE

Incidence refers to the number of new cases that are manifested during a specific time period. For example, the incidence of mental retardation has been estimated at 125,000 births per year (Vitello & Soskin, 1985). Incidence figures are important because they provide a measure of how successful our society is in preventing mental retardation. A decrease in incidence rates of mental retardation would indicate a reduction in the number of new cases of this disorder.

PREVALENCE

Prevalence refers to the total number of persons with mental retardation who are present in a population at a given time. Both incidence and prevalence data are used to project the type and amount of services needed for a given population. Based on the theoretical distribution of the normal curve, roughly 2.3% of the population would be estimated at any point in time to have intelligence scores lower than 2 standard deviations below the mean (one of the criteria for mental retardation). Actual prevalence data have yielded rates somewhat higher than this (closer to 3%). This disparity between estimated and actual prevalence of low IQ scores may be accounted for by the higher than expected incidence of severe mental retardation due to biological causes. There has been considerable debate over the exclusive use of IQ scores to define the prevalence of mental retardation. Mercer (1973) has argued that this approach to classification, in contrast to one that employs adaptive behavior assessments in conjunction with IQ scores, results in a higher number of minority children being identified as mildly mentally retarded. Other professionals have suggested that the 3% figure underestimates the true prevalence of mental retardation, specifically because most prevalence studies use data from community agencies rather than from a total population screening.

To obtain a more refined epidemiological picture of mental retardation, it is useful to look at the prevalence of mental retardation in relation to specific demographic characteristics such as age, sex, and socioeconomic status, all of which have been found to be related to prevalence.

Age. Prevalence of mental retardation varies across age groups. The prevalence rate is lowest for children under 4 years of age. This finding is probably related to the fact that identification of mental retardation in infancy and early childhood is difficult for all but the most severely retarded individuals. For several reasons, the prevalence of mental retardation, especially mild and moderate retardation, increases during the school years. As children enter the school system, widespread testing and identification of children is available. In addition, increasing academic and social demands in the classroom environment reveals problems not likely to be manifested by the children in their home and neighborhood environment. The President's Committee on Mental Retardation (1969) coined the phrase "the six-hour retarded child" to describe children who are considered retarded during the school day, but who are able to function effectively in their neighborhood environments.

Similar explanations account for the decline in the identifiable prevalence of mental retardation with increasing age. Many mildly retarded persons who have had trouble in academic settings are able, upon leaving these settings, to function at least marginally well in vocational and community environments, and thus are no longer identified as mentally retarded. The fact that historically mentally retarded individuals have had shorter lifespans has also led to a decreased prevalence of mental retardation among older adults. This trend toward earlier death, however, has changed as improved medical care has become available.

Socioeconomic Status. Moderate, severe, and profound retardation have fairly similar prevalence rates across socioeconomic groups, although there tend to be slightly higher rates of these levels of mental retardation among low-income families. Mild retardation, however, has been found to be much more prevalent within the lower socioeconomic strata. Some individuals have attributed this finding to the use of intelligence tests that are culturally biased against minority groups (Mercer, 1973). Other factors, however, such as poor nutrition, inadequate health care, impoverished environments, greater life stress, and unstable family situations, also likely account for this greater estimated prevalence. Environmental causes of mental retardation will be discussed in greater detail later in this chapter.

Sex. Researchers report a higher prevalence of mental retardation among males than females, with a reported male-to-female ratio of 1.6:1. Some suggest that this gender difference is most pronounced among the mildly retarded population (Richardson, Katz, & Koller, 1986). Sex differences in prevalence rates among the mildly retarded have been attributed to: the greater vulnerability of the male to biological insult, the higher demands placed by society on males, and the greater proportion of behavior problems among males. Higher prevalence rates of more severe retardation among males may be accounted for by the fact that biological defects associated with the X chromosome are more likely to be manifested by males than females.

EPIDEMIOLOGICAL TRENDS

There are a number of forces currently acting to change the incidence and prevalence of mental retardation. For example, genetic screening and prenatal diagnostic procedures, coupled with an increase in elective abortions, have probably decreased the incidence of babies born with certain types of mental retardation, such as Down's syndrome. At the same time, however, medical technology is saving the lives of "high-risk" infants who would previously not have lived—for example, very low-birth-weight infants among whom there is a high rate of mental retardation. On the other side of the developmental continuum, medical advances have increased the lifespan of individuals with retardation, thus increasing the prevalence rates of mental retardation among the elderly population.

Changes in assessment techniques may also change prevalence figures. Refined medical and psychological methods for assessing development in infants probably increase the prevalence rates of mental retardation among younger children. On the other hand, earlier and more accurate assessment and identification of problems in infancy may result in a reduction in some types of mental retardation, particularly if this assessment leads to earlier placement in prevention and treatment programs.

In general, considerable progress has been made during the past three decades in early educational services directed at preschool-age children and school-age youngsters. Janicki (1988) points out, however, that programs directed toward at-risk families and newborns, such as nutrition services, income assistance, and subsidized health care, have recently been withdrawn for political and economic reasons. It is uncertain what impact this change of services will have. It has been suggested that public policy will play a larger role in determining the incidence and prevalence of mental retardation in the future:

> What will it be like tomorrow? One can only speculate; much of the speculation is dependent upon the future direction of public policies. Fiscal conservatism tends to be associated with decreased resources and diminished programs to help at-risk and needy populations. The continued future availability and enhancement of programs directed toward prevention, early identification and intervention programs for preschoolers, remediation, and special services for adolescents and young adults, work and skill-building programs for adults, and the range of challenging opportunities for elderly persons will be the telling points in terms of defining the composition of tomorrow's population of mentally retarded persons (Janicki, 1988, p. 308).

CLINICAL PICTURE

Providing a clinical picture of a typical person with mental retardation is difficult due to the range of functioning this diagnosis encompasses and the diversity of related disorders that may affect the mentally retarded individual. By definition, a person with mental retardation has significant cognitive deficits as well as deficient adaptive skills. Although considerable training and education may be necessary to facilitate cognitive and behavioral development, the number and types of programs received by different individuals are quite diverse. Moreover, the degree of developmental growth that occurs as a result of programming also varies considerably across recipients. To illustrate this individual diversity, two case descriptions depicting children with different levels of mental retardation are provided.

Case Description 1

Johnny is the 8-year-old son of a young couple. His health history is unremarkable. He was born healthy with no complications following an apparently normal pregnancy and delivery. He had typical childhood ailments but no significant illnesses. In general, Johnny's parents, as well as his pediatrician, felt that Johnny's physical development was normal.

At age 5, Johnny was enrolled in school. At the first parent–teacher conference, Johnny's teacher raised some concerns over Johnny's slow academic progress and suggested that his parents provide him with extra help after school. By the end of the school year, Johnny's teacher informed the parents that because of his lack of achievement, she was recommending that Johnny repeat the first grade. The teacher felt that perhaps with the additional year he would be better able to complete the first grade curriculum. She further recommended a variety of evaluations to assess possible causes for his deficient learning. A medical examination as well as visual and auditory evaluations indicated no physical impairments; however, a psychological evaluation revealed that Johnny's cognitive abilities fell below expectations, given his age. Assessments of intellectual functioning revealed deficiencies in verbal skills, organizational–perceptual skills, and memory abilities. He had an IQ of 65, which placed him in the mildly retarded range of cognitive functioning. Johnny's adaptive skills also fell within the mildly deficient range. Although Johnny displayed skills similar to his peers in terms of motor development and daily living skills, his communication and socialization skills were deficient. Johnny was formally diagnosed as having mild mental retardation.

Following a conference with parents, teachers, and the psychologist, it was decided that Johnny would repeat the first grade as planned, with additional individual assistance provided as necessary. Johnny's Individualized Education Program (IEP) emphasized, however, that he should remain with his class for the majority of the day in order to develop his social skills.

Case Description 2

Sally is a 3½-year-old child who was born prematurely and suffered multiple medical problems postnatally. Though Sally's mother appeared healthy during the beginning of her pregnancy and received good prenatal care, she developed an infection during the second trimester of her pregnancy. Because her infection was not completely controlled by medication, her physician felt it best to induce labor before the infection spread to the baby. Sally was born at 26 weeks, small for her gestational age, weighing 1 pound, 10 ounces. She remained in the hospital for 4 months following birth. During this hospital stay, Sally was treated for a variety of problems including jaundice, bronchopulmonary dysplasia, and intraventricular hemorrhage. She also required several rehospitalizations for treatment of respiratory illnesses.

Because of Sally's medical problems, her mother was referred to a local agency that provided services for infants at risk for developmental delay. Shortly after leaving the hospital, Sally and her mother began to receive weekly visits from a developmental specialist. This consultant worked directly with Sally and also demonstrated to her mother activities that would encourage Sally's development. Sally experienced delays in reaching her developmental milestones. She began walking with assistance at 2 years of age. Approximately 4 months later, she was able to walk independently.

At 3½ years of age, Sally was referred for evaluations to determine her eligibility for a developmental preschool program. At this time, she was found to be small for her age, weighing approximately 15 pounds, with a history of slow weight gain. She was able to walk and to climb on and off furniture. She did not, however, appear able to run. Sally could stack three blocks and place six pegs in a pegboard. Her motor skills were judged to be solid to 19 months with scattered skills assessed at the 22-month level. Sally was able to feed herself and remove her shoes and socks. She had not completed toilet training. Her communication skills were not well developed. She could identify, by pointing, three body parts and could follow simple instructions. Receptively, Sally was at the 19-month level. Expressively, Sally was vocal and could repeat words but had no spontaneous speech. Behaviorally, Sally manifested a short attention span and had great difficulty sitting still. During the evaluation she made loud unintelligible vocalizations, attempted to climb on the table, and threw test materials.

To measure her cognitive abilities, the Stanford-Binet Intelligence Scale (Fourth Edition) was attempted because this assessment begins at the 2 year level. However, Sally was not successful on most of the items, perhaps due to this test's heavy reliance on verbal skills. Therefore, a nonverbal test, the Leiter International Performance Scale, which also begins at the 2-year-level, was administered. Again, Sally was unable to complete the 2-year items, which required matching (color, shape, and form) skills. Next, the Mental Scale of the Bayley Infant Development Assessment, which evaluates mental development from 1 to 30 months, was given. Sally obtained a mental age equivalent of 16 months on this measure. In general, Sally was found to display severe delays in her cognitive and adaptive behavior development. Enrollment in a developmental preschool program was recommended.

COURSE AND PROGNOSIS

As depicted in these case descriptions, some children are identified as at risk for developmental delay at birth due to the presence of biological problems, such as prematurity and postnatal medical complications, and are formally diagnosed as mentally retarded early in their development because of pronounced cognitive and behavioral deficiencies. In contrast, other children may not be identified as having mental retardation until they reach school age. Although the pattern of strengths and weaknesses varies considerably in mildly versus more severely retarded individuals, each manifests, in varying degrees, underlying cognitive deficits and adaptive behavior deficiencies. Although intelligence is a fairly stable trait, the development of skills continues over the lifespan. The course of the mentally retarded individual's development is reflected in his/her acquisition of language, daily-living, socialization, academic, and vocational skills.

Daily-Living Skills

Self-help skill development begins with self-feeding. Persons with profound delays may require considerable assistance before learning to perform this and other self-help activities such as bathing, dressing, toothbrushing, and toileting. It can be anticipated that Sally would learn to perform these basic activities. In contrast to persons with profound retardation, severely retarded persons like Sally generally require only minimal supervision to complete self-help behaviors once these skills are taught. In the domestic arena, severely retarded individuals may learn such skills as putting household items away and wiping a tabletop, while the moderately retarded individual can typically learn to complete tasks, such as setting a table, making a sandwich, and making a bed. Mildly retarded individuals can become independent in even more complex activities, such as meal preparation, house cleaning, and doing laundry. These individuals can also develop basic money skills, but may need assistance with learning to budget. As a person like Johnny develops, he would be expected to reach this level of independence.

Language

Both receptive and expressive language deficiencies are common across all individuals with metal retardation. As indicated in the case studies, Sally had only begun to imitate a few words by age 3, while Johnny had developed functional communication skills. Upon reaching adulthood, profoundly retarded individuals may utilize gestures to indicate needs and, if verbal, may possess a very limited vocabulary and follow only simple instructions. Severely retarded individuals may learn to speak in short sentences and recognize written symbols but probably will not read with comprehension. A person like Sally who is beginning to imitate a few words is likely to develop a basic vocabulary to express her needs and be able to respond to simple questions. Moderately retarded persons can generally carry on a simple conversation while a mildly retarded individual can carry on everyday conversation. Moderately retarded individuals can often learn to read simple material, whereas individuals with mild impairment like Johnny will receive formal instruction in basic academic subjects and learn to read and write.

Socialization

Profoundly retarded individuals engage in isolated play activities but may also learn to participate in highly structured group game activities. Severely mentally retarded individuals may more spontaneously participate in group activities and show a preference for friends, a level which a person like Sally could reasonably achieve. Moderately retarded individuals will interact both cooperatively and competitively with others. They may need assistance in initiating appropriate social activities, however. In contrast, persons with mild mental retardation can more readily plan and carry out social activities and develop lasting friendships, including intimate sexual relationships. A person such as Johnny may have a girlfriend in high school and eventually get married.

Academic Achievement

The focus of educational programming for persons with severe and profound developmental delay is typically upon basic skill training in communication, daily living, and socialization domains. Although they may not develop extensive communication skills, they may learn to utilize alternative communication systems, such as sign language, picture pointing, or computerized communication boards. Individuals like Sally may learn to recognize "survival" signs, such as "stop," "walk," and "poison," but will not learn to read with any proficiency. Severely retarded persons may also learn to identify coins and learn which coins are needed to buy a soft drink from a machine, but they do not typically develop basic addition or subtraction skills. Moderately retarded individuals can learn skills such as adding coins, printing their names, and reading simple instructions. They may also develop more formal, albeit only rudimentary, skills in arithmetic and reading. A mildly retarded individual like Johnny may eventually achieve at the fourth or fifth grade level or higher in terms of reading, writing, and arithmetic. As the case study illustrates, Johnny was experiencing difficulty in school, but with additional instructional assistance he would be expected to achieve considerable academic mastery.

Vocational

Profoundly and severely retarded individuals do not achieve the task persistence and specific job skills necessary for independent employment. When a person like Sally completes her school years, she might receive limited vocational training in a sheltered setting. For individuals with more moderate delays, vocational training and compensated employment opportunities are often provided through sheltered workshops. Such individuals may also enter into supportive employment programs that offer closely supervised training within a community setting, training which is eventually faded out. Through this type of program, adults with mental retardation may hold maintenance and food service jobs in places such as motels and restaurants. Depending on the job market, they are vulnerable to layoffs in adverse economic conditions. A person with mild mental retardation like Johnny will probably receive vocational training as part of his education and therefore be ready to seek employment upon completion of school.

Comment

The prognosis for mentally retarded individuals varies considerably depending upon their cognitive abilities, their adaptive skills, the presence of other disorders (e.g., physical handicaps, sensory deficits, psychiatric disorders), and the quality of their social support systems (i.e., support from family, friends, and professionals). Early intervention and later quality-educational programs increase the likelihood of these individuals reaching their potential. Many persons with mental retardation learn to live independently, while others continue to require varying degrees of social support. Individuals such as Johnny, who are identified as mentally retarded upon entering school, may be able to lose that label upon completion of school if they are able to enter into the workforce and live independently. In contrast, individuals like Sally, who develop only more rudimentary living skills, will require continued training and social support. It should be emphasized, however, that societal expectations concerning the potential development of a person with mental retardation have changed and probably will continue to change over time as medical technologies and educational programs improve.

FAMILIAL AND GENETIC PATTERNS

Although over 200 types of mental retardation have been described in the literature, etiology is specified in less than 50% of the instances in which a person is diagnosed as having mental retardation. The causes of mental retardation can be divided into the two primary categories: organic and psychosocial. Organic causes refer to the presence of a physiological and/or anatomical defect. In contrast, psychosocial causes have roots in the environment in which the individual lives. In this section, both types of causes will be discussed. For a more extensive discussion of the etiology of mental retardation, the reader is referred to Grossman (1983).

Organic Causes

The major organic causes of mental retardation involve central nervous system impairments that are often diagnosed at birth or during early childhood. Organic etiologies account for 15 to 25% of the cases of mental retardation. Generally, the presence of organic etiologies is associated with more severe levels of mental retardation and only rarely with mild retardation. The onset of organic pathology can be during the prenatal, perinatal, and post-natal periods of development; however, organic problems most commonly occur during the prenatal period.

PRENATAL CAUSES

Numerous difficulties can impair the developing fetus during the prenatal period. These include: chromosomal anomalies, recessive and dominant gene disorders, maternal infections, and chemical hazards. Each of these etiological categories will be briefly discussed within this section.

There are multiple chromosomal defects that can produce a variety of mental retardation syndromes. The most common genetic aberration is Down's syndrome. It is an autosomal (non-X-linked) disorder associated with mild to severe impairment. Approximately one out of 1000 live births are cases of Down's syndrome. The prevalence of this syndrome increases dramatically in births to women over the age of 35. In addition to Down's syndrome, other chromosomal anomalies include malformations of the sex chromosomes—for example, fragile X, which is the second leading chromosomal cause of mental retardation. Fragile X syndrome is a condition in which the X chromosome is attentuated. A large number of individuals with this condition are moderately mentally retarded. The incidence rates are presently unavailable; however, this condition may be the second most common diagnosable cause of mental retardation.

Other abnormalities of the sex chromosomes, such as Klinefelter's syndrome and Turner's syndrome, are associated with mild to severe mental retardation. Klinefelter's syndrome, a condition affecting 1 out of 600 live male births, occurs when two or more X chromosomes are paired with a single Y chromosome. Mental retardation is noted in 20% of these cases. Turner's syndrome, a condition affecting 1 in 3000 births, occurs when only one X chromosome is present. Although mental retardation is not typically associated with this syndrome, 18% of children with this syndrome are reported to have intellectual limitations. For further discussion of types of chromosomal abnormalities (there are hundreds of these), the reader is referred to Pueschel and Thuline (1991).

Recessive and dominant gene disorders constitute a second set of prenatal causes of mental retardation. The most common is phenylketonuria (PKU), a recessive genetic problem that affects one in 10,000 live births. The degree of mental retardation associated with this condition is generally severe to profound. The absence of the enzyme phenylalanine hydroxylase results in the affected infant's inability to process phenylalanine, an amino acid in many foods. If the build up of phenylalanine reaches a toxic level, the central nervous system is damaged. Fortunately, with early diagnosis and a modified diet, this damage is not inevitable. Other recessive-gene disorders associated with mental retardation include Maple Syrup Urine Disease, congenital hypothyroidism, and Tay-Sachs disease. Dominant gene disorders include neurofibromatosis, mytonic dystrophy, and craniosynostosis. In general, dominant-gene disorders are not responsible for a large number of cases of mental retardation. [See Abuelo (1991) for further discussion of genetic disorders.]

A third set of factors causally linked to mental retardation in the prenatal period is maternal infections. Risks to the unborn child are typically greatest during the first trimester of pregnancy. One viral infection that has been commonly associated with mental retardation is rubella. Research indicates that fetal infection occurs 50% of the time when the mother has rubella during early pregnancy, and intellectual impairment occurs in half of the infected children. Another condition that can affect the developing fetus through damaging the central nervous system is toxoplasmosis, a protozoan infection carried and transferred to the mother from raw meat and fecal material. Mental retardation results in 85% of live births with this infection. Other common maternal infections associated with mental retardation include cytomegalovirus, syphillis, and AIDS.

In addition to maternal infection, the child is also at risk prenatally as a result of exposure to chemical hazards. Fetal exposure to chemical hazards results from maternal ingestion of a toxic substance. One substance that can have a substantial impact on the developing fetus is alcohol. Fetal Alcohol Syndrome (FAS) results from alcohol consumption during pregnancy with the risk to the fetus being greatest during the first trimester. FAS occurs in one to two of every 1000 births. Mental retardation is accompanied by physical abnormalities, such as a small head, wide-spaced eyes, a flat nose, and a deep upper lip. Other common toxic chemical hazards include drugs such as cocaine, tobacco, radiation, and lead poisoning.

Perinatal Causes

Organic causes of mental retardation are also operative during the perinatal period. For example, cerebral trauma may result from an abnormal labor or delivery. Difficulties may occur as a result of the position of the baby during birth or the length of the labor process. Abnormal fetal positions can create critical pressure on the skull and other complications, such as anoxia, which can cause severe tissue damage to the brain. A precipitous birth may not allow for adequate molding of the head whereas a prolonged labor may place a great deal of pressure on the infant's head. During prolonged labor, the child is at risk for oxygen deprivation if the umbilical cord becomes wrapped around the child's neck or if the placenta detaches from the uterine wall. The severity of impairment manifested in these situations is related to the degree of cerebral trauma that is sustained. In general, these types of perinatal factors account for a only small number of cases of mental retardation.

Prematurity and low birth weight are the most common perinatal factors that place newborns at increased risk for mental retardation. The incidence of prematurity and low birth weight is associated with a variety of maternal factors including: nutritional problems, infections, substance abuse, and medical conditions, such as a thyroid deficiency, chronic diabetes, and anemia. Medical advances have dramatically increased the survival of children born prematurely. Unfortunately, the increased rates of survival, particularly of the extremely premature and very low-birth-weight babies, are associated with a wide variety of perinatal insults, postnatal medical complications, and developmental sequelae. Medical complications include: hydrocephalus, intraventricular hemorrhages, hypoglycemia, hypoxia, and respiratory distress. Research indicates that the prevalence of moderate to severe handicapping conditions for preterm and low-birth-weight infants ranges from 4.5% to 10.1% (McCormick, 1989).

Postnatal Causes

In addition to prenatal and perinatal manifestations, mental retardation can also be caused postnatally, most frequently during the early developmental period by: (1) cerebral trauma associated with head injury and seizure disorders, (2) toxic poisoning, such as from lead and mercury, and (3) infectious diseases, such as meningitis and encephalitis. Meningitis is a condition in which the meninges, membranes that line the brain and spinal cord, become infected and inflamed by a virus or bacteria. This infection can result in increased intracranial pressure, fever, and subsequent neurological damage. Encephalitis is a condition with both primary and secondary forms, which cause inflammation in the brain. Primary encephalitis results from an initial invasion of the brain by infectious agents, such as mumps, herpes simplex, and infectious mononucleosis. Secondary encephalitis results following the infection of another organ. These conditions have debilitating effects primarily in infancy. Despite the numerous postnatal agents that can produce neurological insult, there are relatively few cases of mental impairment associated with damage to the central nervous system during this period.

Psychosocial Causes

Although research has traditionally focused on biological causes of mental retardation, there are a large number of mentally disabled individuals (approximately 75%) who do not manifest an identifiable organic etiology (Weisz, 1990). Typically, these individuals are mildly impaired and are commonly considered to be disabled as a result of psychosocial disadvantage. This type of retardation often occurs in families in which more than one member is mentally handicapped. Zigler and Balla (1982) suggested that this form of mental retardation may be polygenetic in origin, a normal expression of the population gene pool.

Currently, the phenomenon of psychosocially produced mental retardation is most often conceptualized within a multifactorial framework that emphasizes a combination of biological and environmental influences. For example, Whitman, Borkowski, Schellenbach, and Nath (1987), in discussing the correlates and determinants of mental retardation in the children of adolescent mothers, emphasize the influence of an array of socioeconomic and individual factors, including family and community social supports, maternal health, maternal nutritional status, maternal cognitive readiness, maternal personal adjustment, parental education, and parental learning ability. Weisz (1990), noting the importance of social influences on an individual's personal attributes (expectancy of success, outer directedness, and self-concept), stresses that, as a consequence of inadequate social stimulation and a history of failure experiences, a person's motivational orientation can be lowered. This in turn can adversely influence his/her level of cognitive and behavioral functioning.

Research in the behavioral genetics field emphasizes the importance of the combined influence of genetic and environmental factors on individual differences, such as intelligence. A number of investigators have examined the interrelationships between genotypes (the genetic constitution of an individual) and environmental variables (Plomin, DeFries, & Loehlin, 1977; Scarr & McCartney, 1983). Scarr and McCartney (1983) emphasize the importance of *genotype–environment correlations*, that is, relationships between the frequency with which certain genotypes and certain environments occur together. For example, there might be a correlation between an individual's genetic predisposition for low intelligence, and rearing environments that inhibit cognitive development. Plomin, DeFries, and Loehlin (1977) also stress that the expression of an individual's genotype depends in part upon the environment in which he or she is placed. This relationship is referred to as a *genotype environment interaction*. In general, research in this area emphasizes that the genetic make up of individuals can influence the type of environment encountered and that the expression of a genotype can be influenced by these environments.

The complex etiology of mental retardation is also suggested by Baumeister, Kupstas, and Klindworth (1991) in their discussion of the "New Morbidity." This conceptualization emphasizes the linkages between environmental and biological factors. The new morbidity model highlights the dynamic relationship between developmental problems and such factors as drugs, alcohol, low birth weight, prematurity, AIDS, adolescent parenting, and the increasing poverty culture. For example, children from low socioeconomic families are more likely to be born prematurely and as a consequence be more vulnerable to early biological insult. Mental retardation initially caused by such biological problems may subsequently be exacerbated by being raised in a single-parent family in which the mother is an adolescent with few economic, physical, or social resources.

DIAGNOSTIC CONSIDERATIONS

The diagnostic process, guided by the established criteria for defining mental retardation, facilitates the identification and description of mental retardation, establishes an individual's eligibility for services, and may identify causes of a developmental problem. Through this process, an individual's current level of functioning and developmental rate is gauged, and information relevant to remediation and educational planning is provided. In school settings, one outcome of the diagnostic process is the creation of an Individualized Educational Program (IEP) for a child. Through repeated evaluations, this IEP changes as the child develops.

Major Assessment Tools

Historically, intelligence tests have been a central diagnostic tool for identifying mental retardation. Some of the more widely used assessments include the Stanford-Binet, the Wechsler Preschool and Primary Scale of Intelligence-Revised (WPPSI-R), the Wechsler Intelligence Scale for Children-III (WISC-III), and the Wechsler Adult Intelligence Scale-Revised (WAIS-R). The use of IQ tests as a legitimate diagnostic tool has been questioned since the Civil Rights movement of the 1960s, specifically because of the disproportionate number of minority children diagnosed as educable mentally retarded (EMR).

Mercer (1973) suggested intelligence tests were culturally biased and discriminated against minority children who failed to meet the dominant culture's expectations concerning performance in school situations. In order to address this problem, Mercer and Lewis (1978) developed the System of Multicultural Pluralistic Assessment (SOMPA). The SOMPA takes into consideration noncognitive factors that might inhibit a child's performance on IQ tests, including: the child's health history, physical impairments, and social milieu. Emphasis is placed on evaluating adaptive behavior in nonacademic activities in order to determine a child's cognitive capabilities. This assessment battery, although not widely used (due to inadequate standardization and validation procedures), reflects the scientific community's attempt to create culturally fair tests. In addition to issues related to cultural fairness, intelligence tests have also been criticized because of their temporal variations and errors of measurement.

Despite these problems, intelligence tests continue to be employed because they have excellent norms, reliability, and validity. However, due to the current limitations of this diagnostic tool and the complex nature of mental retardation, there is a trend toward employing multidimensional assessment programs in order to better evaluate individual differences in functioning and to facilitate educational programming. Because of concerns regarding the narrow focus of intelligence tests and their use as an exclusive vehicle for defining mental retardation, the American Association of Mental Deficiency (AAMD) has since 1959 emphasized the importance of adaptive behavior in addition to cognitive ability in its definitions of mental retardation. The most widely used assessment tools for examining adaptive behavior include the AAMD Adaptive Behavior Scale and the Vineland Adaptive Behavior Scale. These measures are useful to the extent that the informant who evaluates an individual's adaptive capabilities is an accurate and reliable observer.

Traditional methods of examining cognitive and adaptive abilities also have been supplemented by a thorough examination of the child's developmental history and social environment. Through parent and teacher interviews and evaluations of medical and school records, a broader picture of the child's developmental and medical history is obtained. For example, information is obtained about a child's physical problems, peer interactions, social skills, and emotional problems. These types of data, although sometimes limited in their reliability and validity, can be productively used in conjunction with more formal assessment methods. In addition to developmental histories, environmental assessments also provide valuable information. Influenced by sociological and social developmental theories, the use of this type of assessment recognizes the role of specific environmental arrangements in inhibiting or facilitating development.

One widely used environmental assessment tool is the Home Observation for Measurement of the Environment (HOME) (Caldwell & Bradley, 1978). The HOME is a semistructured observation–interview instrument. This device focuses on the types of physical environments and parenting styles employed in the home setting to promote the cognitive development of the child. The HOME assesses such factors as provision of appropriate play materials, language facilitation, encouragement of social maturity, and stimulation of academic behavior. The scale has good content validity and test-retest reliability (Mitchell, 1985).

Assessment Emphases

Increasingly, the evaluation of mental retardation is taking place within an interdisciplinary, multivariate, and social–developmental framework. Particular attention is being given to early diagnosis and screening. Early assessment has been emphasized because of its implication for early intervention and prevention. Assessment can occur at a number of stages. Prior to conception, genetic screening can be used to provide families with information regarding their carrier status for transmitting genetic defects to their offspring. The process includes a review of the family history as well as chromosomal and biochemical profiles of family members. Currently, a national project to map the human genome is being coordinated by the National Center for Human Genome Research. One outcome of this effort will be the identification and assessment of how genes act to produce mental retardation and how early genetic manipulation might influence healthy development (Wingerson, 1990). This project will undoubtedly have profound influences on the information provided to families in genetic counseling programs.

In addition to preconception genetic screening, prenatal assessments, such as amniocentesis, ultrasonography, amniography, and fetoscopy, can be employed to identify the presence of a fetal defect. Typically, because these procedures are costly and sometimes risky, they are utilized selectively, such as when the mother is 35 years or older, a parent is suspected of being a carrier of a chromosomal defect, or there has been a previous birth of a chromosomally abnormal infant. Screening at this stage enables families to make decisions concerning continuance of the pregnancy, sometimes allows for early prenatal medical intervention to be implemented, and can help the family to emotionally and physically prepare for a child with special needs.

Further assessment can also take place at birth. Newborns are now routinely screened for metabolic disorders that can produce mental retardation and other disabilities. Chromosomal and genetic disorders (e.g., PKU) can be identified and treated in the neonatal period. Early screening also serves to identify children at risk for a developmental disability and to allow social and educational support systems to be developed. In general, however, these very early assessment programs allow for timely identification, treatment, and prevention of biological causes of mental retardation, and are especially useful in cases involving handicapping conditions that are potentially more severe in nature.

Although early diagnosis can identify a child's specific needs, lead to the provision of necessary services, and facilitate interdisciplinary communication among professionals concerning the child's needs, this process can also stigmatize if it creates unrealistic perceptions and unwarranted negative projections by professionals and parents about a child's potential. Professionals in particular need to be sensitive to the effects of labels, candid about their inability to make specific predictions about long-term developmental outcome, and recognize that a handicap is only one defining characteristic of an individual's personality. Zigler and Balla (1982) emphasize the continuing need for flexibility in the diagnostic process due to the fact that individuals, even with similar psychometric profiles, may respond in quite diverse ways to intervention efforts.

In addition to early screening, a comprehensive assessment program needs to examine the individual throughout the developmental period. Current social and behavioral theories emphasize the need for repeated assessments to evaluate the child's changing developmental status and needs, the impact of medical treatments, the appropriateness of class placements, and the effectiveness of educational programs. Rather than view mental retardation as a fixed trait, this approach to assessment captures the dynamic and changing quality of development, as well as it social nature.

This type of perspective is reflected in Vygotsky's (1978) notion of zone of proximal development, which views intelligence not only in terms of the individual's present developmental level, but also in relation to the individual's capacity for new learning. Within this framework, ability is inextricably interrelated to the social context in which learning occurs and is defined in terms of the amount of instruction needed to bring about new learning. This approach to dynamic assessment emphasizes a view of mental retardation as remediable and has more direct implications for designing instructional programs than traditional intellectual assessments. Reflecting this fluid conception of mental retardation and cognitive growth, Feuerstein (1980) utilized cognitive assessments both to gauge an individual's cognitive potential and to structure educational efforts. His program of instrumental enrichment targets for active intervention cognitive processes responsible for poor intellectual performance. Intervention generally focuses on creating appropriate social instructional arrangements. The importance of social context in the diagnostic and educational process is also stressed in current multifactorial models of assessment and treatment. Models such as the one proposed by Whitman, Borkowski, Schellenbach, and Nath (1987) emphasize the need to consider the dynamic and changing social support resources of parents in developing programs for stimulating early development in children at risk for mental retardation. These models are particularly appropriate for families who live in poverty situations.

Current assessment efforts are also increasingly emphasizing the view that mentally retarded persons vary not only in their cognitive functioning, but also in their physical and emotional characteristics and that assessment of these latter domains is critical for the development of effective educational programs. For instance, if a physical handicap accompanies mental retardation, the diagnostic process needs to address how this physical handicap affects learning and how it might influence an individual's eligibility for services. In addition to physical impairments, mental retardation may be accompanied by emotional disturbances, and diagnostic overshadowing can occur. Through diagnostic overshadowing, a diagnosis of mental retardation sometimes excludes the identification and treatment of mental illness. As a consequence, an individual's emotional problems often interfere with educational programming while the emotional disorder goes untreated. In order for effective intervention to be developed for persons with mental retardation, their physical and emotional needs must be actively addressed in addition to their cognitive and behavioral needs.

Summary

During the past three decades, our conceptualizations of mental retardation have undergone profound changes. Current definitions are more holistic, emphasizing the behavioral, emotional, and physical functioning as well as cognitive status of persons with mental retardation and the reciprocal influences between these intrapersonal processes. The role that the environment plays in inhibiting as well as facilitating cognitive development is becoming better understood. As a consequence, more emphasis is being placed on examining physical and social environments in the assessment process and on restructuring these environments during intervention programs. In addition, our knowledge of how biological and environmental factors influence development has led to a more dynamic interdisciplinary approach to assessing and treating mental retardation. Increasing emphasis is also being placed on the early assessment and early treatment of individuals at risk for mental retardation. Finally, the multiplicity of effects that poverty has on both the biological and psychological development of the child is just beginning to be appreciated. As a consequence of all these changes, our assessment and treatment models are becoming increasingly complex.

Acknowledgment   The first two authors were supported in the writing of this chapter by a predoctoral training grant from the National Institutes of Health (Grant Number HD-071184).

Abuelo, D. N. (1991). Genetic disorders. In J. L. Matson & J. A. Mulick (Eds.), *Handbook of mental retardation* (2nd Ed.) (pp. 97–114). Elmsford, NY: Pergamon Press.

American Association on Mental Retardation (1992). *Mental retardation: Definition, classification, and systems of supports* (9th Ed.). Washington, DC: Author.

American Psychiatric Association (1993). *DSM-IV draft criteria*. Washington, DC: Author.

Baumeister, A. A., Kupstas, F. D., & Klindworth, L. M. (1991). *The new morbidity: A national plan of action*. Newbury Place, CA: Sage Publications.

Caldwell, B. M., & Bradley, R. H. (1978). *Home observation for measurement of the environment*. Little Rock: University of Arkansas.

Feuerstein, R. (1980). *Instrumental enrichment: An intervention program for cognitive modifiability*. Baltimore: University Park Press.

Grossman, H. J. (1983). *Classification in mental retardation*. Washington, DC: American Association on Mental Deficiency.

Janicki, M. P. (1988). The changing nature of the population of individuals with mental retardation. In J. F. Kavanagh (Ed.), *Understanding mental retardation: Research accomplishments and new frontiers* (pp. 297–310). Baltimore: Paul H. Brookes.

McCormick, M. C. (1989). Long-term follow-up of infants discharged from neonatal intensive care units. *Journal of the American Medical Association, 261,* 1767–1772.

Mercer, J. R., & Lewis, J. (1978). *SOMPA: Student assessment manual*. New York: Psychological Corporation.

Mercer, J. R. (1973). The myth of 3% prevalence. In R. K. Eyman, C. E. Meyers, & G. Tarjan (Eds.), *Sociobehavioral studies in mental retardation. Monographs of the American Association on Mental Deficiency, 1,* 1–18.

Mitchell, J. V. (Ed.). (1985). *The ninth mental measurements yearbook* (Vol. I). Lincoln, NE: University of Nebraska Press.

Plomin, R., DeFries, J. C., & Loehlin, J. C. (1977). Genotype–environment interaction and correlation in the analysis of human behavior. *Psychological Bulletin, 84,* 309–322.

President's Committee on Mental Retardation. *The six hour retarded child*. Report on a Conference on Problems of Education of Children in the Inner City, August 10–12, 1969. Washington, DC.

Pueschel, S. M., & Thulin, H. C. (1991). Chromosome disorders. In J. L. Matson & J. A. Mulick (Eds.), *Handbook of mental retardation* (2nd Ed.) (pp. 115–138). Elmsford, NY: Pergamon Press.

Richardson, S. A., Katz, M., & Koller, H. (1986). Sex differences in number of children administratively classified as mildly mentally retarded: An epidemiological review. *American Journal of Mental Deficiency, 91,* 250–256.

Scarr, S., & McCartney, K. (1983). How people make their own environments: A theory of genotype → environment effects. *Child Development, 54,* 424–435.

Scheerenberger, R. C. (1987). *A history of mental retardation: A quarter century of promise*. Baltimore: Paul H. Brookes.

Sinclair, E., & Forness, S. (1983). Classification: Educational issues. In J. L. Matson & J. A. Mulick (Eds.), *Handbook of mental retardation*. Elmsford, NY: Pergamon Press.

Vitello, S. J., & Soskin, R. M. (1985). *Mental retardation: Its social and legal context*. New Jersey: Prentice-Hall, Inc.

Vygotsky, L. S. (1978). *Mind in society: The development of higher psychological processes*. Cambridge, MA: Harvard University.

Weisz, J. R. (1990). Cultural–familial mental retardation: A developmental perspective on cognitive performance and "helpless" behavior. In R. M. Hodapp, J. A. Burack & E. Zigler (Eds.), *Issues in the developmental approach to mental retardation* (pp. 137–168). Cambridge: Cambridge University Press.

Whitman, T. L., Borkowski, J. G., Schellenbach, C. J., & Nath, P. S. (1987). Predicting and understanding developmental delay of children of adolescent mothers: A multidimensional approach. *American Journal of Mental Deficiency, 92,* 40–56.

Wingerson, L. (1990). *Mapping our genes: The genome project and the future of medicine*. New York: Penguin Books USA, Inc.

Zigler, E., & Balla, D. (Eds.) (1982). *Mental retardation: The developmental-difference controversy*. Hillsdale, NJ: Erlbaum.

8

Autism: Social Communication Difficulties and Related Behaviors

LYNN KERN KOEGEL,
MARTA C. VALDEZ-MENCHACA,
AND ROBERT L. KOEGEL

DESCRIPTION OF THE DISORDER

There has been considerable progress and development in the diagnosis and treatment of autism over the past several decades. This chapter provides an account of the major findings that have led to our increased understanding of the behavioral manifestations of autism and the development of intervention techniques. Evidence on the etiology and treatment will be reviewed within a framework that explores the possibility that neurological or physiological processes may result in an inappropriate level of social interaction, which in turn leads to disorders in communication and other maladaptive and disruptive behaviors that characterize autism. Understanding this atypical developmental track leads directly to the understanding, treatment, and prevention of many of the severe aspects of autism that are so stigmatizing and disabling to children, adolescents, and adults.

In 1943, Kanner first categorized a perplexing group of eleven children, who could be differentiated from other children with disabilities in terms of their particular combination of idiosyncratic characteristics. To be diagnosed as having autism, children must show abnormal behavior in three related categories according to their developmental level including: (1) a qualitative impairment in reciprocal social interaction; (2) a qualitative impairment in communication; and (3) re-

LYNN KERN KOEGEL, MARTA C. VALDEZ-MENCHACA, AND ROBERT L. KOEGEL • Autism Research Center, Graduate School of Education, University of California, Santa Barbara, California 93106.

Advanced Abnormal Psychology, edited by Vincent B. Van Hasselt and Michel Hersen. Plenum Press, New York, 1994.

stricted, repetitive, and stereotyped patterns of behavior and repertoire of activities and interests. In addition, onset is described in the DSM-IV draft criteria as occurring prior to age 3 (APA, 1987). Because autism comprises such diversity of behavioral characteristics, individuals with autism may appear vastly different based on the extent or degree of involvement within and across the symptoms.

For instance, autistic individuals may be divided in three major subgroups in relation to their cognitive skills. One subgroup is formed by individuals who have intellectual functioning in the retarded range, as measured by standardized IQ tests. It has been estimated that approximately 60% of this population have IQs below 50 (Schopler, 1978). However, some have suggested that these individuals may be more competent than what is revealed in a standardized testing situation.

Another subgroup, made popular in the movie "Rain Man," is characterized by isolated skill areas. These individuals are also termed savant, idiot savant, or autistic savant. Savant skills often surprise people because they appear to be intelligence-independent, which is why the paradoxical term "idiot savant" was coined (Ho, Tsang, & Ho, 1992). This profile often can be seen at a fairly young age in preschoolers with autism who seem to solve difficult puzzles effortlessly. Two of the most common areas in which these individuals excel are music and math calculations. Yet, in spite of remarkable accomplishments in these areas, it is typical for the children to have little appreciation for social recognition for their accomplishments. When these individuals with subjectively reported musical skills are tested systematically by experts, their skills often exceed even the best nondisabled musicians (Applebaum, Egel, Koegel, & Imhoff, 1979), yet they appear to have no special awareness of this superiority, or even any desire to excel above other individuals. While this group of children receive quite a bit of public attention, probably because of uniqueness, they actually make up a small percentage of the children diagnosed as having autism.

The remaining group of individuals with autism have relatively high abilities in areas that require little language use. That is, they function relatively well in daily living skills, but are challenged by situations requiring social communication. Unfortunately, without treatment this deficit will severely limit their ability to be mainstreamed or integrated into work responsibilities or other activities requiring socialization. In spite of such vastly different intellectual scores, individuals in these subgroups are reported as having approximately similar and profound social deficits (Koegel, Frea, & Surratt, in press). This consistency in their difficulties in social area is in accord with the social communicative hypothesis presented earlier. That is, impairment in the use and processing of social stimulation may constitute the common lone characteristic of autism. However, the interaction between the degree of this social impairment and other abilities (e.g., IQ) and skills through a series of social transactions and developmental processes will result in the wide diversity of profiles that characterize this intriguing disability.

In most descriptions of autism, each of the aforementioned behavioral characteristics has been described, and often treated, as a separate entity. However, a recent shift in the field emphasizes the interrelationships among these areas (e.g., Crystal, 1987; Koegel, Camarata, & Koegel, in press). This has led to the hypothesis that autism may involve primary (causal) and secondary (manifestation) behaviors. Within this perspective, a primary crux of autism may be the lack of appropriate social behavior; and because of this lack of an appropriate repertoire for social interaction and stimulation, the individual with autism may develop secondary maladaptive behaviors, such as self-stimulatory behavior, lack of appropriate language development, or tantrums. Some recent studies (Carr & Durand, 1985; Koegel, Koegel, Hurley, & Frea, 1992) have lent support to this hypothesis by demonstrating the interrelationship of these patterns of behavior showing concomitant changes in untreated disruptive behaviors during the treatment of communicative/social behaviors. While reading the following sections describing the three general areas of autism, the reader is encouraged to contemplate how these areas may be related.

Social Interaction

Qualitative impairment in social interaction, which we hypothesize as playing a central role in the disorder, is discussed throughout the lifespan of individuals with autism. Many parents report that, as early as infancy, their children "stiffen up" when they attempt to hold and cuddle them. During their first 5 years, children with autism appear to be unable to form attachments or "bond" in the way typical children do. For example, they may not follow their parents about the house, run to greet them, seek comfort when hurt or upset, or develop routines such as the bedtime kiss-and-cuddle. Further, the lack of eye-to-eye gaze is characteristic of children with autism. While many avoid eye contact, particularly when repeated efforts are made to gain their attention, others do not use eye gaze in a discriminatory way when in need (e.g., wanting attention, or wanting to be picked up, etc.) (Rutter, 1978).

Some of these characteristics may be evident early on, even before the child has been diagnosed or suspected of having autism. For example, in a preliminary study, Adrien and collaborators (1991) reviewed home videotapes of 12 children prior to the age of 2 and before being diagnosed as having autism. Evaluation of these children's behavior, as compared with control subjects, revealed early difficulties in: (1) social interaction (tendency toward isolation, no eye contact, lack of postural adjustment, bad positioning of the head, lack of anticipatory movements, and lack of initiative); (2) emotional differences (deficit of facial expressions, absence of smiles, anxiety to new situations, major emotional lability); (3) visual and auditory behaviors [inappropriate gaze and slow or delayed reactions (hypo- or hyper-reactive)]; (4) disorders of tone and motor behavior (hypotonia, hand flapping, lack of protective movements); and (5) atypical, socially stigmatizing behaviors (such as self-stimulatory behavior and obsessive behavior).

As the child with autism develops, patterns of social problems continue and become more problematic as greater levels of social competence are expected. Children with autism typically do not play spontaneously with other children (Bednersh & Peck, 1986; Wetherby & Prutting, 1984; Koegel, Dyer, & Bell, 1987; Koegel, Firestone, Kramme, & Dunlap, 1974; Dunlap, Koegel, & Egel, 1979) and fail to develop meaningful friendships in adolescence (Haring & Breen, 1992; Koegel, Frea, & Surratt, in press). This limited social network is particularly troubling to parents and others close to the child. In addition, it has important implications for their integration in society, as the range of social experiences that the child or adult is exposed to is significantly limited. Without being actively involved in reciprocal social communicative interactions, the child is unlikely to learn the important social and contextual rules that govern our behavior throughout life.

LYNN KERN
KOEGEL et al.

The communication difficulties of children with autism are closely intertwined with social areas. That is, since most of language is acquired through meaningful social interaction, difficulties in maintaining social interactions result in delayed language acquisition or in inappropriate language use.

Children with autism are often classified into three groups in terms of their language skills: nonverbal, with delayed verbal skills or with language difficulties, and echolalic. About 50% of children with autism develop some type of language, whether it is echolalic or rule-governed (Prizant, 1983). Another group includes those who do not develop verbal language at all (nonverbal). There is also a group of children who develop language but in whom such development is markedly delayed. Another subgroup presents "echolalia," which refers to the repetition by the child of something heard in the speech of others. Echoic utterances are often rigidly reproduced, typically lacking clear evidence of communicative intent (Prizant & Rydell, 1984).

According to parental report, some of those in the nonverbal group develop language during the second year of life, but then cease to continue to use any words. Other nonverbal children are reported to never produce any intelligible words, yet they can make noises, although it is difficult to get these noises under imitative control or to teach them to use the words in a socially meaningful way. Another group of children with autism appear nonverbal in early years, but eventually develop some language that appears to follow developmental language stages in parallel with typically-developing children (Tager-Flusberg, 1990).

Children with echolalia may produce two forms of echolalic responses. "Immediate echolalia" refers to repetition(s) of all or part of an utterance, which are produced either following immediately or a brief time after the production of a model utterance. "Delayed echolalia" refers to utterances repeated at a significantly later time (Prizant & Rydell, 1984). It has been speculated that much of immediate echolalia occurs when the child lacks understanding. Carr, Schreibman, and Lovaas (1975) demonstrated that such children echoed utterances that they did not understand, and answered utterances that they understood. Delayed echolalia still continues to puzzle researchers. It has been theorized that much of delayed echolalia may produce some type of sensory rather than social input for the child (Lovaas, Varni, Koegel, & Lorsch, 1977). This was speculated while children with autism were being observed to engage in repetitive delayed echolalic responses without extinguishing, even when they were alone. In contrast, it has also been suggested that some forms of delayed echolalia (but not all) that occur when children are in the company of familiar people may serve a communicative intent, such as labeling, protesting, or requesting (Prizant & Rydell, 1984). However, while the communicative *intent* may be present, the communicative *social function* usually appears to be absent for all practical purposes.

There are numerous barriers and obstacles encountered by an individual who lacks social communication. While typically-developing infants meet their needs through crying, they soon learn that verbalizations are more efficient and more desirable to a parent, and are able to engage in communicative verbal exchanges that will foster their development of language. However, when verbal skills fail to develop appropriately, failures in communication result in extreme frustration, which may lead the child to revert to early effective forms of communication, such as crying. As children with autism grow up, impairment in linguistic communication results in more restricted social environments and the use of elaborate forms of disruptive behavior to accomplish goals.

Poor social communication skills can be evidenced throughout life, even with adolescents whose language skills are somewhat delayed but sufficient for conversational interaction. Their limited involvement in language interactions results in inappropriate pragmatic behaviors, such as the lack of initiating conversation and responding to the conversation of others (Koegel, Koegel, Hurley, & Frea, 1992), lack of appropriate turn-taking, dysprosody, inappropriate speech detail, perseveration, and preoccupations during conversation (Koegel & Frea, in press; Frea, 1990). When one considers that most individuals do not go through a day without using communicative and associated pragmatic skills, it is obvious that difficulties in this area are especially disabling in developing personal friendships and relationships, and in functioning in social settings, such as school or work, which in turn hinders the flow of the interaction and may precipitate its termination.

Restricted Repertoire of Activities and Interests

The last area of behaviors characteristic to autism is the restricted repertoire of activities and interests. It is likely that the extremely restricted repertoire of activities of these children not only exacerbates their social relationships, but also interferes with the neurological development that may be necessary to overcome the problem. One of the most frequently exhibited behaviors is self-stimulatory behavior (also described as ritualistic behavior, stereotypy, stereotypic behavior, etc.). Self-stimulatory behavior occurs when an individual engages in a repetitive behavior that appears to serve no observable social function. It can be with an object, such as incessantly flipping a twig round and round between the fingers, or repetitively spinning the wheels of a toy truck, or with one's own body parts, such as flipping the fingers in front of the eyes, hand flapping, or body rocking.

It has been theorized that these behaviors provide sensory input for the individual, and while all individuals need sensory input, those with autism obtain it in an inappropriate social manner. It is very likely that the need for sensory stimulation is provided for in typical children through social communicative interactions. While very young children seem to constantly seek attention from their parents and to greatly enjoy games, songs, stories, and other types of social communicative activities, most children with autism do not actively seek such interactions. Without treatment, many can engage in self-stimulatory behavior the entire day.

Aside from the socially stigmatizing effects of these behaviors, it has been shown that learning does not take place when certain types of self-stimulatory behaviors are occurring, since self-stimulatory behavior is incompatible with appropriate responding. However, when self-stimulatory behavior is suppressed, appropriate play increases spontaneously (Koegel, Firestone, Kramme, & Dunlap, 1974; Kern, Koegel, & Dunlap, 1984; Kern, Koegel, Dyer, Blew, & Fenton, 1982).

Another behavior seen in autism is self-injury. Some have theorized that self-injury may be a type of self-stimulatory behavior taken to the extreme (Carr, 1982). These self-injury behaviors appear to have a communicative function (Carr & Durand, 1985). For example, when a teacher instructs a child to engage in a task he does not want to do, he might bang his head against a closed fist as a means of avoiding the task. Likewise, if a child does not want to engage in social interaction, she may pick her skin intensely to the point of drawing blood, which would likely drive the communicative partner away, thus reinforcing the child's inappropriate behavior. While these forms of disruptive behavior may be performed to carry out a social function, they are not perceived by most members of society as a form of social behavior. They are even particularly harmful to the ability of individuals with autism to be accepted in socially integrated settings. Assessing the motivation for these behaviors becomes critical in the treatment of these severe excess behavior problems. Then treatment plans may be developed where the children may be taught socially appropriate behaviors that will serve these same functions.

Another characteristic of autism is the tendency to prefer "sameness" in the environment. An example is a child who wears the same shirt daily and who cries and throws tantrums if the parent tries to put a different shirt on her or him. Similarly, some children with autism may react when an item of furniture is rearranged in the house. This type of preoccupation also can be seen in types of obsessive behavior and irrational fears occasionally exhibited by children with autism. As a whole, these inappropriate behaviors occur in varying degrees but, when present, interfere with common socially acceptable activities in a person's repertoire. Thus, it appears as though the person with autism is exhibiting a very limited and restricted repertoire of activities, and that few of these activities have social components to them.

CLINICAL PICTURE

Jacob. Jacob is a 3½-year-old boy who was brought to a pediatrician who specialized in developmental disabilities. His parents were concerned about his "inability to focus and pay attention." They were also concerned with his sleep difficulties and picky eating. Although his mother had some vaginal bleeding during the second trimester of pregnancy due to partial placenta previa, this problem cleared spontaneously and delivery was normal. His parents reported Jacob's early motor milestones to be age-appropriate. That is, he sat up, crawled, and walked at expected times. They were concerned however, that he did not like to be constrained or confined by adults. For example, he resisted contacts such as holding an adult's hand when crossing the street.

Communicatively, Jacob spoke single words during his first year of life and combined words by 2½ years. However, beginning his first year, his parents reported that he cried easily, became frustrated easily, and often had difficulty keeping to a schedule. They also reported that he was upset by new people and new situations, was withdrawn, and avoided playing with other children. In regard to play activities, they reported that he tended to take his toys apart and to break them down into component parts, then to throw the parts. They also observed that he appeared to have a preoccupation with smelling objects, spinning objects, and twisting his fingers in front of his eyes. Jacob's pediatrician recommended that he be put in a preschool; however, a first visit to a preschool was upsetting to his mother, as he did not participate in any activity but appeared over-aroused and ran about the classroom without focus. At this point Jacob's parents sought further evaluation by a pediatrician specializing in developmental disabilities.

Jacob's new pediatrician immediately recognized the symptoms of autism,

sensory functions, and intrinsic feelings of pain and pleasure, and which controls reward and punishment in learning-habituation and reinforcement, has also been hypothesized as relating to autism. Because this part of the midbrain plays a major role in many interconnections and integration of large areas of functioning, its dysfunction could account for the multitude of disabilities in individuals with autism. (Hetzler & Griffin, 1981; Ornitz, 1985; Damasio & Maurer, 1978).

Similarly, subcortical dysfunction can cause impairments in social, emotional, and language functioning, hemispheric imbalance (relative right-hemisphere over-activation), difficulties in processing novel information, and overarousal. Some researchers have observed differences in auditory brainstem responses in individuals with autism (Gillberg, Rosenhall, & Johansson, 1983; Fein, Skoff & Mirsky, 1981). It is noteworthy that all of these researchers found only a subset of the children who appear to have subcortical abnormalities. Others have found no consistent differences in auditory evoked potentials with subjects who had autism but no mental retardation (Grillon, Courschesne, & Akshoomoff, 1989). Together, these results suggest the possibility that a subpopulation of individuals diagnosed with autism may have subcortical neuroanatomical differences.

More recently, a number of researchers have suggested cerebellar involvement (Ritvo, Freeman, Sheibel, Duong, Robinson, Guthrie, & Ritvo, 1986; Bauman & Kemper, 1985; Courchesne, 1987; Courchesne, Hesselink, Jernigan, & Yeung-Courchesne, 1987). Courchesne [and colleagues (1987)] use magnetic resonance imaging (MRI), a technique considered to yield the most anatomical detail. His work focuses on adults and children whose brains are not likely to be complicated by mental retardation, epilepsy, drug use, postnatal trauma, or disease. Presently, he is pursuing work based on his early findings of size differences between the hemispheres of the cerebellum and decreased or arrested development of specific areas in the cerebellum.

Neurological studies, particularly looking at nystagmus, have found abnormalities (Ritvo, Ornitz, Eviatar, Markham, Brown, & Mason, 1989; Ornitz, 1985; Ornitz, Brown, Mason, & Putnam, 1974) and differences in event-related brain potentials with individuals with autism (Courchesne, Lincoln, Yeung-Courchesne, Elmasian, & Grillon, 1989; Dawson, Finley, Phillips, Galpert, & Lewy, 1988). Such perceptual inconsistency could result in disturbances in relating, language, and communication as a consequence of inconstancy of perception due to faulty modulation of sensory input (Ornitz, 1985).

Neurochemical Factors

Differences in blood serotonin levels, particularly a tendency toward higher levels, have been found in a subgroup of individuals with autism (Campbell, Freidman, DeVito, Greenspan, & Collins, 1974; Ritvo et al., 1984). Serotonergic activity in the brain exerts modulatory effects on many neuronal systems, and has been asserted to affect various physiological functions and behaviors, such as sleep, body temperature, pain, sensory perception, sexual behavior, motor function, neuroendocrine regulation, appetite, learning and memory, and immune response.

Chromosomal and Genetic Patterns

A number of researchers have suggested that there may be some type of chromosomal or genetic factors that are etiologically significant in at least a subgroup of autism. These theories have been based on the greater prevalence of this disability in males than in females, maternal age (Gillberg & Gillberg, 1983; Tsai & Stewart, 1983), identification of a "fragile" site on the X chromosome (fragile-X syndrome) (see August & Lockhart, 1984), a higher than expected incidence of families with multiple cases of autism (Ritvo, Ritvo, & Brothers, 1982), and the far greater incidence of autism in monozygotic than in dizygotic twins (Ritvo, Ritvo, & Brothers, 1982). Finally, some researchers have found an increased incidence of minor physical anomaly as compared to a control group. Some of these differences include low seating of the ears, hypertelorism, syndactylia, high palate, and abnormal head circumference (Walker, 1987). These congenital features also suggest a deviant intrauterine experience.

Conclusion

There are a number of likely reasons for such disparity and contradiction both within and across these organic-based studies. First, children with autism represent an extremely heterogeneous group in terms of the behavior and cognitive and linguistic abilities, which may be related to different areas or processes of neurological dysfunction. Second, some may have delayed brain and neural development, rather than abnormal development, in which case chronologically aged control groups would be irrelevant. Third, many have a history of medically prescribed drug use, anoxia, epilepsy, disease, postnatal trauma, or seizure activity that may result in permanent physiological cerebral damage, and be misinterpreted in tests as true congenital abnormalities. Fourth, some of the equipment utilized in the research lacks adequate sophistication to detect microscopic defects, or metabolic processes, and therefore have focused on gross anatomical correlates. Lastly, there may be exogenous artifacts, particularly in research requiring behavioral responses, as children with autism are classically inconsistent in their responses, and even getting them to attend for the presentation of stimuli may be difficult. In summary, while organic research will most likely reveal the cause of autism in the future, it is very difficult and costly to conduct, and may even yield a multitude of possible causes. However, it seems that because studies yield such variable and conflicting results, careful and precise behavioral descriptions and measurements of the presenting symptoms would allow researchers to search for possible subtypes when analyzing organic factors.

COURSE AND PROGNOSIS

Without treatment, prognosis is poor and individuals with autism are not likely to make much improvement throughout life (DeMeyer, Barton, DeMeyer, Norton, Allen, & Steele, 1973). In contrast, individuals who receive treatment can be expected to improve significantly throughout their lives.

Treatment approaches and theoretical perspectives are closely linked. The recent shift in the conceptualization of autism from a social communicative perspective has had significant implications for the treatment of this disorder. As discussed earlier, this perspective presupposes that social deficits could be the primary impairment in autism, and that avoidance of, or inappropriate engagement in social interactions may be associated with communication difficulties.

These difficulties in efficiently expressing one's needs would, in turn result in inappropriate or disruptive behaviors. Recent studies have documented this inter-relationship between these characteristics of "autistic behavior." Specifically, when exposed to positive and responsive social contexts, attempts for communication may be enhanced, and when communication skills improve, untreated disruptive and self-stimulatory behaviors decrease (Koegel, Koegel, Hurley, & Frea, 1992; Carr & Durand, 1985; Carr, 1977). This integrative view emphasizes three major advances in the treatment of autism that have resulted in significant gains in the quality of life of these individuals. A *first* major breakthrough in the treatment of autism and other severely challenging behaviors has been an attempt to examine the antecedents to, or consequences for, disruptive behaviors, in order to assess the variables that maintain the disruptive behaviors. Such treatment programs replace these disruptive behaviors with appropriate "functionally equivalent" behaviors (O'Neill, Horner, Albin, Storey, & Sprague, 1990). For example, Carr and Durand (1985) identified students who were exhibiting self-injurious behavior, tantrums, and aggression to escape difficult tasks or to seek adult attention. These students were taught to use an appropriate and communicatively equivalent phrase of "I don't understand," or "Am I doing good work?" These communicatively equivalent phrases resulted in reduction or elimination of the disruptive behavior that served the same communicative function. Thus, these and other authors have shown that behavior problems can be reduced or eliminated by teaching communicative phrases that are effective in altering the stimulus conditions that control problems. *Second*, treatment focus has shifted from considering individual target behaviors to a more global approach that treats target behaviors that will result in more widespread gains. Such "pivotal treatment" approaches are conceptually impor-tant, because it is essential to identify target behaviors for treatment that will produce simultaneous changes in many other behaviors, instead of having to treat each behavior individually—a task that would be prohibitively time consuming and expensive and may not allow the person to make socially significant gains. Therefore, researchers have begun to define pivotal behaviors, such as social communication, that seem to be central to wide areas of functioning. Positive changes in pivotal behaviors should have widespread positive effects on many other behaviors and therefore constitute an efficient way to produce generalized behavior improvements (Koegel, Schreibman, Britten, & Laitinen, 1979). *Third*, an increased awareness of the critical role that social context plays in the development of children with autism and other disabilities has propelled a strong movement for mainstreaming and integration into regular education preschools, primary schools, and other community settings. Integration provides opportunities for social and intellectual development that could not occur when children with autism partici-pated in segregated settings with other socially isolated children. In these settings, not only do they have more able peers available to assist them and serve as role models, but they are required to exhibit appropriate behavior, and are challenged to participate in all or part of the regular education curriculum. We are only beginning to experience the social, communicative, and academic benefits that result from integrating children with disabilities into their own community and school environments.

Across the spectrum of autism, regardless of severity, communication is marked by numerous and often severe linguistic and pragmatic skill deficits that affect and limit the ability to integrate and socialize. This can affect interactions with family (Koegel, Koegel, Hurley, & Frea, 1992), adults (Curcio & Paccia, 1987), and peers (Haring, 1993), and the development of friendships (Frea, 1990) in school, work sites, and other community settings. Adding to the difficulty of developing treatment programs for social communication is the issue that, taken as a whole, the literature shows that there is no one "autistic" pattern of communication. To the contrary, communicative acts that are topographically similar may have different communicative functions for different people and in different social contexts (Olley, 1986). Such individual, situational, and contextual differences make treatment and generalization a challenging area of study. However, one common deficit among individuals with autism is the lack of language use to communicate, or the highly limited pragmatic functions of verbal responses. If one considers that much of language development is prompted by the child's motivation to communicate with the outside world, then the inherent difficulties one faces when attempting to communicate with children who are often unmotivated are outstanding.

Such severe lack of desire to attempt to communicate has led some researchers to focus on the general area of *motivating* children with autism to communicate, as a pivotal target behavior. One language development package that has focused on variables proven to improve motivation in other areas is the "Natural Language Treatment" paradigm (Koegel, O'Dell, & Koegel, 1987). This treatment package involves: (a) using stimulus items that are chosen by the individual rather than arbitrarily chosen by the language specialist, varying the stimulus items frequently to prevent boredom, and using age-appropriate items found in the person's natural environment; (b) using natural prompts when necessary, such as repeating the stimulus item rather than manual (physical) prompts; (c) allowing the person to use the stimulus item within a functional interaction rather than unrelated stimulus materials such as picture cards, etc.; (d) rewarding any attempt to communicate, rather than rewarding only approximations or correct responses; and (e) using natural reinforcers (e.g., an opportunity to use the stimulus item), paired with social reinforcers, rather than unrelated tangible reinforcers.

These types of techniques have been very effective in developing an initial lexicon in nonverbal children (Koegel, O'Dell & Koegel, 1987), and have also been expanded to include more complex language skills to assist more communicatively competent individuals (Koegel, Schreibman, Good, Cerniglia, Murphy, & Koegel, 1989). They have been shown to be readily usable by parents with their children (Laski, Charlop, & Schreibman, 1988) and thus can expand the language development activities to occur throughout the day and in the child's natural environment. Similar to other treatment techniques showing an inverse relationship with other behaviors, significant decreases in disruptive behavior were observed by Koegel, Koegel, and Surratt (1992) when Natural Language Paradigm language treatment techniques were being implemented.

Even when individuals become more competent with language and can produce sentences, they may still appear unmotivated or unwilling to use such skills in social communicative contexts where the treatment provider has very little or no control. That is, while children with autism may use language to meet their needs or desires, they still exhibit disruptive behavior to avoid social interactions with others in certain community settings. *Self-management* is a technique that has recently been used to improve communication and related social skills in such cases. Concomitant changes in untreated inappropriate behaviors also occur during self-management. Self-management can be viewed as a pivotal treatment strategy. While most people tend to evaluate their own behavior constantly, people with autism often lack that skill, and learning competent social interactions and other behaviors requires constant self-regulation.

In a study designed to increase social competence of youngsters with autism, Koegel, Koegel, Hurley, and Frea (1992) taught students with autism (who typically became disruptive when others attempted to communicate with them) to self-monitor appropriate answers to questions. An advantage of this technique is that it can be used in community settings without the constant vigilance of an adult or treatment provider, as it relies on the individual with a disability to serve as his or her own treatment provider. In the study we have just mentioned, students monitored and significantly increased their appropriate responding to questions at home and in other community settings without the presence of their treatment providers. Again, all of these students had relatively competent basic communication skills (i.e., good articulation, ability to formulate sentences, good receptive language skills), but actively avoided social communication.

One possibility for this phenomenon is that social interactions may become punishing if they lack a minimum level of fluid or consistent responding, and may result in disruptive behavior. However, by implementing programs that increase the probability of consistent responding, conversational interactions are more coherent and less aversive, and therefore less likely to be associated with escape or avoidance-driven disruptive behavior. Further, increased responding allows the nondisabled communicative partner to adjust to the competency level of the person with a disability, making the entire interaction more reinforcing to the dyad. Although not yet scientifically documented, this possibility is given credence by anecdotal observations of increases in untreated spontaneous utterances while students were self-managing their responses to questions. Other research studies have hypothesized that social skills directly involved in conversation may be part of a relatively large response class so that positive changes in some social skills result in positive changes in other untreated social skills.

For students with autism who appear to be failing to develop any expressive language skills, both sign language and augmentative communication have been effective. The advantage of sign representations for children or adults with severe cognitive impairments is that such symbols are often easier to understand and thus more meaningful than the auditory symbol (word or phrase). And, having some type of communicative system, rather than none, allows more opportunities for academic, vocational, and social development. Nonverbal individuals with autism have been taught sign language and have been able to create new sign combinations that had not been specifically taught to them, thus exhibiting some generative language skills (Carr, Binkoff, Kologinsky, & Eddy, 1978). Other types of augmentative communication devices have included pictorial representations (Lancoini, 1983) and keyboards or other communication aids so the individuals with disabilities can learn to nonverbally express their communicative intent. Alternative communication systems have been found to be particularly effective and critical in the replacement of communicatively motivated challenging behavior (e.g., aggression, throwing tantrums); however, the bulk of assessment and intervention studies have focused on immediate establishment of systems. Because the study of augmentative and alternative communication is still in its infancy, there are questions yet to be answered, concerning the relationship between comprehension and production, the design selection techniques to accommodate the user's level of progress, and the inverse relationship between alternative communication and challenging behavior (Reichle, Mirenda, Locke, Piche, & Johnston, 1992). Further, questions involving acquiring and maintaining motivation to use alternative communication, particularly with adults who may lack repeated exposure and thus reinforcement for its use, still need to be studied (Dattilo & Camarata, 1991). Considering using such systems for prevention of challenging behavior and longitudinal planning for lifespan needs is necessary (Reichle, Mirenda, Locke, Piche, & Johnston, 1992), and is an exciting area for future research (Koegel, Frea, & Surratt, in press).

Closely related to communication is social interaction. Social deficits have been a hallmark of autism since Kanner's first description. Even the technical meaning of the label autism, an extension of the Greek derivative aut(os) meaning "self," connotes the antithesis of social competence. As discussed above, prevailing social philosophy in our country has been gradually shifting from segregating individuals with disabilities such as autism from school and community settings, toward inclusion of all of the nations' citizens, regardless of disability. Therefore, it has become clear that social skills need to be an integral component of any treatment program for individuals with autism for their successful integration into the community.

A number of researchers have successfully improved play interactions with children with autism and their peers in integrated settings. Haring and Lovinger (1989) taught young children to play appropriately and initiate social interactions (e.g., seeking a willing peer, offering toys, sharing, taking turns, etc.) with several different age-appropriate activities. This study took into consideration the play preferences of the student with disabilities and of his peers by having the former seek a child to offer a toy to, who was already playing with a toy that matched his. Other researchers have found that child-preferred activities correlate with the amount of social avoidance behaviors exhibited by individuals with autism, and that such children can be taught to initiate a shift to preferred activities. This, in turn, results in maintained reductions in social avoidance behaviors (Koegel, Dyer, & Bell, 1987). While these studies focused on the child with the disability, other studies (Strain, 1983) have taught peer confederates to initiate social interactions using verbal prompts (e.g., "Come play"), sharing play items, and offering verbal assistance related to play (e.g., pulling a playmate who is seated in a wagon). Through roleplay, peers were also taught to initiate and persevere if their attempts were ignored by the child with a disability (Strain, Shores, & Timm, 1977). While some teacher prompting may be necessary with very young children to maintain high levels of social interaction (Odom, Hoyson, Jamieson, & Strain, 1985), such prompting can be systematically faded with continued social interactions remaining at high levels (Odom, Chandler, Otrosky, McConnell, & Reaney, 1992).

As individuals with autism and their peers mature, recruiting a peer "clique" to interact during recreational and leisure activities has been successful (Haring & Breen, 1992). Such recruiting of peer groups can easily be incorporated into existing school schedules, and results in significant increases in nondisabled teens' social interactions with peers with autism. It is hypothesized that recruiting the entire clique decreases the probability of stigma that may be attached to one peer who would break away from the clique to associate with a peer with a disability. Further, some commitments (e.g., eating lunch with a specific peer) can be rotated, and meeting as a group for discussion sessions can be highly motivating if the entire clique is included.

When those with autism reach adulthood, social integration and social support are critical elements in determining a person's quality of life and are critical components of community integration. Kennedy, Horner, and Newton (1989) described patterns of social contact between persons with severe disabilities living in community-based residential programs, and typical members of local communities, who were not fellow residents or paid to provide services. These longitudinal data, collected over a 2½-year period, showed that such individuals had a limited number of companions who remained part of their social spheres for more than a few months. In fact, the participants were rarely observed to have prolonged contact with anyone other than family members. The authors discuss the possibility that the individuals with disabilities may be perceived as contributing less to people in their social networks. They suggest the need for strategies that increase or equalize the reciprocity in relationships between persons with and without disabilities in order to increase the likelihood of maintaining durable relationships.

To conclude, the social communicative integrative view of autism has contributed to the development of a multifaceted comprehensive approach to treatment. As discussed throughout this section, the importance of social communication skills is foremost in terms of a pivotal behavior, functional communication, and ease of integration. Indeed, researchers, families, professionals, teachers, and others are becoming increasingly aware that intervention should begin at the earliest possible point in time. Evidence has begun to indicate that children are apt to make significantly more progress if specialized services are initiated well before they reach school age (Dunlap, Robbins, Dollman, & Plienis, 1988). It is likely that future research will focus more closely on prelinguistic behaviors that may be precursors to language development, that are not developing typically in very young children. Early intervention is critical when one considers the life development of a child who is rejected by society and peers. Peer acceptance and friendships are critical for healthy development (Koegel, Frea, & Surratt, in press), and children who are stigmatized tend to carry the role of the outcast into adulthood (Dodge, 1983). Further, the social awareness gained by typically developing children and the willingness of the peers to assist with treatment programs have widespread implications for encouraging a more sympathetic and empathetic response from society as well.

An area of concern frequently overlooked when dealing with the individual with disabilities is familial stress related to certain specific subareas of the prognosis. Koegel and colleagues (1992) found higher stress among parents of children with autism than parents in typical families on a number of measures, particularly as to their concern for the well-being of their child after they are no longer able to provide care for him/her. Other areas of parental stress included the level of cognitive impairment and the child's ability to function independently, and the child's ability to be accepted in the community. These and other familial needs are of critical importance in the diagnostic and treatment process (Schreibman, Kaneko, & Koegel, 1991) as social integration in regular communities has become the ultimate goal of intervention.

LYNN KERN
KOEGEL et al.

Because autism has so many behavioral symptoms in common with other disabilities, differential diagnosis may be difficult, or possibly even unnecessary. Yet, three features exhibited in autism are unlikely to occur in other populations: the failure to develop social relationships; language deficits with impaired comprehension, echolalia, and pronominal reversal; and ritualistic or compulsive behavior (Rutter, 1978).

Autism can be differentiated from mental retardation by the splinter skills. That is, while children with mental retardation often exhibit lower abilities in all areas, children with autism typically exhibit some areas of higher functioning relative to other areas. Autism can be differentiated from childhood schizophrenia by age of onset. There is typically a bipolar distribution for children whose disorders begin before the age of three and a second large peak for those in whom disorders are first evident in early adolescence or just before (Rutter, 1978). Autism is most likely congenital and diagnosable prior to 30 months of age (Schreibman & Charlop, 1987).

Finally, although autism may likely be an impairment of social/language skills, it can be differentiated from other language disabilities. For example, language delays in typically developing children often can be associated with chronic otitis media or other hearing loss. While many parents of children with autism initially suspect hearing loss, actual documented evidence of hearing loss is not highly correlated with autism. Some language-delayed children will also show higher receptive than expressive language skills, whereas individuals with autism have depressed abilities in both areas. Other language skills that seem to differ greatly in early language development of children with autism is pronominal reversal, lack of semantic intent in utterances, and echolalic responses. Finally, the numerous differences in pragmatic, social, and other associated behaviors are not as symptomatic in other central language disabilities (also see Bartak, Rutter, & Cox, 1975). For example, self-stimulatory behavior occurs in infancy but not often in young typically developing children, unlike self-stimulatory behavior in autism, which can persist throughout life at high levels.

Next, it is important to briefly discuss some of the difficulties in diagnosis because of the heterogeneity of individuals with autism. As discussed above, the degree of disability and the specific combinations of symptomatology can make the label of "autism" relatively meaningless, and it does not necessarily help to determine a treatment plan. A more functional approach to the diagnosis would be to behaviorally define type and amount of each behavior a particular individual exhibits. As such, communication with other professionals is clearer and more specific treatment plans can then be designed.

SUMMARY

In summary, throughout this chapter we have attempted to point out the significant contributions that the integrative view of autism as a generalized impairment of social communicative functioning has brought to the conceptualization and treatment of this disorder.

Although there is a high probability of organic cause or causes of autism, the specific etiology has yet to be clearly understood. We speculate that the social problems prevalent in autism are both a cause and an effect of the neurological substrate. While we are optimistic that the future holds exciting revelations in this area, the possibility of multiple causes emphasizes the importance of interdisciplinary approaches that carefully and specifically define behavioral characteristics and organic findings so that subtypes can be classified. Those who interact with children with autism are well aware of the vast differences and abilities that are evident within the diagnosis.

The large number of behavioral differences exhibited by children with autism can be greatly stigmatizing in community settings. However, as more efficient and comprehensive treatment techniques are developed, and as opportunities for integration are available, more widespread improvements are occurring. Integration of the very young and participation of typical peers in the treatment process increase our understanding of the disabled and improves the likelihood of their acceptance into society.

Finally, implementing programs that have both social significance and implications for lifespan needs are important considerations. Specific behaviors such as decreasing self-stimulation and tantrums, play, and cooperation have been shown to be most important to subjective observers' global impressions of the person with autism (Schreibman, Koegel, Mills, & Burke, 1981).

While many individuals with autism are still segregated from their peers in regular education classes and other community settings, researchers are gradually accumulating evidence that demonstrates improved functioning in integrated settings (Anderson & Won, 1990). The development of models to create and support stable relationships, and to teach social and communicative behaviors so that people with disabilities can interact in vocational, home, neighborhood, community, and school settings and function independently with a high quality of life is a critical need, which is likely to receive a great deal of attention in the future (Haring, 1993). The current movement toward integration, early intervention, peer involvement in treatment, functional behaviors, and creating stable and meaningful social relationships is definitely a step toward meeting this need to significantly improve the quality of life for those with autism.

ACKNOWLEDGMENTS. Preparation of this manuscript was supported in part by National Institute on Disability and Rehabilitation Research Cooperative Agreement No. G0087CO234 and U.S. Public Health Service Grant MH28210 from the National Institute of Mental Health. The authors would like to thank Tom Haring, Ph.D. and Merith A. Cosden, Ph.D. for their comments and feedback on earlier drafts of this chapter. We would also like to express appreciation to Karen Davidson, M.D., for her assistance with the clinical case descriptions and for her dedication to children with disabilities.

REFERENCES

Adrien, J. L., Faure, M., Perrot, A., Hameury, L., Garreau, B., Barthelemy, C., & Sauvage, D. (1991). Autism and family home movies: Preliminary findings. *Journal of Autism and Developmental Disorders, 21*, 43–49.

American Psychiatric Association. (1993). *DSM-IV draft criteria*. Washington, DC: Author.

Anderson, J., & Won, K. (1990). The influence of participation in regular versus "special" education settings on students with challenging behaviors. Unpublished master's thesis. California State University, Hayward.

Applebaum, E., Egel, A. L., Koegel, R. L., & Imhoff, B. (1979). Measuring musical abilities of autistic children. *Journal of Autism and Developmental Disorders, 3*, 279–285.

Arnold, G., & Schwartz, S. (1983). Hemispheric lateralization of language in autistic and aphasic children. *Journal of Autism and Developmental Disorders, 13*, 129–139.

August, G. J., & Lockhart, L. H. (1984). Familial autism and the fragile-X chromosome. *Journal of Autism and Developmental Disorders, 14*, 197–204.

Bartak, L., Rutter, M., & Cox, A. (1975). A comparative study of infantile autism and specific developmental receptive language disorder: I. The children. *British Journal of Psychiatry, 126*, 127–145.

Bauman, M. L., & Kemper, T. L. (1985). Histo-anatomic observations of the brain in early infantile autism. *Neurology, 35*, 866–874.

Bednersh, F., & Peck, C. A. (1986). Assessing social environments: Effects of peer characteristics on the social behavior of children with severe handicaps. *Child Study Journal, 16*, 315–329.

Bettelheim, B. (1967). *The empty fortress*. New York: Free Press.

Campbell, M., Freidman, E., DeVito, E., Greenspan, L., & Collins, P. J. (1974). Blood serotonin in psychotic and brain damaged children. *Journal of Autism and Childhood Schizophrenia, 4*, 33–41.

Cantwell, D. P., Baker, B. L., & Rutter, M. (1978). Family factors. In M. Rutter & E. Schopler (Eds.), *Autism: A reappraisal of concepts and treatment*, 269–296. New York: Plenum Press.

Carr, E. G. (1977). The motivation of self-injurious behavior: A review of some hypotheses. *Psychological Bulletin, 84*, 800–816.

Carr, E. G. (1979). Teaching autistic children to use sign-language: Some research issues. *Journal of Autism and Developmental Disorders, 4*, 345–359.

Carr, E. G. (1982). Sign Language. In R. L. Koegel, A. Rincover, & A. L. Egel (Eds.), *Educating and understanding autistic children* (pp. 142–158). San Diego: College-Hill Press.

Carr, E. G., & Durand, V. M. (1985). Reducing behavior problems through functional communication training. *Journal of Applied Behavior Analysis, 18*, 111–126.

Carr, E. G., Binkoff, J. A., Kologinsky, E., & Eddy, M. (1978). Acquisition of sign language by autistic children. I: Expressive labelling. *Journal of Applied Behavior Analysis, 11*, 489–501.

Carr, E. G., Schreibman, L., & Lovaas, O. I. (1975). Control of echolalic speech in psychotic children. *Journal of Abnormal Child Psychology, 3*, 331–351.

Chess, S. (1971). Autism in children with congenital rubella. *Journal of Autism and Childhood Schizophrenia, 1*, 33–47.

Chess, S. (1977). Follow-up report on autism in congenital rubella. *Journal of Autism and Childhood Schizophrenia, 7*, 69–81.

Courchesne, E. (1987). A neurophysiological view of autism. In E. Schopler and G. Mesibov (Eds.), *Neurobiological issues in autism*. New York: Plenum Press.

Courchesne, E., Hesselink, J. R., Jernigan, T. L., & Yeung-Courchesne, R. (1987). Abnormal neuroanatomy in a non-retarded person with autism: Unusual findings using magnetic resonance imaging. *Archives of Neurology, 44*, 335–341.

Courchesne, E., Lincoln, A. J., Yeung-Courchesne, R., Elmasian, R., & Grillon, C. (1987). Pathophysiologic findings in nonretarded autism and receptive developmental language disorder. *Journal of Autism and Developmental Disorders, 19*, 1–17.

Crystal, D. (1987). Towards a bucket theory of language disability: Taking account of interaction between linguistic levels. *Clinical Linguistics and Phonetics, 1*, 7–21.

Curcio, F., & Paccia, J. (1987). Conversations with autistic children: Contingent relationships between features of adult input and children's response adequacy. *Journal of Autism and Developmental Disorders, 17*, 81–93.

Damasio, A., & Maurer, R. (1978). A neurological model for childhood autism. *Archives of Neurology, 35*, 777–786.

Dattilo, J., & Camarata, S. (1991). Facilitating conversation through self-initiated augmentative communication treatment. *Journal of Applied Behavior Analysis, 24*, 369–378.

Dawson, G., Finley, C., Phillips, S., & Galpert, L. (1986). Hemispheric specialization and the language abilities of autistic children. *Child Development, 57*, 1440–1453.

Dawson, G., Finley, C., Phillips, S., Galpert, L., & Lewy, A. (1988). Reduced P3 amplitude of the event-related brain potential: Its relationship to language ability in autism. *Journal of Autism and Developmental Disorders, 18,* 493– 504.

Dawson, G., Finley, C., Phillips, S., & Lewy, A. (1989). A comparison of hemispheric asymmetries in speech-related brain potentials of autistic and dysphasic children. *Brain and Language, 37,* 26–41.

Dawson, G., Warrenburg, S., & Fuller, P. (1982). Cerebral lateralization in individuals diagnosed as autistic in early childhood. *Brain and Cognition, 2,* 346–354.

DeMeyer, M. K. (1979). *Parents and children in autism.* Toronto: John Wiley and Sons.

DeMeyer, M. K., Barton, S., DeMeyer, W. E., Norton, J. A., Allen, J., & Steele, R. (1973). Prognosis in autism: A follow-up study. *Journal of Autism and Childhood Schizophrenia, 3,* 199–246.

Dodge, K. A. (1983). Behavioral antecedents of peer social status. *Child Development, 54,* 1386–1399.

Dunlap, G., Dunlap, L. K., Clarke, S., & Robbins, F. R. (1991). Functional assessment, curricular revision, and severe behavior problems. *Journal of Applied Behavior Analysis, 24,* 387–397.

Dunlap, G., Koegel, R. L., & Egel, A. L. (1979). Autistic children in school. *Exceptional Children, 45,* 552–558.

Dunlap, G., Robbins, F. R., Dollman, C., & Plienis, A. J. (1988). Early intervention for young children with autism: A regional training approach. West Virginia, Marshall University.

Egel, A. L., Koegel, R. L., & Schreibman, L. (1980). Review of educational-treatment procedures for autistic children. In L. Mann & D. Sabatino (Eds.), *Fourth review of special education* (pp. 109–150). New York: Grune & Stratton.

Eisenberg, L., & Kanner, L. (1956). Early infantile autism: 1943–1955. *American Journal of Orthopsychiatry, 26,* 55–65.

Fein, D., Skoff, B., & Mirsky, A. F. (1981). Clinical correlates of brainstem dysfunction in autistic children. *Journal of Autism and Developmental Disorders, 11,* 303–315.

Frea, W. D. (1990). Assessing pragmatic deficits in autistic children. Unpublished master's thesis. University of California, Santa Barbara.

Gillberg, C., & Gillberg, I. C. (1983). Infantile autism: A total population study of reduced optimality in the pre, peri-, and neonatal period. *Journal of Autism and Developmental Disorders, 13,* 153–166.

Gillberg, C., Rosenhall, U., & Johansson, E. (1983). Auditory brainstem responses in childhood psychosis. *Journal of Autism and Developmental Disorders, 13,* 181–195.

Grillon, C., Courchesne, E., & Akshoomoff, N. (1989). Brainstem and middle latency auditory evoked potentials in autism and developmental language disorder. *Journal of Autism and Developmental Disorders, 19,* 255–269.

Haring, T. G. (1993). Research basis of instructional procedures to promote social interaction and integration. In S. F. Warren (Ed.), *Advances in mental retardation and developmental disabilities, Volume 5: Research basis of instruction* (pp. 129–164). Baltimore, MD: Paul H. Brookes.

Haring, T. G., & Breen, C. G. (1992). A peer mediated social network intervention to enhance the social integration of persons with moderate and severe disabilities. *Journal of Applied Behavior Analysis, 25, 2,* 319–334.

Haring, T. G., & Lovinger, L. (1989). Promoting social interaction through teaching generalized play initiation responses to preschool children with autism. *Journal of the Association for Persons with Severe Handicaps, 14,* 58–67.

Hetzler, B., & Griffin, J. (1981). Infantile autism and the temporal lobe of the brain. *Journal of Autism and Developmental Disorders, 11,* 317–330.

Hier, D., LeMay, M., & Rosenberber, P. (1979). Autism and unfavorable left-right asymmetries of the brain. *Journal of Autism and Developmental Disorders, 9,* 153–159.

Ho, E. D. F., Tsang, A. K. T., & Ho, D. Y. F. (1992). An investigation of the calendar calculation ability of a Chinese calendar savant. *Journal of Autism and Developmental Disorders, 21,* 315–327.

Kanner, L. (1943). Autistic disturbances of affective contact. *Nervous Child, 2,* 217–250.

Kennedy, C. H., Horner, R. H., & Newton, J. S. (1989). Social contacts of adults with severe disabilities living in the community: A descriptive analysis of relationship patterns. *Journal of the Association for Persons with Severe Handicaps, 14,* 190–196.

Kern, L., Koegel, R. L., & Dunlap, G. (1984). The influence of vigorous vs. mild exercise on autistic stereotyped responding. *Journal of Autism and Developmental Disorders, 14,* 57–67.

Kern, L., Koegel, R. L., Dyer, K., Blew, P. A., & Fenton, L. R. (1982). The effects of physical exercise on self-stimulation and appropriate responding in autistic children. *Journal of Autism and Developmental Disorders, 4,* 399–419.

Koegel, L. K., Koegel, R. L., Hurley, C., & Frea, W. D. (1992). Improving pragmatic skills and disruptive behavior in children with autism through self-management. *Journal of Applied Behavior Analysis, 25, 2,* 341–354.

Koegel, R. L., Camarata, S., & Koegel, L. K. (in press). Aggression and noncompliance: Behavior modification through naturalistic language remediation. In J. L. Matson (Ed.), *Autism in children and adults: Etiology, assessment and intervention*. Sycamore, IL: Sycamore Press.

Koegel, R. L., & Frea, W. D. (in press). Treatment of social behavior in autism through the modification of pivotal social skills, *Journal of Applied Behavioral Analysis*.

Koegel, R. L., Dyer, K., & Bell, L. K. (1987). The influence of child-preferred activities on autistic children's social behavior. *Journal of Applied Behavior Analysis, 20*, 243–252.

Koegel, R. L., Firestone, P. B., Kramme, K. W., & Dunlap, G. (1974). Increasing spontaneous play in autistic children by suppressing self-stimulation. *Journal of Applied Behavior Analysis, 7*, 521–528.

Koegel, R. L., Frea, W. D., & Surratt, A. V. (in press). Self-management as a strategy for modifying problem behavior. In E. Schopler & G. Mesibov (Eds.), *Behavioral issues in children with autism*. New York: Plenum Press.

Koegel, R. L., Koegel, L. K., & Surratt, A. V. (1992). Language intervention and disruptive behavior in preschool children with autism. *Journal of Autism and Developmental Disorders, 22*, 2, 141–154.

Koegel, R. L., O'Dell, M. C., & Koegel, L. K. (1987). A natural language paradigm for teaching nonverbal autistic children. *Journal of Autism and Developmental Disorders, 17*, 187–199.

Koegel, R. L., Schriebman, L., Good, A., Cerniglia, L., Murphy, C., & Koegel, L. K. (1989). *How to teach pivotal behaviors to children with autism: A training manual*. University of California: Santa Barbara.

Koegel, R. L., Schreibman, L., Loos, L. M., Dirlich-Wilhelm, H., Dunlap, G., Robbins, F. R., & Plienis, A. (1992). Consistent stress profiles in mothers of children with autism. *Journal of Autism and Developmental Disorders, 22*, 2, 205–216.

Koegel, R. L., Schreibman, L., Britten, K., & Laitinen, R. (1979). The effect of reinforcement schedule on stimulus overselectivity in autistic children. *Journal of Autism and Developmental Disorders, 9*, 383–397.

Koegel, R. L, Schreibman, L., O'Neill, R. E., & Burke, J. C. (1983). Personality and family interaction characteristics of parents of autistic children. *Journal of Consulting and Clinical Psychology, 16*, 683–692.

Lancoini, G. E. (1983). Using pictorial representations as communication means with low-functioning children. *Journal of Autism and Developmental Disorders, 13*, 87–105.

Laski, K. E., Charlop, M. H., & Schreibman, L. (1988). Training parents to use the natural language paradigm to increase their autistic children's speech. *Journal of Applied Behavior Analysis, 21*, 391–400.

Lovaas, O. I., Varni, J., Koegel, R. L., & Lorsch, N. (1977). Some observations on the non-extinguishability of children's speech. *Child Development, 48*, 1121–1127.

Mahoney, G. (1988). Communication patterns—mothers and mentally retarded infants. *First language, 8*, 157–172.

Odom, S. L., Chandler, L. K., Ostrosky, M., McConnell, S. R., & Reaney, S. (1992). Fading teacher prompts from peer-initiation interventions for young children with disabilities. *Journal of Applied Behavior Analysis, 25*, 2, 307–318.

Odom, S. L., Hoyson, M., Jamieson, B., & Strain, P. S. (1985). Increasing handicapped preschoolers' peer social interactions: Cross-setting and component analysis. *Journal of Applied Behavior Analysis, 18*, 3–16.

Olley, J. G. (1986). The TEACCH curriculum for teaching social behavior to children with autism. In E. Schopler & G. B. Mesibov (Eds.), *Social behavior and autism* (pp. 351–373). New York: Plenum Press.

O'Neill, R. E., Horner, R. H., Albin, R. W., Storey, K., & Sprague, J. R. (1990). *Functional analysis: A practical assessment guide*. Sycamore, IL: Sycamore Press.

Ornitz, E. M. (1985). Neurophysiology of infantile autism. *Journal of the American Academy of Child Psychiatry, 24*, 251–262.

Ornitz, E. M., Brown, M. B., Mason, A., & Putnam, N. H. (1974). Effect of visual input on vestibular nystagmus in autistic children. *Archives of General Psychiatry, 31*, 369–375.

Pitfield, M., & Oppenheim, A. N. (1964). Child-rearing attitudes of mothers of psychotic children. *Journal of Child Psychology and Psychiatry and Allied Disciplines, 5*, 51–57.

Prior, M., & Bradshaw, J. L. (1979). Hemispheric functioning in autistic children. *Cortex, 15*, 73–81.

Prizant, B. M. (1983). Echolalia in autism: Assessment and intervention. *Seminars in Speech and Language, 4*, 63–77.

Prizant, B. M., & Rydell, P. J. (1984). Analysis of functions of delayed echolalia in autistic children. *Journal of Speech and Hearing Research, 27*, 183–192.

Reichle, J., Mirenda, P., Locke, P., Piche, L., & Johnston, S. (1992). Beginning augmentative communication systems. In S. F. Warren & J. Reichle (Eds.), *Causes and effects in communication and language intervention* (pp. 131–156). Baltimore: Paul H. Brookes Publishing Co.

Ritvo, E. R., & Freeman, B. J. (1978). National society for autistic children definition of the syndrome of autism. *Journal of Autism and Childhood Schizophrenia, 8,* 162–169.

Ritvo, E. R., Freeman, B. J., Scheibel, A. B., Duong, T., Robinson, H., Guthrie, D., & Ritvo, A. M. (1986). Lower Purkinje cell counts in the cerebella of four autistic subjects: Initial findings of the UCLA-NSAC autopsy research report. *American Journal of Psychiatry, 143,* 862–866.

Ritvo, E. R., Ornitz, E. M., Eviatar, A., Markham, C. H., Brown, M. B., & Mason, A. (1989). Decreased postrotatory nystagmus in early infantile autism. *Neurology, 19,* 653–658.

Ritvo, E. R., Ritvo, E. C., & Brothers, A. M. (1982). Genetic and immunohematologic factors in autism. *Journal of Autism and Developmental Disorders, 12,* 109–114.

Ritvo, E. R., Freeman, B. J., Yuwiler, A., Geller, E., Yokota, A., Schroth, P., & Novak, P. (1984). Study of fenfluramine in outpatients with the syndrome of autism. *Journal of Pediatrics, 105,* 823–828.

Rutter, M. (1978). On confusion in the diagnosis of autism. *Journal of Autism and Childhood Schizophrenia, 8,* 137–169.

Schopler, E. (1978). On confusion in the diagnosis of autism. *Journal of Autism and Childhood Schizophrenia, 8,* 137–138.

Schreibman, L., & Charlop, M. H. (1987). Autism. In V. B. Van Hasselt & M. Hersen (Eds.), *Psychological evaluation of the developmentally and physically disabled* (pp. 155–177). New York: Plenum Press.

Schreibman, L., & Koegel, R. L. (1975). A christmas tree for Kristin. *Psychology Today, 8*(March), 67.

Schriebman, L., Kaneko, W., & Koegel, R. L. (1991). Positive affect of parents of autistic children: A comparison across two teaching techniques. *Behavior Therapy, 22,* 479–490.

Schriebman, L., Koegel, R. L., Mills, J. I., & Burke, J. C. (1981). Social validation of behavior therapy with autistic children. *Behavior Therapy, 12,* 610–624.

Strain, P. S. (1983). Generalization of autistic children's social behavior change: Effects of developmentally integrated and segregated settings. *Analysis and Intervention in Developmental Disabilities, 3,* 23–24.

Strain, P. S., Shores, R. E., & Timm, M. A. (1977). Effects of peer social initiations on the behavior of withdrawn preschool children. *Journal of Applied Behavior Analysis, 10,* 289–298.

Sullivan, R. C. (1978). The hostage parent. *Journal of Autism and Childhood Schizophrenia, 8,* 233–248.

Tager-Flusberg, H. (1990). Psycholinguistic approaches to language and communication in autism. In E. Schopler & G. B. Mesibov (Eds.), *Communication problems in autism* (pp. 69–87). New York: Plenum Press.

Tsai, L. Y., & Stewart, M. A. (1983). Etiological implication of maternal age and birth order in infantile autism. *Journal of Autism and Developmental Disorders, 13,* 57–65.

Walker, L. J. (1987). Procedural rights in the wrong system: Special education is not enough. In A. Gartner & T. Joe (Eds.), *Images of the disabled, disabling images,* (pp. 97–115). New York: Praeger.

Wetherby, A. M., & Prutting, C. A. (1984). Profiles of communicative and cognitive-social abilities in autistic children. *Journal of Speech and Hearing Research, 27,* 364–377.

Wetherby, A., Koegel, R. L., & Mendel, M. (1981). Central auditory nervous system dysfunction in echolalic autistic individuals. *Journal of Speech and Hearing Research, 24,* 420–429.

Wing, L. (1966). Early childhood autism. Clinical, educational and social aspects. Oxford: Pergamon Press Ltd.

Wing, L. (1976). *Early childhood autism: Clinical, educational and social aspects* (2nd Ed.). Oxford: Pergamon Press.

9

Attention-Deficit Hyperactivity Disorder

Mark D. Rapport

Description of the Disorder

Attention-deficit hyperactivity disorder (ADHD) (American Psychiatric Association, 1987) is the current diagnostic label for children presenting with serious and pervasive problems of attention, impulsivity, and excessive gross motor activity. Previous labels and their approximate dates of use in chronological order include: minimal brain damage (1947 to early 1950s), minimal brain dysfunction (1950s to early 1960s), hyperkinetic reaction of childhood (1968–1979), and attention deficit disorder with or without hyperactivity (1980–1986). Formal diagnostic labels aside, lay persons have nearly always referred to these individuals as simply "hyperactive."

The changes in diagnostic labels over the years have paralleled scientific advances in the study and understanding of the disorder. As indicated above, ADHD was initially thought to be a consequence of brain injury or damage. The original connection between brain damage and behavioral deviance was reported in turn-of-the-century writings (Still, 1902), wherein "classically hyperactive" children with minor physical anomalies and demonstrative organic brain damage were described. The concept was further reified following the 1918 encephalitis epidemics, as the behavioral sequelae in affected children included inattentiveness, gross motor overactivity, aggressiveness, impaired judgment, disruptive conduct, and a range of learning disabilities. Subsequent attempts to validate the concept of minimal brain damage or dysfunction (MBD), however, were unsuccessful. Soft neurological signs were found to be present in a wide variety of childhood

Mark D. Rapport • Department of Psychology, University of Hawaii, Honolulu, Hawaii 96822.

Advanced Abnormal Psychology, edited by Vincent B. Van Hasselt and Michel Hersen. Plenum Press, New York, 1994.

disorders as well as in normal children, and neither a positive history of brain damage nor birth difficulties were evidenced in a majority of children with a history of behavioral problems.

Efforts were subsequently focused on the driven, hyperactive behavior associated with the disorder. Trying to operationalize or define how active was "hyperactive," however, was problematic for a number of reasons. For example, changes in human activity level occur as a function of development and are heavily influenced by a host of environmental factors, such as fatigue, boredom, stimulation level, and personal interest. Measuring gross motor activity also turned out to be an arduous and cumbersome task. Does one count steps taken? How often does one fidget or change positions while seated? What is the frequency of movements in a controlled space, or the speed by which one moves about the environment? As a result, a number of behavior-rating scales were standardized to provide norms for age and gender, and disparate measures of activity level (e.g., pedometers, wrist and leg movement actometers) were developed. Despite these developments, activity level alone simply did not capture the rudimentary nature or core symptomatology associated with ADHD. These children were not only overly active, but experienced multifaceted difficulties while trying to pay attention in classrooms, while interacting with others, and while trying to learn under traditional methods of educational instruction.

By the early 1970s, many were disenchanted with the exclusive focus on gross motor activity, and it was argued that an inability to pay attention and impulsivity were of greater significance in defining the disorder (Douglas, 1980). The radical reconceptualization of the disorder from one focusing on overactive behavior to one of attentional deficits and impulsivity was set forth in the publication of the *Diagnostic and Statistical Manual of Mental Disorders*, Third Edition (DSM-III) by the American Psychiatric Association in 1980. Distinct subtypes of the disorder, one with and one without hyperactivity, were also proposed in the publication although later discarded.

Finally, criteria for defining the disorder were further updated in the publication of the revised version of DSM-III, the DSM-III-R (American Psychiatric Association, 1987). Hyperactivity was reinstated as one of several core symptoms as reflected in the name change to "Attention-Deficit Hyperactivity Disorder" (ADHD). And the disorder was included among three that appeared to overlap with one another under the supraordinate category of "disruptive behavior disorders" occurring in childhood.

EPIDEMIOLOGY

Epidemiology is concerned with the ways in which clinical disorders and diseases occur in human populations and with factors that influence these patterns of occurrence. Three interrelated components of epidemiological research involve: (a) assessing the occurrence of new cases (incidence rate) or existing cases (prevalence rate) of the disorder at a given period of time or within a specific time period; (b) assessing how the disorder is distributed in the population, which may include information concerning geographic location, gender, socioeconomic level, and race; and (c) identifying factors associated with the variation and distribution of the disorder to enable etiological hypotheses to be generated.

Prevalence

Information concerning incidence rate or number of new cases of ADHD in a given time frame is essentially speculative at present. This is because epidemiological studies have not been repeated over sufficiently long time periods using identical populations. The limited information that does exist suggests that incidence of ADHD has increased somewhat over the past several years, which may be due to improved detection and awareness of the disorder, as opposed to any real increase in the number of affected individuals per se.

Current prevalence estimates, on the other hand, indicate that between 3 to 5% of the childhood population has ADHD (Barkley, 1990). These estimates must also be viewed as conjectural, as they are based on parent and teacher rating scale scores in the absence of a clinical interview or knowledge of onset, course, or developmental history of symptoms. Nevertheless, they do indicate that a relatively large number of children exhibit ADHD-like symptoms at home and in school.

Sex Ratio

Prevalence estimates suggest that more males than females are affected with the disorder, with ratios ranging from 3:1 to 6:1 in nonreferred and clinic-referred samples, respectively. The clinic-referred sample estimates may be somewhat inflated, however, due to referral bias. For example, greater numbers of boys are typically referred to outpatient clinics because of inappropriate and especially aggressive conduct. Moreover, most of the rating scales upon which prevalence estimates have been based have not included separate norms for gender. Given that girls differ from boys in many aspects of behavior at various stages of their development, it seems probable that they also manifest an altogether different pattern of behavioral disturbance and thus represent an under-diagnosed population of affected children. Recent evidence supports this supposition, as girls with ADHD have been reported to be more socially withdrawn, have more internalizing symptoms (anxiety and depression), fewer behavioral and conduct problems, and more pronounced intellectual deficits than boys.

Culture and Socioeconomic Status

Rates of ADHD are relatively consistent across cultures, especially when similar diagnostic criteria for defining the disorder are used and rating scale cutoff scores are based on established population norms. Prevalence estimates fluctuate moderately as a function of socioeconomic status (SES) and geographic area, with higher rates associated with lower SES and with urban areas. Various explanations have been offered for these differences, such as social drift and poorer health care and nutrition, but they remain speculative.

CLINICAL PICTURE

Description and Distinguishing Features

The first distinction that should be noted in understanding children with ADHD is that it is not the type or kind of behavior they exhibit that is particularly deviant, but the quantity or degree and intensity of their behavior. That is, they tend to exhibit higher rates of certain behavior and frequently with greater intensity in situations that demand lower rates or more subtle kinds of behavior (e.g., becoming disruptive and behaving inappropriately in school or while interacting with others); and at other times, lower rates of such behavior when higher rates are demanded (e.g., not paying attention and completing academic assignments in the classroom). Overall, they appear to be out of sync with environmental demands and expectations, especially in situations that require careful sustained attention and protracted effort at tasks that are not particularly interesting or stimulating to these children.

Children's behavior must also be viewed in an appropriate developmental context. For example, younger children typically are more active, cannot pay attention to a particular task for a long time interval, and tend to spend less time in making decisions or analyzing problems, compared with older children. Other factors, such as gender and cultural differences, may also play a defining role in determining what constitutes "normality," and it is only when a child's behavior consistently and significantly exceeds these expectations that it is considered deviant.

In ADHD, the developmental behavioral pattern typically observed is associated with an early onset, a gradual worsening of symptoms over time, and an unrelenting clinical course until late adolescence when the child is no longer in school. Most children with ADHD continue to exhibit symptoms of the disorder as adults, the severity of which depends upon a number of factors. As we shall see later in the chapter, many believe that the disorder is inherited and thus present from birth.

A third feature characteristic of children with ADHD is that their behavioral difficulties tend to be pervasive across situations and settings. Most of us have been "hyper" at one time or another, have experienced difficulty concentrating, and have acted impulsively in particular situations. These occurrences tend to be isolated events, and one can usually point to particular environmental circumstances, situations, or contingencies as responsible for, or as contributing factors associated with, the behavior (e.g., feeling ill or having to study for a particularly uninteresting class). The child with ADHD, on the other hand, exhibits this pattern of behavior in most situations and settings, day after day, year after year. A gradual worsening of behavioral and academic difficulties is usually observed as the child grows older. This is because the environment demands that one be able to pay attention, sit still, and control one's impulses for longer periods of time with increasing age. Difficulties are especially conspicuous upon entry into the fourth and seventh grades, when classroom demands and academic assignments become increasingly more complex, take longer to complete, and rely heavily on one's ability to work independently.

Children with ADHD are also known for their "consistently inconsistent" behavior. That is, they tend to behave rather erratically both within and across days, even when their home and school environments are relatively stable. Teachers frequently report, for example, that such children appear relatively settled and able to pay attention and complete academic assignments on some days, although most days are characterized by disruptiveness, inattention, and low work completion rates. Parents report a similar phenomena at home, even among those who are highly skilled in managing their child's behavior. The reasons for the ADHD child's inconsistent pattern of behavior are varied, and as will be discussed, may be related to a complex interaction between brain regulation mechanisms and prevailing environmental stimulation and contingencies.

Primary Symptoms and Diagnostic Criteria

As previously mentioned, the primary symptoms or clinical features of ADHD are developmentally inappropriate degrees of inattention, impulsivity, and gross motor overactivity. The current DSM-III-R (American Psychiatric Association, 1987) diagnostic criteria for ADHD are presented in Table 1 and require a child to exhibit any 8 of the 14 symptoms or behaviors listed under the "A" criterion. Individuals with the disorder generally display some disturbance in each of these areas and in most settings, but to varying degrees. Conversely, signs of the disorder may be minimal or even absent in novel settings (e.g., being examined in a doctor's office, or in a clinical setting), when individualized attention is being given, or under conditions in which stimulation or interest level is relatively high.

Readers may wish to note, however, that the upcoming DSM-IV will reflect additional changes both in the formal name of the disorder and the specific criteria used in arriving at a formal diagnosis. The DSM-IV (1993) planning committee, for example, is currently recommending that children with Attention-deficit Hyperactivity Disorder (ADHD) be subtyped using a three-category classification schema in the upcoming diagnostic nomenclature: ADHD, Predominantly Inattention Type; ADHD, Predominantly Hyperactive-Impulsive Type; and ADHD, Combined Type (see Table 1). The first category will be used to describe those children who were previously diagnosed as ADD without Hyperactivity in the DSM-III-R (1987), and will require children to exhibit at least 6 (from a list of 9) inattentive behaviors for a minimal duration of 6 months, and to a degree that is considered developmentally inappropriate for their age. Moreover, children with ADHD, Predominantly Inattention Type, must not exhibit more than 3 behaviors from a second list of "Hyperactive-Impulsive" items. To meet criteria for the diagnostic subtype category, ADHD, Predominantly Hyperactive-Impulsive Type, children must exhibit a minimum of 4 behaviors (of the 6 listed) from the hyperactive-impulsive symptom list and show no more than 5 of the behaviors listed under the inattentive subtype category. Children meeting diagnostic criteria under both the inattention and hyperactive-impulsive categories will be considered as ADHD, Combined Type. Additional changes recommended by the DSM-IV planning committee include (a) developing a separate symptom list with appropriately worded criteria for adults with ADHD and (b) requiring that symptoms of the disorder be exhibtied pervasively (as opposed to situationally) across settings (e.g., both at home and at school). The DSM-IV planning committee's recommendations were based on extensive field trials and will better reflect the results of empirical field trials and will better reflect the results of empirical studies over the past decade (Lahey, Carlson, & Frick, in press).

At home, inattention is commonly displayed by frequent shifts from one uncompleted activity to another, and a failure to follow through and/or comply with instructions. The impulsivity component is often expressed by acting without considering either the immediate or delayed consequences of one's actions (e.g., running into the street, accident proneness), interrupting the conversation of other household members, and grabbing objects (not with malevolent intent) in the store

TABLE 1. DSM-IV Planning Committee Proposed Diagnostic Criteria for Children with Attention-Deficit Hyperactivity Disorder

A. Either (1) or (2):
   (1) *Inattention*: At least six of the following symptoms of inattention have persisted six months to a degree that is maladaptive and inconsistent with developmental level:
      (a) often fails to give close attention to details or makes careless mistakes in schoolwork, work, or other activities
      (b) often has difficulty sustaining attention in tasks or play activities
      (c) often does not seem to listen to what is being said to him or her
      (d) often does not follow through on instructions and fails to finish schoolwork, chores, or duties in the workplace (not due to oppositional behavior or failure to understand instructions)
      (e) often has difficulties organizing tasks and activities
      (f) often avoids or strongly dislikes tasks (such as schoolwork or homework) that requires sustained mental effort
      (g) often loses things necessary for tasks or activities (e.g., school assignments, pencils, books, tools, or toys)
      (h) is often easily distracted by extraneous stimuli
      (i) often forgetful in daily activities
   (2) *Hyperactivity-Impulsivity*: At least four of the following symptoms of hyperactivity-impulsivity have persisted for at least six months to a degree that is maladaptive and inconsistent with developmental level:

   Hyperactivity
      (a) often fidgets with hands or feet or squirms in seat
      (b) leaves seat in classroom or in other situations in which remaining seated is expected
      (c) often runs about or climbs excessively in situations where it is inappropriate (in adolescents or adults, may be limited to subjective feelings of restlessness)
      (d) often has difficulty playing or engaging in leisure activities quietly

   Impulsivity
      (e) often blurts out answers to questions before the questions have been completed
      (f) often has difficulty waiting in lines or awaiting turn in games or group situations
B. Onset no later than seven years of age.
C. Symptoms must be present in two or more situations (e.g., at school, work, and at home).
D. The disturbance causes clinically significant distress or impairment in social, academic, or occupations functioning.
E. Does not occur exclusively during the course of a Pervasive Developmental Disorder, Schizophrenia or other Psychotic Disorder, and is not better accounted for by a Mood Disorder, Anxiety Disorder, Dissociative Disorder, or a Personality Disorder.

Code based on type:

314.00 *Attention-deficit Hyperactivity Disorder, Predominantly Inattentive Type*: if criterion A(1) is met but not criterion A(2) for the past six months
314.01 *Attention-deficit Hyperactivity Disorder, Predominantly Hyperactive-Impulsive Type*: if criterion A(2) is met but not criterion A(1) for the past six months
314.02 *Attention-deficit Hyperactivity Disorder, Combined type*: if both critera A(1) and A(2) are met for the past six months

Coding note: for individuals (especially adolescents and adults) who currently have symptoms that no longer meet full criteria, "in partial remission" should be specified.

Note: From *DSM-IV draft criteria*, by the American Psychiatric Association, 1993, Washington, DC. Copyright 1993 by the American Psychiatric Association. Reprinted by permission.

while on shopping trips. Problems with overactivity are often expressed by difficulty remaining seated during meals, while completing homework, or while riding in the car, and by excessive movement during sleep.

At school, inattention is usually evidenced by difficulty deploying and maintaining adequate attention (i.e., staying on-task), a failure to complete academic assignments, and deficient organizational and informational processing skills. Impulsivity is expressed in a variety of ways, such as by interrupting others, beginning assignments before receiving (or understanding) complete instructions, making careless mistakes while completing assignments, blurting out answers in class, and having difficulty waiting one's turn in both small-group and organized sport activities. Hyperactivity is frequently manifested by fidgetiness, twisting and wiggling in one's seat or changing seat positions, dropping objects on the floor, and emitting noises or playing with objects during quiet assignment periods. One should be careful to note, however, that all of these behaviors may be diminished or exacerbated by subtle changes in the environment. Teachers will frequently comment, for example, that an identified child with ADHD who is absorbed in a particular activity of high interest value or who is working in a one-on-one situation with an adult can attend for normal time expectations and not move a muscle while doing so. Parents also report that their children with ADHD can sit perfectly still while engaged in high-stimulation activities such as watching movies (e.g., "Star Wars"), and while playing interactive computer or video games. As we will see, this may have a direct bearing on the extant nature of the disorder.

Secondary Symptoms or Associated Features of ADHD

Secondary features are those behaviors and difficulties that occur at a greater than chance frequency in children with a particular disorder, but are not necessary or sufficient to serve as formal diagnostic criteria. Many of these symptoms or behaviors are reported early in the developmental course of the disorder, and may thus represent less prominent features of the disorder. These include affective volatility, lability of mood, temper tantrums, low frustration tolerance, social disinhibition, cognitive impairment with associated learning disability, and perceptual motor difficulties (Barkley, 1990). Other aspects of disturbance or behavioral difficulties may be secondary to, or direct and indirect consequences of, the disorder. For example, disturbed peer and interpersonal relationships, academic underachievement, school failure, decreased self-esteem, depressed mood, and conduct problems are characteristic of many children with ADHD. The presence or absence of attendant aggressive or conduct features is especially important and may be of both diagnostic and prognostic value (Hinshaw, 1987).

Case Description

Brian is a 10-year-old Caucasian male with a history of severely hyperactive and impulsive behavior dating back to his toddler years. Although Brian's mother feels that he was unusually active and more difficult to control than either of his two brothers by the age of 3, it was not until kindergarten that intervention was necessary. During his kindergarten year, Brian's classroom teacher telephoned his mother repeatedly to report that Brian simply could not sit still long enough to complete any of the tasks given to the class. Instead, he would run around the room and try to climb on the window sills and cabinets. He was also unable to play cooperatively with the other children in the classroom due to his "bossiness," inability to take turns and share materials, and increasing frequency of aggressive behavior. Brian fought almost daily with at least one other child in the classroom. On several occasions, he had actually injured another child either accidentally through his quick and impulsive movements, or by design. Brian's mother initially considered her child's unmanageable and increasingly disruptive behavior "a phase" he was going through in response to her recent divorce and the death of her father, with whom Brian had shared a close relationship. Brian's difficulties continued, however, and by the middle of the first-grade year the school indicated that he would require a psychiatric evaluation to determine whether alternative classroom placement and/or treatment was warranted.

Brian was evaluated by a psychiatrist, a psychologist, and a neurologist and was diagnosed as having Attention-deficit Hyperactivity Disorder (ADHD). His physical examination was unremarkable and the neurologic examination revealed no focal abnormalities, although he was felt to have poor fine-motor coordination and to exhibit a "clumsy" way of moving. These abnormalities were not seen in conjunction with any other neurologic symptoms and were thus considered "soft signs."

A semistructured clinical interview (Kiddie-SADS-E; Orvaschel, Puig-Antich, Chambers, Tabrizi, & Johnson, 1982) was administered to Brian's mother, with relevant parts administered to the child. The mother endorsed nearly all items related to a diagnosis of ADHD and oppositional defiant disorder, and several items related to conduct disorder. Conversely, Brian denied having difficulty in most areas of functioning, admitting only to having few or no friends—a phenomenon that he blamed on other children's "not liking him" and "being mean." The K-SADS-E interview also revealed an early onset, developmental history, and clinical course consistent with ADHD.

A broad-band behavior rating scale (i.e., the CBCL, or Child Behavior Check List), and several scales specific to the diagnosis of ADHD (e.g., ADHD Rating Scale, Home and School Situations Questionnaire) were administered to both Brian's mother and the classroom teacher to help quantify the nature and degree of Brian's behavioral difficulties. The pattern of scores on the CBCL showed primary elevation on the "externalizing" dimension of behavioral dysfunction, with factor scores elevated in the clinical range on the narrow-band scales of inattentive, nervous–overactive, aggressive, and unpopular. Scores on the remaining rating scales were consistent with the CBCL, and indicated that Brian experienced significant difficulties both at home and in school, most notably with impulsivity, overactivity, and aggression.

A computerized neuropsychological battery of tests was administered subsequently to Brian. The battery consisted of: (a) the Continuous Performance Test (CPT), a measure of vigilance or sustained attention; (b) the Matching Unfamiliar Figures Test (MUFTy), a measure of behavioral inhibition and cognitive tempo while engaged in visual problem solving; (c) a Paired Associate Learning Test (PAL), a measure of short-term memory; and (d) the Stimulus Equivalence Paradigm (SEP), a measure of higher-order learning and long-term recall. These instruments were administered for two purposes: to help quantify the degree of difficulty Brian experienced in tasks related to school functioning; and to provide a baseline upon which pharmacological intervention could be assessed (Rapport, 1990).

Brian's performance on these tasks indicated that he could not attend to a relatively simple task for even 3 minutes at a time. He was highly impulsive and unorganized in his attempts to solve visually presented problems, and experienced significant difficulties with both short-term memory and long-term recall of learned relationships.

Treatment was started with a stimulant class medication, methylphenidate (MPH), at a dose of 5 mg twice daily. Dosage was increased every other week by 5 mg (twice daily), with clinical response assessed using teacher rating scales administered at the conclusion of each week, and alternative forms of the neuropsychological battery under each dosage. A placebo (nonactive medication) trial was also administered during the last week of the medication trial to help determine whether changes in teacher ratings and test performance were due to active medication as opposed to some other variable such as maturation or practice. Both the classroom teacher and psychological examiner were "blind" to all medication trials. The results of the clinical trials are depicted in Figures 1, 2, and 3.

Brian's performance on the CPT showed considerable improvement under the 5-mg b.i.d. MPH dosage relative to baseline (no medication) conditions. No further improvement was noted under the higher dosages, and in fact, his performance deteriorated moderately (relative to the 5-mg dosage) under 20 mg and reverted to below-baseline levels under placebo (see CPT, Fig. 1). A different pattern of test scores was obtained on the MUFTy. Brian's performance on this instrument improved as a function of increasing dosage in a linear fashion, with optimal performance obtained under the highest dosage (20 mg) before retreating to baseline levels under placebo (see MUFTy, Fig. 1). These findings are not surprising, as children's vigilance is typically optimized with low dosages of psychostimulants, whereas behavioral inhibition (impulsivity) is usually optimized under high dosages (see Rapport & Kelly, 1991).

The next figure in the series summarizes Brian's response to MPH as assessed by the PAL and SEP instruments—both of which tend to have a higher correlation than do the CPT and MUFTy with children's classroom academic performance. As depicted in Figure 2, Brian's short-term memory for learning paired associations and long-term recall of learned relationships was optimally enhanced under the middle-range dosages, 10 mg and 15 mg. Under the higher 20-mg dosage condition, his cognitive performance was compromised and showed a clear decline compared with lower dosages—a phenomenon termed "overfocused state" (Kinsbourne & Swanson, 1979), wherein cognitive efficiency deteriorates as a function of receiving too high a dose of medication.

Brian's classroom teacher completed two rating scales at the end of each week: the Abbreviated Conners Teacher Rating Scales [ACTRS (Werry, Sprague, & Cohen, 1975)] and the recently developed Academic Performance Rating Scale [APRS (DuPaul, Rapport, & Perriello, 1991)]. Teacher ratings on the ACTRS indicate that Brian's classroom behavior was dramatically improved under all active medication conditions compared to both baseline and placebo (see ACTRS, Fig. 3), with optimal change occurring under the higher, 20-mg MPH dosage. The drug-dosage profile pattern thus tends to mirror the MUFTy results (see Fig. 1 for comparison). The APRS academic performance subscale, on the other hand, shows improved classroom performance up to and including the 15-mg dosage, with a subsequent and rather dramatic decline under the higher, 20-mg dosage (see APRS, Fig. 3). These latter results are similar to those obtained on both the PAL and SEP (see Fig. 2 for comparison), and suggest that academic performance and memory yield a somewhat different dose-response profile pattern in some children than do measures of classroom conduct (ACTRS) and impulsivity (MUFTy).

Overall, the higher, 20-mg dosage resulted in greater behavioral improvement and impulse control for Brian, but the results were not compelling enough to warrant compromising his academic performance. As a result, it was recommended that Brian be placed on a 15-mg b.i.d. daily maintenance MPH regimen

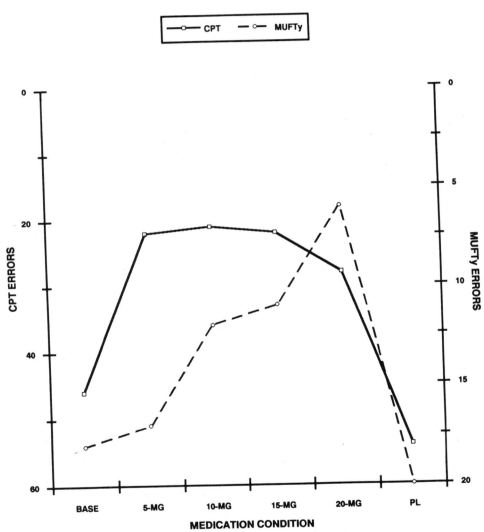

FIGURE 1. Brian's response to four doses of methylphenidate (MPH) contrasted with baseline (no medication) and placebo (PL) conditions on two clinic-based measures: the Continuous Performance Test (CPT) ad the Matching Unfamiliar Figures Test (MUFTy). Improvement (error reduction) is denoted by upward movement on the left (CPT) and right (MUFTy) ordinate for each measure, respectively.

for the remainder of the year. An alternative learning environment was also
recommended, and Brian was placed in a special education classroom with a ratio
of 12 students to 1 teacher and 1 teacher aide (12:1:1 classroom), where he remained
for the next several years. During this time, several behavioral interventions were
tried to further stabilize Brian's behavior and enhance his academic performance.
The most successful of these involved attentional training, based on response cost
procedures (see Rapport, Murphy, & Bailey, 1982), which allowed Brian's daily
MPH dosage to be reduced to 10 mg twice per day [see Hoza, Pelham, Sams, &
Carlson (1992) for a comprehensive discussion of combining treatments for children with ADHD].

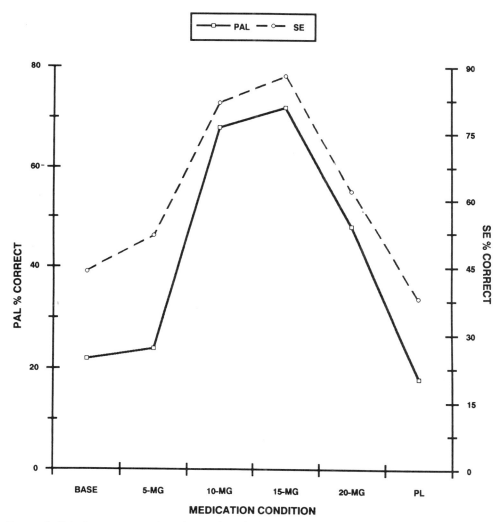

FIGURE 2. Brian's response to four doses of methylphenidate (MPH) contrasted with baseline (no
medication) and placebo (PL) conditions on two clinic-based measures: Paired Associate Learning (PAL)
task and Stimulus Equivalence (SE) Paradigm. Improvement (% correct) is denoted by upward
movement on the left (PAL) and right (SE) ordinate for each measure, respectively.

MARK D.
RAPPORT

Early Childhood

Several well controlled studies indicate that difficulties with attention and overactivity are relatively common among preschoolers (Campbell, 1990; Palfrey, Levine, Walker, & Sullivan, 1985). Only a small subset of these children continues to manifest symptoms characteristic of ADHD, however, by the time they are 4 to 5 years of age, which are in turn, strongly predictive of continued difficulties and a probable clinical diagnosis by ages 6 and 9. Thus, the necessity of considering both

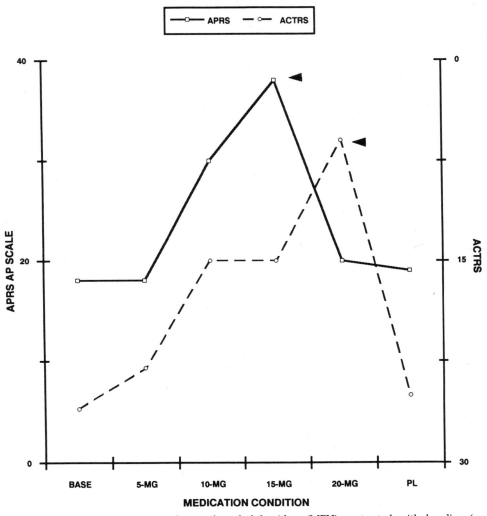

FIGURE 3. Brian's response to 4 doses of methylphenidate (MPH) contrasted with baseline (no medication) and placebo (PL) conditions on two teacher rating scales: the Academic Performance Rating Scale (APRS) and the Abbreviated Conners Teacher Rating Scale (ACTRS). Improvement is denoted by upward movement on the left (APRS) and right (ACTRS) ordinate for each measure, respectively.

the degree *and* duration of behavioral disturbance cannot be overemphasized, especially in very young children.

Parents describe children in this age group who continue to exhibit a durable pattern of ADHD symptoms as always on the go, fearless, restless, continually getting into things, not obeying parental commands, oppositional, highly curious about their environment, and requiring high levels of adult supervision. Other problems, such as perceptual motor difficulties, sleep and eating difficulties, accident proneness, speech and language difficulties, and toilet training difficulties, are reported in a subset of these children. Those with advanced intellectual and cognitive skills and who tend not to be aggressive are generally easier to manage both at home and in preschool settings. Needless to say, the parents (and especially mothers) of these children are under enormous daily stress in their parental roles, the reciprocal interaction of which not infrequently results in psychiatric disability, marital problems, alcoholism, and increased risk for child abuse.

Middle Childhood

Between the ages of 6 and 12 years, children with ADHD continue to demonstrate difficulties with attention, impulsivity, overactivity, and compliance with adult requests. These difficulties are exacerbated after the children enter elementary school, with a subsequent rise in outpatient referral rates owing to two primary factors: the increased familiarity of classroom teachers with age-appropriate norms for behavior; and the increased demands to sit still, pay attention, and engage in increasingly more difficult academic tasks and organized activities for longer periods of time. In some cases, the child will be excused as "immature" by well-meaning school personnel, and forced to repeat the grade or passed marginally with the expectation that the child will magically "mature" over the summer months.

Increasing social and academic demands will impact their already handicapping condition to an even greater extent during these primary school years, and cause the greatest level of stress to already overburdened parents and teachers. Homework assignments add an additional source of conflict to the familial environment, and 25% or more of the children will experience significant difficulties with reading and/or develop other academic skill disorders. Their inattention, impulsivity, and higher-than-normal activity level predestines them to develop poor peer and interpersonal relationships, with a resulting pattern of social isolation and eventual low self-esteem in later years.

Adolescence

One of the prevailing myths about children with ADHD is that they "outgrow" the disorder when they reach adolescence. Follow-up and long-term outcome studies, however, inform us that approximately 80% of children diagnosed as having ADHD in childhood continue to display symptoms of and meet diagnostic criteria for ADHD as adolescents. Primary difficulties with attention/concentration, impulsivity, and difficulty following directions remain, whereas the overactivity component of the disorder diminishes somewhat and shifts into fidgeting and restlessness with increasing age.

Perhaps more unsettling are the findings that between 40% and 60% of adolescents with ADHD also meet diagnostic criteria for conduct disorder (CD)—a disorder characterized by serious and pervasive antisocial behavior. These comorbid adolescents, in turn, are also more likely to engage in substance use (e.g., cigarette) and abuse (e.g., alcohol and marijuana).

One of the strongest predictors during early childhood for becoming a well functioning, stable, successful adult is academic achievement. Follow-up studies on academic outcome during adolescent years, of children with ADHD, particularly those comorbid for CD, have been alarmingly negative. They are significantly more likely to have been suspended or expelled from school, and three times more likely to have failed at least one grade, their standardized achievement test scores are below normal in math, reading, and spelling (Barkley, 1990, p. 119). Of even greater concern is that an estimated 10 to 30% of them quit school and do not graduate with even a high school diploma. Overall, adolescents with ADHD, and especially those carrying a dual diagnosis of CD, represent a population at high risk for a variety of negative outcomes associated with psychiatric disability, and social and adult occupational functioning.

Adult Outcome and Long-Term Prognosis

At least three different clinical models have been postulated concerning the long-term outcome of children with ADHD: developmental delay, developmental decay, and continuous display. The first model presumes that ADHD is primarily a neuromaturational problem and that associated difficulties will eventually diminish with age. The second model holds that the primary symptom picture will worsen with increasing age, and that specific clinical features will be manifested somewhat differently in older children. The third model postulates that the primary symptom picture will continue to be manifested with increasing age to a more or less similar degree of severity, but that, similar to the decay model, the topography of clinical features (e.g., inattention, impulsivity) will change to reflect difficulties related to adolescence and adulthood.

Each of the three outcome models presented above is supported in part by the existing, albeit scant, literature concerning adults diagnosed during childhood as having ADHD. Between 50 and 65% of diagnosed children continue to experience difficulties with core clinical symptoms and related behavioral problems as adults, and only 11% are estimated to be free of any psychiatric diagnosis and to be well functioning adults. These rather bleak estimates are tempered somewhat, when one considers that only about a third of the "normal" population of children are free of psychiatric disability as adults.

Other areas of adult functioning are equally impaired. Relatively few adults with a childhood diagnosis of ADHD go on to complete a university degree program (approximately 5% vs. 41% of control children). A significant minority of them (20 to 25%) continue to display a persistent pattern of antisocial behavior. Poor work records, lower job status, difficulty getting along with supervisors, and overall lower socioeconomic status attainment are common. Greater difficulties with social skills, unstable marriages, and lower self-esteem prevail (Gittelman, Mannuzza, Shenker, & Bonagura, 1985; Weiss & Hechtman, 1986). Conversely, other adults with ADHD appear to function normally and even exceptionally well as adults. The limited evidence available indicates that a supportive, stable family environment, milder ADHD symptoms, higher intelligence, greater emotional stability, and no concomitant conduct disorder and especially aggression during childhood, are the best predictors of positive adult outcome.

ETIOLOGY, FAMILIAL, AND GENETIC PATTERNS

Speculations concerning the cause or causes of ADHD have proliferated in recent years, ranging from brain-based mechanisms to environmental toxins. Although definitive answers remain elusive, recent discoveries suggest several possible factors that may be related to the etiology of ADHD.

Environmental Toxins

A variety of environmental toxins and factors have been suggested as causal or contributing agents to the development of ADHD. The most popular of these include lead (found in elevated levels in the blood), food additives (particularly salicylates, food dyes, and preservatives), sugar, cigarette smoking or alcohol consumption by the mother during pregnancy, and exposure to cool-white fluorescent lighting or radioactive rays emitted from televisions. Although comprehensive coverage of these topics is beyond the scope of this chapter, it is worthwhile to point out that none of the environmental agents have received empirical support as important contributing factors to the development of ADHD in the majority of children.

Neurological and Neurophysiological Factors

Results of routine neurological examinations are usually found to be normal in children with ADHD. Research investigating the presence of neuromaturational signs has been equivocal but generally suggests either nonspecific or no increased frequency of soft signs in this population. Also, as noted previously, the overwhelming majority of children with ADHD do not have histories of brain injury or damage. More recent studies using advanced brain scanning techniques, such as computed tomography (CT) scan analysis, have also failed to reveal differences in brain structure, although preliminary findings using the higher-resolution magnetic resonance imaging (MRI) have been conflicting.

Neurochemical abnormalities, particularly those involving the monoamines, comprising the catecholamines (dopamine and norepinephrine) and the indoleamine, serotonin, have been implicated as potential contributing factors in the pathophysiology of ADHD. The evidence to date remains speculative but suggests a possible selective deficiency in the availability of dopamine and/or norepinephrine.

More promising results have emerged in three recent studies. Lou (1990), using single photon emission computed tomography (SPECT) to measure cerebral blood flow, reported hypoperfusion (reduced) and low neural activity in the striatal and orbital prefrontal regions of children with ADHD, compared with controls, whereas the primary sensory and sensorimotor regions were hyperperfused (overly active). Ongoing studies by Satterfield (1990), using EEG brain electrical activity mapping (BEAM) techniques, have been relatively consistent with Lou's findings in showing abnormality in information processing in the frontal lobes of children with ADHD. Finally, Zametkin et al. (1990), in studying adults who had been hyperactive since childhood, reported reduced glucose metabolism in various areas of the brain, particularly the premotor and superior prefrontal regions—areas known to be associated with the regulation of attention, motor activity, and information processing.

Collectively, these findings implicate a central nervous system mechanism in the development of ADHD, most likely involving connections between the prefrontal areas and the limbic system. The findings are also consistent with speculations concerning a possible selective deficiency in the availability of dopamine and/or norepinephrine. Prefrontal–limbic connections are known to contain relatively high amounts of these neurotransmitters, psychostimulants (the primary pharmacological treatment for children with ADHD) are known agonists of these systems, and the brain areas implicated are thought to underlie several aspects of inattention, behavioral inhibition (impulsivity, executive planning abilities), emotion, and learning. Overall, the findings move us closer to understanding both the pathogenesis and treatment response of children with ADHD.

Genetic Factors and Family Studies

The role of hereditary transmission of ADHD has been investigated in several studies over the past 30 years. Unfortunately, the bulk of this research is uninterpretable because of numerous methodological problems and poorly defined diagnostic groups of children. There are, however, twin studies conducted more recently that indicate a significantly greater concordance for hyperactive symptoms between identical than between fraternal twins, with heritability of ADHD estimated to be 30 to 50%. Thus, genetic factors are likely to play an important role in the development of ADHD, but must be accounted for by something other than a direct genetic model of transmission.

Studies examining the families of children with ADHD represent yet another avenue of inquiry concerning the inheritability of the disorder. Although one cannot completely separate the role of genetics from that of deviant child rearing practices, family studies generally find a significantly higher incidence of ADHD in both the siblings and parents of children with ADHD—especially when both parents have a history of the disorder.

In summary, ADHD is most likely a genetically transmitted condition, the symptomatology of which may be diminished or exacerbated by prevailing environmental conditions. There is also some evidence to indicate that different etiological factors involving pregnancy, birth complications, exposure to lead or drugs, and a variety of central nervous system insults may be the primary culprit in a small subset of these children. The majority, however, have probably inherited the disorder through some yet unknown mechanism, with resulting underactivity of the prefrontal–striatal–limbic regions of the brain.

DIAGNOSTIC CONSIDERATIONS

Diagnosing ADHD represents one of the most difficult endeavors for mental health practitioners. Although a variety of clinic-based laboratory tests (e.g.,

Continuous Performance Test, Matching Familiar Figures Test, specific subtest configurations of intelligence batteries) have been touted as useful diagnostic tools, none has been shown to differentiate children with ADHD from other common pathological conditions of childhood with an acceptable degree of accuracy (Barkley, 1991). Detailed information concerning the child's pre-, peri-, and postnatal history, medical, developmental, and educational history, and family functioning must be obtained—preferably using one of the recently developed structured or semistructured clinical interviews. Onset and course of symptomatology are also essential to the differential diagnostic process, as well as extensive consideration of alternative and/or other existing psychopathological and medical conditions. A variety of broad-band and narrow-band behavior rating scales have been standardized in recent years to help quantify the nature and severity of behavioral disability. They should be used judiciously (see Barkley, 1990; Rapport, in press, for a comprehensive review of assessment of ADHD). Finally, several clinic-based, computerized instruments and observational techniques are currently being evaluated for their sensitivity and specificity in diagnosing ADHD and differentiating it from other forms of childhood psychopathology, but await empirical testing.

SUMMARY

Attention-deficit hyperactivity disorder is considered to be one of the most serious and enigmatic disorders of childhood for which there is no known cure. Our current understanding of ADHD suggests that it is a complex and chronic disorder of brain, behavior, and development, with behavioral and cognitive consequences that pervade multiple areas of functioning.

In the first section of this chapter, ADHD was described and discussed from an historical perspective. The second and third sections, respectively, reviewed recent epidemiological findings and described the clinical picture usually associated with the disorder. In the fourth section, the developmental course associated with ADHD was presented, beginning in early childhood and continuing through adulthood. Etiological, familial, and genetic factors associated with the disorder were described in the ensuing section, followed by a brief summary of diagnostic considerations.

REFERENCES

American Psychiatric Association (1987). *Diagnostic and statistical manual of mental disorders* (3rd ed., rev.). Washington, DC: Author.
American Psychiatric Association (1993). *DSM-IV draft criteria*. Washington, DC: Author.
Barkley, R. A. (1990). *Attention-deficit hyperactivity disorder: A handbook for diagnosis and treatment*. New York: The Guilford Press.
Barkley, R. A. (1991). The ecological validity of laboratory and analogue assessment methods of ADHD symptoms. *Journal of Abnormal Child Psychology, 19*, 149–178.
Campbell, S. B. (1990). *Behavior problems in preschoolers: Clinical and developmental issues*. New York: The Guilford Press.
Douglas, V. I. (1980). Higher mental processes in hyperactive children: Implications for training. In R. Knights & D. Bakker (Eds.), *Treatment of hyperactive and learning disordered children* (pp. 65–92). Baltimore: University Park Press.

DuPaul, G. J., Rapport, M. D., & Perriello, L. M. (1991). Teacher ratings of academic skills: The development of the Academic Performance Rating Scale. *School Psychology Review, 20*, 284–300.

Gittelman, R., Mannuzza, S., Shenker, R., & Bonagura, N. (1985). Hyperactive boys almost grown up. *Archives of General Psychiatry, 42*, 937–947.

Hinshaw, S. P. (1987). On the distinction between attentional deficits/hyperactivity and conduct problems/aggression in child psychopathology. *Psychological Bulletin, 101*, 443–463.

Hoza, B., Pelham, W. E., Sams, S. E., & Carlson, C. (1992). An examination of the "dosage" effects of both behavior therapy and methylphenidate on the classroom performance of two ADHD children. *Behavior Modification, 16*, 164–192.

Kinsbourne, M., & Swanson, J. M. (1979). Models of hyperactivity: Implications for diagnosis and treatment. In R. L. Trites (Ed.), *Hyperactivity in children: Etiology, measurement and treatment implications* (pp. 1–20). Baltimore: University Park Press.

Lahey, B. B., Carlson, C. L., & Frick, P. J. (in press). Attention-deficit disorder without hyperactivity: A review of research relevant to DSM-IV. In T. A. Widiger, A. J. Frances, H. A. Pincus, W. Davis, & M. First (Eds.), *DSM-IV sourcebook, Volume I*. Washington, DC: American Psychiatric Press.

Lou, H. C. (1990). Methylphenidate reversible hypoperfusion of striatal regions in ADHD. In K. Conners & M. Kinsbourne (Eds.), *Attention-deficit hyperactivity disorder: ADHD; clinical, experimental and demographic issues* (pp. 137–148). Munich, Germany: MMV Medizin Verlag.

Orvaschel, H., Puig-Antich, J., Chambers, L. W., Tabrizi, M. A., & Johnson, R. A. (1982). Retrospective assessment of prepubertal major depression with the Kiddie-SADS-E. *Journal of the American Academic of Child and Adolescent Psychiatry, 21*, 392–397.

Palfrey, J. S., Levine, M. D., Walker, D. K., & Sullivan, M. (1985). The emergence of attention deficits in early childhood: A prospective study. *Developmental and Behavioral Pediatrics, 6*, 339–348.

Rapport, M. D. (1990). Controlled studies of the effects of psychostimulants on children's functioning in clinic and classroom settings. In K. Conners & M. Kinsbourne (Eds.), *Attention-deficit hyperactivity disorder: ADHD; clinical, experimental and demographic issues* (pp. 77–111). Munich, Germany: MMV Medizin Verlag.

Rapport, M. D. (1993). Attention-deficit hyperactivity disorder. In T. H. Ollendick & M. Hersen (Eds.), *Handbook of Child and Adolescent Assessment* (pp. 269–291). Boston, MA: Allyn and Baron.

Rapport, M. D., Murphy, H. A., & Bailey, J. S. (1982). Ritalin vs response cost in the control of hyperactive children: A within-subject comparison. *Journal of Applied Behavior Analysis, 15*, 205–216.

Rapport, M. D., & Kelly, K. L. (1991). Psychostimulant effects on learning and cognitive function: Findings and implications for children with attention-deficit hyperactivity disorder. *Clinical Psychology Review, 11*, 61–92.

Satterfield, J. H. (1990). BEAM studies in ADD boys. In K. Conners & M. Kinsbourne (Eds.), *Attention-deficit hyperactivity disorder: ADHD; clinical, experimental and demographic issues* (pp. 127–136). Munich, Germany: MMV Medizin Verlag.

Still, G. F. (1902). The Coulstonian lectures on some abnormal physical conditions in children. *Lancet, 1*, 1008–1012, 1077–1082, 1163–1168.

Weiss, G., & Hechtman, L. (1986). *Hyperactive children grown up*. New York: The Guilford Press.

Werry, J., Sprague, R., & Cohen, M. (1975). Conners Teacher Rating Scale for use in drug studies with children—An empirical study. *Journal of Abnormal Child Psychology, 3*, 217–229.

Zametkin, A. J., Nordahl, T. E., Gross, M., King, A. C., Semple, W. E., Rumsey, J., Hamburger, S., & Cohen, R. M. (1990). Cerebral glucose metabolism in adults with hyperactivity of childhood onset. *The New England Journal of Medicine, 323*, 1361–1366.

10

Conduct Disorder

Marc S. Atkins and Kim Brown

Description of the Disorder

There are many types of conduct problems in children and, as will be noted in this chapter, many factors that impact on the course and outcome of childhood conduct problems. Aggressive behavior, perhaps the most visible of childhood conduct problems, is, in itself, only moderately associated with later antisocial behavior. However, in combination with other behaviors, such as hyperactivity, lying and stealing, and poor peer relations, childhood aggression is clearly and strongly associated with problems in adolescence and adulthood. In fact, this is the case with all factors that contribute to the onset and maintenance of conduct problems. Specifically, this chapter will describe efforts to consider conduct problems in the context of home, school, and peer activities and relationships, and the complex interactions that result.

Conduct disorder is defined in the latest revision of the *Diagnostic and Statistical Manual of Mental Disorders* (DSM-IV) (American Psychiatric Association, 1993) as a "repetitive and persistent pattern of behavior in which either the basic rights of others or major age-appropriate societal norms or rules are violated" (p. E:10). Two distinct types of conduct disorder are defined in DSM-IV: *Childhood onset type* in which at least one conduct problem has been evident prior to age 10, and *Adolescent onset type* in which no conduct problems were evident prior to age 10. Severity of the disorder is also noted as *mild* if there are "few if any conduct problems in excess of those required to make the diagnosis *and* conduct problems cause only minor harm to others" (p. E:11), *moderate* if the "number of problems and effect on others (is) intermediate between 'mild' and 'severe'" (p. E:11), and *severe* if there are "many

Marc S. Atkins and Kim Brown • Children's Seashore House, and University of Pennsylvania School of Medicine, Philadelphia, Pennsylvania 19104.

Advanced Abnormal Psychology, edited by Vincent B. Van Hasselt and Michel Hersen. Plenum Press, New York, 1994.

conduct problems in excess of those required to make the diagnosis, *or* conduct problems cause considerable harm to others, e.g., serious physical injury to victims, extensive vandalism or theft" (p. E:11).

Overt versus Covert Antisocial Behavior

In an extensive review of studies examining childhood antisocial behavior, Loeber and Schmaling (1985a) summarized these findings on a dimension of antisocial behavior ranging from *overt* or confrontative aggression (e.g., fighting, temper tantrums) to *covert* antisocial behavior that occurs outside direct supervision (e.g., theft, truancy, and drug use). In a separate study, Loeber and Schmaling (1985b) described three mutually exclusive subtypes of antisocial behavior: Exclusive Fighter Group (those who fought, but did not steal), Exclusive Theft Group (those who stole, but did not fight), and Versatile Antisocial Group (those who stole and fought).

The validity of this classification was demonstrated through differential relationships with a variety of outcome variables. Early onset of overt behaviors (e.g., aggression, noncompliance), though associated with severity of symptoms (Tolan, 1987), was not highly predictive of long-term outcome. In contrast, early covert activity was strongly associated with worse prognosis (Loeber, 1985). In addition, the versatile antisocial group displayed higher rates of specific types of both covert (e.g., drug use, lying, truancy) and overt (e.g., disobedience, irritability, negativism) antisocial behaviors and, as expected, had the poorest long-term prognosis as compared to the other two groups (Loeber et al., 1985b).

EPIDEMIOLOGY

Conduct disorder is the most common reason for child referrals to mental health clinics. The incidence of conduct disorder within the general population ranges from 3 to 7% for 10-year-old males (Robins, 1991). Discrepancies in the prevalence rate may be due to the absence of explicit diagnostic criteria and to the subjective nature of the assessment measures used. The disorder occurs approximately three times more frequently in males than in females. Surveys of adolescents indicate that approximately 50% admit to theft, 35% admit to assault, 45% admit to property destruction, and as many as 60% admit to engaging in multiple antisocial acts (Kazdin, 1987). Long-term follow-up studies indicate that antisocial behavior is stable over time and across generations with poor long-term prognosis (Loeber, 1991).

CLINICAL PICTURE

John was a 12-year-old male who was seen in an outpatient child psychology clinic for assessment and treatment of a variety of behavior problems including lying, physical aggression toward peers, bullying, noncompliance with adult requests, and poor peer relations. He was described by teachers as being "very bright," but he refused to complete school assignments. Interviews with John, his father, and his teachers revealed extremely high rates of both covert and overt antisocial behaviors by all respondents. His teachers reported that peers described John as being "scary and mean." When unsupervised, he frequently made sexually explicit remarks and gestures to girls in his class and appeared to enjoy the discomfort and fear that resulted. He also was observed to follow students home while threatening to beat them up, and he was observed to abuse neighbors' pets.

John's teachers described him as "sneaky and manipulative." They stated that they rarely caught him acting inappropriately but were constantly hearing from the other students about his aggressive behavior. John's antisocial behavior occurred almost exclusively in unsupervised and unstructured settings, such as on the bus, in the lunch room, and in the boys' bathroom. These impressions were consistent with observational data. For example, while in the hallway during the change of classes, John was observed shoving several students against the wall. During a classroom observation, John was well behaved when supervised; however, as soon as his teacher turned away, he was seen striking a peer.

John's family history included his parents' divorce and a subsequent separation from his mother at 4 years of age. Following the divorce, John was sent to live with his mother, but was returned to his father because of unmanageable behavior. All contact between John and his mother terminated at that time. John's father and stepmother stated that they were unable to control his behavior. They said they attempted to ignore small infractions, while severely punishing more extreme behaviors. Both parents stated that they "blow up" in anger, and have occasionally used harsh physical punishment.

In contrast to John's behavior, which appeared to be coercive and goal directed, Matt's behavior was characterized by an overreactive, impulsive quality. According to his fourth grade teacher, he was a "nice boy" but seemed to "explode" at peers and adults for no good reason. At times Matt's temper outbursts were uncontrollable, and physical restraint was necessary to prevent injury to others. Although educational testing indicated average intelligence, his classroom performance suffered because of his inattention and impulsivity. In addition to his conduct problems, he also met diagnostic criteria for attention-deficit hyperactivity disorder and was prescribed stimulant medication (Ritalin® by CIBA Pharmaceutical Corp.) by his pediatrician.

Peers reported that Matt refused to follow rules when playing games at recess, and that he seemed to cry frequently when he was corrected or didn't get his way. During an observation, he became angry when a student walking down the classroom aisle appeared to bump him accidentally. When the teacher refused to punish the other student, Matt became visibly upset, disrupted the class by shouting, "You never yell at anyone but me," and directed a threat to the other student.

As in John's family history, Matt's parents were divorced before he began school. Matt and his three brothers lived with their father. Their father worked evenings and was therefore often unable to monitor closely his children's behavior. Following several reports of extreme physical punishment, school personnel referred Matt's father for counseling and parent management classes.

Course and Prognosis

There is considerable evidence for the stability of aggressive and antisocial behavior (Loeber, 1991). Nevertheless, most aggressive children do not grow up to be antisocial adults. In fact, it is pre-adolescent *covert* antisocial activities, such as lying, stealing, and truancy, which are predictive of adolescent delinquency rather than aggression, although, as noted previously, it is the occurrence of both which is most predictive of long-term problems (Loeber, 1991). In general, the greater the variety of antisocial behavior, the more varied the settings in which it occurs, and the earlier the onset, the greater the likelihood for adult antisocial behavior (Loeber, 1991).

Poverty is strongly related to pre-adolescent conduct disorder, whereas conduct disorder in adolescence occurs irrespective of family income (Offord, Boyle, & Racine, 1991). Other significant risk factors for childhood conduct disorder are level of family support, marital adjustment of parents, social stress, and parental alcoholism and criminal activity (Farrington, 1991; Tolan, 1988). However, as will be explained later, these are most predictive in tandem rather than in isolation.

Peer Relations

There is a large body of research that demonstrates that social competency is a core deficit for many aggressive children (Coie, Belding, & Underwood, 1988). As compared to nonaggressive children, peer-rejected, aggressive children perceive more hostile intentions from others in ambiguous situations, minimize their perceptions of their own aggressiveness, and exaggerate the aggressiveness of peers (Dodge, Pettit, McClaskey, & Brown, 1986). These social information processing deficits form the basis of a subtyping model distinguishing proactive aggression (e.g., bullying) from reactive aggression (e.g., overreaction to provocation), the latter involving the most severe social cognitive deficits (Dodge & Coie, 1987). In a recent evaluation of this model in a population of juvenile offenders, reactive aggression was associated with aggression toward persons and violent antisocial acts, mediated by deficits in social problem solving. In contrast, proactive aggression correlated more highly with nonviolent crimes and socialized aggression (Dodge, Price, Bachorowski, & Newman, 1990).

Academic Dysfunction

Additional factors impacting on the course and severity of conduct problems involve learning problems and cognitive deficits. Longitudinal investigations revealed that delinquent adolescents had significantly lower IQs in early childhood than nondelinquents (Moffitt & Silva, 1988; White, Moffitt, & Silva, 1989). In addition, high IQ in boys was protective for the development of delinquency, even for those who were at risk by virtue of parental history of antisocial behavior (White et al., 1989). The protection provided by IQ may be related to long-term prospects for school success and the subsequent avoidance of early dropout and delinquency (Feshbach & Price, 1984).

Developmental Pathways

Loeber (1985) has proposed three distinct developmental pathways resulting in delinquency and/or drug use. The *aggressive/versatile* progression begins early in life (e.g., during preschool years) and is characterized by overt aggressive behaviors and noncompliance. At a later age, covert behaviors appear and are followed by violent delinquent acts. The *nonaggressive antisocial* path emerges later in childhood and includes covert nonaggressive behaviors (e.g., lying and stealing). These behaviors are followed by delinquent property offenses. The third developmental path, *exclusive substance abuse*, begins during middle to late adolescence and has no demonstrated history of delinquency or aggression. Recent data indicate that youths in the third developmental path may be experimenting with antisocial activities and are least likely to maintain their antisocial acts into adulthood (Moffitt, 1990). (See Table 1.)

FAMILIAL AND GENETIC PATTERNS

Heredity of Antisocial Behavior

The intractability of antisocial behavior suggests a genetic basis to this constellation of behaviors, although there is dispute as to the strength of this relationship. Several sources of information are used to support the heredity of antisocial behavior. *Family history* is a clear determinant of antisocial behavior in offspring; however, this may be confounded by the social learning occurring in families (Brennan, Mednick, & Kandel, 1991). That is, a history of parental antisocial behavior may suggest a genetic transmission of conduct problems, or the influence of aggressive modeling provided by antisocial parents, or the impact of adult psychopathy on family functioning. In fact, all three are plausible explanations of increased antisocial behavior in offspring and may operate concurrently.

A stronger test of the heredity of antisocial behavior is *twin studies* in which identical twins (MZ) are compared to nonidentical twins (DZ). Several studies have indicated a higher concordance of antisocial behavior among MZ than among DZ twins (Cloninger & Gottesman, 1987). However, MZ twins have a greater reciprocal influence on each other than do DZ twins. This has been shown to account for

TABLE 1. Important and Key Points: Description, Epidemiology, Course, and Prognosis

1. Psychiatric diagnostic criteria (DSM-IV) distinguish between *Childhood onset type* and *Adolescent onset type*, across three categories for severity: mild, moderate, or severe.
2. Children exhibiting both overt antisocial behaviors (e.g., fighting) and covert antisocial behaviors (stealing) had the highest rate of both types of antisocial behaviors and the poorest long-term outcome.
3. Preadolescent covert antisocial behaviors are more predictive of delinquency during adolescence than are overt antisocial behaviors, although it is the occurrence of both which is most predictive of long-term problems
4. Social competency is a core deficit for many aggressive children. Aggressive children who are rejected by peers exhibit social information processing deficits which form the basis of a subtyping model distinguishing proactive aggression (e.g., bullying) from reactive aggression (e.g., overreaction to provocation). Reactive aggression was found to be associated with violent antisocial acts whereas proactive aggression related to socialized aggression.
5. IQ and academic performance are protective for the development of delinquency, possibly by avoiding early school dropout and delinquency.
6. Loeber has described three pathways to antisocial behavior. *Aggressive/Versatile* has the earliest onset and the most extreme antisocial symptomatology. *Nonaggressive Antisocial* emerges later than the Aggressive/Versatile pathway and involves covert antisocial behaviors only. The third path, *Exclusive Substance Abuse*, begins during adolescence and usually does not continue to adulthood.

much of the concordance of later criminality, such that genetic influence appears significant but modest (Carey, 1992).

The third source of evidence for the genetic basis of antisocial behavior is *adoption studies*. In these investigations, the relationship between biological offspring is compared to the influence of the adopted family on the child, to provide independent assessments of genetic and social influences on behavior. Several studies have found a higher concordance of antisocial behavior for biological parent as opposed to adoptive parent (e.g., Brennan et al., 1991). For example, the proportion of adoptees with no convictions as adults significantly decreased from 87% for those whose biological parent had no convictions to 75% for those whose biological parent had three or more convictions (Brennan et al., 1991). However, as Cheyne (1991) notes, these results are limited to property offenses, not violent offenses, to cases in which the biological father had multiple convictions, and to male adoptees. In fact, a purely *biological* explanation might implicate violent acts more than property acts given the high rate of birth complications and minor physical anomalies for those convicted of violent acts (Brennan et al., 1991). Thus, at present, it appears that the genetic basis of antisocial behavior may be significant but modest, or specific to certain antisocial acts in the most extreme offenders. (See Table 2.)

Family Functioning

MATERNAL DEPRESSION

It is well documented that there is a higher rate of maternal depression in families with behavior-problem children than in families without such children (Mash & Johnston, 1990). Does this suggest that maternal depression causes childhood antisocial behavior? Or does antisocial behavior in children cause maternal depression? The answer is that both are probably true. Parents prone to depression are more likely than nondepressed parents to perceive their child negatively and, therefore, to act more negatively toward their child (Lovejoy, 1991). Alternatively, disruptive or aggressive children are often unresponsive to standard discipline. Thus, despite their best efforts, parents will often feel inadequate, frustrated, and depressed, even if they have no prior history of depression (Mash & Johnston, 1990). Indeed, a recent investigation has shown that college students consumed greater amounts of alcohol after viewing videotapes of hyperactive and noncompliant child behaviors (Lang, Pelham, Johnston, & Gerlernter, 1989)—a temptation quite familiar to beleaguered parents.

TABLE 2. Important and Key Points: Genetic Patterns

1. Family history is a clear determinant of antisocial behavior but is confounded by the social learning occurring in families.
2. A higher concordance of antisocial behavior is found in identical twins compared to nonidentical twins. However, after controlling for greater reciprocal influence in identical twins, the genetic influence on antisocial behavior appears modest.
3. Adoption studies suggest that the genetic basis of antisocial behavior may be specific to certain antisocial acts in the most extreme offenders.

Patterson (1982, 1986) has described a pattern of parent–child interactions that provides a "training ground" (Patterson, DeBaryshe, & Ramsey, 1989, p. 329) for teaching a child manipulative and aggressive behaviors. Patterson has shown that families with an aggressive child are characterized by patterns of interaction in which parental responses to an irritable and demanding child alternate between avoiding the child and punishing him harshly. Because in this scenario the child receives consistent attention only when he misbehaves, the child's inappropriate behaviors will continue and often escalate in response to the parent's ineffective management strategies. The parent responds to this by escalating the severity of the subsequent punishment, often to the point of physical punishment. This is doubly unfortunate because, in addition to being an inappropriate and ineffective response to the child's behavior, it is also a model for becoming aggressive when frustrated. Perhaps not unexpectedly, the incidence of parental physical abuse or neglect is strongly predictive of aggressive outcome in children (Dodge, Bates, & Pettit, 1990).

In support of Patterson's "coercive cycle" model, parents of children with conduct disorder often describe their child's early behavior as "irritable" and "uncooperative" (Robins, 1991). In addition, antisocial boys were significantly more likely to continue displaying disruptive behavior after being *mildly* punished than were nonaggressive boys, suggesting that these mild punishers were cues for the child to increase coercive behavior (Patterson, Dishion, & Bank, 1984). Furthermore, parents of aggressive children were twice as likely to respond negatively to their child's behavior and were seven times more likely to hit their child as were parents of nonaggressive children (Patterson, 1982).

Another important element in the coercive cycle is the failure of parents of aggressive children to monitor and supervise their children. This unwillingness or inability to supervise, paired with harsh punishment, is consistent with Patterson's view that parents of aggressive children tend initially to avoid setting limits, and ultimately respond harshly and ineffectively once the child has committed a transgression (Patterson & Stouthamer-Loeber, 1984). In addition, inadequate parental monitoring and supervision become an increasingly important predictor of poor outcome as the child reaches adolescence.

These qualitative differences in family processes also effect nonconflict interactions. For example, conduct-problem children have been shown to be significantly less likely than nonproblem children to be involved in positive interactions with their mothers (Gardner, 1987). This suggests that parents of aggressive children may be ineffective at establishing close emotional bonds with their child as well as ineffective at disciplining maladaptive behaviors. Furthermore, the impact of this coercive cycle often extends beyond the family, as coercive interchanges may become characteristic of the child's interactions with other adults and with peers in school and community settings (Patterson, 1986). (See Table 3.)

DIAGNOSTIC CONSIDERATIONS

Significant advances have evolved from the three latest revisions of DSM, the standard for psychiatric diagnoses in the United States (American Psychiatric

Association, 1980, 1987, 1993). The latest criteria in DSM-IV subsumes Conduct Disorder (CD) under the general rubric of Disruptive Behavior and Attention-deficit Disorders. Specific criteria differentiate between noncompliance and defiance toward authorities (Oppositional Defiant Disorder: ODD), and behavior that violates the rights of others, especially peers (Conduct Disorder: CD). As noted, CD is further subtyped according to whether these behaviors began prior to age 10 (Childhood onset type) or following age 10 (Adolescent onset type). Severity of the disorder is also noted as mild, moderate, or severe.

A diagnosis of CD is made when a youth has displayed a disturbance of conduct for at least 6 months and meets 3 of 15 criteria. As described previously, these criteria represent a wide range of behaviors in terms of symptomatology and severity (e.g., lying, physical cruelty, using a weapon). For youth age 18 or older, CD is not considered if criteria for Antisocial Personality Disorder are met. ODD is viewed as less severe than CD and is not considered if a diagnosis of CD is met. The ODD diagnosis is made when a disturbance of conduct is present for at least 6 months, and 4 of 8 criteria are met (e.g., loses temper, argues with adults, angry and resentful).

Although both CD and ODD criteria are more specific than past diagnostic criteria for these disorders, and were derived from considerable field testing and empirical evaluations, several problems remain. First, it is not clear why overt and covert antisocial acts are combined in CD despite evidence for unique developmental pathways (Loeber, 1991). Second, ODD appears more closely related to Attention-deficit Hyperactivity Disorder than to CD, which argues against the mutual exclusivity of ODD and CD diagnoses (Reeves et al., 1987). Third, although the DSM-IV criteria appear to be superior to prior criteria in DSM-III and DSM-III-R, based on less ambiguous wording of core symptoms, results from the DSM-IV field trials are not yet available to determine interrater reliability (indicating level of agreement among independent diagnosticians) and the degree of independence of categories within the Disruptive Behavior and Attention-deficit Disorders. Low interrater reliability and high concurrence of items across categories plagued DSM-III and DSM-III-R diagnostic criteria for these disorders, which was a primary impetus to revise the criteria (Shaffer et al., 1993; Werry, Methven, Fitzpatrick, & Dixon, 1983). Fourth, as with the DSM-III and DSM-III-R criteria, DSM-IV criteria

TABLE 3. Important and Key Points: Family Functioning

1. Maternal depression and childhood antisocial behavior have reciprocal effects. Parents prone to depression are more likely than nondepressed parents to perceive their child negatively and to act more negatively toward their child. However, parenting a disruptive or aggressive child may also create feelings of inadequacy and frustration in parents.
2. Patterson describes a pattern of coercive parent–child interactions that provide a "training ground" for manipulative and aggressive behaviors. In this cycle, the child learns that the most effective means of getting attention is to act inappropriately, while the parent learns that the only way to stop these behaviors is to overreact and to respond severely to the child.
3. Another important element in the coercive cycle is the failure of parents of aggressive children to monitor and superivse their children. In addition, they also may be ineffective at establishing close emotional bonds with their children.
4. Coercive interchanges often become characteristic of the child's interactions with other adults and peers in school and community settings, thus interfering with academic and social tasks.

are specific but not operationalized. For example, it is not clear how to determine symptom presence or how to resolve differences across sources (e.g., parents and teachers). Especially important in its omission is the lack of specific measurement strategies and cut-off scores for diagnoses. Almost universally, the development of empirically derived, standardized, and explicit diagnostic criteria for childhood antisocial behavior has been advocated for both research and clinical practice (e.g., Quay, Routh, & Shapiro, 1987).

Psychiatric Co-Morbidity

ATTENTION-DEFICIT HYPERACTIVITY DISORDER

Another important issue in the diagnosis of CD is the co-occurrence of other disorders, referred to as co-morbidity. The most prominent concurrent diagnosis with conduct problems is Attention-deficit Hyperactivity Disorder (ADHD). Diagnostic overlap ranges from 30% to 60% depending upon age, sex, and primary symptoms (Szatmari, Boyle, & Offord, 1989). There is considerable evidence that hyperactive children with concurrent aggression represent a distinct subgroup of behavior disordered children (Hinshaw, 1987). For example, boys with co-occurring hyperactivity and delinquency had greater family dysfunction, lower intelligence, and worse school performance as compared to pure groups of hyperactive or delinquent boys (Moffitt, 1990). In addition, social competency may be a core deficit for aggressive/hyperactive boys, as evidenced by higher rates of social information processing biases and a greater risk for future peer problems as compared to boys who are hyperactive only (Johnston & Pelham, 1986; Milich & Dodge, 1984).

DEPRESSION

Another co-morbid factor for conduct problems is depression. Conduct disordered youth high on self-reported depression also reported higher rates of conduct problems and personality problems relative to conduct disordered youth low on depression (Nieminen & Matson, 1989). Surveys of assaultive youth indicate a more than fourfold increase in suicide incidence in this population relative to the general population (Cairns, Peterson, & Neckerman, 1988). As expected, aggressive youth who were suicidal were significantly more depressed than aggressive youth who

TABLE 4.   Important and Key Points: Diagnostic Considerations

1. Psychiatric diagnostic criteria presume that oppositional defiant behavior is a less severe form of conduct disorder, although empirical evaluations suggest that oppositional defiant disorder overlaps more strongly with attention-deficit hyperactivity disorder than with conduct disorder.
2. Problems with diagnostic criteria include low interrater reliability, overlap with other diagnoses, and lack of operationalized criteria.
3. There is considerable evidence that hyperactive/aggressive children represent a distinct subgroup of behavior disordered children with greater dysfunction and greater risk for future problems in social relations.
4. Conduct disordered youth high on self-reported depression had higher rates of conduct and personality problems. These youth are at increased risk of suicide and require careful monitoring.

were nonsuicidal (Pfeffer, Plutchik, & Mizruchi, 1983). Thus, youth who are both depressed *and* aggressive require careful monitoring including possible inpatient hospitalization to forestall the possibility of a suicide attempt. (See Table 4.)

SUMMARY

Childhood conduct problems, characterized by chronic patterns of societal norm violations, represent a serious and seemingly intractable mental health problem. Developmental pathways have been outlined for the multiple factors that impact the course and outcome of childhood conduct problems including type and severity of the problems, initial onset of symptoms, family history and family functioning, academic performance, and peer relations. At present, it is clear that there are multiple pathways to conduct disorder, based on the variety and extremity of antisocial behavior and on the complex interplay of biological and psychosocial factors.

Although much has been learned regarding factors impacting childhood conduct problems, it should be more than obvious that considerably more research is required. Specifically, given the multiplicity of problems and factors that impact long-term outcome, it is likely that future definitions will address specific types of conduct problems maintained by specific factors. The multiple pathways to antisocial behavior illustrate the complexity of childhood conduct disorder and emphasize the importance of considering single factors in the context of real-world concerns. Family, school, and friends each play an important and powerful role in eliciting or maintaining antisocial activities.

REFERENCES

American Psychiatric Association (1980). *Diagnostic and statistical manual of mental disorders*, 3rd Edition. Washington, DC: Author.

American Psychiatric Association (1987). *Diagnostic and statistical manual of mental disorders*, 3rd Edition, Revised. Washington, DC: Author.

American Psychiatric Association (1993). *DSM-IV draft criteria*. Washington, DC: Author.

Brennan, P., Mednick, S., & Kandel, E. (1991). Congenital determinants of violent and property offending. In D. J. Pepler, & K. H. Rubin (Eds.), *The development and treatment of childhood aggression* (pp. 81–92). Hillsdale, NJ: Lawrence Erlbaum.

Cairns, R. B., Peterson, G., & Neckerman, H. J. (1988). Suicidal behavior in aggressive adolescents. *Journal of Clinical Child Psychology, 17*, 298–309.

Carey, G. (1992). Twin imitation for antisocial behavior: Implications for genetic and family environment research. *Journal of Abnormal Psychology, 101*, 18–25.

Cheyne, A. (1991). Bad seeds and vile weeds: Metaphors of determinism. In D. J. Pepler, & K. H. Rubin (Eds.), *The development and treatment of childhood aggression* (pp. 121–136). Hillsdale, NJ: Lawrence Erlbaum.

Cloninger, C. R., & Gottesman, I. I. (1987). Genetic and environmental factors in antisocial behavior disorders. In S. Mednick, T. Moffitt, & S. Stack (Eds.), *The causes of crime: New biological approaches* (pp. 92–109). New York: Cambridge University Press.

Coie, J. D., Belding, M., & Underwood, M. (1988). Aggression and peer rejection in childhood. In B. B. Lahey & A. E. Kazdin (Eds.), *Advances in clinical child psychology* (Vol. 11, pp. 125–158). New York: Plenum.

Dodge, K. A., Bates, J. E., & Pettit, G. S. (1990). Mechanisms in the cycle of violence. *Science, 250*, 1678–1683.

Dodge, K. A., & Coie, J. D. (1987). Social information processing factors in reactive and proactive aggression in children's peer groups. *Journal of Personality and Social Psychology, 53,* 1146–1158.

Dodge, K. A., Pettit, G. S., McClaskey, C. L., & Brown, M. M. (1986). Social competence in children. *Monographs of the Society for Research in Child Development, 51,* (2, Serial No. 213).

Dodge, K. A., Price, J. M., Bachorowski, J., & Newman, J. P. (1990). Hostile attributional biases in severely aggressive adolescents. *Journal of Abnormal Psychology, 99,* 385–392.

Farrington, D. P. (1991). Childhood aggression and adult violence: Early precursors and later-life outcomes. In D. J. Pepler & K. H. Rubin (Eds.), *The development and treatment of childhood aggression* (pp. 31–54). Hillsdale, NJ: Lawrence Erlbaum.

Feshbach, S., & Price, J. (1984). Cognitive competencies and aggressive behavior: A developmental study. *Aggressive Behavior, 10,* 185–200.

Gardner, F. E. (1987). Positive interaction between mothers and conduct-problem children: Is there training for harmony as well as fighting? *Journal of Abnormal Child Psychology, 15,* 283–293.

Gardner, F. E. (1989). Inconsistent parenting: Is there evidence for a link with children's conduct problems? *Journal of Abnormal Child Psychology, 17,* 223–233.

Hinshaw, S. P. (1987). On the distinction between attentional deficits/hyperactivity and conduct problems/aggression in child psychopathology. *Psychological Bulletin, 101,* 443–463.

Johnston, C., & Pelham, W. E. (1986). Teacher ratings predict peer ratings of aggression at 3-year follow-up in boys with attention deficit disorder with hyperactivity. *Journal of Consulting and Clinical Psychology, 54,* 571–572.

Kazdin, A. E. (1987). *Conduct disorders in childhood and adolescence.* Newbury Park, CA: Sage Publications.

Lang, A., Pelham, W., Johnston, C., & Gerlernter, S. (1989). Levels of adult alcohol consumption induced by interactions with child confederates exhibiting normal versus externalizing behaviors. *Journal of Abnormal Psychology, 98,* 294–299.

Loeber, R. (1985). Patterns and development of antisocial child behavior. In G. J. Whitehurst (Ed.), *Annals of child development* (Vol. 3), pp. 77–116. Greenwich, CT: JAI Press.

Loeber, R. (1991). Antisocial behavior: More enduring than changeable? *Journal of the American Academy of Child and Adolescent Psychiatry, 30,* 393–397.

Loeber, R., & Schmaling, K. B. (1985a). The utility of differentiating between mixed and pure forms of antisocial child behavior. *Journal of Abnormal Child Psychology, 13,* 315–335.

Loeber, R., & Schmaling, K. B. (1985b). Empirical evidence for overt and covert patterns of antisocial conduct problems: A metaanalysis. *Journal of Abnormal Child Psychology, 13,* 337–353.

Lovejoy, M. C. (1991). Maternal depression: Effects on social cognition and behavior in parent–child interactions. *Journal of Abnormal Child Psychology, 19,* 693–706.

Mash, E. J., & Johnston, C. (1990). Determinants of parenting stress: Illustrations from families of hyperactive children and families of physically abused children. *Journal of Clinical Child Psychology, 19,* 313–328.

Milich, R., & Dodge, K. A. (1984). Social information processing in child psychiatric populations. *Journal of Abnormal Child Psychology, 12,* 241–490.

Moffitt, T. E. (1990). Juvenile delinquency and attention deficit disorder: Boys' developmental trajectories from age 3 to age 15. *Child Development, 61,* 893–910.

Moffitt, T. E., & Silva, P. A. (1988). IQ and delinquency: A direct test of the differential detection hypothesis. *Journal of Abnormal Psychology, 97,* 330–333.

Nieminen, G. S., & Matson, J. L. (1989). Depressive problems in conduct-disordered adolescents. *Journal of School Psychology, 27,* 175–188.

Offord, D. R., Boyle, M. H., & Racine, Y. A. (1991). The epidemiology of antisocial behavior in childhood and adolescence. In D. J. Pepler & K. H. Rubin (Eds.), *The development and treatment of childhood aggression* (pp. 31–54). Hillsdale, NJ: Lawrence Erlbaum.

Patterson, G. R. (1982). *Coercive family process.* Eugene, OR: Castilia.

Patterson, G. R. (1986). Performance models for antisocial boys. *American Psychologist, 41,* 432–444.

Patterson, G. R., DeBaryshe, D., & Ramsey, E. (1989). Developmental perspective on antisocial behavior. *American Psychologist, 44,* 239–335.

Patterson, G. R., Dishion, T. J., & Bank, L. (1984). Family interaction: A process model of deviancy training. *Aggressive Behavior, 10,* 253–267.

Patterson, G. R., & Stouthamer-Loeber, M. (1984). The correlation of family management practices and delinquency. *Child Development, 55,* 1299–1307.

Pfeffer, C. R., Plutchik, R., & Mizruchi, M. S. (1983). Suicidal and assaultive behavior in children: Classification, measurement, and interrelations. *American Journal of Psychiatry, 140,* 154–157.

Quay, H. C., Routh, D. K., & Shapiro, S. K. (1987). Psychopathology of childhood: From description to validation. *Annual Review of Psychology, 38*, 491–532.

Reeves, J. C., Werry, J. S., Elkind, G. S., & Zametkin, A. (1987). Attention deficit, conduct, oppositional, and anxiety disorders in children: II. Clinical characteristics. *Journal of the American Academy of Child and Adolescent Psychiatry, 26*, 144–155.

Robins, L. N. (1991). Conduct disorder. *Journal of Child Psychology and Psychiatry, 32*, 193–212.

Shaffer, D., Schwab-Stone, M., Fisher, P., Cohen, P., Piacentini, J., Davies, M., Conners, C. K., & Regier, D. A. (1993). The diagnostic interview schedule for children—Revised version (DISC-R): 1. Preparation, field testing, interrater reliability, and acceptability. *Journal of the American Academy of Child and Adolescent Psychiatry, 32*, 643–650.

Szatmari, P., Boyle, M., & Offord, D. R. (1989). ADHD and conduct disorder: Degree of diagnostic overlap and differences among correlates. *Journal of the American Academy of Child and Adolescent Psychiatry, 28*, 865–872.

Tolan, P. H. (1987). Implications of age of onset for delinquency risk. *Journal of Abnormal Child Psychology, 15*, 47–65.

Tolan, P. H. (1988). Socioeconomic, family, and social stress correlates of adolescent antisocial and delinquent behavior. *Journal of Abnormal Psychology, 16*, 317–331.

Werry, J. S., Methven, R. J., Fitzpatrick, J., & Dixon, H. (1983). The interrater reliability of DSM-III in children. *Journal of Abnormal Child Psychology, 11*, 341–354.

White, J. L., Moffitt, T. E., & Silva, P. A. (1989). A prospective replication of the protective effects of IQ in subjects at high risk for juvenile delinquency. *Journal of Consulting and Clinical Psychology, 57*, 719–724.

11

Anxiety Disorders

CYD C. STRAUSS

DESCRIPTION OF THE DISORDERS

Anxiety has been identified as one of the most common, if not the most prevalent, form of psychopathology in childhood and adolescence (Bernstein & Borchardt, 1991). Anxiety can be severe, distressing, and persistent in childhood. In addition, anxiety can interfere significantly with a youngster's adjustment in a range of areas, including school functioning, social adaptation, adjustment in the family, and self-perceptions.

Consequently, anxiety has increasingly become the focus of research and treatment efforts. In particular, research has demonstrated that anxiety can be assessed reliably using structured interviews (Last, Hersen, Kazdin, Finkelstein, & Strauss, 1987; Silverman & Nelles, 1988). The validity of the diagnostic category of anxiety disorders of childhood and adolescence as presented in the *Diagnostic and Statistical Manual of Mental Disorders*, Third Edition, Revised (DSM-III and DSM-III-R: American Psychiatric Association, 1980, 1987) also has been the subject of numerous investigations, with studies on epidemiology, correlates, developmental patterns, and family patterns associated with anxiety disorders. This chapter will present findings from these studies that describe the manifestation of anxiety disorders in childhood and adolescence.

The features of anxiety in childhood and adolescence resemble those found in adults, including physiological symptoms, covert feelings of distress and irrational thoughts, and overt behaviors, such as anxious mannerisms and avoidance behavior. DSM-III-R identifies three anxiety disorder subtypes that arise in childhood and adolescence: separation anxiety disorder, overanxious disorder, and avoidant disorder. Each anxiety disorder subtype is characterized by intense subjective

CYD C. STRAUSS • Center for Children and Families, Gainesville, Florida 32606.

Advanced Abnormal Psychology, edited by Vincent B. Van Hasselt and Michel Hersen. Plenum Press, New York, 1994.

distress and accompanied by maladaptive patterns of thinking and behavior. The specific focus of the anxiety or fear, however, varies for each of the three subcategories.

The first one, *separation anxiety disorder*, is characterized primarily by extreme worry and distress surrounding separation from a major attachment figure or home. There are nine DSM-III-R diagnostic criteria for this anxiety disorder subtype, namely: (1) worry about possible harm befalling major attachment figures or a fear that they will leave and not return; (2) worry that a calamitous event will separate the child from the attachment figure, such as his or her being kidnapped or becoming lost; (3) reluctance or refusal to go to school in order to stay with attachment figures or at home; (4) reluctance or refusal to go to sleep without being near the attachment figure, or to sleep away from home; (5) avoidance of being alone, including, for younger children, following attachment figures around the home, and, for older children, refusal to stay home alone; (6) repeated nightmares involving the theme of separation; (7) complaints of physical symptoms, such as headaches, stomachaches, or vomiting, on school days or in anticipation of separation; (8) excessive distress in anticipation of separation from home or major attachment figure(s); and (9) excessive distress when separated from home or attachment figure(s). Examples include calling parents frequently when away from them or wanting to return home prematurely when away from home. A child must demonstrate a minimum of *three* of these symptoms persistently and unrealistically to be diagnosed as having separation anxiety disorder.

A second anxiety disorder subtype, *overanxious disorder*, refers to generalized anxiety that is not focused on a specific object or situation. Instead, overanxious children are general "worriers." The hallmark of overanxious disorder is excessive or unrealistic worry about future events, which has been found to be characteristic of over 90% of a large sample of clinic children diagnosed with overanxious disorder (Strauss, Lease, Last, & Francis, 1988). Additional diagnostic criteria for overanxious disorder include: excessive concern about the appropriateness of past behavior, overconcern about competence in one or more areas (e.g., social, academic, athletic), somatic complaints, marked self-consciousness, excessive need for reassurance about a variety of concerns, and feelings of tension or an inability to relax. Children with overanxious disorder must show four or more of these symptoms for a period of 6 months or longer to meet the criteria for the disorder.

A child with *avoidant disorder* demonstrates excessive fearfulness and avoidance of social interactions with unfamiliar people. Such shyness interferes with the child's peer relationships. For shyness to be considered pathological in children, it needs to be consistent over time (i.e., a minimum of 6 months) and be present in numerous social settings. Avoidant children do show a desire for social involvement with familiar people, such as family members, in contrast to their discomfort with unfamiliar people.

In addition to these three anxiety disorder subtypes that first appear in childhood or adolescence, youngsters may also be diagnosed with any of the "anxiety disorders" presented as a separate category in the DSM classification system. These diagnoses include generalized anxiety disorder, phobic disorders, panic disorder with or without agoraphobia, obsessive–compulsive disorder, post-traumatic stress disorder, and anxiety disorders not otherwise specified.

Briefly, *generalized anxiety disorder* is characterized by excessive worrying for 6 months or longer, as well as symptoms of motor tension, autonomic hyperactivity, and vigilance and scanning when anxious. There is overlap between this diagnosis and overanxious disorder, but the somatic symptoms required for the generalized

12

Depression

NADINE J. KASLOW, KARLA J. DOEPKE,
AND GARY R. RACUSIN

DESCRIPTION OF THE DISORDER

Cases of despondency and depression in children and adolescents were reported as early as the seventeenth century, and reports on melancholia in youth began to appear by the middle of the nineteenth century. Prior to the 1970s, however, little attention was paid to the phenomenon of depression in children and adolescents. Such paucity of interest can be attributed to suppositions of the era's prevailing classical psychoanalytic theory, which precluded childhood depression due to children's immature superego development and lack of a stable self-concept. Other theorists postulated that children could not tolerate prolonged feelings of dysphoria and thus "masked" their depressive symptoms with myriad emotional and behavioral symptoms. The turning point in the mental health field occurred at the Fourth Congress of the Union of European Pedopsychiatrists held in 1970 in Stockholm, which focused on childhood and adolescent depressive states. These European pedopsychiatrists concluded that depression was a mental disorder found in a significant percentage of troubled children and adolescents and as such deserved study. Increased attention to childhood and adolescent depression in the United States dates back to Schulterbrandt and Raskin's (1977) book, *Depression in Childhood: Diagnosis, Treatment and Conceptual Models*, which detailed findings from a conference sponsored by the National Institute of Mental Health. This group of clinicians and researchers concurred with the European group's conclusion that depression in children and adolescents exists. Their work sparked

NADINE J. KASLOW AND KARLA J. DOEPKE • Department of Psychiatry and Behavioral Sciences, Emory University School of Medicine, Grady Memorial Hospital, Atlanta, Georgia 30335.   GARY R. RACUSIN • Connecticut Mental Health Center, Yale University, New Haven, Connecticut 06516.

Advanced Abnormal Psychology, edited by Vincent B. Van Hasselt and Michel Hersen. Plenum Press, New York, 1994.

research in the areas of diagnostic classification, assessment, description of depressive disorders, their psychosocial and neurobiological sequelae, and treatment outcome. Indeed, over the past 15 years there has been a proliferation of relevant theoretical, clinical, and empirical papers, and depression remains a major focus of child and adolescent psychopathology. This chapter summarizes pertinent literature describing depressive disorders in elementary school children and adolescents, their epidemiology and course, clinical picture, familial and genetic patterns, and diagnostic considerations.

The *Diagnostic and Statistical Manual of Mental Disorders*, Third Edition, Revised (DSM-III-R) (American Psychiatric Association, 1987) provides the standard criteria for diagnosing depression in children and adolescents. These criteria are identical to those of adult depressive disorders, although the DSM-III-R acknowledges age-specific features influencing presentation across the lifespan. A similar stance has been taken in the DSM-IV draft criteria (American Psychiatric Association, 1993). Although data exist supporting the utility of these diagnostic criteria for youth, reservations about the validity of these criteria for children and adolescents have been expressed by developmental psychopathologists (Carlson & Garber, 1986).

According to DSM-III-R and the DSM-IV draft criteria, a spectrum of depressive disorders can be diagnosed depending upon degree of severity and duration. First, major depressive disorder is diagnosed when a child or adolescent exhibits a change from previous functioning in at least five of the following nine symptoms over a single 2-week period: depressed or irritable mood, diminished interest or loss of pleasure in almost all activities (anhedonia), weight change or appetite disturbance, sleep disturbance, psychomotor agitation or retardation, fatigue or loss of energy (anergia), feelings of worthlessness or inappropriate guilt, decreased concentration or indecisiveness, and recurrent thoughts of death or suicidal ideation. At least one of the symptoms must be either a depressed or irritable mood, or anhedonia. According to DSM-III-R criteria, this symptom picture cannot be attributable to a medical condition or reflect the normal reaction to the death of a loved one. The DSM-IV draft criteria also note that this disturbance may not be due to the direct effects of a substance (e.g., drugs of abuse, medication).

Although infants do not manifest depressive symptoms as noted above, Spitz (1946) and Bowlby (1980) described institutionalized infants separated from their primary caretakers as being listless, withdrawn, and weepy, refusing to eat, and having disturbed sleep patterns. These authors termed this syndrome "anaclitic depression," and indeed similar symptom patterns can be observed today in infants separated from primary caretakers, infants who are chronically hospitalized for medical problems, and some infants whose primary caretakers are severely depressed. Age-specific features commonly manifested in depressed preschoolers include angry affect, uncooperativeness, apathy, and a lack of playfulness. The appearance of these symptoms for children in this age group often occurs in response to stressful life events. However, given that prior to age seven children do not use language to effectively communicate affective states, preschoolers are rarely diagnosed as depressed. Therefore, to reach this diagnosis, one must pay attention to children's nonverbal communication. In elementary school children, for instance, common manifestations of depression include depressed appearance, somatic complaints, agitation, separation anxiety, and phobias. Some elementary school children with severe depressions also exhibit mood-congruent auditory hallucinations. Depressed adolescents, on the other hand, exhibit a more classic picture of depression, which is often accompanied by affective lability (grouchiness, social withdrawal), inattention to personal appearance, extreme sensitivity to interpersonal rejection, and acting-out behaviors (negativism, aggression, antisocial behaviors, substance abuse, school problems) (Kutcher & Marton, 1989). Additionally, it is not uncommon for a depressed adolescent to express a dysphoric mood state via suicidal gestures or attempts. Indeed, a significant percentage of suicidal youth meet diagnostic criteria for depression.

For a major depressive episode to be diagnosed, no organic factors should have initiated or maintained the disturbance, and the disturbance must not reflect a normal reaction to the death of a loved one (uncomplicated bereavement). Additionally, the depressive episode should not be superimposed on a psychotic disorder. A major depressive episode may be rated according to severity (mild, moderate, severe), presence of psychotic features such as delusions or hallucinations (severe without psychotic features, severe with mood-congruent psychotic features, severe with mood-incongruent psychotic features), and remission status (not in remission, partial remission, full remission). It is also specified whether the episode is chronic or of the melancholic type.

Children and adolescents who manifest chronic depressive symptoms may meet diagnostic criteria for the second DSM-III-R or DSM-IV draft criteria depressive spectrum diagnosis, dysthymia, formerly termed depressive neurosis. Dysthymia is diagnosed when the child or adolescent exhibits a depressed or irritable mood persisting for a year or longer and is never symptom free for more than a 2-month period. In addition to a chronic depressed or irritable mood, two of the following symptoms must be present, according to DSM-III-R criteria: poor appetite or overeating, insomnia or hypersomnia, low energy or fatigue, low self-esteem, poor concentration or difficulty with decision making, or feelings of hopelessness. However, according to the DSM-IV draft criteria, in addition to chronic depressed or irritable mood, the child or adolescent must exhibit 3 of the following symptoms: low self-esteem, feelings of hopelessness, generalized loss of interest, social withdrawal, chronic fatigue, feelings of guilt, feelings of irritability or excessive anger, decreased productivity, or poor concentration. There must be no evidence of an unequivocal major depressive episode during the first year of the disturbance and no history for manic or hypomanic episodes, and the disorder must not be superimposed on an underlying organic condition or chronic psychotic disorder. Additionally, the DSM-IV draft criteria note that the condition is not due to the direct effects of a substance. For all children and adolescents, their dysthymic disorder is designated as early onset (prior to age 21).

The third, least serious form of a depressive disorder in youth is classified in DSM-III-R and the DSM-IV draft criteria as adjustment disorder with depressed mood. Consistent with the criteria for other adjustment disorders in DSM-III-R, an individual receives this diagnosis when depressed for no longer than 6 months in reaction to an identifiable psychosocial stressor or multiple stressors occurring less than 3 months prior to the onset of depressive symptoms. In such cases, the maladaptive nature of the depressive reaction is indicated by either impaired academic or social functioning, or symptoms exceeding normal, expectable reaction to the stressor(s). The symptom picture is not consistent with any other specific mental disorder and may not represent an uncomplicated bereavement.

Additionally, the DSM-IV draft criteria allow for the specification of acute (symptoms for less than 6 months) versus chronic (symptoms persist for 6 months or longer) adjustment disorders.

Although seasonal affective disorder has been receiving increasing attention as an adult diagnosis, only a few studies examined seasonal affective disorder in children and adolescents (e.g., Rosenthal et al., 1986). Seasonal affective disorder is a condition characterized by recurrent fall and winter depressions remitting (i.e., disappearing) during spring and summer. A seasonal pattern is reflected when there is a temporal relationship between a given 60-day period and the onset of an episode of a recurrent major depression or depressive disorder not otherwise specified. Full remissions of these depressive episodes must also occur within a 60-day period, and the individual must have experienced at least three episodes of mood disturbance in three separate years with at least two of the episodes occurring in consecutive years. Additionally, the seasonal episodes of the mood disturbance must outnumber the nonseasonal episodes by more than a 3:1 ratio. The characteristic symptom picture of seasonal affective disorder includes complaints of fatigue, oversleeping, overeating, and carbohydrate cravings, in addition to more typical depressive features. Some authors (e.g., Weller & Weller, 1991) have noted at least two reasons why seasonal affective disorders are difficult to diagnose in children. *First*, children experience a recurring universal stressor each fall as they begin a new school year. *Second*, due to their young age, many children fail to meet the diagnostic criteria because they have not experienced sufficient prior episodes.

The DSM-III-R also includes a diagnostic category entitled depressive disorder not otherwise specified (NOS). This category encompasses disorders with depressive features that do not meet the criteria for any specific mood disorder or adjustment disorder with depressed mood.

Over 50% of children and adolescents receiving a diagnosis of major depression or dysthymia also meet diagnostic criteria for at least one additional psychiatric disorder (Alessi & Magen, 1988). The presence of more than one diagnosis is termed psychiatric co-morbidity. The most prevalent co-morbid conditions are anxiety disorders and conduct disorders. Additional co-morbid conditions include attention–deficit hyperactivity disorder, eating disorders, obsessive–compulsive disorder, and specific developmental disorders (e.g., Alessi & Magen, 1988). Recently researchers have examined personality functioning in depressed adolescents (e.g., Marton et al., 1989) and have found that a significant percentage of these youth meet criteria for an Axis II personality disorder, most frequently borderline personality disorder. According to Kovacs (1985), such co-morbid disorders complicate the diagnostic and treatment process and may differentially effect the course of the disorders.

EPIDEMIOLOGY

The reported prevalence of depression in children and adolescents varies widely. Indeed, variation is a function of the heterogeneity of populations sampled (age, gender, setting), small sample sizes, inconsistencies in the types of instruments utilized, differences in the number and types of informants, shifting diagnostic criteria, and different methods of defining depression (symptom, syndrome, or disorder) (Fleming & Offord, 1990). To date, no large-scale epidemio-logical studies have been conducted with representative samples of children and adolescents for the explicit purpose of ascertaining prevalence of depressive disorders in youth. Until more methodologically sophisticated studies are undertaken, the extant epidemiological data must be viewed as only a partial picture.

Prevalence of depression increases with age (Angold, 1988). Kashani and Sherman (1988) reviewed prevalence of depression across the age range. Depression in preschoolers is very rare and has been estimated to have a prevalence of less than 1% in the general population. It should be noted, however, that these studies utilized primarily adult criteria for diagnosing depression, and it is conceivable that if more developmentally sensitive criteria are utilized the reported rates of depression in preschoolers may increase. Investigators have found a population prevalence of depression in elementary school children to be 2 to 5%. By mid-adolescence, there appears to be an increase in prevalence rates of major depressive disorder, and epidemiological studies have identified mid- and late adolescence as peak risk periods for the development of depression (e.g., Burke, Burke, Regier, & Rae, 1990). Specifically, in 14- to 16-year-olds, the prevalence rate has been found to be approximately 4 to 5%. Increased rates of depression in adolescents have been attributed to both the biological changes associated with the onset of puberty and differential socialization practices for males and females (e.g., Brooks-Gunn & Warren, 1989).

As opposed to these estimates of the general population, prevalence of depression has been found to be higher in special populations of children and adolescents (Stark, 1990). In clinical samples, prevalence rates have been estimated to be as high as 30% in outpatient clinics and 60% in inpatient psychiatric units. Higher rates of depression are also reported in children evaluated in an educational diagnostic center, children with chronic illnesses, and children whose parents are depressed.

A number of demographic variables appear to influence prevalence rates of mood disorders in youth. The above-noted finding that rates of depression increase with age is modified by an age-by-gender interaction. Specifically, prior to adolescence, there are no gender differences in rates of depression. In adolescence, however, depression is significantly more prevalent in females than in males. Female adolescents report more depressive symptoms, self-consciousness, stressful life events, negative body image, rumination, and low self-esteem than do adolescent males (Allgood-Merten, Lewinsohn, & Hops, 1990; Gjerde, Block, & Block, 1988). By contrast, adolescent males who are dysthymic evidence a more externalizing pattern of personality characteristics, as they are often viewed as disagreeable and antagonistic. This gender gap increases in adulthood.

Although scant relevant literature precludes definitive conclusions, some data suggest that youth from lower socioeconomic backgrounds exhibit more depressive symptomatology than do their counterparts from middle and upper class backgrounds. Moreover, although some studies have found no differences in prevalence of depression across racial groups, other studies have reported race-by-gender differences. Notably, higher rates of depression have been found in African American females than among their Caucasian and/or male peers. Thus, some evidence suggests greater risk for depression among youth residing in socially disadvantaged environments characterized by poverty, lack of adequate resources, and oppression of minorities. Finally, family environment impacts on depression rates (Angold, 1988; Fleming & Offord, 1990), with greater vulnerability to childhood depression associated with parental psychopathology, families in which loss and/ or discord prevail, and significant negative life stressors.

CLINICAL PICTURE

Case Vignette

Ned (not his real name) is an 11-year-old, Caucasian male whose parents recently contacted one of the authors (NJK) regarding their concerns about his mood and behavior following their announcement 8 months earlier of their marital separation and impending divorce. At the initial interview, the parents reported that Ned had become increasingly socially withdrawn and less involved with music and scholastic activities. They stated that this was a significant change from his previous level of functioning, in which he was a popular child who did extremely well in school and excelled in playing the violin. His parents also commented that he seemed sad and unhappy nearly every day, regardless of daily events. He grew profoundly depressed with increased tension between his parents. Reports from Ned's teachers revealed that while his academic performance remained above average, he no longer evidenced enthusiasm about learning and was considerably less active in class and with his peers. At his initial meeting with the clinician, Ned appeared sad and intermittently tearful, made little eye contact, had dull eyes (lacked a gleam in his eyes) and hunched shoulders, spoke quietly and slowly without animation, and moved slowly.

Although Ned's parents and teachers reported that he usually possessed a good sense of humor and was quite playful interpersonally, during initial sessions he appeared to lack a sense of humor and rarely smiled or laughed. In addition to acknowledging feeling unhappy, Ned reported somatic complaints (e.g., headaches) and said that he never felt energetic, but denied other common depressive symptoms, such as stomach aches and sleep or appetite disturbance. He described himself as bored with his friends, and appeared apathetic about scholastic and musical endeavors. The content of his verbal communications revealed a lack of enjoyment in activities typically considered fun by his peers, low self-esteem, and feelings of worthlessness. It was not uncommon to hear him say: "I'm not very smart. I'm ugly. Nobody really likes me. My parents are so wrapped up in their own problems, I'm not sure if they love me." Ned's feelings of helplessness were evidenced both in his reluctance to take initiative and in such verbalizations as: "Why should I bother trying, it doesn't matter what I do. I can never do it good enough." He often communicated his feelings of hopelessness in such statements as, "Things will never get better for our family." He denied, however, any suicidal ideation, attempts, or plans. When meeting with Ned, the therapist often found herself feeling sad, drained of energy, and, at times, helpless. Thus, while she felt considerable empathy for his distress, she often found herself feeling powerless to help him effect change in his life. Concurrent individual and family therapy were recommended in order to help the family cope more effectively with changes associated with divorce and to enable Ned to discuss aspects of the family situation that he found particularly upsetting. Based upon information gleaned from Ned's self-report, from other informants (e.g., parents, teachers), and from the therapist's observations, it appeared that he met DSM-III-R/DSM-IV criteria for major depression, single episode, of moderate severity, and without psychotic features. This diagnosis was based upon the duration of the episode, and the nature and severity of the symptoms.

Kaslow and Racusin (1990) and Racusin and Kaslow (1991) have presented an organizational strategy that more systematically captures the domains of functioning affected by depressive disorders in children and adolescents. These domains include psychological symptomatology and cognitive, affective, interpersonal, family, and adaptive behavior functioning. Using this schema we will highlight briefly depressed youths' functioning in the cognitive, affective, interpersonal, and adaptive behavior domains, and in the neurobiological domain as well. Psychological symptomatology already has been discussed in detail in the section describing depressive disorders in youth. Family functioning will be covered later in the section on familial and genetic patterns.

In terms of their cognitive functioning [for a detailed review, see Kaslow & Racusin (1990)], depressed children and adolescents display deficits in instrumental responding, manifested by a lack of motivation to correctly and efficiently complete tasks and suggesting their belief that their behavior cannot control environmental events. These motivational deficits, behavioral problems, and associated cognitions are typically manifested in feelings of helplessness. Compared to their nondepressed counterparts, depressed youth also have lower self-esteem and perceived competence, and feel more hopeless about their future. Further, these youth often evidence cognitive distortions, most notably a maladaptive attributional style. Specifically, they tend to blame themselves for negative events, and see the causes of these events as stable over time and generalizable across situations (internal-stable-global attributions for negative events). Simultaneously, depressed youth tend to believe and give credit to other people or circumstances for good events, and view the causes of these positive events as unstable over time and specific to the situation (external-unstable-specific attributions for positive events). For example, when a depressed child receives a poor grade on a test, it is not uncommon for that child to think: "I am really dumb." More adaptive attributions to this negative event typically held by nondepressed children may include: "I need to study more for the next test," "The teacher made a stupid test," or "I never was very good at math, but I'm good in other subjects." Further, depressed youth evidence deficits in self-monitoring, self-evaluation, and self-reinforcement. In particular, they are overly focused on negative events to the exclusion of positive events, more influenced by immediate rather than delayed consequences of their actions, set unrealistic expectations for their performance and feel badly about themselves when they fail to meet these standards, and engage in excessive self-punishment and insufficient self-reinforcement.

In the affective domain, depressed youth verbalize a pattern of emotional experiences similar to those reported by depressed adults. Specifically, depressed youth endorse high levels of sadness, anger, self-directed hostility, and shame (Blumberg & Izard, 1985). Nonverbally, as noted above, depressed youth, particularly those on an inpatient psychiatric service, show slow activity (latency, gestures, self movements), flat affect (intonation, facial expressiveness), and outward signs of sadness (e.g., tearfulness) (Kazdin, Sherick, Esveldt-Dawson, & Rancurello, 1985). However, investigators have noted less robust relationships between depression and nonverbal behavior for children than those noted for adults.

In the interpersonal sphere, depressed elementary school children are rated by peers and adults as less likable and attractive, as engaging in fewer positive behaviors, and as being in greater need of therapy than their nondepressed peers

(Mullins, Peterson, Wonderlich, & Reaven, 1986). Depressed youth exhibit relationship deficits with peers, parents, and siblings (e.g., Altmann & Gotlib, 1988; Puig-Antich et al., 1985a). Deficits in this domain tend to persist, even after the child or adolescent has recovered from a depressive episode (Puig-Antich et al., 1985b).

There are some data suggesting that depressed children and adolescents exhibit impairments in adaptive behavior, defined as activities in communication, socialization, and daily living skills. Depressed youth have impaired communication, as they are less verbal within the family system, with their peers, and with authority figures. They are also less able to assert their thoughts, feelings, and needs than are their nondepressed counterparts. As noted above, depressed youth also tend to have significantly impaired socialization. In the area of daily living skills, depressed youth exhibit insufficient attention to self-care and personal hygiene. However, it is interesting to note that psychiatrically hospitalized children with co-morbid mood/anxiety disorders and disruptive behavior disorders exhibit less impaired daily living skills than do youth hospitalized for disruptive behavior disorders (Woolston et al., 1989). It has been hypothesized that the presence of a mood or anxiety disorder tempers the daily living skill impairments associated with disruptive behavior, due to the children's desire to please others and the inhibition of acting-out behavior. These impairments are manifested across settings and relationships.

Finally, considerable strides have been made in the past decade in exploring psychobiological parameters of childhood depression [for a detailed review, see Burke & Puig-Antich (1990)]. Similar to what was reported for depressed adults, cortisol hypersecretion and dexamethasone nonsuppression have been reported in both prepubertal children and adolescents. Other biological markers that have been studied in adults, such as growth hormone secretion, only recently have been examined with children and adolescents. These initial studies suggest that depressed children have hyposecretion of growth hormone in response to an insulin challenge, and there appears to be hypersecretion of a growth hormone during sleep. Of particular interest is the finding that these irregularities in growth hormone secretion persist even upon recovery from the depressive episode. Similar to depressed adults, depressed youth have decreased urinary 3-methoxy-4-hydroxyphenylethyl glycol (MHPG) levels. This finding is consistent with the catecholamine theory of depression, which hypothesizes that norepinephrine levels are decreased in depressed individuals (Weller & Weller, 1991). There is considerable evidence of EEG sleep abnormalities in depressed adults, and thus a number of polysomnography studies have been conducted with depressed youth. These studies reveal virtually no abnormalities in EEG sleep parameters in depressed children prior to puberty. For adolescents, on the other hand, there is evidence of REM (rapid eye movement) abnormalities similar to those found in depressed adults. It has been hypothesized that lack of EEG sleep abnormalities in depressed prepubertal children may be attributed to maturational factors that modify the neuroregulation of the sleep cycle or the neurobiology of the initiation or maintenance of depressive episodes in individuals prior to puberty.

COURSE AND PROGNOSIS

Short-term follow-up and longitudinal studies reveal that children and adolescents diagnosed as depressed may have chronic depressions persisting over time,

and interaction style, yet fail to provide information about specific DSM-III-R symptoms. Each assessment type provides a different window into a child's depressive experience.

Multi-informant assessment refers to gathering information not only from the youth but also from others, such as parents, teachers, peers, and clinicians (Hoier & Kerr, 1988). This topic has received considerable attention in the childhood psychopathology literature during the past decade (e.g., Achenbach, McConaughy, & Howell, 1987), and underscores the need to gather information from multiple sources about multiple domains of functioning. Problematic interinformant agreement and contradictory findings regarding the assessment of depression in children and adolescents is an area of particular concern in the diagnostic process. Some researchers describe acceptable rates of agreement between parent and child reports of the child's depression, whereas others have found minimal correspondence in these reports. Many of the studies reveal that these children describe themselves as being more depressed than portrayed by their parents. However, the opposite trend has been found by other investigators. Kazdin (1988) has speculated that children may deny their depressive symptoms more often than their parents may and thus be more likely to under-report their distress on self-report inventories. The child's age and gender, the varying item content of scales given to different reporters, the nature of the youth's disorder, and the degree and type of parental psychopathology are all factors that appear to contribute to the discrepancy in parents' and children's reports. It is important to note that it is not necessarily the case that one informant is "right" and the other informant "wrong" about the child's psychological status. Rather, the discrepancy in reports may be indicative of the fact that depressed children present differently across settings and with various informants (Kaslow & Racusin, 1990). Initially, it was common practice to classify depressive disorders in youth based upon self-report on a single measure of depressive symptoms. Low correlations between self- and informant reports across types of assessment measures employed, and only moderate concurrence of symptoms across functional domains, have led investigators to utilize assessment batteries measuring a range of symptoms and multiple areas of functioning. This has been accomplished by using various techniques and information from a variety of informants (Kazdin, 1988).

In addition to questions about selection of assessment tools, and how and from whom information is gathered, the diagnosis of mood disorders in youth must take into consideration the demographics and social characteristics of the individual assessed. In particular, it is essential to conduct assessments within a developmental framework. As noted earlier in this chapter, the age of the youth assessed influences significantly the expression of depressive symptoms and of the disorder (Digdon & Gotlib, 1985). For example, a toddler crying relatively easily over a small incident may be considered an age-appropriate expression of distress, whereas this same behavior in an elementary school age child may be indicative of a dysphoric mood state. Age, however, is only one factor in considering a symptom potentially reflective of depression. The toddler who cries frequently may indeed be depressed if inconsolable or unable to play. Thus, labeling a given behavior as a symptom of depression must take into account developmental expressions of the behavior in both normal and depressed youth (Digdon & Gotlib, 1985).

Gender is another demographic variable that may influence the expression and subsequent diagnosis of a depressive disorder. For example, an early adolescent male who reports feeling helpless and behaves in a similar manner may be characterized more quickly as depressed than an early adolescent female who reports similar cognitions and expresses similar behaviors. In the adolescent girl, these cognitions and behaviors may be considered reflective of socialization factors that need to be "teased out" from actual symptoms of depression, whereas in the adolescent male a helpless stance is more readily considered a depressive symptom and generally not reflective of socialization practices.

A third group of demographic characteristics that may influence the manifestation and diagnosis of depressive disorders relates to racial, ethnic, or cultural backgrounds. In the past few years, investigators have begun to examine depression cross-culturally (e.g., Canada, Israel, New Zealand, Spain, Sweden, United States). Due to the paucity of research addressing this question, however, little is known regarding cross-cultural similarities or differences among children and adolescents. The extant data suggest that while there are similarities in the incidence of depressive symptoms cross-culturally, some salient differences in regard to symptom presentation have emerged. For example, Swedish adolescents who are depressed rate themselves as having more feelings of failure, unattractiveness, and self-accusation than do their American counterparts, who were assessed using the same instrument (Larsson & Melin, 1990). In a related vein, while the overall incidence of depression in African American youth appears comparable to that of their Caucasian peers, some researchers (e.g., Politano, Nelson, Evans, Sorenson, & Zeman, 1986) have found that depressed African American youth report less suicidality and dysphoric mood and more acting-out symptoms (e.g., oppositionality) than do their Caucasian peers. There also are some data suggesting that Hispanic American youth endorse significantly more depressive symptoms on a self-report measure than do their non-Hispanic Caucasian peers (Worchel et al., 1990).

Another variable that complicates a clear diagnosis of depressive disorders is physical illness. Some medically ill youth may present with neurovegetative difficulties (e.g., sleep and eating difficulties) and somatic complaints (e.g., stomach aches, headaches). For some of these individuals, such symptoms are indicative of the presence of a mood disorder, whereas for others the symptoms may be a reflection of the disease process or of the iatrogenic effects of medical treatments. Often, these symptoms signal presence of both psychological and physical difficulties. In order to appropriately diagnose mood disorders in medically ill children, a careful and individualized assessment must be conducted (Waller & Rush, 1983). It is not always the case that medically ill children endorse higher levels of symptoms associated with depression than those of their healthy peers. For example, children in whom cancer has been diagnosed often report less depression than do psychiatric patients or normal controls (e.g., Worchel et al., 1988); this is a possible reflection of denial of disease and distress as a coping mechanism.

As noted earlier, high incidence of comorbid depressive and other psychiatric disorders in children and adolescents complicates the diagnostic process. For example, a strong association of depressive disorders with anorexia nervosa and bulimia nervosa has received considerable attention (e.g., Swift, Andrews, & Barklage, 1986). Given that dysphoric mood, irritability, weight loss, sleep disturbance, diminished interest in sex, social withdrawal, and concentration difficulties are integral features of the starvation process and essential symptoms of a depressive syndrome, it is not surprising that the majority of anorexic patients meet diagnostic criteria for major depressive disorder. Presence of these symptoms, however, rather than being indicative of depression, may be more accurately an evidence of semistarvation syndrome. This particularly may be the case in those anorexic individuals who do not express feelings of worthlessness or self-reproach and who are not preoccupied with suicidal ideation or recurrent thoughts of death. Such latter thoughts, though typically observed in depressed patients, are not generally reported by women suffering from anorexia nervosa. Thus, while these individuals might technically meet DSM-III-R/DSM-IV criteria for major depressive disorder, other factors such as the psychobiological effects of starvation and the absence of self-deprecatory thoughts and suicidal ideation call into question a diagnosis of depression.

SUMMARY

Depression as a clinical syndrome can be observed in a significant percentage of children and adolescents in the general population and in a high percentage of clinical samples. Depression "runs in families" (Hammen, 1991), and thus, many depressed children have depressed parents. Although there are many parallels between child/adolescent and adult depression, the unique developmental characteristics of youth result in different manifestations of the disorder at earlier stages of the lifespan. When diagnosing a depressive disorder in a child or adolescent, a clinician must incorporate information obtained from a multitrait, multimethod, and multi-informant assessment. This approach enables the clinician to develop a comprehensive picture of the depressed child's functioning across varying domains. Domains in which depressed youth's functioning may be most impaired and which therefore deserve particular attention include psychological symptomatology, and cognitive, affective, interpersonal, family, adaptive behavior, and neurobiological functioning.

Depression in childhood can be a serious condition interfering with the child's development and functioning, with continued deficits even upon remission from a depressive episode. Depressions in children and adolescents tend to persist over time and to recur and thus necessitate treatment. The limited systematic treatment interventions conducted to date prove that some form of psychosocial or pharmacological treatment is better than no treatment at all in ameliorating depressive symptoms and improving the course of the disorder. Insufficient data preclude supporting the superiority of any given treatment, however, and further research is needed to develop and implement effective interventions.

REFERENCES

Achenbach, T. M., McConaughy, S. H., & Howell, C. T. (1987). Child/adolescent behavioral and emotional problems: Implications of cross-informant correlations for situational specificity. *Psychological Bulletin, 101*, 213–232.

Alessi, N. E., & Magen, J. (1988), Comorbidity of other psychiatric disturbances in depressed, psychiatrically hospitalized children. *American Journal of Psychiatry, 145*, 1582–1584.

Allgood-Merten, B., Lewinsohn, P. M., & Hops, H. (1990). Sex differences and adolescent depression. *Journal of Abnormal Psychology, 99*, 55–63.

Altmann, E. O., & Gotlib, I. H., (1988). The social behavior of depressed children: An observational study. *Journal of Child Psychology, 16*, 29–44.

Ambrosin, P. (1987). Pharmacotherapy in child and adolescent major depressive therapy disorder. In H. Y. Metzler (Ed.), *Psychopharmacology: The third generation of progress* (pp. 1247–1254). New York: Raven.

American Psychiatric Association (1987). *Diagnostic and statistical manual of mental disorders,* 3rd Edition, Revised. Washington, DC: Author.

American Psychiatric Association (1993). *DSM-IV draft criteria.* Washington, DC: Author.

Angold, A. (1988). Childhood and adolescent depression. I. Epidemiological and aetiological aspects. *British Journal of Psychiatry, 152*, 601–617.

Blumberg, S. H., & Izard, C. E., (1985). Affective and cognitive characteristics of depression in 10- and 11-year old children. *Journal of Personality and Social Psychology, 49*, 194–202.

Bowlby, J. (1980). *Attachment and loss: Vol. 3. Loss: Sadness and depression.* New York: Basic Books, Inc.

Brooks-Gunn, J., & Warren, M. P. (1989). Biological and social contributions to negative affect in young adolescent girls. *Child Development, 60*, 40–55.

Burke, K. C., Burke, J. D., Regier, D. A., & Rae, D. S. (1990). Age at onset of selected mental disorders in five community populations. *Archives of General Psychiatry, 47*, 511–518.

Burke, P., & Puig-Antich, J. (1990). Psychobiology of childhood depression. In M. Lewis & S.M. Miller (Eds.), *Handbook of developmental psychopathology* (pp. 327–339). New York: Plenum Press.

Butler, L., Miezitis, S., Friedman, R., & Cole, E. (1980). The effect of two school-based intervention programs on depressive symptoms in preadolescents. *American Educational Research Journal, 17*, 111–119.

Campbell, M., & Spencer, E. K. (1988). Psychopharmacology in child and adolescent psychiatry: A review of the past five years. *Journal of the American Academy of Child and Adolescent Psychiatry, 27*, 269–279.

Carlson, G. A., & Garber, J. (1986). Developmental issues in the classification of depression in children. In M. Rutter, C. E. Izard, & P. B. Read (Eds.), *Depression in young people* (pp. 399–434). New York: Guilford Press.

Digdon, N., & Gotlib, I. H. (1985). Developmental considerations in the study of childhood depression. *Developmental Reviews, 5*, 162–199.

Downey, G., & Coyne, J. C. (1990). Children of depressed parents: An integrative review. *Psychological Bulletin, 108*, 50–76.

Fine, S., Forth, A., Gilbert, M., & Haley, G. (1991). Group therapy for adolescent depressive disorder: A comparison of social skills and therapeutic support. *Journal of the American Academy of Child and Adolescent Psychiatry, 30*, 79–85.

Fleming, J. E., & Offord, D. R. (1990). Epidemiology of childhood depressive disorders: A critical review. *Journal of American Academy of Child and Adolescent Psychiatry, 29*, 571–580.

Gelfand, D. M., & Teti, D. M. (1990). The effects of maternal depression on children. *Clinical Psychology Review, 10*, 329–353.

Gjerde, P. F., Block, J., & Block, J. H. (1988). Depressive symptoms and personality during late adolescence: Gender differences in the externalization-internalization of symptom expression. *Journal of Abnormal Psychology, 97*, 475–486.

Hammen, C. (1991). *Depression runs in families: The social context of risk and resilience in children of depressed mothers.* New York: Springer-Verlag.

Hoier, T. S., & Kerr, M. M. (1988). Extrafamilial information sources in the study of childhood depression. *Journal of the American Academy of Child and Adolescent Psychiatry, 27*, 21–33.

Kahn, J. S., Kehle, T. J., Jenson, W. R., & Clarke, E. (1990). Comparison of cognitive-behavioral, relaxation, and self-modeling intervention for depression among middle-school students. *School Psychology Review, 19*, 195–210.

Kashani, J. H., & Sherman, D. D. (1988). Childhood depression: Epidemiology, etiological models, and treatment implications. *Integrative Psychiatry, 6*, 1–8.

Kaslow, N. J., & Racusin, G. R. (1990). Childhood depression: Current status and future directions. In A. S. Bellack, M. Hersen, & A. E. Kazdin (Eds.), *International handbook of behavior modification and therapy,* (2nd Ed., pp. 649–667). New York: Plenum.

Kaslow, N. J., & Rehm, L. P. (1991). Childhood depression. In R. Morris & T. R. Kratochwill (Eds.), *The practice of child therapy* (2nd ed., pp. 43–75). New York: Pergamon Press.

Kaslow, N. J., & Rehm, L. P., Pollack, S. L., & Siegel, A. W. (1990). Depression and perception of family functioning in children and their parents. *American Journal of Family Therapy, 18*, 227–235.

Kazdin, A. E. (1988). The diagnosis of childhood disorders: Assessment issues and strategies. *Behavioral Assessment, 10,* 67–94.

Kazdin, A. E., Sherick, R. B., Esveldt-Dawson, K., & Racurello, M. D. (1985). Nonverbal behavior and childhood depression. *Journal of American Academy of Child Psychiatry, 24,* 303–309.

Kovacs, M. (1985). The natural history and course of depressive disorders in childhood. *Psychiatric Annals, 15,* 387–389.

Kovacs, M. (1989). Affective disorders in children and adolescents. *American Psychologist, 44,* 209–215.

Kramer, A. D., & Feiguine, R. J. (1981). Clinical effects of amitriptyline in adolescent depression: A pilot study. *Journal of American Academy of Child Psychiatry, 20,* 636–644.

Kutcher, S. P., & Marton, P. (1989). Parameters of adolescent depression: A review. *Psychiatric Clinics of North America, 12,* 895–918.

Larsson, B., & Melin, L. (1990). Depressive symptoms in Swedish adolescents. *Journal of Abnormal Child Psychology, 18,* 91–103.

Lewinsohn, P. M., Clarke, G. N., Hops, H., & Andrews, J. (1990). Cognitive-behavioral treatment for depressed adolescents. *Behavior Therapy, 21,* 385–401.

Marton, P., Korenblum, M., Kutcher, S., Stein, B., Kennedy, B., & Pakes, J. (1989). Personality dysfunction in depressed adolescents. *Canadian Journal of Psychiatry, 34,* 810–813.

Merikangas, K. R., Prusoff, B. A., & Weissman, M. M. (1988). Parental concordance for affective disorders: Psychopathology in offspring. *Journal of Affective Disorders, 15,* 279–290.

Mitchell, J., McCauley, E., Burke, P., Calderon, R., & Schloredt, K. (1989). Psychopathology in parents of depressed children and adolescents. *Journal of the American Academy of Child and Adolescent Psychiatry, 28,* 352–357.

Mullins, L. L., Peterson, L., Wonderlich, S. A., & Reaven, N. M. (1986). The influence of depressive symptomatology in children on the social responses and perception of adults. *Journal of Clinical Child Psychology, 15,* 233–240.

Politano, P. M., Nelson, W. M., Evans, H., Sorenson, S., & Zeman, D. (1986). Factor analytic evaluation of differences between Black and Caucasian emotionally disturbed children on the Children's Depression Inventory. *Journal of Psychopathology and Behavioral Assessment, 8,* 1–7.

Puig-Antich, J., Lukens, E., Davies, M., Goetz, D., Brennan-Quattrock, J., & Today, G. (1985a). Psychosocial functioning in prepubertal major depressive disorders I. Interpersonal relationships during the depressive episode. *Archives of General Psychiatry, 42,* 500–507.

Puig-Antich, J., Lukens, E., Davies, M., Goetz, D., Brennan-Quattrock, J., & Today, G. (1985b). Psychosocial functioning in prepubertal major depressive disorders II. Interpersonal relationships after sustained recovery from an affective episode. *Archives of General Psychiatry, 42,* 511–517.

Puig-Antich, J., Perel, J. M., Lupatkin, W., Chambers, W. J., Tabrizi, M. A., King, J., Goetz, R., Davies, M., and Stiller, R. L. (1987). Imipramine in prepubertal major depressive disorders. *Archives of General Psychiatry, 44,* 81–89.

Puig-Antich, J., Goetz, D., Davies, M., Kaplan, T., Davies, S., Ostrow, L., Asnis, L., Twomey, J., Iyengar, S., & Ryan, N. D. (1989). A controlled family history study of prepubertal major depressive disorder. *Archives of General Psychiatry, 46,* 406–418.

Racusin, G. R., & Kaslow, N. J. (1991). Assessment and treatment of childhood depression. In P. A. Keller & S. R. Heyman (Eds.), *Innovations in clinical practice: A sourcebook* (Vol. 10, pp. 223–243). Sarasota: Professional Resource Exchange.

Rehm, L. P., Kaslow, N. J., & Rabin, A. S. (1987). Cognitive and behavioral targets in a self-control therapy program for depression. *Journal of Consulting and Clinical Psychology, 55,* 60–67.

Reynolds, W. M., & Coats, K. I. (1986). A comparison of cognitive–behavioral therapy and relaxation training for the treatment of depression in adolescents. *Journal of Consulting and Clinical Psychology, 54,* 653–660.

Rosenthal, N. E., Carpenter, C. J., James, S. P., Parry, B. L., Rogers, S. L. B., & Wehr, T. A. (1986). Seasonal affective disorder in children and adolescents. *American Journal of Psychiatry, 143,* 356–358.

Schulterbrandt, J. G., & Raskin, A. (Eds.) (1977). *Depression in childhood: Diagnosis, treatment, and conceptual models.* New York: Raven Press.

Spitz, R. (1946). Anaclitic depression. *Psychoanalytic study of the child, 5,* 113–117.

Stark, K. (1990). *Childhood depression: School-based intervention.* New York: Guilford.

Stark, K. D., Reynolds, W. M., & Kaslow, N. J. (1987). A comparison of the relative efficacy of self-control therapy and a behavioral problem-solving therapy for depression in children. *Journal of Abnormal Child Psychology, 15,* 91–113.

Stark, K. D., Humphrey, L. L., Crook, K., & Lewis, K. (1990). Perceived family environments of depressed and anxious children: Child's and maternal figure's perspectives. *Journal of Abnormal Child Psychology, 18,* 527–547.

Swift, W. J., Andrews, D., & Barklage, N. E. (1986). The relationship between affective disorder and eating disorders: A review of the literature. *American Journal of Psychiatry, 143,* 290–299.

Waller, D. A., & Rush, J. (1983). Differentiating primary affective disease, organic affective syndromes, and situational depression on a pediatric service. *Journal of the American Academy of Child Psychiatry, 22,* 52–58.

Weller, E. B., & Weller, R. A. (1991). Mood disorders. In M. Lewis (Ed.), *Child and adolescent psychiatry: A comprehensive textbook* (pp. 646–664). Baltimore: Williams & Wilkins.

Woolston, J. L., Rosenthal, S. L., Riddle, M. A., Sparrow, S. S., Cicchetti, D., & Zimmerman, L. D. (1989). Childhood comorbidity of anxiety/affective disorders and behavior disorders. *Journal of the American Academy of Child and Adolescent Psychiatry, 28,* 707–713.

Worchel, F. F., Nolan, B. F., Willson, V. L., Purser, J. S., Copeland, D. R., & Pfefferbaum, B. (1988). Assessment of depression in children with cancer. *Journal of Pediatric Psychology, 13,* 101–112.

Worchel, F. F., Hughes, J. N., Hall, B. M., Stanton, S. B., Stanton, S., & Little, V. Z. (1990). Evaluation of subclinical depression in children using self-, peer-, and teacher-report measures. *Journal of Abnormal Child Psychology, 18,* 271–282.

13

Eating Disorders

J. Scott Mizes

Description of the Disorders

In his recent bestselling fiction novel *Bonfire of the Vanities,* Tom Wolfe uses the graphic term "social x-rays" to describe the gaunt, transparent appearance of the high society women who have starved themselves to become thin despite their advancing age. Horror to the middle-aged wife who finds one of her husband's male friends is now married to a younger, and thinner, attractive woman. One does not have to be an observant social scientist to note the culturally endorsed emphasis on thinness, and now increasingly, fitness. The amateur social scientist needs only to take a stroll through daily life to collect numerous examples of the cultural preoccupation with thinness, especially for women: commercials for designer jeans, Virginia Slims cigarettes (targeted toward women), "Lite" foods, the constant running battle between food, body weight, and the bathing suit in the *Cathy* cartoons, and lead articles on check-out stand newspapers boasting a new plan for "Ten Days to Thinner Thighs!" are but a few examples.

Our national quest for thinness is clearly reflected in where we spend our money. Based on industry reports for 1988, over $7 billion was spent on facility-based weight loss programs (Garner & Wooley, 1991). In addition to this, U.S. consumers spent $8 billion at health clubs, $382 million on diet books, and nearly $10 billion on diet soft drinks (Garner & Wooley, 1991). Thus, in 1988 alone, Americans spent in excess of $25 billion on weight loss associated activities or products. Further evidence of the national battle with fat is the high frequency of liposuction, which is a surgical procedure designed to "vacuum" away fat. Lipo-

J. Scott Mizes • Department of Psychiatry, MetroHealth Medical Center, Case Western Reserve University School of Medicine, Cleveland, Ohio 44109.

Advanced Abnormal Psychology, edited by Vincent B. Van Hasselt and Michel Hersen. Plenum Press, New York, 1994.

suction is now the leading cosmetic procedure performed by plastic surgeons, with over 101,000 liposuction procedures undertaken in 1988 (Brownell, 1991). In short, fighting fat SELLS.

The push for this culturally endorsed "fat phobia" comes from societal expectations on what it means to be successful and attractive. In recent years, this push has been further aided by a well intentioned emphasis on weight and diet to reduce the risk of heart disease, and to a lesser extent, cancer. While this additional fitness bent may have had some positive health effects, it may have also provided a "scientific" moral high ground for those who wish to beat the enemy, fat, at all costs. Thus, being overweight changes from merely being unattractive, to moral failure for not taking care of the body that God gave each of us. Several studies show that children as early as kindergarten and grade school judge overweight people as not only less attractive, but also deficient in moral character (Garner & Wooley, 1991). Children describe overweight persons with such terms as "stupid," "lazy," and "sloppy." Adults make similar kinds of judgments, as illustrated by the male bulimic who worried about the effect of his perceived obesity on his effectiveness as a salesman. He assumed that prospective clients would see how sloppy he was in managing his body (i.e., being overweight), and therefore they would surely believe that he would handle their account in a similarly sloppy manner.

This national War Against Fat is one factor in what is termed the "normative discontent" that people, particularly women, have with their own bodies (Rodin, Silberstein, & Striegel-Moore, 1984). Klesges, Mizes, and Klesges (1987) found that 89% of university coeds and 54% of the males had engaged in some type of dieting behavior in the previous 6 months, even though less than 20% could be described as medically overweight. Similarly, 80% of the females and 46% of the males reported using some sort of physical activity to lose weight over the same time frame. This epidemic of dieting and food restriction has led some to speak of the need for treatment of "normal eating" (Polivy & Herman, 1987) because what is "normal" is pathological.

Though a significant national health problem, subclinical weight preoccupation and excessive dieting are not the same as clinically severe eating disorders. However, clinical cases of anorexia nervosa and bulimia nervosa may represent extreme ends on a continuum of disturbed eating. Moreover, our cultural thinness obsession is not the sole reason for the existence of clinical anorexia and bulimia. Medical history has noted the existence of both disorders even though the cultural emphasis on thinness has waxed and waned (Yates, 1989). Bulimia was noted by Galen, a Greek physician, in the second century (Yates, 1989). Anorexia nervosa was noted by Richard Morton in the early 1700s, and other authors described young medieval women who would starve themselves, vomit, and exercise to excess to become acceptable to God. Recently, Stunkard (1990) has presented a translation of four case studies of apparent bulimia nervosa written in the 1930s. Thus, clinical eating disorders were present long before the Jane Fonda Workout tapes, Jordache jeans, and Ultra Slim Fast.

Against this cultural backdrop of weight preoccupation and eating and dieting pathology, what is it that distinguishes clinical bulimia nervosa and anorexia nervosa from subclinical disturbance? In part, it is the extreme nature of certain behaviors and attitudes that occur in less severe form in "normal" women. Additionally, the clinical eating disorders co-occur frequently with other types of psychopathology. Thus, we will discuss the defining characteristics of the eating disorders. Likewise, the frequently occurring secondary psychopathology will be discussed in the Clinical Picture Section.

DIAGNOSTIC CRITERIA

Bulimia Nervosa

The defining features of bulimia nervosa are frequent binge eating and purging behaviors (American Psychiatric Association, 1987). Frequent binge eating is defined as an average of at least two binge episodes per week for at least 3 months. Although many people binge eat at times, it is this frequency and duration criterion that appears to best distinguish clinical bulimia nervosa (Kendler, Mac-Lean, Neale, Kessler, Heath, & Eaves, 1991). Self-induced vomiting is the most common method of purging; use of laxatives for weight control is a secondary strategy. While technically not purging, use of strict weight control methods after bingeing also occurs, including skipping meals or fasting, taking water pills, or vigorous exercise to work off calories. Bulimic women also show a consistent overconcern with body weight and shape. As compared to normal women, this overconcern represents a matter of degree. While normal women on average wish to weigh 11 pounds less than their medically ideal weight, bulimic women want to weigh nearly 18 pounds less (Mizes, 1992).

A brief overview quickly captures the marked disruption in eating that bulimic women experience (see Mizes, 1985). Bingeing and purging one to two times per day is common; however, some patients may have 30–40 bulimic episodes per week. Although binge size varies, it is typical to have 1300 calories in a single binge. To put this into perspective, a normal adult woman eats 1500–2500 calories per day. Preferred binge foods are often cereals, grains, snack foods, and desserts. However, a high frequency binger will binge on almost anything: for example, uncooked oatmeal or raw vegetables. Most bulimic episodes occur while the woman is home alone, and tend to occur in the late afternoon or early evening. However, it is not uncommon for some bulimics to get up at night to binge and purge.

The bulimic's eating episodes are distinguished by the intense emotions that accompany them (Mizes & Arbitell, 1991). Binges are often preceded by strong negative emotions. Feelings of being depressed or "stressed out" are quite common. Since the bulimic sees the preferred binge foods as "forbidden" ones, which will inevitably make her fat, binges are followed by intense feelings of anxiety and guilt, culminating in an overwhelming urge to get rid of the just eaten food. Though purging instantly relieves this urge, the bulimic is often left with lingering feelings of self-disgust and depression.

Bulimic women are also engaged in a daily battle with food and hunger. Most bulimics start each day anew, hoping to hold out as long as they can before giving in and eating. As compared to normal women, they tend to skip or have a very small breakfast and lunch, saving their daily calorie allotment for eating late in the afternoon or evening. Separate from their eating binges, bulimics tend to eat only 70% of what normal women eat in a day (Arbitell & Mizes, 1988).

Anorexia Nervosa

The distinction between normal women who are weight preoccupied and those with anorexia nervosa is much clearer to the untrained observer. The dimension most clearly seen is that of marked weight loss, and the DSM-III-R criterion (American Psychiatric Association, 1987) is weight loss of 15% of the person's "expected weight." Additionally, in women, three consecutive menstrual periods must have been missed, their cessation being due to the loss of the amount of body fat needed to sustain normal menstruation. Despite clearly being markedly underweight, anorectics express an intense fear of gaining weight and becoming fat. The anorectic woman will become highly distraught at gaining even half a pound, and, resolving to lose that half pound, may exercise vigorously or fast for the remainder of the day. The clearest illustration of the intense fear of weight gain is the anorectic's emotional response when asked to eat a forbidden food in a hospital setting. Taking even one bite of a forbidden food such as a doughnut often results in a desperate refusal to eat any more, in crying, and in visible signs of fear, such as shaking like a frightened child, or wide, fearful eyes.

Anorectics also show a marked disruption in their perception of the fatness of their own body. In part this is reflected in their grossly unrealistic desired body weights. They often wish to weigh 30 pounds less than their medically accepted ideal weight, and often their actual weight is a few pounds below this critically low self-ideal weight (Mizes, 1992). Their self-perception of fatness is also reflected in their evaluation that certain body parts are fat, for instance, focusing on their "poochèd out" stomach after having eaten a forbidden food.

Anorexia and Bulimia Nervosa

The diagnostic criteria describe two separate and distinct disorders; however, this may be somewhat of an artificial dichotomy. Though not covered by the formal diagnostic criteria, clinically, anorectics have long been subdivided into "restrictor" versus "bulimic" subtypes. The restrictor anorectic fits the formal diagnostic criteria. Her weight is low, her periods have stopped, and she eats very little, often less than 500 calories per day. This may be supplemented with purging of small amounts of food, and a very rigid and vigorous exercise program designed to work off the few calories from the small amount eaten. For example, one anorectic school teacher, after work, rode her exercise bike a full 8 hours per day. Based on DSM-III-R criteria, the bulimic subtype of anorexia is diagnosed with both disorders. This person shows the full pattern of anorexia as previously described but superimposes chronic bingeing and purging on the clinical picture. Thus, the bulimic anorectic may try to limit her nonbinge food consumption to less than 500 calories per day, but she still struggles with daily eating binges and purging episodes.

The distinction between the two disorders is further clouded by the fact that a given woman may go through phases where she fits the various diagnoses at different points in time (Yager, Landsverk, & Edelstein, 1987). Such overlap in clinical presentation is not surprising. Several authors have suggested that the two disorders are really two faces of one underlying pathology (Fairburn & Garner, 1986; Williamson, 1990): i.e., intense fear of weight gain and disturbance in the personal significance of body weight. For example, cognitive behavioral writers have described very similar core cognitive dysfunctions or unhealthy attitudes for both anorexia (Garner & Bemis, 1982) and bulimia nervosa (Fairburn, 1985; Mizes, 1985). These attitudes include rigid and inaccurate beliefs about food and its effect on body weight, reflected in a mind set of constant "dietary restraint." Dietary restraint is seen in a variety of rigid rules about what is acceptable and unacceptable eating. Examples include not eating before noon, or a complete prohibition against eating certain forbidden foods, such as ice cream. Both disorders are also thought to represent basic disruptions in the criteria used to determine self-esteem. Body weight becomes the most important, if not the exclusive, determinant of self-esteem. Weight becomes critical to self-esteem because the woman believes that others will approve of her more if she is thin (and likewise, she likes herself more). Further, she comes to believe that she demonstrates her psychological strength through her willpower over her body (that is, not eating when hungry).

Changes in the Diagnostic Criteria in DSM-IV

In part due to the diagnostic difficulties noted above, the organization of the diagnostic criteria for eating disorders has been modified in DSM-IV (American Psychiatric Association, 1993). Anorexia nervosa has been reorganized into two subtypes: a restricting type, and a binge-eating/purging type. Thus, persons formerly diagnosed with anorexia and bulimia under DSM-III-R will now be diagnosed with anorexia nervosa, binge/purge type. Similarly, the new criteria for bulimia nervosa reflect two subtypes. The first is bulimia nervosa, purging type, and it describes persons who binge eat and purge via self-induced vomiting, laxatives, or diuretics. The nonpurging subtype of bulimic utilizes inappropriate compensatory behaviors such as fasting, excessive exercise, or abuse of diet pills, but does not use the purging methods described previously.

After a great deal of debate in the professional community, a new eating disorder will be listed as a "provisional diagnosis requiring further study." This disorder, binge-eating disorder (BED), is very similar to bulimia nervosa in that its prominent feature is repeated binge episodes in which there is a subjective sense of loss of control and marked distress about the binge eating. However, in BED, neither purging nor extreme compensatory behaviors is present. Although BED can be present in normal weight persons, it is envisioned as occurring mostly in moderately to severely overweight persons. Due to its provisional status in DSM-IV, BED is listed as a specific example of the diagnosis Eating Disorder Not Otherwise Specified, rather than being a diagnosis in its own right.

MEDICAL COMPLICATIONS

Bulimia Nervosa

Bulimics often have physical problems that range from the relatively benign to the potentially very serious (Mitchell, Specker, & de Zwaan, 1991; Mizes, 1993). These problems occur due to dieting and modestly low weight, and as a consequence of purging. The most common serious problem is low potassium in the body, due to the effects of purging. Low potassium results in a condition called hypokalemia, and the most common result is muscle weakness and chronic fatigue. However, in severe hypokalemia, there can be irregular heartbeats and even complete stoppage of the heart.

Although there can be severe medical complications, these are the exception rather than the rule. The most common problems are sore or burning throat, puffy cheeks near the jaw, cavities in the teeth, wearing away of the enamel on the insides of the teeth, constipation, coldness in the arms and legs, irregular periods, dry skin, and hair breakage. Some bulimics become dehydrated—occasionally, enough to cause a serious medical problem. Dehydration may lead to feeling dizzy upon standing up, and marked fluid retention after food is eaten and purging has temporarily stopped. The resulting puffy wrists and ankles often activate the bulimic's fear of gaining weight, so she breaks down and quickly starts purging again.

It appears that most bulimics have adequate health. In one study, 2% of bulimics had very low potassium levels, 8% had mildly low potassium, 8% had heartbeat irregularities, 13% had dental problems, 18% had irregular periods, and 8% reported having puffy cheeks (Jacobs & Schneider, 1985). Bulimics may show changes in their body's metabolic rate due to their semistarvation state. Two preliminary studies have found that bulimics have lower resting metabolic rates than normal women (Bennett, Williamson, & Powers, 1989; Detzer et al., 1989).

Anorexia Nervosa

It is a rare parent or family member of an anorectic who is not frightened by the real risk of death in anorexia nervosa. Many families have seen or are aware of the TV movie dramatization of the story of the singer Karen Carpenter, and her eventual death due to anorexia nervosa. Not to minimize the severe health problems, it is nonetheless impressive how many anorectics can have precariously low weight, but continue to function well in basic job and life roles. Even more amazing is that they continue to push themselves in vigorous exercise.

The medical effects of chronic starvation have been extensively studied (Keys, Brozek, Henschel, Michelsen, & Taylor, 1950). These effects have been documented in groups of male volunteers who were starved down to a predetermined level under carefully controlled conditions. These volunteers developed most of the medical and psychological symptoms seen in anorexia nervosa. Of note is that these men became preoccupied with food, and in some cases developed bulimia.

Starvation-related effects seen in anorexia nervosa have been described in several articles (for example, Kaplan & Woodside, 1987). To the lay person, the most obvious effect is the "concentration camp" appearance; that is, being gaunt, emaciated, and lacking skin color. Many anorectics have dry skin and thinning hair, and some have a yellowish cast to their skin. Low blood pressure and very slow heart rate is common, as are irregular heartbeats. Gastrointestinal distress, such as stomach pain, feeling bloated, quickly feeling full, and constipation, is common. This is likely due to a general slowing of the digestive processes throughout the gastrointestinal tract. In part due to the loss of body fat, anorectics often easily feel cold, particularly in the arms and legs. They may also have a lowered body temperature as the body attempts to conserve energy. Patients report general muscle weakness, in part due to the loss of muscle tissue, but also because of dehydration and loss of potassium, particularly if they are purging. Despite being chronically tired, many anorectics have insomnia problems, and many lose their interest in sex.

The effects on mood and personality are also pronounced. Depression due to starvation alone is common, although some patients show rapidly shifting emotions. Obsessive thoughts and compulsive behaviors concerning food are frequently noted. Because anorectics have difficulties in higher level thinking, it is almost impossible to reason with the severely emaciated ones. They also have difficulty in concentrating and are easily distracted.

EPIDEMIOLOGY

Estimates of the prevalence of bulimia nervosa have changed, largely due to a change toward more stringent diagnostic criteria. The suggested prevalence rates of 20% in high-risk populations generated much alarm. More recent estimates, which use stricter criteria, put prevalence at 1% of adolescent and young adult women (Fairburn, Phil, & Beglin, 1990). A recent study identified the current prevalence of ever having had bulimia nervosa as 2.8%, and the lifetime risk of eventually developing bulimia nervosa as 4.2% (Kendler et al., 1991). The current prevalence of bulimia nervosa and bulimia-like syndromes was 5.7%, and the lifetime risk was 8.0%.

Bulimia nervosa is most often a disorder of females, though it does occur in males. For example, a recent study of university students found that 0.3% of males reported current bulimia nervosa, as compared to 2.2% of the females (Pyle, Neuman, Halvorson, & Mitchell, 1991). In general, approximately 10 to 13% of bulimics are male. Conventional wisdom indicates that bulimia nervosa was increasing. For example, the risk for bulimia nervosa appears to be higher for women born after 1960 (Kendler et al., 1991). However, there is some evidence that prevalence of bulimia may have peaked, and may now be declining (Pyle et al., 1991).

Since anorexia nervosa is rare, studies of anorectics have been primarily investigations of incidence per year, and have focused on identified anorectics (i.e., case registers or hospital treatment records) rather than general population samples. Most studies estimate the incidence per year between 0.37 and 1.60 cases per 100,000 people, though one study stands out at 4.06/100,000 (Szmukler, 1985). Estimates of the community prevalence of anorexia nervosa vary from 0.1% to 0.7% (Strober, 1991). As with bulimia nervosa, anorexia-like syndromes exist, and tentative estimates suggest that 5% of adolescent and young adult women may have some form of subclinical anorexia nervosa (Szmukler, 1985). Anorexia, like bulimia, is primarily a female problem, though male anorectics do exist. It is estimated that the ratio of females to males is 10–20 to 1 (Yates, 1989).

Incidence of anorexia is often thought to be rising, as at least two studies assessing the same geographic areas in the 1960s and then again in the 1970s found a nearly twofold increase in incidence (Szmukler, 1985). However, a recent follow-up study of one of these areas found that the incidence was level between the mid-1970s and mid-1980s (Willi, Giacometti, & Limacher, 1990). There did appear to be an increase in the number of cases of both bulimia and anorexia.

Traditionally, the eating disorders have been thought to occur mainly in the better-educated, more achievement oriented, higher socioeconomic status groups.

For example, one of the anorexia incidence studies found that the disorder was found exclusively in the middle and upper economic levels (Jones, Fox, Babigian, & Hutton, 1980). Female medical students appear to have a higher incidence of eating disorders, and university women may have a higher incidence of bulimia than working women (Yates, 1989). There is also evidence that anorexia nervosa is more common in adolescent girls attending private school than in those attending public school (Szmukler, 1985). In contrast to these findings, a recent well executed community study did not find any relationship between the prevalence of bulimia and the participants' educational level, income, occupation, or the education or occupation of their parents (Kendler et al., 1991).

Both anorexia and bulimia nervosa tend to occur mainly in Caucasian populations. African-Americans may comprise only 2 to 3% of all cases of anorexia nervosa (Andersen & Hay, 1985). Fewer African-Americans than Caucasians suffer from bulimia nervosa (Gray, Ford, & Kelly, 1987). This difference does not appear to be due to socioeconomic differences between African-Americans and Caucasians. It has been suggested that the difference is due to less strict expectations regarding women's weight in the African-American culture. Bulimia has also been found to be more common in Caucasian women as compared to Asian-American women (Nevo, 1985).

CLINICAL PICTURE

Associated Psychopathology

Both anorexia and bulimia can occur in a given patient in the absence of other major psychological problems. Indeed, there is reason to suspect that there are far more anorectics and bulimics than our experience in treatment settings would lead us to anticipate. These persons may function reasonably well in terms of fulfilling major life roles, despite suffering from the ravages of their eating disorder. However, these "pure" anorectics and bulimics may have strong tendencies toward patterns of psychological characteristics that fill out the overall clinical picture. Further, the eating disorders can co-occur with other psychiatric conditions, with some disorders more likely to be seen. Whether or not these other disorders co-occur in the eating disorders at a rate higher than in other psychiatric conditions is a matter of considerable debate, and there are few clear answers. Most studies are of eating disordered patients who seek treatment, and they may have an overall greater level of life problems than anorectics and bulimics who do not seek treatment. Also, the referral pattern of specific research and treatment centers may alter the picture of the co-occurring disorders, because they may attract more difficult patients, or ones with particular combinations of disorders.

GENERAL PSYCHOLOGICAL CHARACTERISTICS

Bulimics are frequently sensitive to interpersonal rejection, uncomfortable in social situations, have high personal expectations for achievement or performance, and have problems in self-regulation (Yates, 1989) For example, Mizes' (1985) theoretical model suggests that bulimics are excessively concerned about approval from others in order to feel good about themselves, base their self-esteem on high external performance criteria rather than on internal self-acceptance, and have basic self-control deficits.

Like bulimics, anorectics often feel very socially insecure and may be perfectionistic with very high expectations for achievement and performance. However, the anorectic tends to be more withdrawn, experiencing an inhibition of emotional expression and spontaneity. She also will often be more compliant, and may have more difficulty making up her own mind (Yates, 1989). A crucial difference is that the anorectic will often vigorously deny that her eating and weight are a problem, while the bulimic will hopelessly admit that her eating behavior is out of control. Thus, anorectics are very unwilling to accept treatment, and they are much more distrustful regarding others' motives regarding their eating and weight. The anorectic's starvation and malnutrition results in another major difference. It contributes substantially to her becoming more withdrawn, depressed, feeling fatigued and physically not well, being obsessed with thoughts about food, and having a rigid and concrete thinking style.

BULIMIA NERVOSA AND OTHER PSYCHOPATHOLOGY

Bulimia nervosa appears to co-occur with depressive disorders, chemical dependency, anxiety disorders, and personality disorders (Mitchell et al., 1991). Bulimics experience dysphoria (mild depression) as well as clinically severe major depression. It is clear that the disruption of frequent bingeing and purging results in periods of modest depression in many bulimics. Also, bulimia and clinical depression can co-occur.

Frequent occurrence of alcohol and substance abuse in bulimics has been observed. Conversely, a high frequency of eating disorders has been found in those who abuse substances (Jonas, Gold, Sweeney, & Pottash, 1987). For example, cocaine tends to reduce appetite and result in weight loss. A substance abusing bulimic may find her bulimic symptoms lessening while using cocaine. However, after stopping its use, she becomes frightened by the eating and weight gain that occurs, and this worsens her bulimic symptoms.

Though it has been only recently examined, many bulimics also have problems with anxiety disorders (Mitchell et al., 1991). Given bulimics' difficulties with social discomfort and concerns about approval from others, it is not surprising that social phobia may be particularly common. Other anxiety disorders occur as well, including simple phobias, agoraphobia, and obsessive–compulsive disorder. There is much discussion about histories of physical and sexual abuse in bulimics, which suggests the possibility of posttraumatic stress disorder, though this has not yet been examined.

Bulimia also tends to be associated with personality disorders (Mitchell et al., 1991). Although a variety of personality disorders can occur in bulimia, there is some suggestion that hystrionic personality disorder may be the most likely. Hystrionics tend to be very emotional, overly concerned with physical attractiveness, seek to be the center of attention, seek constant approval and reassurance, tend to be impulsive, and tend to have strained superficial interpersonal relationships. Much attention has been given to the combination of bulimia and borderline personality disorder because of evidence that the two together are very difficult to treat (Garner et al., 1990). The combination of bulimia and borderline personality disorder is particularly challenging because borderlines have marked instability in their emotions, marked impulsivity as evidenced by spending sprees, shoplifting, or sexual acting out, frequent suicidal threats, and self-mutilation such as cutting their wrists.

ANOREXIA NERVOSA AND OTHER PSYCHOPATHOLOGY

Less is known about the disorders that may co-occur with anorexia nervosa. Although all the eating disorder subtypes show a moderate frequency of borderline and dependent personality disorders (Mitchell et al., 1991), there is some suggestion that anorectics may be more likely to have one of the DSM-III-R cluster C "anxious–fearful" diagnoses. Avoidant (Piran, Lerner, Garfinkel, Kennedy, & Brouillette, 1988) and obsessive–compulsive personality (Wonderlich, Swift, Slotnick, & Goodman, 1990) are the most common. Persons with avoidant personality are socially withdrawn and have few close relationships. They tend to feel very uncomfortable socially and fear the evaluations of others. They also tend to be very timid and are hesitant to involve themselves in activities unless they are sure that things will go well and that they will be well received by others. Obsessive–compulsives are dominated by a pervasive perfectionism and fear of making a mistake or having something go wrong. They tend to have overly strict standards about how well things should be done, and have detailed rules, rituals, and schedules that regiment their daily activities. They are often overly devoted to work or what they "should" be doing, and often have restricted emotional expression that allows for little enjoyment, relaxation, and spontaneity.

The personality diagnoses that co-occur in persons with both anorexia and bulimia are more unclear. Similar to pure bulimics, bulimic anorectics tend to have more of the dramatic, emotional, and erratic DSM-III-R Cluster B diagnoses; however, they tend more toward borderline rather than histrionic personality disorders (Piran, Lerner, Garfinkel, Kennedy, & Brouillette, 1988). On the other hand, other research has suggested that this group has more avoidant personality diagnoses representative of the anxious–fearful cluster C diagnoses (Wonderlich et al., 1990), which is more similar to pure anorectics. A high frequency of the odd–eccentric cluster A personality disorders has also been suggested, with a higher occurrence of schizoid and schizotypical disorders (Kennedy, McVey, & Katz, 1990). It is of note that both these personality disorders are characterized by social withdrawal and a lack of close relationships, as well as tight, restricted emotionality, showing a similarity to the avoidant and obsessive–compulsive features described for pure anorectics.

Similar to bulimia, anorexia nervosa has also shown an association with depression (Swift, Andrews, & Barklage, 1986). Depression can occur as a clinical problem independent of anorexia, or can be a direct result of the effects of starvation and weight loss. Many estimates suggest that approximately 25 to 50% of anorectics are depressed. For reasons that are not clear, bulimic anorectics tend to be more depressed than the pure restrictor anorectics.

Anxiety disorders have also been observed in anorexia. Though research is sparse, anorectics may be very likely to suffer from obsessive–compulsive disorder (Hudson, Pope, Jonas, & Yurgelun-Todd, 1983). Obsessive–compulsive disorder is distinct from obsessive–compulsive personality. While the obsessive–compulsive personality is excessively perfectionistic and rigid, the person with obsessive–compulsive disorder is overwhelmed with purposeless compulsive rituals or obsessive, meaningless thoughts that dominate the day. Common rituals include compulsive hand washing (often several hundred times a day), or compulsive checking, such as having to repeatedly check to be sure the stove and lights are turned off to the extent that the person has little time for other activities. The opposite association has also been reported. Female obsessive–compulsives have shown a higher than expected rate of a history of anorexia nervosa (Kasvikis, Tsakiris, Marks, Basoglu, & Noshirvani, 1986).

CASE EXAMPLES

1. Donna was a 25-year-old, white, single woman who came from an affluent family in an exclusive suburb. Her father and mother were both prominent professionally, and were involved socially with an exclusive tennis club. Both parents were weight conscious, and Donna grew up listening to frequent discussions of dieting and "bad" foods at meals. Interestingly, her elderly grandmother (who was underweight) worried about her own weight, and would often fuss with Donna about her weight. Both parents seemed very concerned about "appearances" and achievement. For example, when the mother learned of about Donna's eating disorder, she wanted to keep it a secret to make sure that Donna could still get into a "good" college. For her education, Donna had gone to private girls' schools, and then entered college at a prestigious university. After working a few years in the business world to satisfy her father, she had gone back to school to enter a less lucrative profession that she truly enjoyed.

Donna, who was diagnosed as bulimic, began bingeing and purging when she was a freshman in high school. At the initial interview, she was binge eating and vomiting about three times per day. Binges usually occurred in the late afternoon and early evening, and the episodes would often last up to 90 minutes. A typical binge might be a salad, a box of cereal, and a box of cookies. She was constantly dieting and on most days would only eat lunch. She also took one over-the-counter diet pill daily. Donna was 5 feet, 4 inches tall and weighed 118 pounds. The medically ideal weight for her was 131 pounds; her goal was to weigh 110 pounds. The approximate cutoff weight for anorexia nervosa was 111 pounds. Physically, she had puffy cheeks, occasional fluid retention in her hands and feet, dizziness upon standing, and frequent coldness. Her periods were regular, though they had stopped while she was a college sophomore. Although she had very high expectations for herself and was often self-critical, she did not report depression or any other specific psychological disorder.

2. The original contact for Jeri (age 17) came from her father. He called, very upset, describing the extensive weight loss in his daughter over the past few months. Also, she skipped meals and ate very little at the meals she did eat with the family. Mealtime had degenerated into a battle between Jeri and her parents, as they tried to either force or "sweet talk" her into eating. Her parents had taken her to a well known clinic and hospital for a physical evaluation to determine the cause of her weight loss and lack of periods. No medical reason was found, and none of the physicians who saw Jeri suspected anorexia nervosa.

Jeri was brought to the initial interview against her wishes, and she was very angry and initially did not want to talk. Eventually, she described her eating pattern. She ate a light breakfast a couple of mornings a week, mainly to "get her parents off her back." At school, she would eat only an apple, and at home, dinner was usually a salad. Jeri denied vomiting and use of laxatives or water pills for weight control. Although always athletic, her exercise behavior had recently increased dramatically. She exercised primarily to reduce the guilt she felt after eating. Her parents had become increasingly concerned when she began getting up very early in the morning to go walking, in addition to 1–2 hours of heavy exercise later in the day. They were also worried because Jeri would not let anything interrupt her rigid exercise routine. Jeri was 5 foot 6 inches tall, and a typical hyperlate pre-anorexia weight for her was 130 pounds. She now weighed 100 pounds, which was an ideal weight in her eyes. The medically expected weight for her was 137 pounds, and the cutoff for anorexia was 116 pounds. She had never had a period, even when at normal weight. Her physical symptoms included feeling cold in her arms and legs, dizziness upon standing, and chronic tiredness.

Jeri graduated from high school with a straight 4.0 average. Nevertheless, she was very worried about how she was going to do in college. She worried that she might get a "B," and that her parents would no longer be proud of her, despite their reassurances. Interpersonally, she was quiet, saw herself as boring, and worked very hard to "say the right thing" so that others would like her. She saw herself as not all that popular and not very attractive, despite having been the homecoming queen during her senior year in high school.

COURSE AND PROGNOSIS

The average age for bulimia nervosa to begin is about 21, with a standard deviation of ±6 years (Kendler et al., 1991). A recent summary of the course and prognosis of bulimia nervosa (Herzog, Keller, Lavori, & Sacks, 1991) suggests that it is a chronic disorder that tends to wax and wane. Even when the person improves, there may be a persistent preoccupation with eating and body weight. However, this may be true for bulimics whose disorders are severe enough so that they have sought treatment. For those with less severe disturbance, bulimia may tend to eventually get better with time. In one study of bulimics who had received outpatient treatment, approximately 70% had recovered at least once within 3 to 4 years. However, most of those who recovered did so in the first year. Unfortunately, among those who recovered, over 60% relapsed within a year. Even after recovery, about one third continued to have problems with chronic dieting or compulsive exercise.

Factors associated with a poor outcome are chemical abuse, borderline personality disorder (Garner et al., 1990), and more severe body image disturbance (Freeman, Beach, Davis, & Solyom, 1985). Interestingly, although depression has sometimes been related to poor outcome, more frequently it is not related to outcome. In general, duration of the disorder, frequency of bingeing and purging, and history of anorexia have not been associated with outcome.

The average age of onset for anorexia appears to be earlier than that for bulimia. It begins at about age 17, with a standard deviation of ±3 years (Willi et al., 1990). Theander (1985) has recently summarized the research on outcome in anorexia, and presented the longest period of observation, on average, of over 30 years. Looking at outcome after 24 years, one finds that 76% of the anorectics had recovered. However, most of these recoveries were in the first 12 years. Even among those who recover, there tends to be a persistent preoccupation with weight and dieting. In the first 5 years of the study, 8% of the anorexics had died. However, more recent studies have found lower initial death rates, perhaps due to recent improvements in treatment, at least in terms of increasing the anorectic's weight. The long-term outcome after 30 years for a quarter of the anorectics was dismal, with 6% continuing to have severe symptoms, and 18% dying, two thirds from anorexia, the others from suicide. Little is known about the factors associated with poor outcome. Those who have had anorexia for a long time were older when it began, have lower weight, suffer severe body image disturbance, or who binge and purge, tend to have a poorer outcome (Theander, 1983).

FAMILIAL AND GENETIC PATTERNS

Strober and Humphrey's (1987) recent summary suggests that bulimics and anorectic bulimics have more distressed family relationships than do pure anorectics. Bulimics' families tend to show a more pronounced lack of parental affection, and display more open hostility, isolation among family members, and lack of emotional support. However, families of both anorectics and bulimics have more problems than normal families. They tend to have more conflict and hostility, tend to respond to the patient's emotions as if they were unimportant, and tend to not operate as a close-knit supportive family. They also tend to become overinvolved with the daughter's personal business and meddle. Examples of the latter (known as "enmeshment") include the parents' responding to the daughter's successes and failures as if they were their own, or not allowing the daughter to make her own decisions and thereby learn from her own successes and mistakes. The pattern of more problems in the bulimic groups, as compared to pure anorectics, is seen in the parents as well. There is some suggestion that they have more alcoholism, more problems due to impulsivity, and are more likely to be obese.

Although many eating disordered families are psychologically unhealthy, many families seem to have no more problems than normal families. Some of the problems in these families may be a reaction to having an ill daughter. For example, the overinvolvement and anger expressed by parents of anorectics may be due to the terror of watching their daughter waste away and their desperate attempt to do anything to make her eat. Parents are often angry as they watch their daughter doing this to herself for reasons they cannot understand, while completely disrupting the family emotionally and often financially. Also, it is very difficult for parents to watch all their normal parental hopes and dreams for their child seemingly go down the drain. Even in those families that had problems prior to the beginning of the eating disorder, little is known about what specific characteristics of these problems led to the daughter developing an eating disorder rather than some other problem.

Eating disorders tend to run in families, and this may suggest that there is a genetic risk that is inherited [for a summary, see Strober (1991) and Scott (1986)]. Alternatively, it may be because all the members of the family are exposed to the same unhealthy attitudes about eating and weight. Teasing out the genetic portion requires elaborate studies of twins, though studies of the family members of eating disorder patients provides clues. Family members of anorectics are more likely to have an eating disorder. For example, 3 to 10% of sisters of anorectics develop anorexia themselves. Also, among female identical twins where one has anorexia, her twin will have anorexia 44 to 50% of the time. Among nonidentical, fraternal female twins (who are no more alike genetically than normal sisters), anorexia occurs in both only 7% of the time. One of the best studies on the genetic contribution to eating disorders is an investigation of the occurrence of bulimia by Kendler et al. (1991). Though most studies have too few twins to give firm answers, this investigation assessed over 2000 female twins. Among the identical twins, both had bulimia nervosa 29% of the time; this occurred only 9% of the time for the fraternal twins. It was estimated that 55% of the inherited risk for bulimia came from genetic factors alone.

DIAGNOSTIC CONSIDERATIONS

Although the diagnostic criteria for anorexia and bulimia nervosa have been refined over time, problems remain. For bulimia nervosa, one of the biggest problems is that there is no clear definition of a binge. To a certain extent it is like current efforts to define obscenity: no one can clearly define it, but everyone "knows it when they see it." The problem is important, since a fair number of bulimics will purge after eating a very small amount of a forbidden food, such as one cookie. The bulimic may clearly see this as a binge, as evidenced by her need to get rid of it. However, most other people would not see this as even mild overeating, much less a binge. When women are asked to describe their own eating behavior, the term binge tends to relate more to a sense of loss of control rather than an amount of food eaten (Beglin & Fairburn, 1992). Loss of control was perceived if the woman thought she could not stop herself from starting to eat, or could not stop once eating began. Although focus on loss of control allows for consumption of small amounts of food to be considered binges, the term is still most likely to be used to describe clear instances of overeating in which there is a perceived loss of control.

The diagnostic criterion of weight loss of 15% below "expected weight" for anorexia is problematic because it is not clear what defines expected weight. Expected weight depends on variables such as level of physical maturity relative to age (such as for adolescents), frame and body build, and normal tendency to be underweight, normal or overweight. A rough approximation of expected weight can be inferred from standard "ideal" weight tables. The Metropolitan weight tables of 1959 and 1983 and the 1978 DHEW weight tables are the most frequently used to determine ideal weight. However, these tables specify very different ideal weights. The 1978 DHEW tables have the highest ideal weights, while the 1959 Metropolitan tables have the lowest. The net result is that there are huge differences on whether a person is classified as underweight, normal, or overweight, depending on the table used (Pyle, Mitchell, & Eckert, 1986).

Others have questioned the usefulness of the weight tables at all, noting that they do not account for differences in ideal weight due to slow versus early physical maturation in adolescents, or failure to grow due to malnutrition. Also, they do not give a precise measurement of the loss of lean muscle, which represents a serious health risk (Drewnowski & Garn, 1987). The tables also do not reflect the loss of percent of body fat. Thus, some have recommended using the body mass index (BMI = weight in kilograms divided by height in meters, squared) because it is a practical estimate of amount of body fat (Williamson, 1990). For adults, a BMI between 20 and 25 is considered healthy, and a cutoff of 16 for anorexia has been suggested. The tables also do not account for differences in what is a normal weight for a specific person, regardless of what the tables say. This is increasingly important due to recent evidence that a person's tendency to be relatively thin, of normal weight, or overweight is about 66% due to genetic factors (Stunkard, Harris, Pedersen, & McClearn, 1990). Thus, for two women who are both 5 feet, 6 inches tall and age 24, normal weight may differ; for one, it may be 125 pounds, and for the other, 160 pounds.

The concept of body image distortion has long been graphically illustrated in textbooks by illustrations of a gaunt woman looking into a mirror, only to see a fat woman in the reflection. Body image distortion is one of the diagnostic criteria for anorexia, and implied for bulimia in terms of overconcern with body weight and shape. Although there have been numerous studies of body image distortion using a variety of techniques to measure it, the area has been plagued by inconsistent results (Cash & Brown, 1987). Eating disorder patients sometimes show body image distortion; sometimes they do not (Mizes, 1991). Further, normal women sometimes suffer body image distortion. Some have even suggested that the concept of body image distortion be abandoned (Hsu & Sobkiewicz, 1991). Traditionally, body image distortion has been seen as having two components: a tendency to misperceive actual body size (as illustrated by the mirror example above), and negative attitudes about one's body and weight. In general, studies of misperception of body size have been contradictory, while those of negative body attitudes have more consistently indicated the disturbance in eating disorders (Cash & Brown, 1987). Recently, Mizes (1992) has suggested that the disturbance in anorexia and bulimia can be described in terms of subjective weight dissatisfaction (the difference between actual weight and preferred ideal weight) and unrealistic preferred ideal weight (the difference between "medically" ideal weight and preferred weight). Bulimics tend to show both weight dissatisfaction and unrealistic preferred ideal weight. Anorectics tend to have extremely low and unrealistic preferred ideal weights, but little weight dissatisfaction. This is because their actual weight is often within a few pounds of their preferred ideal weight. Until the concept of body image distortion or disturbance is clarified, this part of the diagnosis will remain murky.

Summary

It is often said that you can never be too rich or too thin. While others will have to comment on the pitfalls of excess money, the disorders of anorexia and bulimia nervosa clearly show the horrible price to be paid for either being too thin, or desiring to be too thin. In large part the price is psychological, characterized by declining self-esteem, increased insecurity, the torment of the constant preoccupation with food and body weight, and increasing isolation and withdrawal as the person's life becomes more and more dominated by the eating disorder. The price is often also physical, and in the extreme case of anorexia nervosa, the price can be death. Many a woman who is "watching her weight" has commented that she wished she could be anorectic. This is usually a naive, though understandable, desire to be able to show the apparent self-control of the anorectic. What these individuals do not appreciate is that anorectics are anything but in control. Rather, they have become enslaved to their fears about food and body weight, and ultimately, their own fears about their personal worth.

The phrase "never too rich or too thin" succinctly captures the unhealthy cultural attitudes that create risk factors for the development of anorexia and bulimia nervosa. Though it is not entirely clear what variables cause eating disorders, it is clear that our cultural "fat phobia" and pursuit of thinness are not the sole causes of these disorders. Apparently, a variety of psychological and/or genetic factors are also associated with the development of eating disorders. We are in the early phases of defining clearly what constitutes anorexia and bulimia, and there have been important advances in the past 15 years. Important progress is also being made regarding the "core" psychopathology of the eating disorders, as well as the associated psychological conditions. As these issues become clarified, we will be able not only to understand the causes of eating disorders, but to improve the available treatments as well.

REFERENCES

American Psychiatric Association. (1987). *Diagnostic and statistical manual of mental disorders*, 3rd Edition, Revised. Washington, DC: Author.

American Psychiatric Association (1993). *DSM-IV draft criteria*. Washington, DC: Author.

Andersen, A. E., & Hay, A. (1985). Racial and socioeconomic influences in anorexia nervosa and bulimia. *International Journal of Eating Disorders, 4*, 479–487.

Arbitell, M. R., & Mizes, J. S. (1988). *Typographical and descriptive variables in bulimia nervosa: A controlled comparison*. Paper presented at the Southeastern Psychological Association Convention, New Orleans.

Beglin, S. J., & Fairburn, C. G. (1992). What is meant by the term "binge"? *American Journal of Psychiatry, 149*, 123–124.

Bennett, S. M., Williamson, D. A., & Powers, S. K. (1989). Bulimia nervosa and resting metabolic rate. *International Journal of Eating Disorders, 8*, 417–424.

Brownell, K. D. (1991). Dieting and the search for the perfect body: Where physiology and culture collide. *Behavior Therapy, 22*, 1–12.

Cash, T. F., & Brown, T. A. (1987). Body image in anorexia nervosa and bulimia nervosa. *Behavior Modification, 11*, 487–521.

Detzer, M. J., Leitenberg, H., Poehlman, E., Rosen, J. C., Hiser, J., Wolf, J., Catalano, P. M., & Tyzbir, E. D. (1989). *Resting metabolic rate in bulimia nervosa*. Poster presented at the 23rd Annual meeting of the Association for Advancement of Behavior Therapy, Washington, DC.

Drewnowski, A., & Garn, S. M. (1987). Concerning the use of weight tables to categorize patients with eating disorders. *International Journal of Eating Disorders, 6*, 639–646.

Fairburn, C. G. (1985). A cognitive–behavioral treatment of bulimia. In D. M. Garner & P. E. Garfinkel (Eds.). *Handbook of psychotherapy for anorexia nervosa and bulimia* (pp. 160–192). New York: Guilford.

Fairburn, C. G., & Garner, D. M. (1986). The diagnosis of bulimia nervosa. *International Journal of Eating Disorders, 5*, 403–419.

Fairburn, C. G., Phil, M., & Beglin, S. J. (1990). Studies of the epidemiology of bulimia nervosa. *American Journal of Psychiatry, 147*, 401–408.

Freeman, R. J., Beach, B., Davis, R., & Solyom, L. (1985). The prediction of relapse in bulimia nervosa. *Journal of Psychiatric Research, 19*, 349–353.

Garner, D. M., & Bemis, K. M. (1982). A cognitive–behavioral approach to anorexia nervosa. *Cognitive Therapy and Research, 6*, 123–150.

Garner, D. M., & Wooley, S. C. (1991). Confronting the failure of behavioral and dietary treatments for obesity. *Clinical Psychology Review, 11*, 729–780.

Garner, D. M., Olmsted, M. P., Davis, R., Rockert, W., Goldbloom, D., & Eagle, M. (1990). The association between bulimic symptoms and reported psychopathology. *International Journal of Eating Disorders, 9*, 1–15.

Gray, J. J., Ford, K., & Kelly, L. M. (1987). The prevalence of bulimia in a black college population. *International Journal of Eating Disorders, 6,* 733–740.

Herzog, D. B., Keller, M. B., Lavori, P. W., & Sacks, N. R. (1991). The course and outcome of bulimia nervosa. *Journal of Clinical Psychiatry, 52*(10 Suppl), 4–8.

Hsu, L. K. G., & Sobkiewicz, T. A. (1991). Body image disturbance: Time to abandon the concept for eating disorders? *International Journal of Eating Disorders, 10,* 15–30.

Hudson, J. I., Pope, H. G., Jonas, J. M., & Yurgelun-Todd, D. (1983). Phenomenologic relationship of eating disorders to major affective disorder. *Psychiatry Research, 9,* 345–354.

Jacobs, M. B., & Schneider, J. A. (1985). Medical complications of bulimia: A prospective evaluation. *Quarterly Journal of Medicine, 54,* 177–182.

Jonas, J. M., Gold, M. S., Sweeney, D., & Pottash, A. L. C. (1987). Eating disorders and cocaine abuse: A survey of 259 cocaine abusers. *Journal of Clinical Psychiatry, 48,* 47–50.

Jones, D. J., Fox, M. M., Babigian, H. M., & Hutton, H. E. (1980). Epidemiology of anorexia nervosa in Monroe County, New York: 1960–1976. *Psychosomatic Medicine, 42,* 551–558.

Kaplan, A. S., & Woodside, D. B. (1987). Biological aspects of anorexia nervosa and bulimia nervosa. *Journal of Consulting and Clinical Psychology, 55,* 645–653.

Kasvikis, Y. G., Tsakiris, F., Marks, I. M., Basoglu, M., & Noshirvani, H. F. (1986). Past history of anorexia nervosa in women with obsessive–compulsive disorder. *International Journal of Eating Disorders, 5,* 1069–1075.

Kendler, K. S., MacLean, C., Neale, M., Kessler, R., Heath, A., & Eaves, L. (1991). The genetic epidemiology of bulimia nervosa. *American Journal of Psychiatry, 148,* 1627–1637.

Kennedy, S. H., McVey, G., & Katz, R. (1990). Personality disorders in anorexia nervosa and bulimia nervosa. *Journal of Psychiatric Research, 24,* 259–269.

Keys, A., Brozek, J., Henschel, A., Michelsen, O., & Taylor, H. L. (1950). *The biology of human starvation.* Minneapolis: University of Minnesota Press.

Klesges, R. C., Mizes, J. S., & Klesges, L. M. (1987). Self-help dieting strategies in college males and females. *International Journal of Eating Disorders, 6,* 409–417.

Mitchell, J. E., Specker, S. M., & de Zwaan, M. (1991). Comorbidity and medical complications of bulimia nervosa. *Journal of Clinical Psychiatry, 52*(10 Suppl), 13–20.

Mizes, J. S. (1985). Bulimia: A review of its symptomatology and treatment. *Advances in Behavior Research and Therapy, 7,* 91–142.

Mizes, J. S. (1991). Validity of the Body Image Detection Device. *Addictive Behaviors, 16,* 411–417.

Mizes, J. S. (1992). The Body Image Detection Device versus subjective measures of weight dissatisfaction: A validity comparison. *Addictive Behaviors, 17,* 125–136.

Mizes, J. S. (1993). Bulimia nervosa. In A. S. Bellack & M. Hersen (Eds.), *Handbook of behavior therapy in the psychiatric setting* (pp. 311–327). New York: Plenum.

Mizes, J. S., & Arbitell, M. R. (1991). Bulimics' perceptions of emotional responding during binge-purge episodes. *Psychological Reports, 69,* 527–532.

Nevo, S. (1985). Bulimic symptoms: Prevalence and ethnic differences among college women. *International Journal of Eating Disorders, 4,* 151–168.

Piran, N., Lerner, P., Garfinkel, P. E., Kennedy, S. H., & Brouillette, C. (1988). Personality disorders in anorexic patients. *International Journal of Eating Disorders, 7,* 589–599.

Polivy, J., & Herman, C. P. (1987). Diagnosis and treatment of normal eating. *Journal of Consulting and Clinical Psychology, 55,* 635–644.

Pyle, R. L., Mitchell, J. E., & Eckert, E. D. (1986). The use of weight tables to categorize patients with eating disorders. *International Journal of Eating Disorders, 5,* 377–383.

Pyle, R. L., Neuman, P. A., Halvorson, P. A., & Mitchell, J. E. (1991). An ongoing cross-sectional study of the prevalence of eating disorders in freshman college students. *International Journal of Eating Disorders, 10,* 667–678.

Rodin, J., Silberstein, L., & Striegel-Moore, R. (1984). Women and weight: A normative discontent. In T. B. Sonderegger (Ed.), *Psychology and gender: Nebraska symposium on motivation* (pp. 267–307). Lincoln, NE: University of Nebraska Press.

Scott, D. W. (1986). Anorexia nervosa: a review of possible genetic factors. *International Journal of Eating Disorders, 5,* 1–20.

Strober, M. (1991). Family-genetic studies of eating disorders. *Journal of Clinical Psychiatry, 52*(10 Suppl), 9–12.

Strober, M., & Humphrey, L. L. (1987). Familial contributions to the etiology and course of anorexia nervosa and bulimia. *Journal of Consulting and Clinical Psychology, 55,* 654–659.

Stunkard, A. (1990). A description of eating disorders in 1932. *American Journal of Psychiatry, 147,* 263–268.

Stunkard, A. J., Harris, J. R., Pedersen, N. L., & McClearn, G. E. (1990). The body-mass index of twins who have been reared apart. *New England Journal of Medicine, 322,* 1483–1487.

Swift, W. J., Andrews, D., & Barklage, N. E. (1986). The relationship between affective disorder and eating disorders: A review of the literature. *American Journal of Psychiatry, 143,* 290–297.

Szmukler, G. I. (1985). The epidemiology of anorexia nervosa and bulimia. *Journal of Psychiatric Research, 19,* 143–153.

Theander, S. (1983). Research on outcome and prognosis of anorexia nervosa and some results from a Swedish long-term study. *International Journal of Eating Disorders, 2,* 167–174.

Theander, S. (1985). Outcome and prognosis in anorexia nervosa and bulimia: Some results of previous investigations, compared with those of a Swedish long-term study. *Journal of Psychiatric Research, 19,* 493–508.

Willi, J., Giacometti, G., & Limacher, B. (1990). Update on the epidemiology of anorexia nervosa in a defined region of Switzerland. *American Journal of Psychiatry, 147,* 1514–1517.

Williamson, D. A. (1990). *Assessment of eating disorders: Obesity, anorexia, and bulimia nervosa.* New York: Pergamon Press.

Wonderlich, S. A., Swift, W. J., Slotnick, H. B., & Goodman, S. (1990). DSM-III-R personality disorders in eating-disorder subtypes. *International Journal of Eating Disorders, 9,* 607–616.

Yager, J., Landsverk, J., & Edelstein, C. K. (1987). A 20-month follow-up study of 628 women with eating disorders, I: Course and severity. *American Journal of Psychiatry, 144,* 1172–1177.

Yates, A. (1989). Current perspectives on the eating disorders: I. History, psychological and biological aspects. *Journal of the American Academy of Child and Adolescent Psychiatry, 28,* 813–828.

III

Adult and Older Adult Disorders: Introductory Comments

The past several years have witnessed a dramatic upsurge of clinical and investigative interest in the epidemiology, prevention, assessment, and treatment of adult disorders. The increased activity in this area is partly attributable to improvements in the primary classification system utilized to diagnose these problems: the *Diagnostic and Statistical Manual of Mental Disorders* (DSM). Since inception of the more empirically derived DSM-III in 1980, and its improved capabilities for nosological precision and prediction, adult research efforts have burgeoned. In addition to this, the growing awareness of the need to consider psychological, biological, and environmental factors in psychopathology has: (1) greatly expanded the range of specialty areas (e.g., neurology, biochemistry, endocrinology) involved in the study of the various disorders, and (2) underscored the need for interdisciplinary approaches that consider the multiple and complex factors responsible for their occurrence.

Chapters in this part of the book cover the major adult and older adult disorders. In Chapter 14, Paul M. G. Emmelkamp and Patricia van Oppen review the major anxiety disorders, including: simple and social phobias, panic disorder, generalized anxiety disorder, obsessive-compulsive disorder, and posttraumatic stress disorder. Case illustrations of assessment and intervention approaches for each of the aforementioned difficulties are provided. Lynn P. Rehm and Paras Mehta discuss current strategies and issues in the assessment and treatment of depression (Chapter 15). Further, they underscore the importance of a biopsychosocial perspective in studying this problem. Schizophrenia, one of the most disabling psychiatric disturbances, is covered by Patrick McGuffin and Randall L. Morrison (Chapter 16). These authors provide an overview of psychosocial and pharmacologic treatments, in addition to a discussion on major etiological theories.

Substance use disorders are the most common group of psychiatric disorders in the United States. In Chapter 17, Timothy J. O'Farrell outlines heuristic evalua-

271

tion and remediation strategies that have found utility with alcohol and drug problems. Judith V. Becker and Meg Kaplan, in Chapter 18, discuss the two categories of sexual problems: sexual dysfunctions and sexual deviations. The authors document research confirming the efficacy of various treatment techniques with these disorders. In Chapter 19, Donald A. Williamson, Susan E. Barker, and Staci Veron-Guidry define psychophysiological disorders as physical or medical problems influenced by psychological factors, such as stress, emotion, and personality. They review clinical and research findings pertaining to the three most prevalent difficulties under this rubric: headache, insomnia, and essential hypertension. Finally, Gerald Goldstein covers organic mental disorders (Chapter 20). This category includes the constellation of severely disabling conditions caused by impairment of brain functions. Delirium, dementia, amnesia, and other syndromes that alter personality, mood, or anxiety level also are reviewed.

14

Anxiety Disorders

Paul M. G. Emmelkamp and Patricia van Oppen

Introduction

The purpose of this chapter is to discuss the description, epidemiology, clinical features, course and prognosis, familial and genetic patterns, and differential diagnosis of anxiety disorders. The various anxiety disorders (i.e., specific phobia, panic disorder with and without agoraphobia, social phobia, generalized anxiety disorder, obsessive–compulsive disorder, and posttraumatic stress disorder) will be dealt with separately.

Specific Phobia

Description of the Disorder

One of the most widespread anxiety disorders is the specific or simple phobia. The term specific phobia refers to a broad scale of phobias associated with different stimuli. Specific phobias are restricted to specific situations. According to the diagnostic criteria of DSM-IV (American Psychiatric Association, 1993), specific phobia should be diagnosed in the case of a persistent excessive or irrational fear of a circumscribed stimulus (object or situation), which is avoided, or endured with intense anxiety. The fear or the avoidance behavior has to interfere significantly with the person's normal life.

The fear-related stimulus of specific phobia has to be different from panic disorder/agoraphobia or social phobia stimuli and unrelated to the content of the

Paul M. G. Emmelkamp • Department of Clinical Psychology, Academic Hospital, 9713 EZ Groningen, The Netherlands.   Patricia van Oppen • Department of Psychiatry, Valeriuskliniek, 1075 BG Amsterdam, The Netherlands.

Advanced Abnormal Psychology, edited by Vincent B. Van Hasselt and Michel Hersen. Plenum Press, New York, 1994.

PAUL M. G.
EMMELKAMP
and PATRICIA
VAN OPPEN

obsessions of obsessive–compulsive disorder or the trauma of posttraumatic stress disorder.

The most common clinically seen specific phobias are: fear of animals (zoophobia), fear of heights (acrophobia), fear of confinement (claustrophobia), and fear of injury and/or blood. Phobia of animals or insects can involve any animal or insect, but mostly seen are phobias of spiders, dogs, cats, snakes, and birds (pigeons).

Epidemiology

In the last decade, several epidemiological studies investigated the prevalence rate of simple phobia according the DSM-III (Bland, Orn, & Newman, 1988; Burnam et al., 1987; Karno et al., 1987; Myers et al., 1984; Robins et al., 1984; Wittchen, 1988). These data are presented in Table 1. Specific phobia is the most common anxiety disorder. The mean lifetime prevalence of specific phobia is just over 10%.

Clinical Picture

Angela is a 29-year-old unmarried woman. She is employed in a large business firm. Since several years she has had a flight phobia. She particularly fears a crash. Angela avoids to go by plane. Besides this phobia, she has a cat and insect phobia, but the latter phobias do not restrict her life. Angela does not know how these phobia developed. The anxiety increased over the years. Recently, she received a promotion and her new job requires several far away trips; therefore, she is now seeking treatment for her flight phobia.

Specific phobia can lead to intense panic and extreme avoidance of the specific situations. In some cases, this might have severe consequences such as when a blood phobic avoids medical treatment. Rarely are the fears strong enough to motivate individuals to refer themselves for treatment. When specific phobics do seek treatment, it is often because they anticipate that circumstances will force confrontation with a dreaded cue stimulus (McGlynn & McNeil, 1990).

TABLE 1. Prevalence Rate of Anxiety Disorders

Authors/Study	Total phobia (%)	Agoraphobia (%)	Panic disorder (%)	Social phobia (%)	Specific phobia (%)	Obsessive–compulsive disorder (%)
Robins et al. (1984) Myers et al. (1984)						
New Haven	7.8	3.5	1.4	—	6.3	2.6
Baltimore	23.3	9.0	1.4	—	20.4	3.0
St. Louis	9.4	4.0	1.5	—	6.8	1.9
Karno et al. (1987) Burnam et al. (1987)	11.7	—	1.5	—	8.0	2.1
Wittchen (1988)	13.9	5.7	2.4	—		2.0
Bland et al. (1988)	8.9	2.9	1.2	1.7	7.2	3.0

It is remarkable that there exists a selection of objects or situations that specific phobics fear. Surprisingly, some phobias never occur, like gun phobias, mixer phobias, car phobias, mower phobia, hammer phobia, etc. The preparedness theory attempts to explain this phenomenon. According to this perspective, most phobias are based on a genetic disposition or preparedness to develop fear of those objects and situations (e.g., snakes, spiders, enclosed places) that were threatening to our prehistorical ancestors. Although a number of experimental laboratory studies have been conducted to test this theory, results are inconclusive (Merkelbach, van den Hout, & van der Molen, 1989).

When specific phobics are confronted with the phobic object or situation, this immediately induces extreme distress and panic. When the phobic stimulus is away, the anxiety decreases. Confrontation with the phobic stimuli leads to a sympathetically mediated increase in blood pressure and heart rate. However, blood-injury phobics show a very short sympathetic activation followed by a parasympathetic activation (a drop in heart rate and/or blood pressure) (Thyer, Himle, & Curtis, 1985).

The gender incidence of animal, flying, and blood-injury phobias is higher for women than for men (Marks, 1987). The majority of the specific phobics are women (Myers et al., 1984).

There is a considerable overlap between anxiety and affective syndromes. This overlap is not seen for specific phobics. Only 9% of patients with specific phobia reported past depressive episodes (Monroe, 1990).

Course and Prognosis

In young children (2–6 years), simple phobias (mostly fears of animals) often improve "spontaneously" without any treatment. Those with phobias that continue into adulthood seldom recover spontaneously. Age at onset varies, but Sheehan, Sheehan, and Michiello (1981) reported a mean age of 19.6 years in various studies. The mean onset age for animal phobia and blood-injury phobia is about 8 years, 12 years for dental phobia, and 20 years for claustrophobia (Öst, 1987).

Specific phobias are especially responsive to behavioral treatment. However, there may be problems in arranging exposure for less approachable stimuli (e.g., storms) (Marks, 1987).

Familial and Genetic Patterns

Clearly there are familial influences on fears during childhood and adulthood. Positive correlations have been found routinely between the fears of children and their mothers (Barrios & Hartmen, 1987). The influence of mothers' and siblings' fears on the fears of children is probably greater among younger than among older children (McGlynn & McNeil, 1990). Familial influences also might be relatively stronger among children from lower socioeconomic strata. These data suggest that social learning factors are important in the development of specific phobias.

The concordances of blood-injury phobias and animal phobias were higher among monozygotic than among dizygotic twins (Torgersen, 1979). Blood-injury phobics have more relatives with similar problems than other phobics do. Among blood phobics, about 60% had first-degree relatives who were also blood phobic; this is three to six times more frequently than panic disorder, obsessive–

compulsive disorder, and agora-, social, dental, or animal phobics (Marks, 1987; Öst, 1992).

Diagnostic Considerations

In general, the diagnosis of specific phobia provides little difficulty. For the differential diagnosis, it is important that the fear is unrelated to agoraphobia, social phobia, posttraumatic stress disorder, and obsessive–compulsive disorder. A specific phobia can be a part of another anxiety disorder. For example, a patient with obsessive–compulsive problems also had an AIDS phobia. She had many cleaning rituals and obsessional concerns with germs and contamination. One of her obsessional concerns pertained to the fear of developing AIDS. In this case, the diagnosis of specific phobia should not be made. Further, anxiety related to a severe trauma is not diagnosed as specific phobia but may be associated with posttraumatic stress disorder. Finally, the fear of being scrutinized by other persons or feeling embarrassed is not referred to as specific phobia but as social phobia.

PANIC DISORDER

Description of the Disorder

Panic disorder is characterized by recurrent unexpected panic attacks. A panic attack is a discrete period of intense fear or discomfort. According to DSM-IV, attacks: (1) do not occur immediately before or after exposure to a situation that nearly always causes anxiety, and (2) are not the result of situations in which the person is the focus of others' attention (as in social phobia). During a panic attack, four of the following symptoms occur: shortness of breath (dyspnea), dizziness or unsteady feelings, palpitations (tachycardia), trembling or shaking, sweating, choking, nausea or abdominal distress, depersonalization or derealization, paresthesias, (hot) flushes or chills, chest pain or discomfort, fear of dying, and fear of losing control. These symptoms should not be due to any organic factor, such as amphetamine or caffeine intoxication or hyperthyroidism. DSM-III-R (American Psychiatric Association, 1987) differentiated among mild, moderate, and severe panic attacks. A severe panic disorder indicates at least eight panic attacks over the preceding month. In mild panic disorder, there has been at most one attack during the preceding month or all attacks were in fact limited-symptom attacks. The moderate panic disorder is in between mild and severe.

Many panic patients tend to avoid situations or activities that trigger panic attacks. Although avoidance behavior may prevent a person from having a panic attack, it usually leads to a very restricted lifestyle. A diagnosis of panic disorder with agoraphobia is made when the complaints meet the criteria of panic disorder and those of agoraphobia as well.

DSM-IV distinguishes between agoraphobia in connection with panic disorder and agoraphobia without a history of panic attacks. Agoraphobia as connected with panic disorder is described as a fear to be in places or situations from which it is difficult to escape, or in which there is no help at hand in case of a panic attack. In agoraphobia without panic disorder, there is a fear of suddenly emerging symptoms that may cause embarrassment to the person or make him or her in need of help, such as losing control over bladder or bowel, vomiting, depersonalization or derealization, and dizziness. This fear leads to avoidance of a number of situations, such as walking, standing in a queue, being in a large shop, mall, or crowded and busy streets, traveling in public transport, and driving a car.

Epidemiology

Panics are occasionally experienced by nearly 30% of the adult population, but most of these attacks are only mildly distressing (Norton, Cox, & Malan, 1990). An important difference between nonclinical panickers and panic patients is that the latter group responds with anxiety to the physical sensation whereas the former group does not.

The mean lifetime prevalence rate of panic disorder is 1.6%, and of agoraphobia about 4% in the community surveys summarized in Table 1. It should be noted that the prevalence figure of agoraphobia and panic disorder is somewhat unreliable due to the definitions used in the particular interview employed in the Epidemiology Catchment Area Study. Agoraphobia was found to be more prevalent than panic disorder. Agoraphobia and panic disorder constitute about 50 to 80% of the phobic patients seen in clinical practice. Both disorders are much more common among females than among males.

Clinical Picture

Jeanet (28 years of age) is referred for anxiety complaints, which have prevented her from doing her job in the past year. For 5 years, she has been suffering from panic attacks and symptoms of breathlessness, palpitations, and dizziness. She is afraid of having a heart attack. Over the past six months, she has had attacks on the average of 12 a month, characterized by a sudden increase of panic, which subsides after about 15 minutes. The attacks predominantly occur in crowded situations: crowded streets, shopping malls, and supermarkets. Recently, the patient has not been going out of the house on her own; she needs to be accompanied by a friend. Sometimes, at home, she becomes panicky without any apparent reason.

Although the somatic symptoms of panic attacks are well defined, the cognitive concomitants of patients may vary from patient to patient. A number of panic patients' fears are focused on the somatic consequences: They fear a heart attack, a stroke, or fainting. When patients' fears concern psychic loss of control, the anxiety centers around patients' belief that they are possibly going mad, often as a result of the depersonalization and derealization a patient may experience during a panic attack. Finally, a number of panic patients are afraid of criticism from other people reacting to their panic attack.

A number of investigators suggest that biological mechanisms may predispose subjects to experience panic attacks. Although it has been found that panic patients are characterized by heightened levels of activation in autonomic measures (e.g., heart rate, skin conductance), the significance of this for the development of panic disorder remains unclear. Such heightened physiological arousal may be the result of anxiety elicited by the laboratory situation, rather than evidence of a biological vulnerability. Further, rather than being a causative agent, the physiological activation can be secondary to the development of panic attacks.

PAUL M. G.
EMMELKAMP
and PATRICIA
VAN OPPEN

Why some individuals with recurrent panic attacks develop agoraphobia while others do not is as yet not really understood. The acute and intense experience of anxiety is held responsible for the tendency to escape, which is characteristic of the panic attack. It has been suggested that the severity of panic attacks and catastrophic cognitions associated with them determine whether patients will maintain a panic disorder without avoidance behavior or develop agoraphobia. Comparisons between patients having panic disorder with agoraphobia and those having panic disorder without agoraphobia have found few consistent disparities between groups.

Over half of the panic patients with or without agoraphobia also qualify for another anxiety disorder or depression (de Ruiter et al., 1989). There is considerable symptom overlap between panic disorder and generalized anxiety, which suggests that the differences between generalized anxiety and panic are more quantitative than qualitative. Agoraphobia and panic appear to be associated with depression and hypochondriasis. The rate of primary major depression is about 30%, while the range for secondary depression is 30 to 53% (Lesser, 1988). It is questionable whether depressive symptoms should be viewed as an independent disorder or as merely the result of the severe restrictions imposed on one's life when one has a panic disorder. The somatic complaints and preoccupations may be related to hyperventilation, which can result in heart palpitations, chest pains, sweating, and lightheadedness; these may play a causal role in provoking a panic attack. A hyperventilation attack with the concomitant bodily sensations often is accompanied by severe anxiety, which by itself may provoke hyperventilation in the future. This fear of panic may lead to avoidance of a number of situations, which ultimately may result in agoraphobia. In a number of patients, abnormalities in the vestibular system are involved; but how many of the panic patients this applies to is unclear (Jacob et al., 1989).

Alcohol abuse is common among panic patients. In a sample of panic patients with agoraphobia gathered from the Epidemiologic Catchment Area Study, nearly 30% qualified for the diagnosis of alcohol abuse or dependence (Himle & Hill, 1991). Patients with agoraphobia without panic attacks are less likely to also have an alcohol problem.

Most panic patients report catastrophic cognitions related to physical sensations during panic attacks. Patients with chest pain, breathlessness, numbness and tingling, blurred vision, and choking typically have thoughts about having a brain tumor, heart attack, or a stroke. Other patients have thoughts about the psychosocial consequences of their anxiety. For example, depersonalization is often related to thoughts about losing control, acting foolishly, and going crazy.

Agoraphobia is significantly more likely to be diagnosed among women than among men. The preponderance of agoraphobia in women may be due to psychosocial factors such as sex-role stereotyping, or biological factors (e.g., sex hormones). As yet, there is no convincing evidence for either a social learning or a biological interpretation of the sex difference in prevalence of agoraphobia (Emmelkamp, 1982; Hedlund & Chambless, 1990).

It has been suggested that the intimate relationship of agoraphobic patients with their partner may be of critical importance in the development and maintenance of agoraphobic symptoms (Hafner, 1982). Controlled studies, however, found that agoraphobics and their partners tend to be comparable to happily married individuals in terms of marital adjustment, intimacy, and relationship needs (Arrindell & Emmelkamp, 1986).

Although agoraphobics have been found to be more socially anxious, more externally controlled, and more introverted than controls, it is unclear whether these are premorbid personality features or whether these personality characteristics are merely the result of the panic and agoraphobic complaints. The same applies to the finding that nearly 20% of agoraphobics qualify for the diagnosis of avoidant personality disorder (Brooks, Baltazar, & Munjack, 1989).

Course and Prognosis

The mean age of onset of agoraphobia is approximately 28 years (Mannuzza, Fyer, Liebowitz, & Klein, 1990). In a large series of clinical patients, agoraphobia started mainly between ages 17 and 29, but with a few (16%) it started only after age 40 (Lelliott, McNamee, Marks, 1991). It has been suggested that agoraphobia has its precursor in separation anxiety in childhood; however, there is little evidence to substantiate such clinicians' claims (van der Molen et al., 1989).

Although agoraphobics may have their good days and their bad days, in only a few persons will agoraphobia remit spontaneously after a year. Treatment consisting of *in vivo* exposure is effective in nearly 75% of agoraphobics. Panic can be effectively treated by cognitive-behavior therapy and tricyclic antidepressants. If patients discontinue medication, relapse is the rule rather than the exception.

Familial and Genetic Patterns

Reich and Yates (1988) found the rate of panic disorder to be higher among the relatives of panic patients (9.3%) than among the relatives of social phobics (1.3%) and of controls (0%). A family history of agoraphobia has been reported to be more common in panic patients with agoraphobia than in patients with uncomplicated panic disorder (Harris et al., 1983; Noyes et al., 1986). Torgersen (1983) found a significantly higher concordance rate for agoraphobia and panic disorder in monozygotic twins than in dizygotic twins. Taken together, these results suggest that genetic factors play some role in panic disorder.

Diagnostic Considerations

Clinicians need to be attuned to the possibility of co-morbid alcohol dependence among panic patients. Since a number of panic patients do not report alcohol problems spontaneously, sensitive questioning is needed.

Although a number of agoraphobics appear to have specific phobias as well, closer scrutiny may reveal that these phobias are actually part of the agoraphobic symptomatology and the result of a panic attack in particular situations. A close temporal relationship between a panic attack and fear in a particular situation may alert clinicians to the possibility that the phobia developed in the context of a panic attack. It is also important to realize that most specific phobias develop at a relatively young age. In a number of patients, however, specific phobias, such as fear of heights and fear of enclosed spaces, may exist long before the onset of their first panic attack (de Ruiter et al., 1989), in which case an additional diagnosis of specific phobia is justified. Panic should be distinguished from hypochondriasis, which is characterized by a persistent conviction and fear of having a serious disease. Panic patients are usually less concerned about having a serious disease between panic attacks.

Some social phobics avoid the same situations as agoraphobics. Agoraphobia can be differentiated from social phobia by detailed inquiry into the reasons people avoid certain situations. With social phobics, anxiety is triggered by the fear of criticism and (negative) evaluation. The fear is not for the symptoms as such, but for possible scrutiny by other people. In agoraphobia (with panic), the fear involves having a panic attack or losing control. There is also some difference in the physical symptoms experienced. With social phobics, blushing is common, whereas difficulty in breathing, dizziness, and weakness in limbs are more characteristic somatic symptoms of agoraphobics.

SOCIAL PHOBIA

Description of the Disorder

In DSM-IV, "social phobia" is described as a persistent fear of one or more social or performance situations in which the person is exposed to possible scrutiny by others, and fears to behave in a way that will be humiliating and embarrassing. Social phobics are anxious when confronted with the feared situation, and those situations will generally be avoided or endured only with intense anxiety, if avoidance is impossible. The avoidance behavior interferes with occupational or social functioning. The fear must be unrelated to panic disorder or to somatic disorders. As an example, fear of trembling that results from Parkinson's Disease does not justify a diagnosis of social phobia.

In DSM-III, social phobia was described as a persistent irrational fear of one specific social situation: Fears for more than one social situation were classified as "avoidant personality disorder" rather than as social phobia. In DSM-IV, fear of several social situations is classified as "social phobia" with the addition "generalized type."

Epidemiology

Results of epidemiological studies are summarized in Table 1. The 6-month prevalence rate is less than 2%. Social phobia is less prevalent than agoraphobia. Both in community surveys (Bourdon et al., 1988) and in clinical samples there appears to be an equal sex ratio.

Clinical Picture

John is 20-year-old male who is extremely bothered by social phobia. At first sight, the complaints look like agoraphobia. He does not leave the house and is afraid of going to shops because it makes him anxious. On inquiry it appears that it is not so much a matter of fear of a panic attack, but rather, a fear of what other people might think of him. He is very discontented about his appearance although there is nothing wrong with it. And he is preoccupied with the idea that everybody finds him stupid. Recently, he would not dare to open the door or to answer the phone. He is still living with his mother, who takes care of shopping and such things. When his mother has visitors, which happens rarely, he remains in his room. As a child, John was very withdrawn and always had a feeling of not belonging. For a brief period, he worked at a warehouse; however, when his boss made a very critical remark once, he did not return to work. Since that time his complaints have worsened.

The essential feature of social phobia is "a marked or persistent fear of one or more social or performance situations in which the person is exposed to possible scrutiny by others and fears that he or she may do something or act in a way that will be humiliating or embarrassing." A number of social phobics experience fear in any social situation; however, in other patients, fears are limited to specific situations. For example, some patients fear that their hands may tremble when writing or holding a cup in front of others. Others may be afraid of blushing or of eating in public places. Most social phobics have difficulty with at least two different situations, and nearly half feel anxious in three or more situations.

Holt, Heimberg, Hope, and Liebowitz (1992) distinguished four different situational domains of social phobia: (1) formal speaking and interaction, (2) informal speaking and interaction, (3) observation by others, and (4) assertion. Seventy-five percent of the social phobics experienced anxiety in more than one domain. Nearly all social phobics had significant problems in the formal speaking/ interaction domain, which corroborates the clinical impression that public speaking anxiety is prevalent among social phobics.

Although earlier research suggested that social phobics lacked adequate social skills, more recent studies do not support this as far as specific interpersonal behaviors such as eye contact and length of speaking time are concerned (Monti et al., 1984). Cognitive factors, such as negative self-statements and irrational beliefs, appear to be more important (Sanderman et al., 1987). Social phobics display considerably more negative self-statements in social contacts than non-anxious persons. Further, they tend to evaluate their own (social) behavior in an excessively negative way and selectively attend to negative experiences in social situations.

Although alcohol abuse and dependence is often a problem in social phobics, the prevalence is less among social phobics than among panic patients (Himle & Hill, 1991). However, social phobics with concurrent alcohol abuse are more anxious than social phobics without an alcohol problem (Schneier et al., 1989). Retrospective studies focusing on the antecedent factors of social phobia have found problematic relationships with parents—relationships lacking in emotional warmth, and marred by rejection and overprotection (Arrindell et al., 1983).

Course and Prognosis

The onset of social phobia is usually in adolescence (around the age of 18), which is much earlier than the mean age of onset in agoraphobia. When patients report both alcohol abuse and social phobia, the social phobia precedes the onset of the alcohol problem in nearly all cases (Schneier et al., 1989). The prognosis for patients treated with cognitive and behavior therapy is relatively good (Scholing & Emmelkamp, 1990).

Familial and Genetic Patterns

Few systematic studies exist. Reich and Yates (1988) found a higher prevalence of social phobia (6.5%) among the relatives of social phobics than among the relatives of panic patients (0.4%). However, this study provides only meager evidence of a genetic disposition, since environmental factors can account equally well for the differences obtained. Torgersen (1988) garnered some support in twin studies for a genetic contribution to social fears in normals; however, twin studies with social phobics are lacking.

Diagnostic Considerations

Social phobia is distinguished from the shyness and social anxiety that many individuals experience by the intensity of the fears and the abnormal avoidance of the social situations involved. There is considerable overlap among social phobia, panic disorder, and generalized anxiety. Rather than being considered as distinct diagnostic categories, phobic symptoms are better viewed as lying in a number of different continua. The actual primary diagnosis depends on the predominant features in a particular patient.

Many social phobics meet criteria for avoidant personality disorder; and it is questionable whether social phobia and avoidant personality disorder are two separate categories (Scholing & Emmelkamp, 1990). Actually, in DSM-III-R, six out of the seven criteria for the avoidant personality disorder overlap with criteria for generalized social phobia. However, there is some evidence that individuals with an avoidant personality disorder are less socially skilled and more socially anxious than social phobics. It has been suggested that individuals with an avoidant personality disorder are more accepting of their limitations in social situations than social phobics without this personality disorder.

Social phobia may, in a number of cases, be related to dysmorphophobia and difficult to distinguish from this disorder. In other cases, the diagnosis of dysmorphophobia rather than social phobia is more appropriate. In DSM-III-R, dysmorphophobia is not classified among the anxiety disorders but among the somatoform disorders. Patients qualify for the diagnosis of dysmorphophobia when they are preoccupied with a presumed physical anomaly of their body, with no objective basis. Most dysmorphophobics experience anxiety in social contacts and tend to avoid these situations. Marks and Mishan (1988) found that most dysmorphophobics had to cope with social anxiety and avoidance behavior as a result of the disorder.

GENERALIZED ANXIETY DISORDER

Description of the Disorder

Generalized anxiety disorder (GAD) is defined in DSM-IV as excessive or unrealistic anxiety and worry about a number of events or activities for a period of 6 months or more. Although a patient may have "good days" without much worrying, there should be more "worry days" than days that the individual is not bothered by these concerns. Most worries of generalized anxiety patients involve anxious apprehension with respect to finances, work, interpersonal problems, accidents, or illnesses and health issues.

GAD, which before its introduction in DSM-III, was known as free-floating anxiety, has poor diagnostic reliability and is not easily distinguished from other anxiety disorders. Many patients with GAD also meet criteria for another anxiety disorder, usually social or simple phobia (Barlow et al., 1986). Most panic patients, agoraphobics, obsessive–compulsives, and social phobics present symptoms that belong to the generalized anxiety cluster. There is further symptom overlap with depression. Breslau and Davis (1985) found that many depressed persons had concomitant symptoms of GAD, and they questioned the utility of the category of generalized anxiety.

Epidemiology

Generalized anxiety is very common in the general population. It is probably the most frequent anxiety disorder in the community. Yet, most patients do not seek treatment other than that provided by their general practitioner (Edelmann, 1992).

Clinical Picture

> Judith is a 34-year-old woman with two children, who has sought treatment because of anxiety complaints. In fact, she has felt anxious as long as she can remember. She describes herself as the worrying type. In elementary school, she was afraid of being teased; and during her adolescence she hardly went out because she thought other people would not like her anyway. As a child, she was afraid of accidents, thunder, and being home alone. These fears have persisted over the years. Since she got married, she has been constantly worried about financial matters although her husband has a well-paid job. Since she had children, she has been constantly afraid that they might meet an accident or be taken away by strangers. Further, Judith cannot stand loud noises and she is very frightful. She makes a very tense impression and startles at the sound of a telephone. The immediate reason for referral is that her eldest son (12 years old) has to go to school by bike, but she would not allow this until now because she is afraid of him having an accident. This has led to a severe row with her husband, who thinks she is too overprotective.

Worry is the central characteristic of GAD. However, before meeting full criteria, persons also need to have a number of anxiety symptoms. Three out of the following symptoms are required: (1) restlessness or feeling keyed up or on edge, (2) being easily fatigued, (3) difficulty concentrating, (4) irritability, (5) muscle tension, and (6) sleep disturbance.

Most generalized anxiety patients are seen by general practitioners, who usually prescribe tranquilizing drugs. Few patients are referred to clinical psychologists or psychiatrists.

Some have argued that generalized anxiety should not be considered a separate anxiety disorder. According to these investigators, the difference between GAD and other anxiety disorders, particularly panic disorder, is more quantitative than qualitative. There is some evidence, however, that generalized anxiety can be differentiated from panic on physiological measures. Hoehn-Saric and McLeod (1988) have suggested that generalized anxiety is associated with an inhibition in some sympathetic systems. Panic patients had higher EMG and higher heart rate than generalized anxiety patients when tested in the laboratory (Barlow et al., 1984). Other differences between panic disorder and GAD are the sudden onset in panic patients in contrast with the more gradual onset in generalized anxiety and a presumably genetic component in panic disorder, which has not been found in GAD.

Barlow (1988) has contended that GAD is the end result of a process in which multiple etiological factors are involved. According to Barlow, generalized anxiety patients have a biological vulnerability and experience external stressors (life events and daily hassles) as uncontrollable and unpredictable, eventually culminating in a spiral of worrying. Although this model has some appeal, it is far from proven yet. There is some evidence that generalized anxiety patients are characterized by selective processing of emotional stimuli. Mathews and his colleagues have consistently shown that selective attentional attraction to threat cues is characteristic of generalized anxiety patients (Mathews, 1990).

Course and Prognosis

The onset of generalized anxiety is usually earlier than in panic disorder and, as a rule, slow and gradual. However, this picture is based on GAD patients seen by clinicians. Whether the same applies to generalized anxiety patients who are not referred to clinicians is unclear. No reliable data exist on the prognosis of treated and untreated patients with GAD.

Familial and Genetic Patterns

There is no evidence of a genetic component in GAD (Torgersen, 1983, 1986). Family studies do not reveal a higher prevalence of generalized anxiety among family members of generalized anxiety patients than among family members of controls (Anderson, Noyes, & Crowe, 1984).

Diagnostic Considerations

Given the symptom overlap with mood disorders, such as major depression and dysthymia, and with anxiety disorders (e.g., agoraphobia, panic disorder, obsessive–compulsive disorder, and social phobia), the diagnosis of GAD often presents problems, even for the experienced clinician. An important diagnostic difference is the focus of the worries. Panic patients are primarily concerned over having a panic attack. They report catastrophic cognitions associated with disastrous consequences primarily related to malfunctioning of their own body. Social phobics are primarily concerned about social evaluation and criticism from others and obsessive–compulsives about contamination, harming, etc. In contrast, generalized anxiety patients worry excessively about minor and often futile things and are not primarily concerned about bodily symptoms. However, a number of generalized anxiety patients are concerned about social evaluation and criticism, thus blurring a clearcut difference with social phobics. In such cases, the degree of avoidance of social situations may help in differentiating between social phobia and GAD. Although patients with generalized anxiety tend to avoid a number of situations, the avoidance is less focused than in the case of social phobia, agoraphobia, and simple phobia.

Description of the Disorder

Either recurrent obsessions or compulsions have to occur for a diagnosis of obsessive–compulsive disorder (OCD). Essential for the diagnosis of OCD is that the complaints cause marked distress, are time-consuming (take more than an hour), or interfere with the social or work functioning. The content of the obsession or compulsion must be unrelated to any other Axis I disorder.

Obsessions are repetitive, recurring thoughts, ideas, images, or impulses that are experienced as intrusive. The person recognizes that the obsessions are the product of his or her own mind. Obsessions are experienced as senseless or repugnant, which the patient attempts to ignore or suppress.

Compulsions, on the other hand, are repetitive, apparent, purposeful behaviors that are performed according to certain rules, or in a stereotyped fashion. Compulsions have the function of neutralizing or preventing discomfort and/or anxiety.

Epidemiology

About 10 years ago, the prevalence of OCD in the general population was estimated at 0.05% (Emmelkamp, 1982). However, in recent years, community surveys (Bland et al., 1988; Burnam et al., 1987; Karno et al., 1987; Myers et al., 1984; Robins et al., 1984; Wittchen, 1988) have shown a relatively high prevalence rate of OCD. The lifetime prevalence rate of different surveys is presented in Table 1. The mean lifetime prevalence of OCD was 2.4%. In these community surveys, the prevalence of OCD was slightly higher among females than among males.

Clinical Picture

Sophia, a 30-year-old unmarried woman, has been suffering from compulsive checking and obsessions. Over the past month, she also felt very depressed. She had an apartment of her own but lived with her parents as a result of her fear of losing control over her behaviors. When leaving home, she had to return several times to check the gas, taps, doors, and windows repeatedly. In addition, her father had to check everything in order to make sure that she did not do anything wrong. Apart from this checking, she suffered from obsessions. She had the idea that she would do some horrible things on purpose and that other people would be harmed. For example, she had to check letters over and over again because she was afraid that she would write down Stupid Mrs. X instead of Dear Mrs. X. She developed her obsessive–compulsive problems at age 26, shortly after her boyfriend broke up their relationship. Soon after her complaints started, she was unable to perform her job. She worked in a day-care center and her obsessions concerned doing irresponsible things in her job. She had never had any checking compulsions or obsessions before, but she used to be very perfectionistic. She hardly had any relationships apart from her parents.

Obsessions are mostly accompanied by rituals or compulsions. A majority (nearly 80%) of the obsessive–compulsive patients have obsessions as well as compulsions. A minority of such patients suffer from obsessions only, most often harming obsessions. Patients with harming obsessions are afraid of harming

PAUL M. G.
EMMELKAMP
and PATRICIA
VAN OPPEN

others (e.g., by strangling) and avoid ropes and sharp objects—such as knives, scissors, pieces of glass—or being alone with young children or helpless elderly people. A few are only concerned about harming themselves (e.g., by committing suicide). Patients with only rituals are seen very rarely. Generally, the obsessions are anxiety-inducing and the performance of compulsions leads to anxiety reduction.

The most common compulsions involve "cleaning" and "checking." Less common complaints are compulsive slowness, orderliness, hoarding, buying, and counting. A person who suffers from compulsive hoarding collects all kinds of things and may have cupboards full with old bills, notes, hundreds of pairs of shoes, and underwear. These objects are not used, but the patient is afraid of throwing them away because they may come in handy one day. Compulsive buying implies that the person has a strong inclination to buy a wide variety of items. Compulsive counting often accompanies checking and washing. In some patients, this counting is the main problem. In a number of patients, neutralizing thoughts have the same function as rituals, that is, the undoing of the harmful effects of the obsession.

Two types of avoidance behavior are distinguished: active and passive avoidance. The obsessive–compulsive person avoids stimuli that might provoke anxiety and discomfort (passive avoidance). Active avoidance refers to the motor component of obsessive–compulsive behavior (e.g., cleaning and washing) in case the passive avoidance failed (Emmelkamp, 1982). Examples of passive avoidance are people with checking compulsions who avoid situations that provoke their rituals, such as being alone, driving a car, using matches, or being the last one going to bed. Individuals with a cleaning or washing obsession take many precautions to avoid contaminations. When obsessions are related to death, people avoid all kinds of situations that suggest the notion of death, such as reading papers (obituaries), watching TV, and going to a funeral.

There exists considerable co-morbidity between OCD and other disorders. For example, depression and OCD overlap with one another. Depression is a frequent complication of OCD. Studies of co-morbidity suggest that about 75% of obsessive–compulsive patients report major depression (Black & Noyes, 1990). The obsessive–compulsive symptoms often worsen during the depressed mood and severe depression may influence the prognosis badly (Marks, 1987). Transition from obsession to depression occurs three times more often than the opposite direction (Marks, 1987). There is also a considerable overlap between OCD, phobias, and other anxiety disorders. Rasmussen and Tsuang (1986) found that 58% of 100 obsessive–compulsive patients had a lifetime prevalence of simple phobia, social phobia, or panic disorder. The frequency of personality disorders among obsessive–compulsives is high. The obsessive–compulsive personality seems overrepresented among obsessive–compulsive patients. According to DSM-III, an obsessive–compulsive personality was reported in over half of OCD patients. There is also a marked history of anorexia nervosa in women with OCD (Kasvikis et al., 1986). Although it has been suggested that OCD is often associated with the Gilles de la Tourette syndrome, Rasmussen and Tsuang (1986) reported only a 5% incidence of Tourette's syndrome in patients with OCD; this is consistent with our own clinical observation. Previously, many investigators suggested that OCD and schizophrenia were related; however, longitudinal studies have not found an increased incidence of schizophrenia either in obsessive–compulsive patients or in their relatives (Black & Noyes, 1990).

The gender ratio among patients was nearly 1:1 (Marks, 1987). Checking, however, is more prevalent among males, while washing and cleaning are more common among females (Hoekstra, Visser, & Emmelkamp, 1989). These investigators provide some evidence that the type of obsessive–compulsive behavior is related to the tasks for which the individual is responsible.

Course and Prognosis

Mean age of onset is 20 to 25 years with 10% starting before age 10, and 9% starting after age 40 (Black, 1974; Emmelkamp, 1990). The age at onset among males (20 years) is earlier than among females (25 years) (Minichiello, Baer, Jenike, & Holland, 1990). Data from this study revealed that cleaners had a later age of onset than checkers.

The age of consultation between onset of illness and the time of the first visit to a clinician is about 10 years. Thus, the age of obsessive–compulsive patients at first treatment is about 30 years (Yaryura-Tobias & Neziroglu, 1983). Sometimes the onset of OCD is immediate; typically, however, problems arise insidiously over several years.

If the obsessive–compulsive patients do not get adequate treatment, the disorder tends to have a chronic, fluctuating course. Treatment of choice consists of behavior therapy, namely, *in vivo* exposure plus response prevention. Where this treatment is given, approximately 75% of the patients have displayed improvement and about 25% of the patients have remained unchanged on self-ratings of obsessive–compulsive symptoms, anxiety, and depression (Marks, 1987).

Familial and Genetic Patterns

Some previous family investigations observed from 4% to 15% obsessive–compulsive traits and/or symptoms among relatives of patients with OCD (see review by Torgersen, 1988). Studies showed that relatives of obsessive–compulsives have an increased risk of developing an anxiety disorder. They also showed that relatives of phobic patients have an increased risk of getting OCD. More recently, Rasmussen and Tsuang (1986) found that 5% of the parents of probands with OCD met the criteria for OCD.

Twin studies indicate that OCD seems to be influenced by genetic factors, although environmental factors also have an important role in their development.

Diagnostic Considerations

Certain obsessive thoughts should not be diagnosed as OCD (e.g., the worrying in GAD and the obsessive concern with one's own health in hypochondriasis).

It is not always simple to distinguish agoraphobia from OCD, especially when the OCD patient avoids situations that are characteristic of avoidance in agoraphobics, such as going outdoors. However, the evoking stimuli of obsessive–compulsives differ from those of agoraphobics. And when passive avoidance fails, exposure will lead to compulsions in OCD. Although an obsessive–compulsive patient may avoid going outdoors, the reason for this avoidance is totally different from that of an agoraphobic. Agoraphobic patients are often afraid of having a panic attack; obsessive–compulsive patients may avoid going outdoors out of fear of contamination or in order to prevent checking rituals when he/she has to leave the house.

Depression is very common in people with obsessions and compulsions. In most cases, the depression is secondary to the obsessive–compulsive disorder, which is not surprising considering the severity of the complaints. When obsessive thoughts are part of a depressive episode and disappear when the depression subsides, the diagnosis of depression is more appropriate than the diagnosis OCD. Similarly, obsessions as part of a psychotic episode are not classified as OCD. Hallucinations and delusions need to be differentiated from obsessions. The main diagnostic question here is whether the person recognizes that his/her thoughts or ideas are unreasonable.

Obsessive–compulsive traits are differentiated from OCD in that they are ego-syntonic, rarely provoke resistance, and are seldom accompanied by compulsions. In OCD patients, symptoms are ego-dystonic and usually provoke resistance; compulsions are very common.

When patients have tics, these are diagnosed as tic disorder. Tics are seen as involuntary behaviors, whereas compulsions are intentional behaviors (Emmelkamp, 1990).

POST-TRAUMATIC STRESS DISORDER

Description of the Disorder

Post-traumatic stress disorder (PTSD) is characterized by a number of stress symptoms that are the result of exposure to a recognizable stressor of sufficient magnitude to evoke stress in almost anyone. Characteristic symptoms include: (1) reexperiencing of the trauma (e.g., flashbacks), and intrusive thoughts related to the traumatic event (e.g., nightmares); (2) avoidance of stimuli related to the trauma (e.g., psychogenic amnesia), and numbing symptoms (e.g., constricted affect and feelings of detachment); and (3) indices of increased tension (e.g., sleep disturbance, irritability and anger, difficulty in concentrating, exaggerated startle response, hypervigilance). The symptoms are the result of extreme stress following a trauma, such as rape, assault, severe accident, aircrash, natural disasters, and war atrocities. Although this disorder previously has been described as "war neurosis," KZ-syndrome, " shell shock," or traumatic neurosis, it was not until 1980 that it was recognized as a specific diagnostic category in DSM-III.

Epidemiology

In the ECA study, the prevalence of PTSD was estimated at about 1% (Helzer, Robins, & McEnroy, 1987), although this figure is probably an underestimation. In a large representative sample of Vietnam veterans, the incidence of PTSD was 15% and 8.5% and the lifetime prevalence 30.9% and 26.9% for males and females, respectively (Kulka et al., cited in Keane, Litz, & Blake, 1990). Similar figures were reported for crime victims: 27.8% lifetime prevalence and 7.5% incidence (Kilpatrick et al., 1987). Thus, PTSD appears to be a common disorder among persons who have undergone a severe trauma.

> Diana (22 years old) works behind the desk at a bank. One day, a disguised man appeared at her desk with a gun and threatened to kill her if she would not immediately hand over all the money to him. It was ruled, according to the bank's regulations, that Diane provided the attacker with the money. After this event, she stayed at home for a couple of days. The manager had to coerce her to resume her activities, after a few days. In the course of a month, she reported being sick because of an increase in complaints. She had inexplicable attacks of anger at home as well as at work. Several times at night she suffered from nightmares, wherein she was being threatened or being followed by a man with a balaclava. She would awaken totally perspiring. Her relationship with her boyfriend was negatively influenced by this course of events. He became much like a stranger to her. Upon seeing violent scenes on television, she became extremely anxious, which was also the case upon seeing men on mopeds (the bank robber disappeared on a moped). Diana does not go to work, out of fear of being attacked again. Over the past year, the office had been robbed three times. Apart from this, she no longer watches television, out of fear of being confronted with violence; she reads only the sports pages of the newspaper for the same reason.

Immediate stress reactions are common and normal after a traumatic event. These symptoms include nightmares, heightened startle responses, or dissociative reactions; they frequently disappear without any treatment.

A number of studies suggest that PTSD is associated with drug and alcohol abuse; these findings, however, are primarily based on Vietnam veterans. Although alcohol and drug abuse may occur in other PTSD sufferers (e.g., rape victims), this is more often the exception than the rule. Although many factors appear to be involved in the etiology of PTSD (including biological and psychological vulnerability, social support, and coping style), one factor seems to be the most important: the severity of the trauma (Keane, Litz, & Blake, 1990). Generally, the degree of exposure to the stressor, the duration of the traumatic event, and the degree of the life threat are all directly related to the severity of the disturbance.

Course and Prognosis

Little is known about the course of PTSD, since longitudinal studies are lacking. However, recent developments in cognitive-behavior therapy look promising, especially for combat- and crime-related PTSD (Emmelkamp, 1993). Long-term follow-up investigations are needed before firm statements regarding the prognosis can be made.

Familial and Genetic Patterns

Few studies have addressed this issue. Davidson et al. (1985) found among Vietnam veterans a lower prevalence of family disorder in PTSD than in major depression and GAD. The most common disorders of PTSD family members were alcohol/drug abuse (60%) and other anxiety disorders (22%). Although Foy, Resnick, Sipprelle, and Carroll (1987) reported a higher prevalence of family psychopathology among Vietnam veterans with PTSD than among Vietnam veterans without PTSD, they found that under conditions of high combat exposure, the

PAUL M. G.
EMMELKAMP
and PATRICIA
VAN OPPEN

influence of familial disposition was negligible. As noted earlier, a history of family psychopathology alone does not prove any genetic contribution. If there is a vulnerability, this may be genetically determined, psychologically determined, or a coeffect of both genetic and psychological influences.

Diagnostic Considerations

Although PTSD is one of the few disorders in which an etiological agent (traumatic event) is part of the diagnostic criteria, a traumatic event by itself is an insufficient basis to warrant the diagnosis of PTSD. For every sufferer of a traumatic event with PTSD, there are many more persons who have undergone the same trauma but do not qualify for the diagnosis of PTSD.

Generally, the diagnosis of PTSD does not offer special difficulties. In some cases, depression may be more in the forefront of the clinical picture, and the PTSD symptomatology may be overlooked. In other instances, the distinction from GAD can be difficult. In contrast with GAD, PTSD patients do not worry about the future; rather, they worry about the past, and the (cognitive) avoidance and numbness of feelings are not characteristic of GAD. Further, PTSD can be distinguished from adjustment disorder by the reexperiencing of the traumatic event and by the severity of the stressor.

SUMMARY

Since the introduction of DSM-III in 1980, considerable research has been conducted regarding characteristics and clinical features of anxiety disorders. As a result of these efforts, reliable data are now available on such issues as onset age, co-morbidity, and prevalence of the various anxiety disorders.

The onset age varies across the different anxiety disorders. Co-morbidity seems to be a frequent phenomenon in the general population and even more common in clinical samples. Many patients of one anxiety disorder qualify for another anxiety disorder as well. Depression and alcohol abuse are often co-morbid disorders, especially in panic patients and social phobics.

Epidemiological studies have revealed that anxiety disorders are much more frequent among the general population than once thought. Actually, anxiety disorder is the most prevalent disorder among females and the second most prevalent disorder among males.

Few long-term follow-up studies have been conducted on course and prognosis of anxiety disorders. Consequently, our knowledge regarding the natural course of untreated anxiety disorders is limited (Wittchen & Essau, 1989). Generally, spontaneous remission is infrequently found in the various anxiety disorders (Wittchen, 1991). A number of long-term follow-up studies with obsessive–compulsives and agoraphobics reveal that the positive results of behavioral treatment are maintained up to 6 and 9 years. Long-term follow-up studies with respect to the other anxiety disorders and to other treatment approaches are lacking.

The role of genetic factors is still unclear. Although there is some evidence for a genetic contribution, especially in panic disorder, further investigations are needed before more definitive conclusions can be reached. It is now a well-established finding that there is a higher family prevalence of anxiety disorders than would be expected by chance (Torgersen, 1988). However, results of such family studies have to be qualified. First, there is a serious risk of overdiagnosis when carrying out family studies in an unblind fashion. Second, such studies provide meager evidence of a genetic disposition, since environmental factors can account equally well for the differences found.

REFERENCES

American Psychiatric Association (1987). *Diagnostic and statistical manual of mental disorders*, 3rd Edition, Revised. Washington, DC: Author.

American Psychiatric Association (1993). *DSM-IV draft criteria*. Washington, DC: Author.

Anderson, D. J., Noyes, R. J., & Crowe, R. R. (1984). A comparison of panic disorder and generalized anxiety disorders. *American Journal of Psychiatry, 141*, 572–575.

Arrindell, W. A., & Emmelkamp, P. M. G. (1986). Marital adjustment, intimacy and needs in female agoraphobics and their partners: A controlled study. *British Journal of Psychiatry, 146*, 405–414.

Arrindell, W. A., Emmelkamp, P. M. G., Monsma, A., & Brilman, E. (1983). The role of perceived parental rearing practices in the aetiology of phobic disorders: A controlled study. *British Journal of Psychiatry, 143*, 183–187.

Barlow, D. H. (1988). *Anxiety and its disorders*. New York: Guilford Press.

Barlow, D. H., Cohen, A. S., Waddell, M. T., Vermilyea, B. B., Klosko, J. S., Blanchard, E. B., & DiNardo, P. A. (1984). Panic and generalized anxiety disorders: Nature and treatment. *Behavior Therapy, 15*, 431–449.

Barlow, D. H., DiNardo, P. A., Vermilyea, B. B., Vermilyea, J., & Blanchard, E. B. (1986). Co-morbidity and depression among the anxiety disorders: Issues in diagnosis and classification. *Journal of Nervous and Mental Disease, 174*, 63–72.

Barrios, B. A., & Hartmen, D. P. (1987). Fears and anxieties. In E. J. Mash & L. G. Terdal (Eds.), *Behavioral assessment of childhood disorders* (pp. 196–262). New York: Guilford Press.

Black, A. (1974). The natural history of obsessional neurosis. In H. R. Beech (Ed.), *Obsessional states*. London: Methuen.

Black, A. & Noyes, R. (1990). Co-morbidity of the obsessive compulsive disorder. In J. D. Maser, & C. R. Cloninger, (Eds.), *Comorbidity of mood and anxiety disorders* (pp. 463–543). Washington: American Psychiatric Press.

Bland, R. C., Orn, H., & Newman, S. C. (1988). Lifetime prevalence of psychiatric disorders in Edmonton. *Acta Psychiatrica Scandinavica, 77*, 24–32.

Bourdon, K. H., Boyd, J. H., Rae, D. S., Burns, B. J., Thompson, J. W., & Locke, B. Z. (1988). Gender differences in phobias: Results of the ECA Community Survey. *Journal of Anxiety Disorders, 2*, 227–241.

Breslau, N., & Davis, G. C. (1985). Further evidence on the doubtful validity of generalized anxiety disorder. *Psychiatry Research, 16*, 177–179.

Brooks, R. B., Baltazar, V., and Munjack, D. J. (1989). Co-occurrence of personality disorders with panic disorder, social phobia, and generalized anxiety disorder: A review of the literature. *Journal of Anxiety Disorders, 3*, 259–285.

Burnam, M. A., Hough, R. L., Escobar, J. I., Karno, M., Timbers, D. M., Telles, C. A., & Locke, B. Z. (1987). Six-month prevalence of specific psychiatric disorders among Mexican Americans and non-hispanic whites in Los Angeles. *Archives of General Psychiatry, 44*, 687–694.

Davidson, J., Swartz, M., Stork, M., Krishman, R. R., & Hammett, E. (1985). A diagnostic and family study of posttraumatic stress disorder. *American Journal of Psychiatry, 142*, 90–93.

de Ruiter, C., Rijken, H., Garssen, B., van Schaik, A., & Kraaimaat, F. (1989). Comorbidity among the anxiety disorders. *Journal of Anxiety Disorders , 3*, 57–68.

Edelmann, R. J. (1992). *Anxiety: Theory, research and intervention in clinical and health psychology*. Chichester: Wiley.

Emmelkamp, P. M. G. (1982). *Phobic and obsessive–compulsive disorders*. New York: Plenum Press.

Emmelkamp, P. M. G. (1990). Obsessive compulsive disorder in adulthood. In M. Hersen & C. G. Last (Eds.), *Handbook of child and adult psychopathology* (pp. 221–234). New York: Pergamon.

Emmelkamp, P. M. G. (1993). Behavior therapy with adults. In S. Garfield & A. Bergin (Eds.), *Handbook of psychotherapy and behavior change* (4th Ed.). New York: Wiley.

Foy, D. W., Resnick, H. S., Sipprelle, R. C., & Carroll, E. M. (1987). Premilitary, military, and postmilitary factors in the development of combat-related stress disorders. *The Behavior Therapist, 10*, 3–9.

Hafner, J. (1982). The marital context of the agoraphobic syndrome. In D. L. Chambless & A. J. Goldstein (Eds.), *Agoraphobia: Multiple perspectives on theory and treatment.* (pp. 77–118). New York: Wiley.

Harris, E. L., Noyes, R., Crowe, R. R., & Chaudry, D. R. (1983). A family study of agoraphobia: Report of a pilot study. *Archives of General Psychiatry, 40*, 1061–1064.

Hedlund, M. A., & Chambless, D. L. (1990). Sex differences and menstrual cycle effects in aversive conditioning: A comparison of premenstrual and intermenstrual women with men. *Journal of Anxiety Disorders, 4*, 221–231.

Helzer, J. E., Robins, L. N., & McEnroy, M. A. (1987). Post-traumatic stress disorder in the general population. *The New England Journal of Medicine, 317*, 1630–1634.

Himle, J. A., & Hill, E. M. (1991). Alcohol abuse and the anxiety disorders: Evidence from the Epidemiologic Catchment Area Survey. *Journal of Anxiety Disorders, 5*, 237–245.

Hoehn-Saric, R., & McLeod, D. R. (1988). The peripheral sympathetic nervous system: Its role in normal and pathologic anxiety. *Psychiatric Clinics of North America, 11*, 375–386.

Hoekstra, R. J., Visser, S., & Emmelkamp, P. M. G. (1989). A social learning formulations of the etiology of obsessive–compulsive disorders. In P. M. G. Emmelkamp, W. T. A. M. Everaerd, R. W. Kraaimaat, & M. J. M. van Son (Eds.), *Fresh perspectives on anxiety disorders.* Lisse: Swets and Zeitlinger.

Holt, C. S., Heimberg, R. G., Hope, D. A., & Liebowitz, M. R. (1992). Situational domains of social phobia. *Journal of Anxiety Disorders, 6*, 63–77.

Jacob, R. G., Lilienfeld, S. O., Furman, J. M. R., Durrant, J. D., & Turner, S. M. (1989). Panic disorder with vestibular dysfunction: Further clinical observations and description of space and motion phobic stimuli. *Journal of Anxiety Disorders, 3*, 117–130.

Karno, M., Hough, R. L., Burnam, A., Escobar, J. I., Timbers, D. M., Santana, F., & Boyd, J. H. (1987). Lifetime prevalence of specific psychiatric disorders among Mexican Americans and non-hispanic whites in Los Angeles. *Archives of General Psychiatry, 44*, 695–701.

Kasvikis, G. Y., Tsakiris, F., Marks, I. M. Basoglu, M., & Noshirvani, H. F. (1986). Past history of anorexia nervosa in women with obsessive–compulsive disorder. *International Journal of Eating Disorders, 5*, 1069–1075.

Keane, T. M., Litz, B. T., & Blake, D. D. (1990). Post-traumatic stress disorder in adulthood. In M. Hersen & C. G. Last (Eds.), *Handbook of child and adult psychopathology.* New York: Pergamon Press.

Kilpatrick, D. G., Saunders, B. E., Veronen, L., Best, C. L., & Von, J. M. (1987). Criminal victimization: Lifetime prevalence, reporting to police, and psychological impact. *Crime and Delinquency, 33*, 479–489.

Kulka, R. A., Sehlenger, W. E., Fairbank, J. A., Hough, R. L., Jordan, B. K., Marmar, C. R., & Weiss, D. S. (1988). *National Vietnam veterans readjustment study (NVVRS): Description, current status, and initial PTSD prevalence estimates.* Washington, DC: Veterans Administration.

Lelliott, P., McNamee, G., & Marks, I. (1991). Features of agora-, social, and related phobias and validation of the diagnoses. *Journal of Anxiety Disorders, 5*, 313–322.

Lesser, I. M. (1988). The relationship between panic disorder and depression. *Journal of Anxiety Disorders, 2*, 3–15.

Mannuzza, S., Fyer, A. J., Liebowitz, M. R., & Klein, D. F. (1990). Delineating the boundaries of social phobia: Its relationship to panic disorder and agoraphobia. *Journal of Anxiety Disorders, 4*, 41–59.

Marks, I. M. (1987). *Fears, phobias, and rituals. Panic, anxiety and their disorders.* New York: Oxford University Press.

Marks, I. M., & Mishan, J. (1988). Dysmorphophobia: A pilot study of behavioural treatment in disturbed bodily perception. *British Journal of Psychiatry, 152*, 674–678.

Mathews, A. (1990). Why worry? The cognitive function of anxiety. *Behavior Research and Therapy, 28*, 455–468.

McGlynn, F. D., & McNeil, D. W. (1990). Simple phobia in adulthood. In M. Hersen & C. G. Last (Eds.), *Handbook of child and adult psychopathology* (pp. 197–208). New York: Pergamon.

Merkelbach, H., van den Hout, M. A., & van der Molen, G. M. (1989). The phylogenetic origin of phobias: A review of the evidence. In P. M. G. Emmelkamp, W. T. A. M. Everaerd, F. W. Kraaimaat, & M. J. M. van Son (Eds.). *Fresh perspectives on anxiety disorders.* Lisse: Swets and Zeitlinger.

Minichiello, W. E., Baer, L., Jenike, M. A., & Holland, A. (1990). Age of onset of major subtypes of obsessive–compulsive disorder, *Journal of Anxiety Disorders, 4*, 147–150.

Monroe, S. M. (1990). Psychosocial factors in anxiety and depression. In J. D. Maser & C. R. Cloninger

(Eds.), *Comorbidity of mood and anxiety disorders* (pp. 463–543). Washington, DC: American Psychiatric Press.

Monti, P. M., Boice, R., Fingeret, A. L., Zwick, W. R., Kolko, D., Munroe, S., & Grunberger, A. (1984). Midi-level measurement of social anxiety in psychiatric and non psychiatric samples. *Behaviour Research and Therapy, 22,* 651–660.

Myers, K. M., Weissman, M. M., Tischler, G. L., Holzer, C. E. III., Leaf, P. J., Orvaschel, H., Anthony, J. C., Boyd, J. H., Burke, J. D., Kramer, M., & Stoltzman, R. (1984). Six-month prevalence of psychiatric disorders in three communities. *Archives of General Psychiatry, 41,* 959–967.

Norton, G. R., Cox, B., & Malan, J. (1992). Non-clinical panickers. A critical review. *Clinical Psychology Review, 12,* 121–139.

Noyes, R., Crowe, R. R., Harris, E. L., Hamra, B. J., McChesney, C. M., & Chaudry, D. R. (1986). Relationship between panic disorder and agoraphobia: A family study. *Archives of General Psychiatry, 43,* 227–232.

Öst, L-G. (1987). Age of onset in different phobias. *Journal of Abnormal Psychology, 96,* 223–229.

Öst, L-G. (1992). Blood and injection phobia: Background and cognitive, physiological, and behavioral variables. *Journal of Abnormal Psychology, 101,* 68–74.

Rasmussen, S. A., & Tsuang, M. T. (1986). Clinical characteristics and family history in DSM-III obsessive–compulsive disorder. *American Journal of Psychiatry, 143,* 317–322.

Reich, J., & Yates, W. (1988). Family history of psychiatric disorders in social phobia. *Comprehensive Psychiatry, 29,* 72-75.

Robins, L. N., Helzer, J. E., Weissman, M. M., Orvaschel, H., Gruenberg, E., Burke, J. D., & Regier, D. A. (1984). Lifetime prevalence of specific psychiatric disorders in three sites. *Archives of General Psychiatry, 41,* 949–958.

Sanderman, R., Mersch, P. P., van der Sleen, J., Emmelkamp, P. M. G., & Ormel, J. (1987). The rational behavior inventory (RBI): A psychometric evaluation. *Personality and Individual Differences, 8,* 561–569.

Schneier, R., Martin, L. Y., Liebowitz, M. R., Gorman, J. M., & Fyer, A. J. (1989). Alcohol abuse in social phobia. *Journal of Anxiety Disorders, 3,* 15–23.

Scholing, H. A., & Emmelkamp, P. M. G. (1990). Social phobia: Nature and treatment. In H. Leitenberg (Ed.), *Handbook of social and evaluation anxiety* (pp. 269–324). New York: Plenum Press.

Sheehan, D. V., Sheehan, K. E., & Michiello, W. E. (1981). Age of onset of phobic disorders: A reevaluation. *Comprehensive Psychiatry, 22,* 544–553.

Thyer, B. A., Himle, J., & Curtis, J. C. (1985). Blood-injury-illness phobia: A review. *Journal of Clinical Psychology, 41,* 451–459.

Torgersen, S. (1979). The nature and origin of common phobic fears. *British Journal of Psychiatry, 134,* 343–351.

Torgersen, S. (1983). Genetic factors in anxiety disorders. *Archives of General Psychiatry, 40,* 1085–1089.

Torgersen, S. (1986). Childhood and family characteristics in panic and generalized anxiety disorders. *American Journal of Psychiatry, 143,* 630–632.

Torgersen, S. (1988). Genetics. In C. G. Last, & M. Hersen (Eds.), *Handbook of anxiety disorders* (pp. 159–170). New York: Pergamon Press.

van der Molen, G. M., van den Hout, M. A., van Dieren, A. C., & Griez, E. (1989). Childhood separation anxiety and adult-onset panic disorders. *Journal of Anxiety Disorders, 3,* 97–106.

Wittchen, H. U. (1988). Natural course and spontaneous remissions of untreated anxiety disorders. In I. Hand & H. U. Wittchen (Eds.), *Panic and phobias* (Vol.2). New York: Springer.

Wittchen, H. U. (1991). Der langzeitverlauf unbehandelter Angststörungen (Follow-up of untreated anxiety disorders). *Verhaltenstherapie, 1,* 273–282.

Wittchen, H. U., & Essau, C. A. (1989). Comorbidity of anxiety disorders and depression: Does it affect course and outcome? *Psychiatry and Psychobiology, 4,* 315–323.

Yaryura-Tobias, J. A., & Neziroglu F. A. (1983). *Obsessive–compulsive disorders: Pathogenesis-diagnosis-treatment.* Basel: Marcel Dekker.

15

Depression

Lynn P. Rehm and Paras Mehta

Description of the Disorder

Disorders of mood include various syndromes of depression and of mania, separately and in combination. These are ordinarily distinguished from anxiety syndromes, although the boundaries between depression and anxiety are not distinct and much overlap in symptoms exists. The term "affective disorders" is sometimes applied to depression, mania, and the anxiety disorders. Although the mood disorders are characterized as disturbances of mood, which range from profound sadness to grandiose elation, the syndromes include symptoms in cognitive, behavioral, and somatic domains as well.

Among the mood disorders there is a great deal of heterogeneity in symptomatology. The distinction between normal, sad, and elated states, and pathological states of depression and mania is itself complex. Symptoms overlap with other disorders and co-morbid diagnoses are common. Differential diagnosis from anxiety disorders, certain personality disorders, and schizophrenia is often difficult. To make sense out of the complex phenomena involved, many different syndromes have been defined and many distinctions made among subtypes of mood disorders. Distinctions have often been based on theoretical models of etiology.

Our discussion of the mood disorders will follow the classification scheme of the *Diagnostic and Statistical Manual of Mental Disorders*, Third Edition, Revised (DSM-III-R) (American Psychiatric Association, 1987). We will also describe some additional categorizations, including changes that will be incorporated in DSM-IV (American Psychiatric Association, 1993). A diagnostic system evolves over time, and definitions of disorders and boundaries between them change. We will

Lynn P. Rehm and Paras Mehta • Department of Psychology, University of Houston, Houston, Texas 77204-5341.

Advanced Abnormal Psychology, edited by Vincent B. Van Hasselt and Michel Hersen. Plenum Press, New York, 1994.

LYNN P. REHM
and PARAS
MEHTA

comment on some of these changes. The DSM system attempts to make distinctions among disorders based on observed co-occurrence of symptoms without invoking putative cause. Nevertheless, there are a number of causal assumptions that underlie the DSM system, and we will attempt to make these explicit. We will also critique the DSM and point out the ways in which it is at times arbitrary and inexact.

Our conceptualization of this chapter approaches the issues of etiology from a biopsychosocial perspective. We assume that biological variables, psychological variables, and environmental variables interact in various ways to produce the mood disorders. While the importance of each set of variables may vary from one syndrome to another, all three sets contribute to each disorder. Within a disorder the contributions of biology, psychology, and environment may vary tremendously from case to case. Many theories of etiology are posed within single dimensions of causality (biological theories, psychological theories, or environmental theories) and are often pitted against one another (e.g., the biological versus the psychological explanation). Two dimensional diathesis-stress models posit interactions between either biological or psychological predispositions and life stress. We will try to maintain a three-dimensional view, which acknowledges interaction between biology and psychology, as well as the interactions of both with the environment.

Although we want to stress interaction among etiological factors from the biopsychosocial perspective, sections of the chapter will highlight different contributing causes. In the "Familial and Genetic Pattern" section, we review evidence for biological contributions. The "Diagnostic Considerations" section contains most of our discussion of psychological models, and the "Epidemiology" and "Course of the Disorder" sections of the chapter will highlight social, environmental, or life stress factors. Each section shows how various components fit with the biopsychosocial perspective.

Description of the mood disorders is dependent on the many diagnostic distinctions made by DSM-III-R and other nosological systems. To begin with, it is useful to distinguish among mood per se, mood syndromes, and mood disorders. Mood refers to the normal affective states experienced by all people on a day-to-day, hour-to-hour, or even moment-to-moment basis. It is important to note that mood is a normal part of human existence and a contrast, in either degree or quality, to syndrome or disorder. As a syndrome, extreme mood states are part of a constellation of symptoms remaining relatively stable over a longer period of time. An episode of depression or mania is diagnosed when a set of symptoms, including altered mood, exists for a relatively enduring period. A specific mood disorder is diagnosed based on the pattern of mood syndromes over the person's past history. Many different mood disorders have been defined historically and distinguished from each other. Among the most important is the distinction between unipolar and bipolar mood disorders.

Unipolar and Bipolar Mood Disorders

Emil Kraepelin (1921) first made the distinction manic–depressive illness and dementia praecox (schizophrenia). The distinction was made on the basis of syndrome, course, and prognosis. Manic–depressive disorder was seen as encompassing recurrent syndromes of depression, mania, or both, and as episodic with relatively complete recovery between episodes. In contrast, schizophrenia was viewed as having a chronic, deteriorating course. DSM-II adopted Kraepelin's distinction, but also included neurotic depression, which was defined as a less severe, though often more chronic, depressive syndrome than manic–depression.

In the late 50s, Leonhard (1957) and others began arguing that recurrent episodes of depression only should be distinguished from disorders that included both episodes of mania and depression. The distinction was based on differences in age of onset, genetics, and depressive symptomatology as well as course. Unipolar disorder (deviation toward only one pole of the mood spectrum) was broadened to include some of what earlier was considered neurotic depression. Bipolar disorder (deviation toward both manic and depressive poles) was a narrower category than Kraepelin's manic–depressive category. DSM-III incorporated the unipolar–bipolar distinction, basing the diagnoses solely on the history of at least one manic episode occurring with depressive episodes.

Syndromes of Depression and Mania

The DSM-III-R criteria for depression and mania are shown in Table 1. A pervasively sad mood was a required criterion symptom in DSM-III. DSM-III-R recognizes an alternate form of mood disturbance, anhedonia. Anhedonia is the inability to experience emotion, particularly pleasure. Apathy predominates and expression of affect is blunted and "flat." Other affective states can coexist with sadness, including anxiety and anger. Anxiety is so common in depressive disorders as to make differentiation from anxiety disorders (particularly generalized anxiety disorder) difficult. A combined depression–anxiety disorder has been proposed for DSM-IV. Especially among children and adolescents, sadness is often accompanied by irritability or an angry mood.

Somatic symptoms include sleep and appetite disturbances, psychomotor agitation/retardation, decreased energy, and loss of libido. Insomnia is a common symptom, but hypersomnia also is seen in depression. Middle or terminal insomnia (waking up in the middle of the night or early morning, and inability to return to sleep) is distinguished from initial insomnia. Loss of appetite is more common than increased appetite, and each may be assessed by corresponding changes in weight. Feeling slowed down and "energyless" is common. Agitation involves anxious, unproductive hyperactivity and, if present, is often noticeable in an interview where the patient fidgets or paces while reporting his complaints. Loss of libido, like many of the other symptoms above, may have cognitive and behavioral components as well as somatic dysfunction).

Depressive episodes associated with bipolar disorder are often marked by anhedonia, middle or terminal insomnia, and motor retardation. In contrast, unipolar depressions are often marked by anxiety, agitation, and initial insomnia. Syndromes with hypersomnia and weight gain are sometimes called atypical depression and may be treated with different medications.

Other symptoms include impaired cognitive functioning, depressive ruminations, and in extreme cases, psychotic features. Impaired cognitive function includes inability to concentrate and indecisiveness. Depressive thinking is unrealistically negative and biased, and has been described as the cognitive triad (Beck, 1972) of negative view of self, world, and future. A depressed person is overly self-critical and perceives him- or herself as guilty, worthless, and helpless. The world is perceived as a full of loss, and lacking in obtainable gratification. The future looks hopeless. Preoccupation with death and suicidal ideation may be the result of perceptions of hopelessness. Psychotic symptoms, hallucinations, or delusions may be present in very severe episodes. The content of the delusions or hallucinations in a depressive episode is typically mood congruent (i.e., the content reflects themes of guilt, persecution, punishment, ruin, and disaster).

Apathy and lack of motivation felt in depression are reflected in psychomotor retardation and lowered activity level. Other behavioral symptoms of depression include social withdrawal and lack of communication with others. Interpersonal relationships may be disrupted in various ways from increased dependency to irritable hostility. The typical mood in mania is described as elevated, expansive, or euphoric. Irritability is common here as well, and mood may be very labile or, paradoxically, even depressed. In contrast to depression, the content of manic thinking is often grandiose, ranging from unrealistic self-confidence to delusions of grandeur. Other forms of delusion occur but are usually congruent with elevated mood (e.g., delusions of persecution based on belief that others are jealous). Hallucinations are infrequent and are predominantly auditory.

Cognitive functioning is also impaired in manic episodes. The person may feel that her/his thoughts are accelerated (described as 'flight of ideas'), and this may be

TABLE 1. DSM-III-R Criteria for Major Depressive and Manic Episodes

MAJOR DEPRESSIVE EPISODE

A. At least 5 of the following symptoms have been present during the same 2-week period and represent a change from previous functioning; at least one of the symptoms is either (1) depressed mood, or (2) loss of interest or pleasure. (Do not include symptoms that are clearly due to a physical condition, mood-incongruent delusions or hallucinations, incoherence, or marked loosening of associations.)
   1. depressed mood (or can be irritable mood in children and adolescents) most of the day, nearly every day, as indicated either by subjective account or observation by others
   2. markedly diminished interest or pleasure nearly every day (as indicated either by subjective account or observation by others)
   3. significant weight loss or weight gain when not dieting (e.g., more than 5% of body weight in a month), or decrease or increase in appetite nearly every day (in children, consider failure to make expected weight gains)
   4. insomnia or hypersomnia nearly every day
   5. psychomotor agitation or retardation nearly every day (observable by others, not merely subjective feelings of restlessness or being slowed down)
   6. fatigue or loss of energy nearly every day
   7. feelings of worthlessness or excessive or inappropriate guilt (which may be delusional) nearly every day (not merely self-reproach or guilt about being sick)
   8. diminished ability to think or concentrate, or indecisiveness, nearly every day (either by subjective account or as observed by others)
   9. recurrent thoughts of death (not just fear of dying), recurrent suicidal ideation without a specific plan, or a suicide attempt or a specific plan for committing suicide
B. 1. It cannot be established that an organic factor initiated and maintained the disturbance
   2. The disturbance is not a normal reaction to the death of a loved one (uncomplicated bereavement)
C. At no time during the disturbance have there been delusions or hallucinations for as long as 2 weeks in the absence of prominent mood symptoms (i.e., before the mood symptoms developed or after they have remitted)
D. Not superimposed on schizophrenia, schizophreniform disorder, delusional disorder, or psychotic disorder NOS

(Continued)

reflected in pressured speech. In mild cases, thinking is experienced as more fluid and creative. In more severe cases thinking may become confused and the person may have difficulty in concentration, and be easily distracted.

Behaviorally, a grandiose outlook may result in poor judgment with negative social consequences, such as precipitous business decisions, gambling, spending sprees, or hypersexuality. The distinction between a full manic episode and a lesser hypomanic episode is often made on the basis of negative social consequences in mania. Hypomania may actually be associated with high levels of productivity and gregarious sociability. Activity level is increased in either form of episode, and need for sleep is decreased often to only 2 or 3 hours per night.

A formal diagnosis in DSM-III-R assumes that episodes of mood disorder are distinct periods of changed mood. For depression, a minimum duration of 2 weeks is specified. Organic causes need to be ruled out, and psychotic symptoms must occur only during the mood episode to rule out other psychotic diagnoses. DSM-IV adds a criterion specifying that the mood disturbance also must cause marked distress or significant impairment in social or occupational functioning. The reason for the addition was a concern that the diagnosis was overinclusive in the general population by diagnosing individuals who met minimal criteria but were not concerned or impaired by the symptoms.

TABLE 1. (*Continued*)

MANIC EPISODE

Note: A "Manic Syndrome" is defined as including criteria A, B, and C below. A "Hypomanic Syndrome" is defined as including criteria A and B, but not C, i.e., no marked impairment.

A. A distinct period of abnormally and persistently elevated, expansive, or irritable mood

B. During the period of mood disturbance, at least three of the following symptoms have persisted (four if the mood is only irritable) and have been present to a significant degree:
1. inflated self-esteem or grandiosity
2. decreased need for sleep, e.g., feels rested after only 3 hours of sleep
3. more talkative than usual or pressure to keep talking
4. flight of ideas or subjective experience that thoughts are racing
5. distractibility, i.e., attention too easily drawn to unimportant or irrelevant external stimuli
6. increase in goal-directed activity (either socially, at work or school, or sexually) or psychomotor agitation
7. excessive involvement in pleasurable activities that have a high potential for painful consequences, e.g., the person engages in unrestrained buying sprees, sexual indiscretions, or foolish business investments

C. Mood disturbance sufficiently severe to cause marked impairment in occupational functioning or in usual social activities or relationships with others, or to necessitate hospitalization to prevent harm to self or others

D. At no time during the disturbance have there been delusions or hallucinations for as long as 2 weeks in the absence of prominent mood symptoms (i.e., before the mood symptoms developed or after they have remitted)

E. Not superimposed on schizophrenia, schizophreniform disorder, delusional disorder, or psychotic disorder NOS

F. It cannot be established that an organic factor initiated and maintained the disturbance. Note: Somatic antidepressant treatment (e.g., drugs, ECT) that apparently precipitates a mood disturbance should not be considered an etiologic organic factor

DSM-III-R makes the distinction between bipolar disorder and depressive disorder (unipolar depression). The essential feature of bipolar disorder is the presence of at least one episode each of mania and depression. Episodes of depression alone, without a history of mania, are classified as major depressive disorder—either single or recurrent. Exclusions of manic or hypomanic episodes are necessary for diagnosis of a depressive disorder. Specific bipolar episodes are classified as depressed, manic, or mixed, depending upon the nature of symptoms. Bipolar syndromes that show only hypomanic episodes are sometimes referred to as bipolar IIs. Some authorities classify individuals with only depressive episodes but with bipolar relatives as bipolar IIIs, on the assumption that their underlying biochemistry and medication response will be similar to that of bipolar patients. DSM-IV formally recognizes the bipolar II diagnosis by adding criteria for a hypomanic episode.

DSM-III-R also includes milder, but more persistent forms of bipolar and unipolar syndromes termed cyclothymia and dysthymia. Cyclothymia is defined by numerous episodes of hypomania and numerous periods of depressed mood that do not meet the criteria of major depressive episode. This pattern must extend over a minimum of 2 years. Dysthymia also is defined as having a minimum duration of 2 years during which depression never remits for more than 2 months. Depression is less severe than in major depression, but at least two of the criteria for major depressive episode should be present over the course of the disorder. Dysthymia and cyclothymia were formerly classified as personality disorders because of their long durations and often early onsets.

DSM-IV focuses on issues of severity and course of episodes in several ways. Major depressive disorder is now separated into single episode and recurrent subtypes, and bipolar I is separated into subtypes based on the nature of the most recent episode: single manic episode and most recent episode either hypomanic, manic depressed, or unspecified. New sections on course specifiers identify rapid cycling (4 episodes of any kind in 12 months), seasonal pattern (regular seasonal onsets and remissions outnumbering other episodes), and postpartum onset (applicable to major depressive disorder, bipolar I, bipolar II, or acute psychotic disorder). Longitudinal course specifiers differentiate (1) single and recurrent episodes, (2) with or without antecedent dysthymia or cyclothymia, and (3) with or without full interepisode recovery. Minor depressive disorder (less than 4 symptoms) and recurrent brief depressive disorder (less than 2 weeks) will be added to the DSM-IV appendix for further study.

Other Diagnostic Distinctions

Former versions of the DSM included diagnostic distinctions based on putative cause. One such distinction is between endogenous and exogenous or reactive depressions. Endogenous depressions are presumed to be caused by internal biological mechanisms, in contrast to reactive depressions, which are seen as reactions to external events. Endogenous depressions are believed to be more severe, to be characterized by predominant somatic symptoms, and to be more medication-responsive. Reactive depressions are seen as milder and often self-limiting, as being characterized by more psychological symptoms, and as being responsive to psychotherapy. Endogenous depression is essentially a negative diagnosis since it is based on an absence of an identifiable external cause. Since this determination is unreliable and is an unsatisfactory basis for a diagnosis, the distinction was not included in the DSM-III.

The DSM-III-R does, however, specify a subtype of major depressive disorder, the melancholic type, which parallels endogenous depression. Based on current symptomatology, melancholic type is defined by symptoms of anhedonia, diurnal variation with depression worse in the morning, early morning insomnia, loss of appetite or weight, psychomotor agitation or retardation, no premorbid personality disorder, and previous good response to antidepressant medication (seen as evidence for a biological base). The melancholic type distinction is difficult to support empirically. It is confounded with severity and the definition is partly circular (i.e., a pharmacologically responsive subtype is defined in terms of previous pharmacological response). The biological component of depression is complex, polygenic, and variable in the risk it imparts. The expression of biologic vulnerability depends on environmental and psychological factors. As such, any distinction between internally versus externally caused, biological versus psychological types of depression, is overly simplistic.

In DSM-IV, 2 additional subtypes of depression besides melancholia are included under the heading of cross-sectional symptom features. Atypical features are characterized by mood reactivity and 2 symptoms out of a list including: significant weight gain or increase in appetite, hypersomnia, leaden paralysis, and long-standing pattern of interpersonal rejection sensitivity. With catatonia is a symptom feature characterized by such symptoms as motoric immobility, purposeless excessive activity, extreme negativism or mutism, movement peculiarities, echolalia, or echopraxia.

Postpartum depression or mania is another diagnosis based on putative causation. Although some controversy remains, the idea that biological events associated with childbirth cause postpartum mood disorders is poorly supported. Childbirth is associated with a variety of physical and psychosocial stresses and changes in life patterns. Depression or mania in the postpartum period may be at least partly stress-induced. The DSM-III-R takes the position, therefore, that a separate category for postpartum mood disorders is not necessary. DSM-IV has reinstated Postpartum Onset, however, as a course specifier.

Death of a loved one may be followed by a condition that is similar to a depressive episode; however, it is excluded from the mood disorders in DSM-III-R. Labeled "uncomplicated bereavement," it is assumed that grief is a natural and normal depressive reaction. From a biopsychosocial perspective, death of a loved one can be viewed as a form of psychosocial stressor or loss. It is not clear why this form of stress or loss should be different from others in producing normal versus abnormal depression. In some cases, duration, severity, and symptomatology are sufficient to warrant intervention, so that the distinction may be quite arbitrary. DSM-IV adds 2 new diagnostic categories based on presumed etiology. Secondary mood disorder due to a medical condition assumes that some medical conditions cause mood disorders directly, i.e., the depression is not merely a reaction to the stress of being ill. Substance-induced mood disorder is associated with intoxication, withdrawal, or cessation of use. Again, the assumption is that the depression is not merely a response to the stressors and life events involved in substance abuse.

LYNN P. REHM
and PARAS
MEHTA

The Epidemiologic Catchment Area (ECA) program of The National Institute of Mental Health (NIMH) is the major source of epidemiologic data in the United States (Regier et al., 1988). Data from all five sites were used to calculate 1-month and lifetime prevalence of the mood disorders. One-month prevalence refers to the number of new and continuing cases identifiable in a 1-month period. Lifetime prevalence is the number of people who will develop the disorder during their lifetime. Estimates for all affective disorders were 5.1% and 8.3%; for major depressive episode, 2.2% and 5.8%; for manic episode, 0.4% and 0.8%; and for dysthymia, 3.3% and 3.3%. Mood disorders are the most prevalent psychiatric disorders after anxiety disorders.

Risk of affective disorders in general is about twice as high in females than in males. While this conclusion has been supported for unipolar depression in a number of studies, data for bipolar depression are less conclusive. In bipolar disorder, estimates of the prevalence vary from equal for the sexes to slightly higher rates for women. Many explanations have been offered for the sex differences in prevalence of affective disorders. These range from suggestions that criteria may be biased or that reporting biases may make depression more likely to be endorsed by women, to sex-linked genetic explanations, to differences in sex role socialization that make women more psychologically vulnerable to depression.

Findings from the ECA program suggest that risk for depression is greater for people born in more recent decades. Incidence of depression is highest for young people, especially from ages 25 to 34. A recent study of depression in adolescence (Lewinsohn, 1991) indicates that its is about twice as prevalent in girls than boys between the ages 14 and 18, with prevalence rates much higher than for the general adult population.

Unipolar depression is considered to be more prevalent among lower socioeconomic classes, and bipolar disorder in the higher socioeconomic class. While increased prevalence of unipolar depression in lower SES can be attributed to environmental stressors, increased prevalence of bipolar disorder in the upper SES is often attributed to reporting bias and unreliable diagnosis. Among higher socioeconomic classes, bipolar disorder may be diagnosed over schizophrenia, whereas lower SES individuals may be more likely to receive the diagnosis of schizophrenia. Higher rates of depression in urban versus rural areas are often found, but these differences are probably attributable to socioeconomic and stress factors.

The relationship between depression and marital status is complex. Among men, rates of depression are higher for single and divorced individuals, but among women rates are higher for married persons. Differences seem to relate to different stress and support factors for men and women. For example, among married women, depression is lower for women with a job outside the home. Presumably this is because the job offers an additional source of gratification. Job status, housekeeping duties, and marital satisfaction also contribute to the differences (Radloff, 1975).

Findings of the ECA program suggest that prevalence rates for mood disorders are fairly equal across racial and ethnic groups in the United States. There are relatively few cross-cultural studies, and those that exist are hard to interpret because of differences in methodology. The data available suggest that depression is common in comparable rates around the world. Sex differences seem to be the same in industrialized countries, but perhaps less discrepant in less developed countries (Nolen-Hoeksema, 1987).

CLINICAL PICTURE

Case Description

Six months ago Dan, 32, was hospitalized for depression after he informed his half-brother that he was considering suicide. For several months before this, following a breakup with his girlfriend, he had been feeling increasingly depressed and unable to handle the demands of his daily life. Prior to his hospitalization, Dan complained that he did not derive pleasure from anything he did. He was constantly fatigued and felt slowed down in his activities. Dan was quite worried about his health, citing difficulty getting to sleep at night and loss of appetite resulting in unplanned weight loss. He told his half-brother that he felt worthless, guilty about things that he had done or not done for the family, and that he saw no hope for improvement in his life in the future.

As a child Dan was close to his mother, who also suffered from bouts of depression. He was the only child of his father's second marriage with a much older half-brother. His mother was hospitalized several times for depression during Dan's childhood, and she died when he was 12 of what may or may not have been an intentional overdose of sleeping medication. His father was never close and became even more distant and critical of Dan after his mother's death. Although Dan did well in school his grades always fell short of his father's expectation.

Dan went off to college and felt a new experience of independence, acceptance for his accomplishments, and self-confidence. However, he had to drop out of school to care for his father who was disabled following a stroke. For the last several years he has been living with his aging father, who recently has undergone a bypass surgery and needs constant attention. His brother provides minimal financial support but does not participate in taking care of the father.

A typical day for Dan prior to his hospitalization started at 5 in the morning, when he woke up to give his father his medications and ended at midnight, making sure that the kitchen was clean. During the day he attended to his father's complaints and constant demands for attention. Despite his handling of his father's demands, Dan described himself as incompetent and unable to reach his own standards for performing even the simplest tasks. Although he would occasionally admit resentment for having to take care of his father, he also said at times that he was grateful to do it, because otherwise his life would be meaningless.

During his hospitalization, Dan was diagnosed as experiencing major depressive disorder as an exacerbation of a longtime dysthymia. He was started on one of the new heterocyclic antidepressants, which improved his energy, mood, and sleep. With help from a therapist he negotiated with his brother for additional assistance in caring for the father, giving him more time for himself and the possibility of looking for a job outside the home.

Therapy after hospitalization began with efforts to increase Dan's activities and social interactions outside the family. As he made more contacts with people, therapy focused on his skills in certain social situations and proceeded to examine the ways in which he interpreted the behavior of others as rejecting and critical. His relationship with his father has been discussed as a source of his feelings about himself and his assumptions about his tendency to put the needs of others over any needs of his own. He has begun to question these assumptions and test them in his new relationships. Dan has found a job and is making progress in forming friendships while sharing responsibilities for his father's care with his half-brother.

COURSE AND PROGNOSIS

Part of the definition of mood disorders is that they are considered to be relatively constant over fairly long time periods. The DSM-III-R requires that an episode of depression last a minimum of 2 weeks. While no minimum duration is specified for an episode of mania, it is usually measurable at least in days. Time course, including age of onset, duration, and spacing of episodes, varies among disorders; differences in time course may be part of the validation of the distinction between two disorders (i.e., if they have different time courses, they are seen as different disorders).

Angst et al. (1973), in a prospective study of 400 patients with mood disorder, demonstrated differences in the time course of unipolar disorder, bipolar I, and bipolar II (hypomania only). There were significant differences in the age of onset among the three groups. Average age of onset for unipolar disorder was 45, whereas for bipolar I disorder it was 28, and for bipolar II, 32. About half of bipolar disorders occurred before age 30, but only about a fourth of unipolar depression cases occurred by age 30. About 64% of bipolar I and 80% of bipolar II disorders began with a depressive episode. The first manic episode occurred later for bipolar II. The average durations of unipolar and bipolar I episodes were 5.3 and 4.4 months respectively. Bipolar I had the shortest interval between the onset of two consecutive episodes (2.5 years), as compared to 4.7 years average for unipolar disorder.

Stress and Depression

Many psychological and biological theories of depression posit vulnerability factors that interact with life stress to produce an episode of the disorder. Stress is often defined in terms of major life events as occurrences that require major readjustment in the person's life. Stress can therefore result from adverse events, such as loss of a job or the exit of an important other (person) in the individual's life. But stress can also result from positive events that require major readjustment, such as moving one's residence or a change of jobs. Stress can accumulate over a period of time to increase vulnerability to depression and other psychological and physical disorders. It can also be the precipitating factor for the origination of an episode. Stressful life events have also been associated with increased risk of relapse after treatment and with increased risk of suicide attempts (Nezu & Roman, 1985). The role of negative life events has been frequently demonstrated in the etiology of unipolar depression, and recently Ellicot, Hammen, Gitlin, Brown, and Jamison (1990) have documented the relationship between stressful life events and bipolar depressive and manic episodes.

In addition to major life events, minor events that occur on a daily basis may also be important in depression. Daily mood is affected negatively by adverse events and positively by pleasant events. This is true for normal and clinical populations. Changing daily minor life events is the basis for therapy interventions as described below under diagnostic considerations.

Depression is often a recurring disorder. A past episode of depression represents a risk factor for the development of subsequent episodes of depression. This suggests that factors responsible for the first episode may be different from the ones for the subsequent episodes. Life events may be less important or lesser events may precipitate later episodes. Depression itself creates problems by interfering in adequate performance in many areas of life. Depression can produce events that are stressful and thus, negative life events and depression may be reciprocally related.

FAMILIAL AND GENETIC PATTERNS

Family Studies

Depression is known to run in families. The problem is to separate out the biological effects of genetics from the psychological effects of family environments. In general there is a higher risk of having an affective disorder among the relatives of a unipolar/bipolar patient as compared to the relatives of a normal control person. Data from the NIMH Collaborative Study of the Psychobiology of Depression (Andreasen, 1987) indicate that unipolar depression is common among first-degree relatives of both unipolar and bipolar patients, but relatives of unipolar patients have higher rates of unipolar disorder than bipolar disorder. These data have been taken as an indication that the two disorders run relatively true in families, or that the rarer bipolar disorder may be a more severe form of the same genetic vulnerability. Bipolar patients have severely and less severely afflicted relatives while unipolar patients have mostly less severely afflicted relatives.

The NIMH Epidemiological Catchment Area study (Regier et al., 1988) showed that individuals in the younger age ranges have an earlier age of onset and an increased rate of affective illness. These facts are inconsistent with a purely genetic explanation. This "cohort effect" may be attributable to methodological artifact, or to increasing social, financial, and environmental stressors in a rapidly changing world along with increasing psychological emphasis on individual responsibility (Seligman, 1989).

Twin Studies

Monozygotic twins (MZ) are genetically identical while dizygotic twins (DZ) share on an average 50% of the genetic material. Since pairs of twins usually have similar environments, comparing MZ and DZ twins allows a measure of the effect of genetics with environment held constant. If affective disorders have a genetic component, an MZ twin of a unipolar/bipolar patient is more likely to have the disorder than a DZ twin. Data from the Danish twin study (Bertelsen, Harvald, & Hauge, 1977) indicate that rates of concordance (co-occurrence) for MZ and DZ twins for bipolar probands were 79% and 24%, respectively. Corresponding rates for unipolar patients were 54% and 19%, respectively. This is indicative of a strong genetic component for affective illness, especially for bipolar disorders. However, it also demonstrates that genetics do not provide the entire answer to cause of mood disorder since a large percentage of risk is not accounted for by common genes.

Adoption Studies

Even though twin studies provide strong evidence for genetic bases of affective disorders, they do not rule out the contribution of the environmental factors. MZ twins may be reared as more alike and DZ twins as more different. Adoption studies attempt to tease apart the genetic from the environmental influences by comparing the biological with the adoptive parents of patients. If environment is more important, then adoptive parents would be more likely to have a mood disorder. If genetics are more important, then biological parents would have higher rates of mood disorder. Mendlewicz and Rainer (1977) studied 29 bipolar adoptees. Thirty one percent of the biological parents of these patients had bipolar disorders, as compared to 12% of the adoptive parents. The higher risk of affective illness in biological parents of bipolar adoptees is comparable to the risk in parents of nonadopted bipolars (26%). This suggests a strong genetic component in bipolar illness.

Mode of Genetic Transmission

If there is a genetic basis of affective disorders, the ultimate goal would be to identify the particular genes and the specific mode of transmission. Hints of specific modes of transmission have been stronger in bipolar than unipolar disorder. Winokur, Clayton, and Reich (1969) suggested a sex-linked connection to the X-chromosome for bipolar illness. The higher risk for female first-degree relatives of bipolar patients and the low rate of father-to-son transmissions were suggestive of a dominant X-linked illness. This effect has proven to be weak and suggestive that only some component of the transmission may be sex linked.

Egeland et al. (1987) studied genetic patterns in a large sample from the Old Order Amish, an ideal population to study because of the ability to identify and locate relatives of patients in a stable society. They appeared to show the contribution of a single gene, dominant transmission on a specific gene for bipolar disorder. As more data were collected, however, this effect became increasingly doubtful.

At present, the mode of transmission for both bipolar and unipolar disorder is best seen as the sum of many genetic factors that accumulate to create differences in risk for disorder. Expression of genetic risk may depend on other factors including psychosocial vulnerability and environmental stressors.

DIAGNOSTIC CONSIDERATIONS

Comorbidity

When making practical treatment decisions, a number of diagnostic issues need to be taken into account. Depression is often comorbid with other disorders. For example, it is frequently encountered along with alcoholism or other substance abuse. Clinical lore suggests that the primary disorder (i.e., the one that occurred first), needs to be the primary target of treatment. It is assumed that treating the primary disorder will also affect the secondary disorder. This is based on the idea that the primary depressed person may be self-medicating her depression with alcohol, and the primary alcoholic may be depressed over the consequences of her alcoholism. In practice it may be difficult to determine a sequence of occurrence, and practical issues (such as need for detoxification) may take precedence in treatment.

Anxiety is also frequently seen in conjunction with depression. The DSM system may in fact be making artificial distinctions among problems of dysphoric affect that blend along a continuum. Problematic anxiety may precede depression in the history of many depressed persons. Medication choice may be predicated on the predominance of depressive or anxious symptoms. Psychological approaches may deal with combined themes or techniques—for example, identifying cognitive distortions concerning loss and danger, or combining social skills training and relaxation training.

Depression in conjunction with medical disorders is common, and while it may be secondary to the medical condition, it should not be ignored. Depression is a negative prognostic sign for recovery and rehabilitation, so that treatment for depression can be a useful adjunct to medical treatment. While few controlled studies exist, psychotherapy for depression in conjunction with cancer treatment or cardiac rehabilitation has the potential to be very helpful.

Personality disorders are typically seen as a complicating factor in the treatment of depression or any other Axis I disorder. Developing a working collaboration may take more effort, relationship issues may be more prominent in therapy, and therapy may take longer in order to deal with maladaptive interpersonal styles and chaotic interpersonal relationships. Empirical evidence for the efficacy of treatments for depression in the presence of personality disorders is sparse, and more attention to this form of comorbidity would advance the field. The so-called personality disorders should be looked at in terms of extremes on basic dimensions of personality, in terms of personality styles or dimensions relevant to depression or other psychopathology proneness, or in terms of more basic levels of behavioral analysis of skill deficits and excesses.

Severity

Severity is another issue of diagnostic and treatment planning significance. Hospitalization may be required for severe depression or mania. In mania, hospitalization may be necessary to protect the person and others around this person from the adverse social consequences of poor decision making and impulsive behavior. In depression the reasons for hospitalization are more likely to be deterioration in self-care or protection from suicide. Suicide is a risk in both unipolar and bipolar forms of depression, and it is important to note that risk increases during the period when the person appears to be recovering from an episode of depression. Medication management is also a reason for hospitalization. Research on psychotherapies with inpatients is beginning to appear (e.g., Miller, Norman, Keitner, Bishop, & Dow, 1989) and suggests that it can be a useful adjunct in the hospital, especially if maintained on an outpatient basis after discharge.

There is some evidence that more severe depressions respond better to pharmacotherapy, while moderate depressions respond equally or better to psychotherapies (Elkin et al., 1989). People with more severe depressions may comply better with medication regimens while moderately depressed subjects are less likely to drop out of psychotherapy interventions. Combinations of pharmacotherapy and psychotherapy have been found to be superior to either pharmacotherapy alone or psychotherapy alone, in a few studies but not so in others.

Medication may be necessary or useful in severe depression to energize the patient sufficiently to take advantage of psychotherapeutic intervention, and sequencing may be a useful strategy. Psychotherapies appear to have the advantage over pharmacotherapy in prevention of relapse or recurrence, though recurrence is frequent in either form of treatment.

Diagnostic Subtypes

Diagnostic subtypes, such as the distinctions made by the DSM system, have significance for choice of treatment among medications, but less for choice of psychotherapies. Bipolar disorders are generally considered to be largely biological in origin, and lithium salts (e.g., lithium carbonate) are the usual treatment of choice, sometimes enhanced by other medications. Lithium has a prophylactic effect in preventing future episodes of depression and mania and is prescribed as a maintenance treatment over long periods of time. Little attention has been given to bipolar disorder in the psychotherapy literature, and most studies assessing the efficacy of psychotherapy exclude bipolars. Psychological treatments that are offered in practice are typically aimed at social support for patients and/or family members concerning the consequences of the disorder, and medication education and management.

The possibility of more specific treatment of bipolar disorders via psychotherapy is beginning to be examined by psychotherapy researchers. Psychotherapies effective in treating unipolar depressive episodes may also be effective in treating bipolar depressive episodes. Psychotherapy strategies targeting manic episodes have not been developed to date. Recent evidence indicates that bipolar episodes, like unipolar episodes, are often preceded by stress (Ellicott et al., 1990). Psychotherapies aimed at coping skills and stress reduction could be useful in reducing episodes. Evidence for such prophylactic effects in unipolar depression should be cause for exploring similar effects in bipolar disorder.

Unipolar depression is treated by a wide variety of medications, including the tricyclic antidepressants, newer heterocyclic antidepressants, and monoamine oxidase inhibitors (MAOIs). The efficacy of the tricyclics, such as amitriptyline (Elavil), or imipramine (Tofranil), for treating many forms of unipolar depression is well established in the research literature. The tricyclics seem to have special advantage for the more severe depressions. They have the disadvantage of some unpleasant side effects and the danger of precipitating manic episodes in bipolar I and II patients. The heterocyclics, such as bupropion (Welbutrin) or fluoxetine (Prozac), seem to have fewer side effects and less danger of inducing a manic episode. The MAOIs, such as isocarboxazid (Marplan) or tranylcypromine sulfate (Parnate), are usually reserved for tricyclic nonresponders because of severe dietary restrictions that must be followed by patients taking these medications. MAOIs may have special advantage for treating atypical depressions (i.e., those involving increased appetite and sleep).

Dysthymia is a particular diagnostic problem in terms of recommended treatment. Dysthymia is seen by some as a biologic disorder difficult to treat with antidepressant medications. On the other hand it may be viewed as a problem of chronic pessimism, low self-esteem, and poor coping skills, akin to the personality disorders. Skill-oriented psychotherapies may be useful if they take into account the same concerns that are relevant to personality disorder co-morbidity. Unfortunately, the dysthymia distinction has generally not been studied as a distinct population in the psychotherapy literature.

Psychotherapy Strategies

Psychotherapy is often the treatment preferred by patients and may be recommended for individuals who do not tolerate the side effects of antidepressant medications. Psychotherapy may be indicated instead of, or in addition to, medication for individuals who are dealing with significant life events or interpersonal problems, or who have a history of poor coping skills.

A number of psychotherapy strategies have been assessed and have proven effective in treating nonpsychotic, nonbipolar depression. Five general psychotherapy strategies can be identified in the psychotherapy research literature: (1) reinforcement, (2) social skill, (3) learned helplessness, (4) self-management, and (5) cognitive therapies. Logically, the rationales and targeted symptoms could be considered a basis for making recommendations for specific individuals. That is, it would make sense to match the individual patient to the psychotherapy that best targets the person's deficits. Empirical evidence for matching strategies is weak at best (e.g., Rehm, Kaslow, & Rabin, 1987; Zeiss, Lewinsohn, & Munoz, 1979). Most therapies are actually complex programs targeting multiple symptoms, and the programs may have more commonalities than differences. Matching psychotherapies with patient strengths may actually be a better matching strategy, since available evidence suggests that individuals with skills and attitudes consistent with therapy approaches do better in those therapies (Rude & Rehm, 1991).

REINFORCEMENT

Reinforcement strategies are based on the behavioral rationale that depression can be seen as a deficiency in reinforcement for important response chains in the person's life. This approach is most closely associated with the work of Peter Lewinsohn (1974), who defines depression as a response to a loss or lack of response-contingent reinforcement. When behavior decreases due to nonreinforcement, the other symptoms of depression, such as low self-esteem or feelings of fatigue, follow as secondary sequelae. Lewinsohn argues that there are three primary reasons for such a condition of nonreinforcement: (1) reinforcement is not available from the person's environment, as in lack of employment opportunities or loss of a significant figure in the person's life; (2) the person lacks essential skills to obtain reinforcement, such as job skills or interpersonal skills requisite to satisfying interpersonal relations; and, (3) reinforcement is available, but the person is not able to experience it, as when social anxiety interferes with otherwise rewarding interpersonal relationships.

Each of these three conditions leads to a different therapy strategy. Deficient reinforcement in the environment leads to a strategy of encouraging the person to engage in new or old behaviors that lead to reinforcement. Behaviors are identified that are potentially reinforcing and the person develops a schedule of increasing these behaviors. For example, the person who has lost a significant friend might be encouraged to increase activities that used to be reinforcing before meeting the friend or to increase similar activities with other friends. The purpose would be to reengage the person with reinforcing social activities.

The therapy strategy for lack of important social skills would be some form of skill training. For example, job skill programs, assertiveness training, or communication skill training might be recommended. This form of therapy strategy overlaps with the next section, where additional alternatives will be described. If the identified deficit is interfering social anxiety, it follows logically that an anxiety reduction program, such as relaxation training or systematic desensitization, would be recommended.

Lewinsohn and his colleagues have developed a "Pleasant Event Schedule" (PES) (MacPhillamy & Lewinsohn, 1974, 1982) to assess the therapy strategy that best fits the individual's pattern of depression. The PES consists of a lengthy list of events that many people find reinforcing. Subjects indicate the degree to which the event would be potentially reinforcing to them, and the frequency with which the event has occurred in the last month. Scores of reinforcement potential, activity level, and obtained reinforcement are useful in choosing the appropriate therapy strategy.

It should be noted, however, that a study of matching by this strategy (Zeiss, Lewinsohn, & Munoz, 1979) did not find it useful. Subjects who were theoretically mismatched did just as well as subjects who were theoretically matched. In recent years, the therapy strategies have been combined into a larger therapy program targeting a series of behavioral deficits. The program has been demonstrated to be effective in group, individual, and self-help formats (Brown & Lewinsohn, 1984).

SOCIAL SKILLS

Social skill approaches share the general assumption that depressed individuals suffer from deficiencies in social skill. A variety of deficiencies and conceptions of depression are involved. Gotlib and Colby (1987) make a general case for depression as an interpersonal phenomenon. Several researchers have taken the approach that depression occurs in the context of a marital relationship and have employed marital communication skill training as a therapeutic approach (e.g., Beach & O'Leary, 1986; McLean & Hakstian, 1979). Deficits in problem-solving skills are posited by Nezu, Nezu, and Perri (1989) to be central to depression. Klerman, Weissman, Rounsaville, and Chevron (1984) developed a dynamically oriented "Interpersonal Psychotherapy" predicated on the idea that depression is based on disturbances in interpersonal relationships.

Each of these interpersonal approaches has implications for assessment and treatment matching. Marital dissatisfaction, interpersonal loss or conflict, and problem-solving deficits are constructs that are associated with their own assessment domains. It is entirely consistent with the biopsychosocial model to assess the interpersonal environment and the person's skills in interacting with that environment.

LEARNED HELPLESSNESS

The learned helplessness theory of depression has gone through several revisions (Abramson, Seligman, & Teasdale, 1978; Alloy, Clements, & Kolden, 1985; Seligman, 1975). The basic concept of learned helplessness is that depressed people have acquired a belief that they are incapable of affecting important outcomes in their lives (i.e., outcomes are independent of their actions). Drawing such a helpless conclusion typically follows a major aversive event. The likelihood of drawing a helpless conclusion is heightened if the person has a depressogenic attributional style. This psychological diathesis consists of a predisposition to conclude that negative events are due to internal, stable, and global causes. That is, the adverse event is due to something about oneself, is due to something that is true about oneself now and continuing into the future, and is due to something about oneself that is true in all or many circumstances. If adverse events occur because of internal, stable, global causes, the person feels helpless to control future outcomes. In its most recent form (Alloy, Clements, & Kolden, 1985), the theory states that helplessness leads to hopelessness about the future which, in turn, produces depression.

Although the learned helplessness theory has not led to a specific form of therapy, Seligman (1981) argues that four therapy strategies are consistent with the theory. First, environmental enrichment could be used to put the person in an environment that is more controllable, allowing the person to regain a sense of control over outcomes. Second, skill training might be used to realistically increase the person's control in specific areas, for instance, job or interpersonal skills. Third, resignation training might be appropriate in situations where the helplessness is based on an unrealistically hopeless goal. The tactic is to help the person resign himself or herself to a more appropriate and attainable goal. Finally, the fourth strategy is attribution retraining, whereby the person is made aware of their depressogenic attributional style and is taught to make more optimistic causal attributions for failures and successes.

SELF-MANAGEMENT

The self-control model of depression (Rehm, 1977) was intended to be an integrative model bringing together cognitive and behavioral elements under the framework of Kanfer's (1970) model of self-control. The model suggests that depression or depression proneness can be thought of in terms of one or more deficits in self-control behavior. Specifically, depression involves: (1) selective attention to negative events to the relative exclusion of positive events; (2) selective attention to the immediate as opposed to the long-term outcomes of behavior; (3) the setting of stringent, perfectionistic self-evaluative standards; (4) depressive attributions for successes and failures; (5) insufficient contingent self-reward; and (6) excessive self-administered punishment.

Several scales have been developed that assess the deficits identified by the model to determine whether the program might be appropriate. The Self-Control Questionnaire was developed by Rehm and his colleagues (Fuchs & Rehm, 1977) to assess all of the depressive deficits hypothesized by the model. The scale has been used primarily as an outcome measure in therapy studies. Rosenbaum's (1980) Self-Control Schedule (also referred to as the Learned Resourcefulness Scale) was developed as a more general measure of self-control behavior. It has been found to be an indicator of good prognosis in cognitive–behavioral treatments generally. Good prognosis is related to scoring in the direction of good self-control skills, not in the direction of deficits to be remediated.

Specific components of the model may be assessed by other scales. Self-evaluation and attributions can be assessed by self-esteem and attributional style measures. Heiby (1982) has published a Self-Reinforcement Questionnaire and

Lewinsohn, Larson, and Munoz (1982) developed the Cognitive Events Scale as a means to assess self-reinforcing thoughts.

COGNITIVE THERAPY

Aaron Beck's (1972) cognitive therapy is based on a cognitive model of depression and psychopathology generally. It assumes that depression is the product of negative distortions of events in daily life. For Beck, the primary components of depression are the *cognitive triad*: (1) a negative view of self, (2) a negative view of world, and (3) a negative view of the future. Distortions occur when people view their world through the filter of depressive schemata, which are organized sets of assumptions and rules about the world stored in memory and accessed during depressive episodes. Interpretive *automatic thoughts* occur at the edge of awareness and lead to negative affect.

Several typical forms of negative distortion are identified. *Arbitrary inference* involves the automatic assumption that one is to blame for any negative life event. *Selective abstraction* occurs when the person focuses on minor negative information in an otherwise positive situation. A third example is *inexact labeling*, where the person attaches a negative label to an experience and then reacts emotionally to the label.

Therapy is aimed at helping the patient to identify negative automatic thoughts and challenge them rationally and empirically. Gradually, as automatic thoughts are identified, the negative underlying assumptions and rules of the depressive schemata become apparent and can be challenged and modified by similar means.

Several instruments have been developed to assess negative automatic thoughts and underlying assumptions. The Automatic Thoughts Questionnaire (Hollon & Kendall, 1980) was developed to assess the symptomatic thoughts experienced by depressed persons on a daily basis. The Dysfunctional Attitudes Scale (Weissman & Beck, 1978) was developed to assess more basic assumptions presumed to reflect depression vulnerability. While both seem to reflect depressive symptoms, Miranda and Persons (1986) found that formerly depressed people score much higher on the Dysfunctional Attitudes Scale when a mild negative mood has been induced. Their interpretation of this finding is that depression-prone people access alternative depressive schemata when in a depressed mood. "Affect priming," as this procedure has come to be called, is a promising assessment technique for assessing cognitive vulnerability to depression and perhaps the suitability of cognitive therapy.

SUMMARY

A biopsychosocial approach to depression takes into account biological, psychological, and environmental factors in etiology, maintenance, symptomatology, underlying mechanisms, and intervention. While different subtypes of depression may represent different loadings of these factors, all three factors may have some contribution to each individual's depression in a unique combination and interaction. We need more comprehensive theoretical approaches to understanding depression that take into account both biological and psychological diatheses as they interact with stress. We need a better understanding of the processes whereby these factors interact reciprocally over the development, course and treatment of depression.

313

DEPRESSION

REFERENCES

Abramson, L. Y., Seligman, M. E. P., & Teasdale, J. D. (1978). Learned helplessness in humans: Critique and reformulation. *Journal of Abnormal Psychology, 87,* 32–48.

Alloy, L. B., Clements, C., & Kolden, G. (1985). The cognitive diathesis-stress theories of depression: Therapeutic implications. In S. Reiss & R. R. Bootzin (Eds.), *Theoretical issues in behavior therapy* (pp. 379–410). Orlando, FL: Academic Press.

American Psychiatric Association. (1987) *Diagnostic and statistical manual of mental disorders,* 3rd Edition, Revised. Washington, DC: Author.

American Psychiatric Association (1993). *DSM-IV draft criteria.* Washington, DC: Author.

Andreasen, N. C., Rice, J., Endicott, J., Coryell, W., Grove, W. M., & Reich, T. (1987). Familial rates of affective disorder. A report from the National Institute of Mental Health Collaborative Study. *Archives of General Psychiatry, 44,* 461–469.

Angst, J., Bastrup, P., Grof, P., Hippius, H., Poldinger, W., & Weiss, P. (1973). The course of monopolar and bipolar psychoses. *Psychiatrica, Neurologica, and Neurochirurgia, 76,* 489–500.

Beach, S. R. H., & O'Leary, K. D. (1986). The treatment of depression occurring in the context of marital discord. *Behavior Therapy, 17,* 43–49.

Beck, A. T. (1972). *Depression: Causes and treatment.* Philadelphia: University of Pennsylvania Press.

Bertelsen, A., Harvald, B., & Hauge, M. (1977). A Danish twin study of manic depressive disorders. *British Journal of Psychiatry, 130,* 330–351.

Brown, R. A., & Lewinsohn, P. M. (1984). A psychoeducational approach to the treatment of depression: Comparison of group, individual, and minimal contact procedures. *Journal of Consulting and Clinical Psychology, 52,* 774–783.

Egeland, J. A., Gerhard, D. S., Pauls, D. S., Sussex, J. N., Kidd, K. K., Allen, C. R., Hostetter, A. M., & Housman, D. (1987). Bipolar affective disorders linked to DNA markers on chromosome II. *Nature, 325,* 783–787.

Elkin, I., Shea, M. T., Watkins, J. T., Imber, S. D., Sotsky, S. M., Collins, J. F., Glass, D. R., Pilkonis, P. A., Leber, W. R., Docherty, J. P., Fiester, S. J., & Parloff, M. B. (1989). National Institute of Mental Health treatment of depression collaborative research program: General effectiveness of treatments. *Archives of General Psychiatry, 46,* 971–982.

Ellicot, A., Hammen, C., Gitlin, M., Brown, G., & Jamison, K. (1990). Life events and course of bipolar disorder. *American Journal of Psychiatry, 147,* 1194–1198.

Fuchs, C. Z., & Rehm, L. P. (1977). A self-control behavior therapy program for depression. *Journal of Consulting and Clinical Psychology, 45,* 206–215.

Gotlib, I. H., & Colby, C. A. (1987). *Treatment of depression: An interpersonal systems approach.* New York: Pergamon Press.

Heiby, E. M. (1982). A self-reinforcement questionnaire. *Behaviour Research and Therapy, 20,* 397–401.

Hollon, S. D., & Kendall, P. C. (1980). Cognitive self-statements in depression: Development of an automatic thoughts questionnaire. *Cognitive Therapy and Research, 4,* 383–397.

Kanfer, F. H. (1970). Self-regulation: Research, issues and speculations. In C. Neuringer & J. L. Michael (Eds.), *Behavior modification in clinical psychology* (pp. 178–220). New York: Appleton-Century-Crofts.

Klerman, G. L., Weissman, M. M., Rounsaville, B. J., & Chevron, E. S. (1984). *Interpersonal psychotherapy of depression.* New York: Basic Books.

Kraepelin, E. (1921). *Manic-depressive insanity and paranoia.* Edinburgh, Scotland: Livingstone.

Leonhard, K. (1957). *Aufteliung der Endogenen Psychosen* (4th Ed.). Berlin: Akademieverlag.

Lewinsohn, P. M. (1974). A behavioral approach to depression. In R. M. Friedman & M. M. Katz (Eds.), *The psychology of depression: Contemporary theory and research.* (pp. 157–185) New York: John Wiley and Sons.

Lewinsohn, P. M. (1991). *Depression in adolescents.* Paper presented at the 99th meeting of the American Psychological Association, San Francisco.

Lewinsohn, P. M., Larson, D. W., & Munoz, R. F. (1982). The measurement of expectancies and other cognitions in depressed individuals. *Cognitive Therapy and Research, 6,* 437–446.

MacPhillamy, D. J., & Lewinsohn, P. M. (1974). Depression as a function of levels of desired and obtained pleasure. *Journal of Abnormal Psychology, 83,* 651–657.

MacPhillamy, D. J., & Lewinsohn, P. M. (1982). The Pleasant Events Schedule: Studies on reliability, validity, and scale intercorrelation. *Journal of Consulting and Clinical Psychology, 50*, 363–380.

McLean, P. D., & Hakstian, A. R. (1979). Clinical depression: Comparative efficacy of outpatient treatments. *Journal of Consulting and Clinical Psychology, 47*, 818–836.

Mendlewicz, J., & Rainer, J. D. (1977). Adoption studies in manic–depressive illness. *Nature, 268*, 327–329.

Miller, I. W., Norman, W. H., Keitner, G. I., Bishop, S. B., & Dow, M. G. (1989). Cognitive–behavioral treatment of depressed inpatients. *Behavior Therapy, 20*, 25–47.

Miranda, J., & Persons, J. B. (1986). *Relationship of dysfunctional attitudes to current mood and history of depression.* Paper presented at the 20th meeting of the Association for the Advancement of Behavior Therapy, Chicago, Illinois.

Nezu, A. M., & Ronan, G. F. (1985). Life stress, current problems, problem-solving and depressive symptoms: An integrative model. *Journal of Consulting and Clinical Psychology, 53*, 693–697.

Nezu, A. M., Nezu, C. M., & Perri, M. G. (1989). *Problem-solving therapy for depression: Theory research and clinical guidelines.* New York: John Wiley & Sons.

Nolen-Hoeksema, S. (1987). Sex differences in unipolar depression: Evidence and theory. *Psychological Bulletin, 101*, 259–282.

Radloff, L. (1975). Sex differences in depression: The effects of occupation and marital status. *Sex Roles, 1*, 249–265.

Regier, D. A., Boyd, J. H., Burke, J. D., Jr., Rae, D. S., Myers, J. K., Kramer, M., Robins, L. N., George, L. K., Karno, M., & Locke, B. Z. (1988). One-month prevalence of mental disorders in the United States: Based on five Epidemiological Catchment Area sites. *Archives of General Psychiatry, 45*, 977–986.

Rehm, L. P. (1977). A self-control model of depression. *Behavior Therapy, 8*, 787–804.

Rehm, L. P., Kaslow, N. J., & Rabin, A. S. (1987) Cognitive and behavioral targets in a self-control therapy program for depression. *Journal of Consulting and Clinical Psychology, 55*, 60–67.

Rosenbaum, M. (1980). A schedule for assessing self-control behaviors: Preliminary findings. *Behavior Therapy, 11*, 109–121.

Rude, S., & Rehm, L. P. (1991). Cognitive and behavioral predictors of response to treatments of depression. *Clinical Psychology Review, 11*, 493–514.

Seligman, M. E. P. (1975) *Helplessness: On depression, development and death.* San Francisco: W.H. Freeman.

Seligman, M. E. P. (1981). A learned helplessness point of view. In L. P. Rehm (Ed.), *Behavior Therapy for depression: Present status and future directions.* New York: Academic Press.

Seligman, M. E. P. (1989). Research in clinical psychology: Why is there so much depression today? In I. S. Cohen (Ed.), *The G. Stanley Hall Lecture Series* (Vol. 9). Washington, DC: American Psychological Association.

Weissman, A. N., & Beck, A. T. (1978). *Development and validation of the Dysfunctional Attitude Scale.* Paper presented at the 12th annual convention of the Association for the Advancement of Behavior Therapy, Chicago.

Winokur, G., Clayton, P. J., & Reich, T. (1969). *Manic–depressive disease.* St. Louis, MO: Mosby.

Zeiss, A. M., Lewinsohn, P. M., & Munoz, R. F. (1979). Nonspecific improvement effects in depression using interpersonal skills training, pleasant activity schedules, or cognitive training. *Journal of Consulting and Clinical Psychology, 47*, 427–439.

16

Schizophrenia

Patrick W. McGuffin
and Randall L. Morrison

*Most diseases can be separated from one's self and seen
as foreign intruding entities. Schizophrenia is very
poorly behaved in this respect. Colds, ulcers, flu, and
cancer are things we get. Schizophrenic is something
we are. It affects the things we most identify with as
making us what we are.*

*If this weren't problem enough, schiz comes on
slow and comes on fast, stays a minute or days or
years, can be heaven one moment, hell the next,
enhance abilities and destroy them, back and forth
several times a day and always weaving itself
inextricably into what we call ourselves. It can
transform only a small corner of our lives or turn the
whole show upside down, always giving few if any
clues as to when it came or when it left or what was
us and what was schiz.*

(M. Vonnegut, 1975, p. ix)

Description of the Disorder

Schizophrenia is an extremely disabling disorder, which presents with a wide
range of disruptive symptoms and leads to a significant loss in ability to function
independently. Its prognosis is generally poor and its course tends toward progressively more disabled functioning over time. Schizophrenia has been observed
for more than 3000 years. In the time that the disorder was recognized, it had been

Patrick W. McGuffin • Hahnemann University, Philadelphia, Pennsylvania 19102-1192. Randall
L. Morrison • Response Analysis Corporation, Princeton, New Jersey 08542.

Advanced Abnormal Psychology, edited by Vincent B. Van Hasselt and Michel Hersen. Plenum Press, New
York, 1994.

PATRICK W.
McGUFFIN and
RANDALL L.
MORRISON

attributed to various causes, including satanic possession. More recently, empirically based theories regarding schizophrenia began to develop.

Emil Kraeplin developed the term *dementia praecox* in 1898, to differentiate between manic–depressive illness and other major psychoses. The disorder described by the term dementia praecox, indicating the disruption of perceptual and cognitive processes and early onset of the disorder, would later be known as schizophrenia. Persons who suffered from dementia praecox tended to have a progressively worsening level of functioning. Their decline in functioning was generally permanent, unlike manic–depressive illness, which had periods of normal functioning interrupted by short-duration manic–depressive symptoms.

The term *schizophrenia* was coined by Eugen Bleuler, in 1908. Bleuler's choice of the term schizophrenia (meaning "split mind" in Greek) was an attempt to focus on the symptomatic nature of the illness, rather than its course. Bleuler intended the term to reference the inability of the schizophrenic person to maintain goal-directed behavior and integrated thinking. Despite popular lore, "schizophrenia" does not refer to multiple personality.

Schizophrenia costs the United States approximately $50 billion per year in lost productivity, treatment costs, and public assistance funds. Persons with schizophrenia occupy over 30% of the total number of beds in psychiatric hospitals (Keith, Regier, & Rae, 1991).

While the economic cost of schizophrenia is readily ascertained, the emotional cost to individuals with schizophrenia and their families is impossible to adequately measure. Approximately 10% of persons with schizophrenia commit suicide; approximately 20% make suicide attempts. These attempts do not tend to occur during psychotic periods, but just as symptoms begin to clear. The rate of suicides among schizophrenics is staggering, when one considers that the suicide rate among the general population is less than 0.05% (Maxmen, 1986).

Even though individuals with schizophrenia appear to be at high risk for causing harm to themselves, there is no evidence that they present any significant risk to others. Evidence indicates that persons with schizophrenia tend to commit fewer crimes than the general population, although they are more frequently victims of crimes.

Symptom Presentation

Schizophrenia typically first develops in young adulthood, although earlier or later onset can occur. Onset can be either rapid or gradual and can occur in individuals with no prior evidence of mental illness as well as in persons who have had long-standing difficulties. In most cases, the manifestation of psychotic symptoms begins after a gradual deterioration of social functioning and personal hygiene, and the development of flat or inappropriate affect (Maxmen, 1986). Those cases with slower onset tend to have a more negative prognosis than those cases in which schizophrenic symptoms develop rapidly (Harris, 1984).

Diagnosis of schizophrenia, based on the *Diagnostic and Statistical Manual of Mental Disorders*, Third Edition, Revised (American Psychiatric Association, 1987), requires that an individual exhibit a minimal number of symptoms out of a broad range of symptoms that have been found to be indicative of schizophrenic disorders. Owing to the heterogeneity among symptoms, the illness can appear quite differently across patients. Minimal criteria required for the diagnosis include psychotic symptoms and a deterioration in adaptive functioning. These symptoms must have been present for at least 6 months and must not be superimposed on a mood disorder. Additionally, the symptoms cannot be secondary to any known organic factor. The specific types of psychotic symptoms and the particular changes in adaptive functioning can vary significantly between individuals.

The most obvious schizophrenic symptoms include hallucinations, delusions, and thought disorder (frequently referred to as *positive symptoms* [Andreason & Olsen, 1982]). *Hallucinations* are sensory perceptions based on no external reality. The most frequent type of hallucinations seen in schizophrenia are auditory. With auditory hallucinations, the patient generally reports voices making statements to him/her. The voices will often comment on the individual's behavior. At times the voices are reported to give commands to the individual. The command hallucinations may tell the individual to harm him/herself or others. Consequently, it is important during clinical evaluation to ask the patient about the content of auditory hallucinations, as well as any intention to act upon them.

Olfactory, tactile, and visual hallucinations may also occur, but are extremely rare. When these other types of hallucinations do occur, they generally co-occur with auditory hallucinations. Whenever nonauditory hallucinations are reported, consideration must be given to the possibility that they are the result of some organic factor. This must be clarified before a diagnosis of schizophrenia can be made.

Delusions represent false beliefs that develop out of a misinterpretation of environmental events. These include grandiose delusions ("an exaggerated sense of one's importance, power, knowledge, or identity" [APA, 1987, p. 396]), persecutory delusions (a person's belief that others are trying to harm, cheat, or conspire against him/her [APA, 1987]), and delusions of reference (belief that external events or people "have a particular and unusual significance" [APA, 1987, p. 396]). Other types of delusions include thought insertion and thought withdrawal (belief that thoughts are being put into or taken out of the patient's brain) and thought broadcasting (belief that others can hear the patient's thoughts).

Thought disorders are disturbances in the organization or the content of an individual's thoughts. One example is flight of ideas, where a person's verbalization quickly shifts from topic to topic. Although the content of the patient's verbalization may seem to be completely illogical, there is a connection between topics that are being discussed. Conversely, in looseness of association, a person's verbalizations will switch from one unrelated topic to another, without any apparent recognition of the absence of logic in the statements.

Other examples of thought disorder are perseveration, echolalia, and neologisms. Perseveration involves repetition of the same word or phrase over and over. Echolalia refers to the repetition of those words or phrases that another person has spoken. Neologisms are words that are invented by a person, which have idiosyncratic meaning to that person.

In addition to the positive symptoms described above, persons with a diagnosis of schizophrenia must display *negative symptoms*, which result in decreased role functioning. Negative symptoms include social withdrawal, loss of adaptive personal and social skills, flat affect, attentional impairment, poverty of speech (statements appear normal, but convey very little information), increased speech latency (abnormally long period of time taken to respond to another person's statement or question), and negative motor symptoms (maintaining bizarre postures, passively allowing one's body to be manipulated by others, catatonic stupor [no response to or interaction with the external environment]).

The complete DSM-III-R diagnostic criteria are listed in Table 1.

PATRICK W.
McGUFFIN and
RANDALL L.
MORRISON

In the new edition of the *Diagnostic and Statistical Manual of Mental Disorders*, DSM-IV, most diagnostic criteria for schizophrenia remain unchanged. However, some changes in language as well as minor alterations in the criterion level for symptom presentation have been made.

According to DSM-IV, the active phase of schizophrenia must be of at least 1 month's duration, not 1 week, as stated in DSM-III-R. Additionally, while DSM-III-R specifies that the symptoms cannot be due to organic factors, DSM-IV rephrases this to state that symptoms cannot be due to drugs or a medical condition.

The most significant difference between the 2 editions of DSM regarding the diagnostic criteria for schizophrenia is in the classification of course. The DSM-IV course descriptions refer to the continuity of symptom presentations, not the duration of symptoms, as is done in DSM-III-R. DSM-IV provides 8 different descriptions of course of the disorder which fall into 3 general categories (continuous, episodic, and in remission). The continuous category replaces both the chronic and subchronic categories in DSM-III-R. The DSM-IV episodic categories replace the 2 acute exacerbation categories in DSM-III-R. The DSM-IV episodic categories differ in the type of symptom presentation that occurs in the time period between psychotic episodes. During this time period, there may or may not be any negative symptoms. If negative symptoms do persist during this time period, they may remain stable in their intensity or they may progress.

DSM-IV allows for classifying an individual as being in either full or partial remission, but only after a single episode. Persons with multiple episodes would receive one of the episodic classifications.

If an individual meets none of the previously listed course criteria, DSM-IV provides the option of "other pattern." Also, if the individual's course is of less than one year's duration, DSM-IV provides a classification which indicates that.

EPIDEMIOLOGY

Prevalence

Schizophrenia is a rare disorder, with studies indicating a rate of occurrence ranging from 0.2 to 1.0% of the world population (APA, 1987). The incidence of

TABLE 1. Diagnostic Criteria for Schizophrenia

A. Presence of characteristic psychotic symptoms in the active phase: either (1), (2), or (3) for at least one week (unless the symptoms are successfully treated):

   (1) Two of the following:

      (a) delusions
      (b) prominent hallucinations (throughout the day for several days or several times a week for several weeks, each hallucinatory experience not being limited to a few brief moments)
      (c) incoherence or marked loosening of associations
      (d) catatonic behavior
      (e) flat or grossly inappropriate affect

   (2) bizarre delusions (i.e., involving a phenomenon that the person's culture would regard as totally implausible, e.g., thought broadcasting, being controlled by a dead person)

   (3) prominent hallucinations (as defined in (1)(b) above) of a voice with content having no apparent relation to depression or elation, or a voice keeping up a running commentary on the person's behavior or thoughts, or two or more voices conversing with each other

(Continued)

TABLE 1. *(Continued)*

B. During the course of the disturbance, functioning in such areas as work, social relations, and self-care is markedly below the highest level achieved before onset of the disturbance (or, when the onset is in childhood or adolescence, failure to achieve expected level of social development).

C. Schizoaffective Disorder and Mood Disorder with Psychotic Features have been ruled out, i.e., if a Major Depressive or Manic Syndrome has ever been present during an active phase of the disturbance, the total duration of all episodes of a mood syndrome has been brief relative to the total duration of the active and residual phases of the disturbance.

D. Continuous signs of the disturbance for at least six months. The six-month period must include an active phase (of at least 1 week, or less if symptoms have been successfully treated) during which there were psychotic symptoms characteristic of schizophrenia (symptoms in A), with or without a prodromal or residual phase, as defined below.

Prodromal phase: A clear deterioration in functioning before the active phase of the disturbance that is not due to a disturbance in mood or to a psychoactive substance use disorder and that involves at least two of the symptoms listed below.

Residual phase: Following the active phase of the disturbance, persistence of at least two of the symptoms noted below, those not being due to a disturbance in mood or to a psychoactive substance use disorder.

Prodromal or Residual Symptoms:

(1) marked social isolation or withdrawal
(2) marked impairment in role functioning as a wage-earner, student, or homemaker
(3) markedly peculiar behavior (e.g., collecting garbage, talking to self in public, hoarding food)
(4) marked impairment in personal hygiene and grooming
(5) blunted or inappropriate affect
(6) digressive, vague, overelaborate, or circumstantial speech, or poverty of speech, or poverty of content of speech
(7) odd beliefs or magical thinking, influencing behavior and inconsistent with cultural norms, e.g., superstitiousness, belief in clairvoyance, telepathy, "sixth sense," "other can feel my feelings," overvalued ideas, ideas of reference
(8) unusual perceptual experiences, e.g., recurrent illusions, sensing the presence of a force or person not actually present
(9) marked lack of initiative, interests, or energy

Examples: Six months of prodromal symptoms with one week of symptoms from A; no prodromal symptoms with six months of symptoms from A; no prodromal symptoms with one week of symptoms from A and six months of residual symptoms.

E. It cannot be established that an organic factor initiated and maintained the disturbance.

F. If there is a history of Autistic Disorder, the additional diagnosis of Schizophrenia is made only if prominent delusions or hallucinations are also present.

Classification of course. The course of the disturbance is coded in the fifth digit:

1—Subchronic. The time from the beginning of the disturbance, when the person first began to show signs of the disturbance (including prodromal, active, and residual phases) more or less continuously, is less than 2 years, but at least six months.

2—Chronic. Same as above, but more than two years.

3—Subchronic with Acute Exacerbation. Reemergence of prominent psychotic symptoms in a person with a subchronic course who has been in the residual phase of the disturbance.

4—Chronic with Acute Exacerbation. Reemergence of prominent psychotic symptoms in a person with a chronic course who has been in the residual phase of the disturbance.

5—In Remission. When a person with a history of Schizophrenia is free of all signs of the disturbance (whether or not on medication), "In Remission" should be coded. Differentiating Schizophrenia in remission from no mental disorder requires consideration of overall level of functioning, length of time since the last episode of disturbance, total duration of the disturbance, and whether prophylactic treatment is being given.

0—Unspecified.

Reprinted with permission from *Diagnostic and Statistical Manual of Mental Disorders*, Third Edition, Revised. Copyright 1987 American Psychiatric Association.

schizophrenia is generally consistent across different cultures. The most common age of onset is between 15 and 35 years, although onset during childhood or later adulthood does occur.

Gender Issues

Schizophrenia occurs equally among males and females. The age of onset of schizophrenia, however, is later among women. Men with schizophrenia tend to be hospitalized more often than women and show a more deteriorating course of illness. Women with schizophrenia are more likely to be married than their male counterparts and to have higher premorbid sexual and social functioning. Women are more likely to be parents. Men with schizophrenia are more likely to display antisocial behavior, although men and women display equivalent rates of assaultive behavior. Women with schizophrenia are more likely to report depressive symptoms, to have troubled relationships, and to display self-destructive behavior (McGlashan & Bardenstein, 1990).

Sociodemographic Issues

The prevalence of schizophrenia is greater in lower socioeconomic groups. There is a belief that this is related to the tendency for those persons with schizophrenia to drift downward to lower socioeconomic class due to the deterioration in adaptive functioning (and related difficulty maintaining employment), which is part of the schizophrenic disorder. While there is face validity to this belief, there is also some thinking that poverty and its related environmental hardships may play a causative role in the development of schizophrenia. Persons within the lower socioeconomic classes have limited access to medical care, particularly prenatal care, and this may result in a range of difficulties during pregnancy and delivery. Additionally, this limited access to medical care may increase the likelihood that infants and children will not receive treatment for infectious disorders, which are thought to play a role in the inception of schizophrenia (Knight, 1985; Tsuang, Faraone, & Day, 1988).

Other Risk Factors

Several factors have been found to be correlated with the development of a schizophrenic disorder. There is evidence of a high incidence of social phobia, obsessive–compulsive disorder, and panic attacks in persons who later develop schizophrenia (Tien & Eaton, 1992). These findings coincide with clinical presentations of schizophrenia, as one often observes social withdrawal (that would also occur in social phobia) in persons with schizophrenia. Further, feelings of panic are reported by many people who have schizophrenia. Obsessions and compulsions are also often seen in schizophrenia. Consequently, the presence of obsessive–compulsive disorder in some persons who later develop a schizophrenic disorder is not surprising.

Also, the marital status of an individual appears to be related to the development of schizophrenia. Married men appear to have the lowest incidence of schizophrenia. Relative to married men, unmarried men have almost a 50 times greater incidence of schizophrenia. Unmarried women have a 14 times higher incidence of schizophrenia than do married men. While being married appears to be correlated with lower incidence of schizophrenia, the incidence rates vary between married men and married women, with married women having a 2.4 times higher incidence of schizophrenia than do their male counterparts (Tien & Eaton, 1992).

Being actively employed is negatively correlated with the development of schizophrenia. In addition, the more years of education an individual has, the less likely the development of schizophrenia. These are both logical, in that schizophrenia involves a deficit in role functioning. Therefore, the ability to remain successful in school or maintain gainful employment would indicate adequate role functioning and would be contraindicators for a diagnosis of schizophrenia.

CLINICAL PICTURE

When Dan first began to suffer from schizophrenia, our family thought it was just a case of teenage blues. We sent him off to college. By the time he began attacking the refrigerator for reading his mind and threatening family members for using the word "right," we had learned to recognize the disease.

He never took his medicine once he was away from us. Gradually he began working less and coming home more often for "visits." Each time he finally began breaking things, and we once more brought the drafting table, suitcases, and sometimes cockroaches back home. Eventually, he would be reaccepted by a hospital, and we sat with heavy hearts while heaving sighs of relief. (Piercey, 1985, p. 155).

Initial Presentation

Schizophrenic symptoms can present either abruptly or gradually. Approximately 25% of patients will have an abrupt onset, with a predominance of positive symptoms (Maxmen, 1986). Generally, the active phase of the disorder (when positive symptoms predominate) is preceded by a prodromal phase, where the individual's social, occupational, and personal functioning deteriorates. The length of this prodromal phase varies. As stated above, prognosis is worse in those cases where there is an extended prodromal phase, with gradual and progressive deterioration over an extended period of time.

The psychotic symptoms (hallucinations, delusions, etc.) that are predominant during the active phase generally result in referral for treatment. The individual is often an unwilling patient, however. Family members will often play an active role in convincing the patient to obtain treatment.

The following case describes the factors leading up to a patient's first hospitalization due to a schizophrenic disorder, as well as some brief personal history.

CASE DESCRIPTION

William was the youngest of three children raised in a middle-class neighborhood. He was an average student who had a small group of friends. He did not participate in any organized extracurricular activities. He graduated from high school and began working at a department store while living at his parents' home.

When William originally began working, no problems were reported. He appeared to be performing adequately in his job. He tended to spend most of his nonworking hours at his parents' home.

By the fall after William's graduation, however, some problems began to develop. William began to have difficulty sleeping and concentrating. He began to call in sick for work and became more and more withdrawn. He later started hoarding food in his bedroom and in his pockets. By the end of December, William had stopped attending to his personal hygiene.

One night in January, William began yelling at his mother, accusing her of spying on him. He became very loud and threatening, frightening his parents. William's father called the police and they transported William to the local hospital. William was admitted to the hospital's psychiatric unit.

On presentation to the hospital, William was delusional and extremely agitated. He stated that he worked for the CIA and that his hospitalization was a plot to silence him. William stated that the government wanted him hospitalized because he knew the truth behind the assassination of John F. Kennedy.

William made continual threats to the hospital staff, threatening them with malpractice suits if they treated him. He was extremely loud and argumentative, but he did not become physically violent.

While William's case presents an individual with rapid onset of symptoms and relatively good premorbid functioning, other persons might present differently. Another case example will make this clear.

Denise was raised in multiple foster homes. She was moved from foster home to foster home, due to her disruptive behavior and her social withdrawal (she would either have no interactions with others or behave in such a way as to bother others and draw attention to herself). Denise did poorly at school, both academically and socially. She had no close friends and spent most of her free time alone. Due to socially inappropriate behavior and acting-out behavior, Denise was placed in a residential facility at age 16. In her early twenties, Denise began to report auditory hallucinations. She also displayed paranoid thinking, reporting that people in her day program were attempting to poison her and that staff were plotting to keep her from getting well. Denise remained in hospitals almost continuously for the next 20 years, interrupted only occasionally by attempts to place her in supervised community housing. These community placements failed, due to the same behaviors Denise displayed when she was a child.

In the hospital, Denise ignored her personal hygiene almost completely. She would bathe and change clothing only when she was coaxed to do so by hospital staff. Even with coaxing, Denise would not always agree to bathe. Denise made frequent inappropriate sexual advances toward other patients and staff, but was easily directed to stop. She would not willingly participate in psychotherapy or any other therapeutic activities at the hospital. The only way to have her participate in these activities was to make privileges contingent on her compliance with these activities. Various medication regimens were tried with Denise, but none was able to adequately address her negative symptoms. Additionally, she would frequently display loud, disruptive, and threatening behavior when she was frustrated. She frequently stated that the hospital staff were working to keep her in the hospital.

COURSE AND PROGNOSIS

Course

The course of schizophrenia is highly variable but generally includes a series of acute episodes interspersed with residual phases. During the residual phases, the individual might be able to function at some minimal level (live independently or with supervision, work in a low-level position in a competitive workplace or in a therapeutic workshop, etc.). The degree of impairment often increases with each subsequent residual phase.

Once a person develops schizophrenia and becomes involved with the mental health system, a rather typical course of treatment follows. In virtually all cases, the patient is treated pharmacologically. This is a relatively recent treatment option, as the first use of neuroleptic medication for the treatment of schizophrenia occurred in 1952. Since that time, a number of *antipsychotic medications* have been developed that are beneficial in the treatment of schizophrenia, although they have a greater impact on reducing positive symptoms of schizophrenia, as opposed to negative symptoms.

The use of antipsychotic medications has allowed patients with schizophrenia to remain out of hospital for longer periods of time than was possible prior to the advent of these medications. Antipsychotic medications have allowed the treatment of many patients to take place in outpatient settings, rather than require the individuals to be treated in hospitals. The ability of antipsychotic medication to control the bizarre positive symptoms of schizophrenia has also improved patients' ability to maintain homes and jobs within the community.

Antipsychotic medications have the tendency to produce side-effects, however. These include dry mouth, constipation, blurred vision, photosensitivity, sedation, weight gain, sexual dysfunction, drug-induced parkinsonism, and tardive dyskinesia (Davis, Barter, & Kane, 1989). The latter two side-effects listed (drug-induced parkinsonism and tardive dyskinesia) result in a range of bizarre body movements, including tremor, rigidity, bizarre tongue movements, and lip smacking. Tardive dyskinesia is generally irreversible. Drug-induced parkinsonism, on the other hand, can be effectively controlled through the use of antiparkinsonian medication in most cases (Baldessarini & Cole, 1988).

In spite of the side-effects that can be produced by antipsychotic medications, these medications have resulted in a much more positive outcome for persons with schizophrenia than was possible prior to the discovery of these medications. While side-effects do occur, most patients are able to tolerate them, and adjustments in medication dosage can often decrease the severity of the side-effects.

Various *psychosocial treatments* have been found to be effective in the treatment of schizophrenia, when they are combined with pharmacological treatments. *Milieu Therapy* focuses on "group and social interactions . . . rules and expectations . . . viewing patients as responsible human beings . . . patients' involvement in setting goals . . . freedom of movement . . . informality of relationships with staff, and interdisciplinary participation and goal-oriented, clear communication" (Liberman & Mueser, 1989, p. 800). The theoretical modalities utilized within a milieu can fall anywhere within the wide range of psychological treatment theories.

One model of milieu therapy that is based on learning theory and has been used successfully in the hospital treatment of persons with schizophrenia is *Social Learning Therapy* (Paul & Lentz, 1977). Social Learning Therapy utilizes token reinforcement (Ayllon & Azrin, 1965) to impact on all aspects of the patients' lives (physical appearance and hygiene, housekeeping chores, appropriate interpersonal behavior, and participation in educational programs). Specific instruction is given to patients as to what behaviors they are expected to display. As time passes, higher behavioral expectations are made of the patients. This treatment model has resulted in a high rate of discharge and a low rate of recidivism, relative to traditional hospital treatment (Paul & Lentz, 1977). It has been especially beneficial in treating individuals who, due to the severity of their symptoms, have not been previously able to leave the hospital (Liberman & Mueser, 1989). Social Learning Therapy has also been found to be beneficial in community treatment programs.

The *Fountain House Model* was developed by a group of former patients as a means for providing themselves with a support system that would help them to deal with day-to-day problems and develop to their highest potential. Persons involved in Fountain House programs see themselves as "members," not "patients." The members develop both social and work activities for themselves and work to help each other develop work skills. Fountain House programs are able to find employment for its members within a range of companies, from small firms to large corporations. The majority of Fountain House members who work within these companies are successful in maintaining employment and remaining out of hospital (Beard, Propst, & Malamud, 1982).

While Social Learning Therapy uses token economies to reward patients who display appropriate social skills, and Fountain House programs provide many opportunities for members to participate in social activities, many patients cannot exhibit socially skilled behavior due to the absence of requisite interpersonal skills from their behavioral repertoire. Given that "social dysfunction is a hallmark of schizophrenia" (Morrison & Bellack, 1984, p. 247), the importance of patients developing appropriate social skills cannot be overstated. As a result, considerable emphasis has been placed on *social skills training* for patients with schizophrenia.

Morrison and Bellack (1984) describe a social skills training program that consists of five elements: (1) instructions, (2) modeling, (3) role play, (4) feedback and positive reinforcement, and (5) homework (Morrison & Bellack, 1984). In this model, the therapist/trainer tells the patient what he/she should do in a particular situation (instruction) and shows the patient how to exhibit the particular skill (modeling). Once the patient has received the instruction and seen the desired behavior being modeled, he/she practices the new skill with the therapist/trainer (role play). Following the role play, the therapist/trainer tells the patient what he/she did correctly in the role play and what still needs to be worked on (feedback and positive reinforcement). Following this feedback, the patient will complete multiple repetitions of the role play, in order to provide the patient with multiple learning opportunities. The final step in the social skills training program is for the patient to be given a homework assignment to practice the skill in real-life situations before the next training session. It has been found that this approach results in improvement in the particular skills being trained and that these new skills are maintained over time. It has also been shown that improving social skills results in lower recidivism rates among persons with schizophrenia (Bellack, Turner, Hersen, & Luber, 1984; Hogarty, Anderson, Reiss, Kornblith, Greenewald, Javna, & Madonia, 1986).

Very frequently, social skills deficits in patients are seen to have negative impact on family interactions. The chronic nature of schizophrenia, the disruptive symptoms of the disorder, and the impact these have on the patient's social interactions can place so much stress on the family that family members are unable to provide adequate support and assistance to the patient (Anderson, Reiss, & Hogarty, 1986). While in certain households, the patient's limited social skills can have negative impact on the family, there are also patients who live in households where other family members have social skills deficits as well. These social skills deficits within the family often result in a high level of conflict between family members. Studies indicate that patients who live in homes with high levels of conflict (high expressed emotion, or EE), tend to have a high level of symptom reoccurrence and rehospitalization (Davison & Neale, 1990). For these reasons, an area of growing interest in the treatment of schizophrenia is the importance of *family therapy* for the family of the patient with schizophrenia. Like milieu therapy, family therapy can be based on any of a number of psychological theories. Family therapy, regardless of theoretical basis, has been found to be beneficial in reducing patient relapse rates. Family therapy has reduced rehospitalization rates from approximately 50% (the typical rate for patients receiving standard aftercare) to as low as 6 to 19% when "supportive and behavioral therapies that employ educational and skill-building methods" are employed (Liberman & Mueser, 1989, p. 795).

As stated above, supportive and behavioral family therapy related to schizophrenia initially involves education of the family about schizophrenia. Family members are taught that schizophrenia is the result of normal life stress impacting on a person with a biological predisposition for the disease. The family often needs to know that the patient's symptoms are typical presentations of the disorder and are not intentional efforts to upset family members. The family also needs to be informed about the patient's prognosis, the typical course of the disorder, and the treatment.

In addition to learning the important facts about schizophrenia, the family also needs to learn what role they can play in the control of symptoms and in helping the patient to remain out of the hospital. In particular, they need to learn about the role that conflict and overinvolvement can play in the patient's symptom status, and to be trained in methods of conflict resolution. The method for training family members in conflict resolution follows that of social skills training outlined above. The family is given instruction, sees appropriate conflict resolution modeled, participates in role plays, receives feedback and positive reinforcement, and is given homework assignments. The topics that are role played originally are not related to the family specifically, but rather are neutral situations that are unlikely to produce strong emotional responses in any of the family members. As training progresses, more emotionally volatile topics are addressed.

As noted previously, there is evidence that improving the family's methods for dealing with conflict can have a significant positive impact on the patient's symptoms and ability to remain out of the hospital. Hogarty et al. (1991) found that patients who participated in both family treatment and social skills training, in addition to receiving medication, had the lowest rate of relapse when compared with patients who received medication alone or medication and either one of the two additional treatments over a 2-year period (no relapse during year one and 25% relapse by year two).

A therapy method that addresses a wide range of issues, including conflict resolution, social interaction, behavior change, and personal insight is *group therapy*. Group therapy can be based on any psychological theory and can take place in both inpatient and outpatient settings. Group therapy is often unstructured, with the concerns and behaviors of the group members on any given day determining the activities of the group on that day. Some groups, however, are structured with specific goals to be achieved through participation in the group. Group therapy tends to be most beneficial when it is focused on practical, day-to-

PATRICK W.
McGUFFIN and
RANDALL L.
MORRISON

day problems. Group therapy targeting the improvement of work and social functioning is generally more effective than individual therapy. This is felt to be due to the social experience inherent in group therapy and the modeling of appropriate social and work behaviors by peers within the group context (Liberman & Mueser, 1989).

Prognosis

The prognosis for a person with schizophrenia is guarded, at best. As is evident above, many patients will never completely return to their premorbid level of functioning; their level of functioning will generally decrease with each subsequent residual phase. Studies have indicated that between 20% and 30% of persons with schizophrenia will be able to lead relatively normal lives (e.g., work competitively, live independently, remain out of hospital). The majority of individuals will have a much less promising course, with 20 to 30% continuing to experience moderate symptoms and 40 to 60% remaining significantly impaired for the rest of their lives (Grebb & Cancro, 1989).

Several variables have a positive impact on an individual's prognosis, however. These include adequate social functioning prior to onset of symptoms, rapid onset of symptoms, family history of a mood disorder, and confusion as a presenting symptom. Those persons with a less positive prognosis would tend to have a poorer premorbid level of functioning, a more gradual onset of symptoms (with gradually increasing deficits in independent functioning), and a presentation that is more heavily loaded for negative, rather than positive symptoms (Kaplan & Sadock, 1989).

FAMILIAL AND GENETIC PATTERNS

No single causative factor has been found for schizophrenia. There is evidence that biological, environmental, or psychosocial factors can all play a role in the development of schizophrenic symptoms.

Genetic factors appear to play a role in the etiology of schizophrenia, given that risk of developing schizophrenia is higher among relatives of persons with schizophrenia. Ninety percent of persons with schizophrenia, however, have no first-degree relatives with the disorder. Studies of the prevalence of schizophrenia among twins have shown a higher incidence of the disorder based on the degree of genetic similarity between siblings. Among monozygotic twins, the likelihood that one twin will develop schizophrenia when his/her twin has the disorder is strikingly higher than the rate found in the general population (44% versus 1%). The rate in dizygotic twins is much lower (21%), but still higher than the rate for the general population. Siblings who are neither monozygotic or dizygotic twins have a 7% likelihood of developing schizophrenia when a sibling has the disorder, showing a correlation that decreases as the level of similarity between siblings decreases (see Table 2).

Adoption studies have also indicated that genetics play a role in the development of schizophrenia. In one study, children of schizophrenic mothers, who were adopted or put into foster care at birth, were compared with a control group of children who were adopted at the same time and in the same locale. None of the control group were diagnosed as having schizophrenia when evaluated more than 35 years later; however, 16.6% of the children of schizophrenic mothers were diagnosed as having schizophrenia. In addition, 66% of the children of schizophrenic mothers had some psychiatric diagnosis, although this was true of only 18% of the control children (Heston, 1966). These findings suggest that even when children are removed from the potentially disruptive home environment that parents with schizophrenia might be expected to provide, the incidence of schizophrenia among these children is still higher than that found in the general population.

While there is evidence of a likely genetic role in the development of schizophrenia, it is clear that genetics alone do not produce the disorder. If genetics were sufficient to produce schizophrenia, the rate of schizophrenia in monozygotic twins would be 100% whenever one twin had schizophrenia (as monozygotic twins have identical genes). Clearly, genetics play a role in the development of schizophrenia, but other factors are necessary for the appearance of the disorder in individuals with a genetic predisposition.

Among other possible factors that might produce schizophrenia in those who are at risk for the disease, the role of familial factors (other than genetics) has been considered. Specifically, *expressed emotion* (EE) has been investigated for its etiologic significance in the development and exacerbation of schizophrenic symptoms. Expressed emotion is a measure of involvement and criticism among family members. Families with high EE tend to be intrusive and overly involved in the patient's life and tend to be highly critical. Studies have indicated that persons with schizophrenia whose families display high EE tend to have higher rates of relapse of schizophrenic symptoms and poor prognosis. While this correlation exists, no causal relationship has been found (Halford, Schweitzer, & Varghese, 1991).

Other Theories of Schizophrenia

Various etiological theories of schizophrenia have arisen over the years. As is true with most areas of psychopathology, early theories were based on the psychodynamic model. *Psychodynamic theories* hold that schizophrenia is the result of a child's failure to develop positive interpersonal relationships during childhood or of traumatic events that occur during a person's childhood. These theories have fallen into disrepute over the years, as research has not produced supporting

TABLE 2.   European Family and Twin Studies of Schizophrenia, 1920–1978

	Percent with definite diagnosis of schizophrenia (by relationship to schizophrenic subject)
Spouses	1.00
Children	9.35
Siblings	7.30
Monozygotic twins	44.30
Dizygotic twins	12.08
Half sibling (reared by common parent)	2.94
Nieces/nephews	2.65
Grandchildren	2.84
First cousins	1.56

Source: Gottsman, McGuffin, & Farmer (1987).

PATRICK W.
McGUFFIN and
RANDALL L.
MORRISON

evidence (Davison & Neale, 1990; McGlashan, 1984; Mueser & Berenbaum, 1990). Still, they are important from a historical perspective.

As part of the psychodynamic theory of schizophrenia, the concepts of the *schizophrenogenic mother* and the *double-bind* relationship between a mother and child have been widely discussed as having a causal role in the development of schizophrenia. The schizophrenogenic mother is seen as one who, through her cold and dominant style and her tendency to be rejecting, overprotective, and fearful of intimacy, produces schizophrenia in her children. The double-bind theory postulates that the individual with schizophrenia developed the disorder secondary to an intense relationship with another person (often the mother), where the other person gives conflicting messages to the individual (i.e., mother stiffens when son hugs her and then complains when the son withdraws the hug).

As stated above, controlled studies examining psychodynamic theories of schizophrenia have not produced data to support them. The psychodynamic theory of schizophrenia has, therefore, been generally discounted throughout the scientific community.

The *biochemical theory* of schizophrenia states that neurotransmitter activity plays a significant role in its development. This theory is based, in part, on the impact that biological treatments (medication) have on schizophrenic symptoms, as well as the side effects that medications produce. Patients receiving medication to treat their psychotic symptoms often show side effects that mimic Parkinson's disease. Parkinson's disease is known to be caused by low levels of the neurotransmitter *dopamine*. Since medication decreases symptoms of schizophrenia and at the same time produces symptoms that are correlated with low levels of dopamine, it is theorized that schizophrenia is related to high levels of dopamine and that dopamine levels must be lowered (through medication) in order to control the schizophrenic symptoms. The impact of medication on positive symptoms (i.e., hallucinations and delusions), however, is more obvious than on negative symptoms (i.e., apathy, withdrawal, flat affect). While antipsychotic medications are often effective in treating positive symptoms, they tend to be less effective in minimizing negative symptoms. The dopamine theory, therefore, appears to provide some useful information relative to patients' positive symptoms but has a weaker relation to negative symptoms (Stahl & Wets, 1988).

While there is evidence of a correlation between excess dopamine activity and schizophrenia, there is no proof of causality. It is unclear whether excess dopamine activity occurs prior to or subsequent to the onset of schizophrenic symptoms.

Another biological theory that has received much attention over the last decade is the possible role of *brain pathology* in the development of schizophrenia, particularly when the negative symptoms are the most prominent. Post mortem studies of individuals with schizophrenia, as well as CAT scans and PET scans, have provided evidence of brain abnormalities among schizophrenic individuals. These examinations have provided evidence that suggests possible brain atrophy among persons with schizophrenia. Evaluation of neurological functioning has also shown decreases in frontal cortical functioning among this population. One theory is that the brain pathology found among persons with schizophrenia is the result of infection during pregnancy, which causes abnormal fetal development. This is an area of continuing research.

A theory that takes into consideration various aspects of biological theories, as well as the impact of environmental factors, is the *diathesis-stress theory*. The diathesis-stress model states that the individual who develops schizophrenia is born with a genetic predisposition to developing schizophrenia, but does not develop the disorder unless he/she is subjected to stress (Zubin & Spring, 1977). The stress can come from any source (family, traumatic event, etc.); however, the theory does not state that the stress itself can bring on schizophrenic symptoms. This is an important point, given the long-held, but discounted belief that schizophrenia is the result of bad parenting. As stated above, research has not supported the theory that schizophrenia is caused by child–parent conflicts or particular parenting styles.

The diathesis-stress theory is valuable in its explanation of the interaction between biology and environment (Liberman, Marshall, Marder, Dawson, Nuechterlein, & Doane, 1984). This theory recognizes the evidence that biology seems to play a role in schizophrenia, but has not been shown to be sufficient to cause the disorder. This model recognizes that, on the one hand, stress has a role in the development of symptoms but that, on the other hand, not all persons who are exposed to similar stressors develop schizophrenia.

DIAGNOSTIC CONSIDERATIONS

Given the heterogeneity of symptoms that may be present and the fact that various disorders share common symptoms with schizophrenia, diagnosis may be extremely difficult. The diagnostic interview, therefore, is very important in determining: (1) symptoms of schizophrenia, (2) other possible diagnoses, and (3) symptom precipitants.

When conducting a diagnostic interview, the interviewer can ask a series of questions that address the patient's complaints and his/her understanding of the events that lead to the need for such an interview. One method that has been seen as valuable in diagnostic interviewing is the use of a structured interview, such as the Schedule for Affective Disorders and Schizophrenia (Endicott & Spitzer, 1978) or the Diagnostic Interview Schedule (Robins, Helzer, Croughan, & Ratcliff, 1981). Structured interviews provide a series of specific questions that have been developed to provide consistency in those questions that are asked before determining a person's diagnosis. They also facilitate comparability between individuals who are diagnosed as having schizophrenia by different interviewers at different times.

Regardless of method used to conduct a diagnostic interview, there are several questions that must be answered before a diagnosis of schizophrenia can be made. These questions will determine whether: (1) the patient displays symptoms within the schizophrenia diagnostic framework, (2) the particular symptoms are also seen in other disorders, (3) any symptoms are present which preclude a diagnosis of schizophrenia, and (4) the symptoms are secondary to some known organic factor.

The easiest of the above questions to address, although not always the easiest to answer, is the issue of organicity. Simply put, schizophrenia cannot be diagnosed if it is secondary to an organic disorder. If there is a known history or current evidence of an organic disorder that may be producing the symptoms, then either a diagnosis reflecting this must be given, or it must be shown that while an organic disorder could be producing the symptoms, there is evidence that it is not. Also, if there is evidence of current or recent substance abuse, the possibility that the substance may account for the symptoms must be considered. In this case, diagnosis should probably be deferred until the patient's system has been cleared of the substance.

When there is no clear evidence that a specific organic factor might be causing the patient's symptoms, it may not be obvious that organic factors need to be considered. However, if the patient reports hallucinations other than auditory (visual, olfactory, etc.), the patient should receive a neurological evaluation to rule out any organic disorder. Regardless of the particular symptoms that a patient displays, the possible presence of an organic disorder must be ascertained before the diagnosis of schizophrenia can be given.

In addition to evaluating the possibility of a specific organic disorder causing the patient's symptoms, one must also determine if the symptoms fall within the diagnostic framework of schizophrenia. The most obvious symptoms seen in schizophrenia are those that indicate an impairment in reality testing. These include delusions, hallucinations, incoherence, catatonia, and inappropriate affect. These can be assessed by questioning the patient as well as by observing the patient and interviewing family members. At times, the patient will not report any problems; however, observations by others will indicate that the patient's reality testing is significantly impaired.

The patient must display, in addition to the positive symptoms listed above, negative symptoms in order to receive a diagnosis of schizophrenia. These symptoms include social withdrawal, decreased academic or work functioning, impaired self-care, and marked lack of initiative. These symptoms are present during the active stage of schizophrenia and tend to continue during the residual (inactive) stage of the disorder.

After determining that the individual shows an impairment in reality testing and a marked decrease in functioning (socially, academically, etc.) that is not secondary to organic factors, one must determine that these symptoms are of sufficient duration to meet criteria for a diagnosis of schizophrenia. If the patient displays psychotic symptoms, but the symptoms have been present for only a brief period of time (less than 1 month), there have been no prodromal symptoms, and the patient has been under significant stress, schizophrenia would not be diagnosed. In this case, either a brief reactive psychosis or a psychotic mood disorder would be diagnosed, the latter being considered if a major depressive or manic syndrome is present.

If a patient reports nonbizarre delusions (related to real-life events or situations) of at least 1 month duration, there is no evidence of hallucinations, and no bizarre behaviors are observed, then the diagnosis of delusional disorder would be made.

When psychotic symptoms co-occur with major depressive or manic symptoms, and the mood symptoms are present during the majority of psychotic symptoms (although the psychotic symptoms are present for at least 2 weeks when there are no prominent mood symptoms), then schizoaffective disorder would be diagnosed.

When psychotic symptoms have lasted for more than 1 month, mood symptoms are not predominant, social and/or occupational functioning is markedly impaired, but the total duration of the illness is less than 6 months (including prodromal, active, and residual phases), schizophreniform disorder is diagnosed. The duration of the disorder is what distinguishes schizophreniform disorder from schizophrenia. Only when the disorder is longer than 6 months in duration can the diagnosis of schizophrenia be made.

In many patients, it may be difficult to distinguish between diagnoses of schizophrenia and bipolar disorder. There are several symptoms found in both disorders. For example, the elevated, expansive mood often seen in persons with bipolar disorder can be confused with the grandiose or paranoid delusions often seen in persons with schizophrenia. Additionally, delusions and/or hallucinations can occur in bipolar disorder, although they must occur in the presence of mood symptoms or, if they occur independently, they must last no longer than 2 weeks. Both schizophrenia and bipolar disorder also result in marked impairment of functioning. The important distinction to make in these cases is the presence of mood symptoms, which would be indicative of bipolar disorder but would rule out a diagnosis of schizophrenia. Obtaining a thorough history of both the patient and the patient's family is generally very helpful in determining a diagnosis of bipolar disorder, as persons with bipolar disorder will generally have evidence of prior mood disorders as well as history of mood disorders among family members.

Several studies have spoken of the difficulty in differentiating schizophrenia from other major mental illnesses. It has been found that when a structured assessment of patient symptoms is conducted, the majority of hospital patients who were originally diagnosed as having schizophrenia in fact suffered from mania (Abrams, Taylor, & Gaztanaga, 1974). In one sample of patients (Taylor & Abrams, 1975), none of the patients originally diagnosed with schizophrenia were found to have the disorder upon reevaluation.

It has been equally difficult to distinguish between schizophrenia and schizo-affective disorder (Kendall & Gourlay, 1970). Given the various diagnostic criteria used throughout the world, it has been found that patients who meet one definition of schizophrenia will often meet another criterion for schizoaffective disorder (Brockington & Leff, 1979).

These examples point out the difficulty in making a diagnosis of schizophrenia and the existence of several disorders that share many of the same symptoms. Much care must be taken in reaching a correct diagnosis so that the patient may receive the most appropriate treatment. Further investigation of the symptoms found in schizophrenia and the varying responses to treatment of individuals with different symptom clusters may help to improve the ability to develop a diagnosis with confidence, and thereby improve the efficacy of treatment.

SUMMARY

While it is a relatively rare disorder, schizophrenia is extremely disabling to the sufferer and disruptive to the lifestyle of both the individual and his/her family. Schizophrenia is a disease of uncertain etiology, apparently having both biological and environmental determinants. Familial patterns of occurrence exist, but a purely genetic basis for the disorder has not been proven. Additionally, there is evidence that critical or argumentative family interactions, as well as overinvolvement by family members in the patient's life, can play a role in relapse rates of persons with schizophrenia.

Outcomes for schizophrenia are generally not positive. Very few persons with schizophrenia are able to return to a level of functioning comparable to that which existed prior to the onset of the disorder. At particular risk for a negative prognosis are those patients who have a gradual, progressive onset of the disorder and a preponderance of negative symptoms. The reason for this is not yet known, nor is there a clear understanding of why some persons will display more positive symptoms, and others more negative ones. Various theories have been developed as to the cause of particular symptom types, including structural abnormality in the brain (Turner, Toone, & Brett-Jones, 1986) and variation in the sensitivity or number of dopamine receptors (Berrios, 1985). It has also been suggested that schizophrenia may, in fact, be "a heterogeneous group of disorders" (Andreason & Olsen, 1982, p. 789) and that patients with prominent positive symptoms may require a different treatment from that of patients with mostly negative symptoms (Andreason & Olsen, 1982). Continuing research in the area of positive and negative symptoms, their causes, and most effective treatment will likely provide important information regarding how best to treat all patients with schizophrenia.

Regardless of the relative presentation of positive or negative symptoms, treatment of schizophrenia almost always involves the use of antipsychotic medications. These medications have been shown to be effective in controlling the positive symptoms that often precipitate hospitalization. Antipsychotic medications may produce side effects that can lead to noncompliance in the patient. Side effects range from dryness of mouth to the presence of tremors and bizarre bodily movements of tardive dyskinesia. While a great number of persons with schizophrenia have been benefitted by medication and have managed to remain out of hospital and maintain involvement in social and occupational activities because of it, some patients may undergo multiple hospitalizations and spend years in hospitals, unable to function adequately in community settings. Hopefully, future research will provide some methods for distinguishing patients who respond positively to pharmacological interventions from those who do not. Then, perhaps, more effective treatments for nonresponders can be developed.

In addition to pharmacological treatment of schizophrenia, several psychosocial treatments have been shown to be effective. Behavioral treatment, used to address both the high frequency of disruptive behaviors and the deficit functioning level of persons with schizophrenia, has been effective in improving patients' self-control as well as their self-care and independent functioning. Rates of aggressive behavior, levels of independent self-care, and degree of participation in therapeutic and work activities have all been positively affected by the use of behavioral interventions.

One particular behavioral strategy, social skills training, has been successful in remediating social deficits so frequently seen in schizophrenic persons. Through the use of structured role-play tasks and repeated practice of realistic social situations, persons with schizophrenia have become better able to deal with interpersonal conflicts and to initiate and maintain conversations, thereby minimizing the social withdrawal frequently observed in the disorder.

Behavioral family therapy, addressing methods for dealing with interpersonal conflict, the difficulties inherent in having a person with schizophrenia in the family, and the level of interpersonal involvement among family members, has been shown to decrease the rate of relapse among patients. By teaching methods for decreasing tension within the family and for dealing with conflict appropriately, the level of anxiety decreases, making the family environment more pleasant.

There is evidence that the most effective treatment of schizophrenia involves a combination of pharmacological and psychosocial treatment. Hogarty, Goldberg, and Schooler (1974) reported that psychosocial treatment is most effective in patients who are already stabilized on antipsychotic medications. There is also evidence that an additive effect is present when both pharmacological and psychosocial treatments are utilized. Patients who are receiving antipsychotic medication are more tolerant of psychosocial interventions and show more benefit from them. Patients who are receiving psychosocial treatment are also more compliant with their medication regimens (Strang, Falloon, Moss, Razani, & Boyd, 1981). It also has been reported that patients who, through family therapy, are able to decrease the level of stress within the family, often require lower dosages of antipsychotic medications (Falloon & Liberman, 1983).

Even with these various treatments, the prognosis for those with schizophrenia continues to be guarded. Research continues in an attempt to improve treatment outcome and to gain further information regarding etiologic factors. As more investigative endeavors are carried out, it is hoped that a more promising prognosis will result.

REFERENCES

Abrams, R., Taylor, M. A., & Gaztanaga, P. (1974). Manic-depressive illness and paranoid schizophrenia. *Archives of General Psychiatry, 31*, 640–642.

American Psychiatric Association. (1987). *Diagnostic and Statistical Manual of Mental Disorders*, 3rd Edition, Revised. Washington, DC: Author.

American Psychiatric Association (1993). *DSM-IV draft criteria*. Washington, DC: Author.

Anderson, C. M., Reiss, D. J., & Hogarty, G. E. (1986). *Schizophrenia and the family*. New York: Guilford Press.

Andreason, N. C., & Olsen, S. (1982). Negative vs. positive schizophrenia: Definition and validation. *Archives of General Psychiatry, 39*, 789–794.

Ayllon, T., & Azrin, N. H. (1965). The measurement and reinforcement of behavior of psychotics. *Journal of Experimental Analysis of Behavior, 8*, 357–383.

Baldessarini, R. J., & Cole, J. O. (1988). Chemotherapy. In A. M. Nicholi (Ed.), *The new Harvard guide to psychiatry* (pp. 481 –533). Cambridge: The Belknap Press of Harvard University Press.

Beard, J. H., Propst, R. N., & Malamud, T. J. (1982). The Fountain House model of psychiatric rehabilitation. *Psychosocial Rehabilitation Journal, 5*, 47–59.

Bellack, A. S., Turner, S. M., Hersen, M., & Luber, R. F. (1984). An examination of the efficacy of social skills training for chronic schizophrenic patients. *Hospital and Community Psychiatry, 35*, 1023–1028.

Berrios, G. E. (1985). Positive and negative symptoms. *Archives of General Psychiatry, 42*, 95–97.

Brockington, I. F., & Leff, J. P. (1979). Schizo-affective psychosis: definitions and incidence. *Psychological Medicine, 9*, 91–99.

Davis, J. M., Barter, J. T., & Kane, J. M. (1989). Antipsychotic Drugs. In H. I. Kaplan & B. J. Sadock (Eds.), *Comprehensive textbook of psychiatry* (5th ed.) (pp. 1591–1626). Baltimore: Williams & Wilkins.

Davison, G. C. & Neale, J. M. (1990). *Abnormal psychology*. New York: Wiley.

Endicott, J., & Spitzer, R. L. (1978). A diagnostic interview: The schedule for affective disorders and schizophrenia. *Archives of General Psychiatry, 35*, 837–844.

Falloon, I. R. H., & Liberman, R. P. (1983). Behavioral family interventions in the management of chronic schizophrenia. In W. R. McFarlane (Ed.), *Family therapy in schizophrenia* (pp. 117–137). New York: Guilford Press.

Gottsman, I. I., McGuffin, P., & Farmer, A. E. (1987). Clinical genetics as clues to the "real" genetics of schizophrenia. (A decade of modest gains while playing for time.). *Schizophrenia Bulletin, 13*, 23–48.

Grebb, J. A., & Cancro, R. (1989). Schizophrenia: Clinical features. In H. I. Kaplan & B. J. Sadock (Eds.), *Comprehensive textbook of psychiatry* (5th ed.) (pp. 757–777). Baltimore: Williams & Wilkins.

Halford, W. K., Schweitzer, R. D., & Varghese, F. N. (1991). Effects of family environment on negative symptoms and quality of life of psychotic patients. *Hospital and Community Psychiatry, 42*, 1241–1247.

Harris, J. G. (1984). Prognosis in schizophrenia. In A. S. Bellack (Ed.) *Schizophrenia: Treatment, management, and rehabilitation* (pp. 79–112). Orlando, FL: Grune & Stratton.

Heston, L. L. (1966). Psychiatric disorders in foster home reared children of schizophrenic mothers. *British Journal of Psychiatry, 112*, 1103–1110.

Hogarty, G. E., Goldberg, S. C., & Schooler, N. R. (1974). Drug and sociotherapy in the aftercare of schizophrenic patients. *Archives of General Psychiatry, 31*, 609–618.

Hogarty, G. E., Anderson, C. M., Reiss, D. J., Kornblith, S. J., Greenwald, D. P., Javna, C. D., & Madonia, M. J. (1986). Family psychoeducation, social skills training, and maintenance chemotherapy in the aftercare treatment of schizophrenia. *Archives of General Psychiatry, 43*, 633–642.

Hogarty, G. E., Anderson, C. M., Reiss, D. J., Kornblith, S. J., Greenwald, D. P., Ulrich, R. F., Carter, M., & EPICS Research Group (1991). Family pyschoeducation, social skills training, and maintenance chemotherapy in the aftercare treatment of schizophrenia, II: Two-year effects of a controlled study on relapse and adjustment. *Archives of General Psychiatry, 48*, 340–347.

Kaplan, H. I., & Sadock, B. J. (1989). *Comprehensive textbook of psychiatry* (5th ed.). Baltimore: Williams & Wilkins.

Keith, S. J., Regier, D. A., & Rae, D. S. (1991). Schizophrenic disorders. In L. N. Robins & D. A. Regier (Eds.), *Psychiatric disorders in America* (pp. 33–52). New York: Free Press.

Kendell, R. E., & Gourlay, J. (1970). The clinical distinction between affective psychoses and schizophrenia. *British Journal of Psychiatry, 117*, 261–266.

Knight, J. G. (1985). Possible autoimmune mechanisms in schizophrenia. *Integrative Psychiatry, 3*, 134–143.

Liberman, R. P., Marshall, B. D., Marder, S. R., Dawson, M. E., Nuechterlein, K. H., & Doane, J. A. (1984). The nature and problem of schizophrenia. In A. S. Bellack (Ed.), *Schizophrenia: Treatment, management, and rehabilitation* (pp. 1–34) Orlando, FL: Grune & Stratton.

Liberman, R. P., & Mueser, K. T. (1989). Schizophrenia: Psychosocial treatment. In H. I. Kaplan & B. J. Sadock (Eds.) *Comprehensive textbook of psychiatry* (5th ed.) (pp. 792–806). Baltimore: Williams & Wilkins.

Maxmen, J. S. (1986). *Essential psychopathology*. New York: Norton.

McGlashan, T. H. (1984). The Chestnut Lodge follow-up study. II. Long-term outcome of schizophrenia and the affective disorders. *Archives of General Psychiatry, 41*, 586–601.

McGlashan, T. H., & Bardenstein, K. K. (1990). Gender differences in affective, schizoaffective, and schizophrenic disorders. *Schizophrenia Bulletin, 16*, 319–329.

Morrison, R. L., & Bellack, A. S. (1984). Social skills training. In A. S. Bellack (Ed.), *Schizophrenia: Treatment, management, and rehabilitation* (pp. 247–279). Orlando, FL: Grune & Stratton.

Mueser, K. T., & Berenbaum, H. (1990). Psychodynamic treatment of schizophrenia: Is there a future? *Psychological Medicine, 20*, 253–262.

Paul, G. L., & Lentz, R. J. (1977). *Psychosocial treatment of chronic mental patients*. Cambridge: Harvard University Press.

Piercey, B. P. (1985). First person account: Making the best of it. *Schizophrenia Bulletin, 11*, 155–157.

Robins, L. N., Helzer, J. E., Croughan, J., & Ratcliff, K. S. (1981). National Institute of Mental Health Diagnostic Interview Schedule: Its history, characteristics, and validity. *Archives of General Psychiatry, 38*, 381–389.

Stahl, S. M., & Wets, K. M. (1988). Clinical pharmacology of schizophrenia. In P. Bebbington & P. McGuffin (Eds.), *Schizophrenia: The major issues* (pp. 135–156). Oxford, England: Heinemann Professional Publishing Ltd.

Strang, J. S., Falloon, I. R. H., Moss, H. B., Razani, J., & Boyd, J. L. (1981). The effects of family therapy on treatment compliance in schizophrenia. *Psychopharmacology Bulletin, 17*, 87–88.

Taylor, M. A., & Abrams, R. (1975). Manic-depressive illness and good prognosis schizophrenia. *American Journal of Psychiatry, 132*, 741–742.

Tien, A. Y., & Eaton, W. W. (1992). Psychopathologic precursors and sociodemographic risk factors for the schizophrenia syndrome. *Archives of General Psychiatry, 49*, 37–46.

Tsuang, M. T., Faraone, S. V., & Day, M. (1988). Schizophrenic disorders. In A. M. Nicholi (Ed.), *The new Harvard guide to psychiatry* (pp. 259–295). Cambridge: The Belknap Press of Harvard University Press.

Turner, S. W., Toone, B. K., & Brett-Jones, J. R. (1986). Computerized tomographic scan changes in early schizophrenia—preliminary findings. *Psychological Medicine, 16*, 219–225.

Vonnegut, M. (1975) *The Eden express*. New York: Praeger.

Zubin, J., & Spring, B.J. (1977). Vulnerability: A new view of schizophrenia. *Journal of Abnormal Psychology, 86*, 103–126.

17

Substance Abuse Disorders

Timothy J. O'Farrell

Description of the Disorder

This chapter discusses serious psychological problems that can arise in relation to the use of certain substances. These substances are called psychoactive substances because they can be used to affect moods, thinking, and behavior. In most societies, use of certain substances to modify mood or behavior is regarded as normal and appropriate, and such use may be a valued part of the culture. Customary and social drinking of alcohol as a beverage with meals or to enhance interaction at social gatherings is one example. The ritual use of peyote (a drug obtained from the mescal cactus that produces a variety of vivid visual hallucinations) for religious purposes by Indians in Mexico and the Southwestern United States is another. Further, some psychoactive substances are used for medical purposes under a physician's prescription to relieve pain or decrease anxiety, or for other appropriate medical purposes. Therefore, this chapter is concerned not with these and other normal and appropriate uses of psychoactive substances, but rather with use that is considered pathological largely due to the negative behavioral effects. Table 1 lists major classes of psychoactive substances that are commonly subject to problematic use. The criteria for determining problematic use of such substances is considered next.

Criteria for Diagnosing a Substance Use Disorder

The most widely accepted clinical description of substance abuse disorders is contained in the fourth edition draft criteria of the *Diagnostic and Statistic Manual of Mental Disorders* (DSM-IV) (American Psychiatric Association, 1993). In DSM-IV,

Timothy J. O'Farrell • Department of Psychiatry, Harvard Medical School, Boston, Massachusetts 02115, and Veterans Affairs Medical Center, Brockton and West Roxbury, Massachusetts 02401.

Advanced Abnormal Psychology, edited by Vincent B. Van Hasselt and Michel Hersen. Plenum Press, New York, 1994.

substance abuse problems are classified under the general heading of Substance-Related Disorders, which includes problems with alcohol and other drugs.

The essential feature of substance-related disorders, as described in DSM-IV is "a maladaptive pattern of substance abuse, leading to clinically significant impairment or distress" (APA, 1993). In DSM-IV, problems with substance use can be described as *substance dependence* or *substance abuse*, depending on the seriousness of the problem and on specific diagnostic criteria. Although in most cases, a separate diagnosis is made for each specific problematic substance (e.g., alcohol dependence, cocaine abuse), DSM-IV diagnostic criteria are stated in general terms that apply to all of the substances listed in Table 1.

SUBSTANCE DEPENDENCE

At least 3 of the 7 symptoms listed in Table 2 must be present for the diagnosis of substance dependence. To qualify for the diagnosis, at least 3 of these symptoms must have persisted for at least 1 month, or must have occurred in the same month (APA, 1993).

A final point is that DSM-IV further specifies substance dependence as occurring (1) *With Physiological Dependence* if there is evidence of tolerance or withdrawal (i.e., either item 1 or 2 in Table 2 is present) or (2) *Without Physiological Dependence* if there is no evidence of tolerance or withdrawal (i.e., neither item 1 nor 2 in Table 2 is present). Since the results of withdrawing from substance use varies according to the substance (e.g., alcohol versus heroin), DSM-IV also provides specific criteria for the characteristic withdrawal syndrome and symptoms that occur after stopping or sharply reducing substance intake after a period of prolonged and heavy use. This emphasis on specifying physical dependence in DSM-IV represents a minor modification to DSM-III and DSM-III-R (APA, 1980, 1987).

SUBSTANCE ABUSE

Less severe substance use problems that do not meet the criteria for substance dependence may be classified as substance abuse problems. In DSM-IV, substance abuse is a residual category for noting maladaptive patterns of substance use that have never met the criteria for substance dependence for the specific substance under consideration. The maladaptive pattern of use is indicated by at least one of

TABLE 1. Classes of Psychoactive Substances

1. Alcohol
2. Amphetamine (e.g., "speed")
3. Cannabis (e.g., marijuana)
4. Cocaine
5. Hallucinogens (e.g., LSD)
6. Inhalants (e.g., glue sniffing)
7. Nicotine
8. Opioids (e.g., heroin, morphine)
9. Phencyclidine (PCP, e.g., "angel dust")
10. Sedatives, hypnotics (e.g., barbiturates) or anxiolytics (e.g., Valium®, Xanax®)

the following: "(1) recurrent substance use resulting in a failure to fulfill major role obligations at work, school, or home (e.g., repeated absences or poor work performance related to substance use; substance-related absences, suspensions, or expulsions from school; neglect of children or household); (2) recurrent substance use in situations in which it is physically hazardous (e.g., driving an automobile or operating a machine when impaired by substance use); (3) recurrent substance-related legal problems (e.g., arrests for substance-related disorderly conduct); (4) continued substance use despite having persistent or recurrent social or interpersonal problems caused or exacerbated by the effects of the substance (e.g., arguments with spouse about consequences of intoxication, physical fights)" (APA, 1993). Examples of situations in which a diagnosis of psychoactive substance abuse would be appropriate (APA, 1987, p. 169) include:

1. A college student binges on cocaine every few weekends. These periods are followed by a day or two of missing school because of "crashing." There are no other symptoms.
2. A middle-aged man repeatedly drives his car when intoxicated with alcohol. There are no other symptoms.
3. A woman keeps drinking alcohol even though her physician has told her that it is responsible for exacerbating the symptoms of a duodenal ulcer. There are no other symptoms.

PROBLEMS WITH MORE THAN ONE SUBSTANCE

Among patients seeking help for substance use disorders, many individuals have problems that involve the use of more than one substance. When an individual's problems meet the criteria for more than one psychoactive substance use disorder, multiple diagnoses are made. The case of Jack Smith described later in this chapter provides an example of an individual with multiple substance use disorders.

Another type of case involving problems with multiple substances is diag-

TABLE 2. DSM-IV Diagnostic Criteria for Substance Dependence

1. Tolerance, as defined by either of the following:
   a. need for markedly increased amounts of the substance to achieve intoxication or desired effect
   b. markedly diminished effect with continued use of the same amount of the substance
2. Withdrawal, as manifested by either of the following:
   a. the characteristic withdrawal syndrome for the substance (as specified in DSM-IV)
   b. the same (or closely related) substance is taken to relieve or avoid withdrawal symptoms
3. The substance is often taken in larger amounts or over a longer period than was intended.
4. A persistent desire or unsuccessful efforts to cut down or control substance use.
5. A great deal of time is spent in activities necessary to obtain the substance (e.g., visiting multiple doctors or driving long distances), use the substance (e.g., chain-smoking), or recover from its effects.
6. Important social, occupational, or recreational activities given up or reduced because of substance use.
7. Continued substance use despite knowledge of having had a persistent or recurrent physical or psychological problem that was likely to have been caused or exacerbated by the substance (e.g., current cocaine use despite recognition of cocaine-induced depression, or continued drinking despite recognition that an ulcer was made worse by alcohol consumption).

Reprinted with permission from the *DSM-IV Draft Criteria*. Copyright 1993 American Psychiatric Association.

nosed as *polysubstance dependence*. This diagnosis is reserved for noting a period of at least 6 months during which the person was repeatedly using substances from at least three of the categories (not including nicotine) listed in Table 1, but no single substance predominated. During this period, the dependence criteria of Table 2 were met for psychoactive substances as a group but not for any specific substance (APA, 1993).

Table 3 summarizes important and key points about the definitions and characteristics of psychoactive substance use disorders.

EPIDEMIOLOGY

Epidemiological data on substance use disorders presented here are from the Epidemiologic Catchment Area Study (ECA) (Robins & Regier, 1991). The ECA was a large-scale study of almost 20,000 Americans sponsored by the National Institute of Mental Health to determine the prevalence of psychiatric disorders in the United States and the factors that are associated with elevated risk for these disorders. The ECA study data on substance use disorders were chosen because they provide an estimate of the prevalence of diagnosed disorders, and not just a description of the patterns and problems of substance use. Although the ECA data are based on interviews conducted in the early 1980s and on diagnostic criteria from the DSM-III (APA, 1980) rather than the DSM-III-R or DSM-IV (APA, 1987, 1993), they represent some of the best data available. Other sources will be cited when ECA estimates may be misleading.

Prevalence of Substance Use Disorders

OVERALL PREVALENCE RELATIVE TO OTHER PSYCHIATRIC DISORDERS

Table 4 presents ECA data on prevalence of substance use disorders in the United States throughout the lifetime of persons interviewed in the ECA study and for the year prior to being interviewed (Anthony & Helzer, 1991; Helzer, Burnham,

TABLE 3. Important and Key Points about Definitions of Psychoactive Substance Use Disorders

1. Psychoactive substance can be used to affect moods, thinking, and behavior. When serious negative behavioral effects occur from the use of such substances, these serious psychological problems are call *substance-related disorders*.
2. Ten classes of substances that can lead to psychoactive substance disorders are: (1) alcohol; (2) amphetamines (e.g., "speed"); (3) cannabis (e.g., marijuana); (4) cocaine; (5) hallucinogens (e.g., LSD); (6) inhalants (e.g, glue sniffing); (7) nicotine; (8) opioids (e.g., heroin morphine); (9) phencyclidine (PCP, e.g., "angel dust"); (10) sedatives, hypnotics (e.g., barbiturates), or anxiolytics (e.g., Valium®, Xanax®).
3. Essential features of the disorder are a maladaptive pattern of substance use leading to clinically significant impairment or distress.
4. *Substance dependence* is diagnosed if the person has had at least three of seven specific symptoms which must have occurred within the same twelve-month period.
5. *Substance abuse* is diagnosed for less severe problems that have never met the criteria for substance dependence but involve continued use despite adverse consequences or recurrent physically hazardous use (e.g., driving while intoxicated).

TABLE 4. Prevalence of Substance Use Disorders in the United States[a]

	Lifetime	Past year
Alcohol abuse/dependence	13.76%	6.80%
Drug abuse/dependence	6.19%	2.67%
Any substance use disorder[b]	17.00%	NI[c]

[a]These prevalence data are taken from the Epidemiologic Catchment Area study data as presented by Helzer, Burnham, and McEvoy (1991) and by Anthony and Helzer (1991).
[b]Includes individuals with alcohol abuse/dependence and/or drug abuse/dependence. Prevalence for combined substance use disorder category is less than combined prevalence for alcohol and drug problems because some individuals had both alcohol and drug problems.
[c]No information; information was not provided in the reports of the Epidemiologic Catchment Area Study.

& McEvoy, 1991). Alcoholism is the second most prevalent psychiatric disorder, next only to phobia (lifetime prevalence = 14.3%). However, when alcohol and drug problems are considered together, then substance use disorders are the most frequent (17% lifetime prevalence) psychiatric disorders (Robins, Locke, & Regier, 1991).

Due to methodological concerns, some have questioned whether the prevalence rates for alcoholism in the past year might be an overly high estimate. These "past year" figures are important since they estimate the number of people during any year who are affected by alcoholism. As indicated in Table 4, each year nearly 7% of U.S. adults were estimated to have a problem with alcoholism with nearly 12% of men and about 2% of women affected (Helzer et al., 1991). More conservative methods showed 4.5% overall (8.13% of men and 1.16% of women) with an alcoholism problem in the past year. By either estimate, alcoholism is a major problem in the United States with 4.5 to 7% of the population (8 to 12% of men and 1 to 2% of women) being actively symptomatic in the past year (Helzer et al., 1991, p. 93).

RELATIVE PREVALENCE OF DIFFERENT TYPES OF SUBSTANCE USE DISORDERS

What types of substance use disorders were experienced by the 17% of the ECA sample who had such a disorder? Table 5 indicates that nearly 11% had only alcohol problems, about 3% had only drug problems, and about 3% had problems involving both alcohol and drugs. Another way to look at this same question is presented in Figure 1. Nearly 65% of those with substance use disorders suffered only from alcoholism, while the remaining 35% were split fairly evenly between those with drug problems only and those with both alcoholism and drug problems.

Among those with drug problems, lifetime prevalence rates of drug abuse/

TABLE 5. Lifetime Prevalence of Alcohol and/or Drug Disorders

Alcohol abuse/dependence *only*	10.73%
Drug abuse/dependence *only*	3.24%
Both alcohol abuse/dependence and drug abuse/dependence	3.03%

dependence disorder varied considerably in the ECA study, depending on the type of drug. Figure 2 shows 6.2% of adults have experienced at least one drug disorder. Cannabis (marijuana) abuse/dependence was the most frequently diagnosed disorder affecting an estimated 4.4%. Other disorders affected less than 2% of the population. Two points must be considered when evaluating the prevalence rates in Figure 2. *First*, these rates, which apply to all adults, do not reflect the rates of disorder in specific subgroups of the U.S. population. For example, among young men (age 18–29) the lifetime prevalence of a drug abuse/dependence disorder is 15.06%, over two and one half times the rate for the general population. *Second*, the ECA study data were collected in the early 1980s and do not reflect the increased use and abuse of some drugs (e.g., cocaine) during the mid-1980s. Of the total U.S. population age 12 and older, 2.9% were "current users" of cocaine in 1985, a figure which dropped to 1.5% in 1988 and 0.9% in 1991 according to the National Household Survey on Drug Abuse (U.S. HHS, 1992).

Factors Related to Higher Risk for Substance Use Disorders

ECA data (Robins & Regier, 1991) showed that substance use disorders were more common among men than women. Five times as many men as women are affected by alcoholism and nearly twice as many men as women experience drug disorders. People who have completed fewer years of education and the unmarried

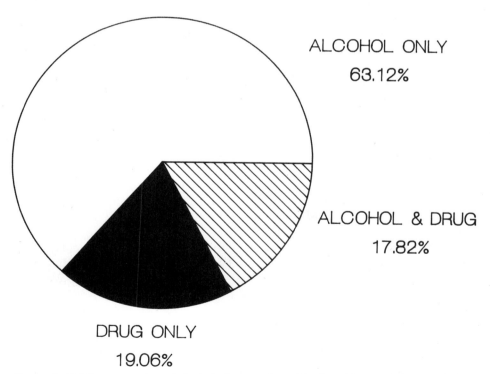

FIGURE 1. Relative proportion of alcohol, drug, and combined problems for those with lifetime diagnosis of substance use disorder.

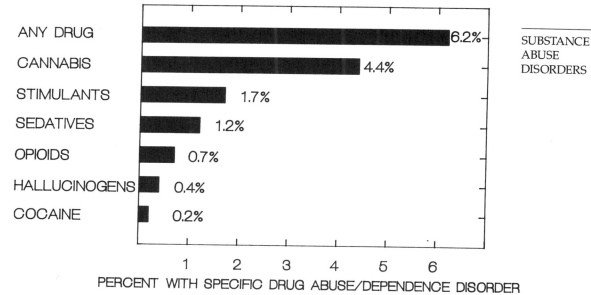

FIGURE 2. Lifetime prevalence of specific drug abuse/dependence disorders.

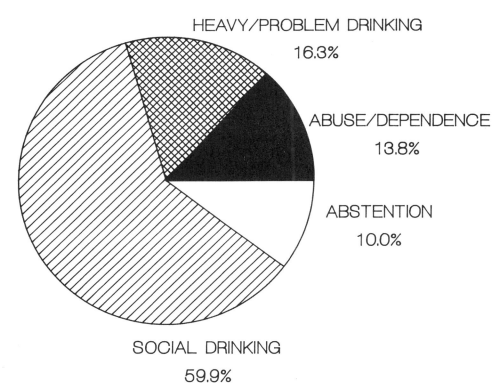

FIGURE 3. Lifetime drinking pattern in the Epidemiologic Catchment Area study.

(particularly those who have experienced more than one separation or divorce) are more likely than more educated and married persons to experience alcoholism or drug problems. Age also is a significant risk factor with younger people more likely to experience drug problems (age 18–29) and alcoholism (age 18–44). It should be remembered that the association between these factors and higher rates of substance use disorder does not necessarily mean that these factors cause or are caused by the substance use disorder.

Another type of risk factor, the extent of use of the substance, also was examined in the ECA study. Substance exposure is a prerequisite for developing a substance use disorder (Helzer et al., 1991). Therefore, it is interesting to examine alcohol consumption patterns and frequency of illicit drug use in relation to the prevalence of substance use disorders. Figure 3 presents ECA study data on lifetime drinking patterns. Lifelong abstainers account for 10% of the U.S. population. Another 60% are social drinkers who deny both heavy consumption and alcohol-related problems. The most interesting group is *heavy or problem drinkers*, defined in the ECA study as "those who reported seven or more drinks at least one evening a week for several months (or daily for 2 weeks or more) and/or one or more lifetime drinking problems" (Helzer et al., 1991). The prevalence rate of alcoholism among these heavy drinkers was 48.5%, nearly four times the general population rate. Regarding drug problems, people who have ever used illicit drugs have a three times greater chance of having a drug disorder. Further, 54% of those who use illicit drugs daily for 2 weeks or more had a lifetime diagnosis of drug abuse/dependence nearly nine times the rate for the general population.

Table 6 summarizes important and key points about the epidemiology of psychoactive substance use disorders.

CLINICAL PICTURE

The clinical picture of substance use disorders seen in treatment centers has become more varied and complicated in the past decade. Patients in their forties

TABLE 6. Important and Key Points about the Epidemiology of Psychoactive Substance Use Disorders

1. Substance use disorders are the most prevalent type of psychiatric disorder in the United States, with 17% of adults in the Epidemiologic Catchment Area study having experienced this disorder in their lifetime.
2. This same study indicated that in the past year, 4.5 to 7% of the U.S. population (8 to 12% of men and 1 to 2% of women) experienced a substance use disorder.
3. Of those in the general population with substance use disorders, over 60% have problems with alcoholism, while the remaining cases are about evenly divided between those with drug problems and those with combined alcoholism and drug problems. Many treatment centers have a higher proportion of patients with both alcoholism and drug problems.
4. Factors related to higher risk for substance use disorders are:
   a. male gender
   b. less education, dropout from high school or college
   c. unmarried; separated or divorced more than once
   d. younger age
5. Heavy and repeated use of the substance is a controllable risk factor for substance use disorders.

with primarily alcohol problems still are seen in treatment centers. Such patients used to comprise the largest segment of the treatment population. More recently, a greater number of younger patients have sought help and these patients tend to have problems with multiple substances. Therefore, two cases from the author's experience will be described briefly to illustrate these different types of patients.

The Case of Frank Johnson

Case identification. Frank Johnson was a 45-year-old, unemployed, white male accountant. He was the father of six children, ages 13 to 21. He had been separated from his wife for 5 months when admitted to the medical service of a large veterans' hospital.

Presenting complaints. Mr. Johnson's complaints were difficulty sleeping, tenseness, depression, chest pains, and excessive alcohol use of 1–2 quarts of rum daily for 4½ months prior to admission. Given his history of serious heart problems, he was admitted to the medical service for detoxification from alcohol and close monitoring of his cardiac status.

Events leading to hospitalization. These were: (a) his oldest son had a court hearing following an arrest for theft, (b) after a heated argument with his wife about the son's difficulties, the wife had initiated a court petition for legal separation, and (c) he had thoughts of suicide including an idea of purchasing a gun for this purpose.

Earlier history. Frank began drinking at age 15 at parties during high school but did not feel it was a problem then or later during military service and college. Around age 30, his work as an accountant began to involve increased drinking with clients and associates. At age 36, when the patient had his first heart attack, his physician advised him to stop drinking, a warning that went unheeded. During the next 6 years, he suffered more cardiac problems and a ruptured disk that required a spinal fusion. Drinking continued to increase. Despite the extensive history of heavy drinking, both Frank and his wife dated onset of what they considered a drinking problem to the period when at age 42, after suffering the health problems, he lost his job due to company reorganization, and his oldest son was arrested. Frank's drinking escalated to a quart or more per day of rum. On occasion he became verbally abusive and threatening to his wife, especially when they argued about the oldest son's problems or Frank's excessive drinking.

About 18 months prior to the present hospital admission, Frank again suffered serious chest pain. When his physician diagnosed possible alcoholic cardiomyopathy, he entered a 7-day detoxification program. He did not drink and attended Alcoholics Anonymous (AA) sporadically for 6 weeks after this first alcoholism treatment, but resumed drinking after an argument with his wife. The patient found a new job and resumed heavy drinking. After an incident in which the patient became extremely abusive and threatening, the couple separated just prior to their 25th wedding anniversary and remained living apart for 2 months. Six months after their reconciliation and approximately 5 months prior to the present admission, Mr. Johnson quit his job after his boss told him he should get help for his drinking problem. The couple again separated. The patient continued to drink daily up to 2 quarts of rum on many days. He became increasingly depressed over the separation from his wife and children, worked at a new job, and continued drinking very heavily, until the events (described above) that immediately preceded his admission to the hospital.

Assessment. Medical evaluation revealed elevated liver enzymes without liver pathology and a history of coronary artery disease complicated by alcoholic cardiomyopathy. The Time-Line drinking interview showed that he had spent 80% of the days in the previous year drinking 1–2 quarts of rum daily. He had experienced blackouts and severe shakes and sweats when trying to stop drinking on his own. On the Michigan Alcoholism Screening Test (MAST), he received a very elevated score of 47, indicating multiple and serious consequences from alcohol abuse. A diagnostic interview was conducted by a psychiatrist in response to the patient's complaints of depression, sleep disturbance, and suicidal ideation and his request for antidepressant medication. The psychiatrist concluded that *alcohol dependence* was the primary diagnosis and that the "depression" and other complaints were caused by the alcohol problem and did not represent an affective disorder for which an antidepressant would be helpful. Finally, an evaluation of the marital relationship was conducted.

Reviewing the assessment and history materials indicated a number of antecedents that had been associated with alcohol consumption. For each antecedent, the short-term consequence of the drinking had brought some temporary improvement, but the longer-term consequences had been to create or exacerbate serious life problems. The following analysis was presented to Mr. Johnson and he concurred with this formulation of factors involved in his drinking:

(a) He was a rigid, perfectionist individual who experienced considerable anxiety and both mental and physical (muscular) tension in response to daily life events. After his first episode of chest pain, he became fearful when he experienced muscular tension that this might lead to a heart attack. Alcohol relieved the tension and his fears about a heart attack in the short run but exacerbated his heart problem leading to alcoholic cardiomyopathy in the long run.

(b) Business-related social drinking with clients and associates seemed to help these relationships initially. As time went on, he developed a reputation as a heavy drinker that contributed to his loss of two jobs. Drinking helped relieve his distress over this job instability but cost him his current job when he had to enter the hospital for alcoholism treatment.

(c) Marital conflict clearly contributed to the drinking, which brought temporary escape from the feelings of frustration, anger, and loss associated with these conflicts. Eventually, drinking led to increasingly more frequent and severe outbursts at his wife that led to police intervention, marital separation, and finally a legal separation.

(e) The losses experienced led to feelings of depression, sadness and guilt, at first relieved by, and later seriously increased by, the alcohol. When intoxicated, he had made one suicidal gesture, and serious suicidal ideas continued to frighten the patient when he was abstinent.

(f) He had become physically dependent on alcohol, and some of his drinking was done to ward off withdrawal symptoms.

Treatment. After detoxification from alcohol and repeated testing to insure his cardiac condition was stable, Frank entered a 4-week inpatient alcoholism treatment program. This was followed by outpatient aftercare treatment that included couples' counseling. At 5 years posthospital discharge, the patient remained continuously abstinent and employed, with stable cardiac functioning. The couple's marriage had stabilized. No separation had occurred.

The patient's high degree of motivation for change certainly was an important factor in the success of the treatments used. He had lost his job, seriously risked his health, considered suicide, and nearly lost his family when he entered the hospital for detoxification, all because of his drinking. The inpatient treatment bolstered his desire for change and increased his motivation by providing specific methods he could use to cope with his drinking and other problems. The outpatient treatment reinforced sobriety directly and indirectly by reducing marital conflicts that had been one threat for continued sobriety. The interested reader is referred to Hester and Miller (1989) for more information on current methods for treating alcoholism.

The Case of Jack Smith

Case identification. Jack Smith was a 36-year-old, unemployed, white male surveyor technician. He was the father of two preschool age children. He had been separated from his wife for 4 months at the time of his admission to the alcohol and drug treatment program of a large veterans' hospital.

Presenting complaints. Mr. Smith's complaints at time of admission were that he had been drinking up to a quart of vodka daily for the past 4 months and taking morphine 200 milligrams intravenously on a daily basis for the past 2½ months. Given the quantity of his substance intake and past history of blackouts and severe tremors, he was judged to be physically dependent on both alcohol and morphine. Therefore, he was admitted for a 5-day medical detoxification program to help him withdraw from his alcohol and morphine safely.

Events leading to hospitalization. These were: (a) he had been unemployed due to a job layoff for over a year, (b) his house had been foreclosed on by a bank due to nonpayment of his mortgage, (c) his wife had insisted he leave due to his substance abuse, and (d) when feeling depressed about the loss of his family, job, and house, he had tried unsuccessfully to kill himself through drinking a large amount of vodka and inhaling paint solvent until he passed out.

Early history. Jack began drinking at age 15 in high school, when he drank heavily on weekends and smoked marijuana. On a number of occasions, he and some friends inhaled paint solvent together. On one occasion, he blacked out briefly when he deeply inhaled the solvent. This experience scared him and his friends. He stopped the inhalant abuse and did not return to it until the incident just prior to admission described above.

Jack had been a very nervous child and adolescent, who experienced periods of strong anxiety when confronted with new social or achievement situations. His father was a recovering alcoholic. His parents had been separated during his preschool years, a time of marked financial and emotional insecurity for Jack and his mother and brother.

When Jack graduated high school he enrolled at the local community college. The new social and academic challenges made him very anxious and his weekend drinking increased to nearly daily drinking to make him feel more comfortable. Eventually, he began missing classes, got behind in his school work, and then dropped out of school.

He joined the Army and decided not to drink. He remained abstinent through basic training. When sent to an Army technical school far from home for training as a surveyor technician, he began drinking heavily on a daily basis. It was not long before he entered a 28-day Army alcohol rehabilitation program, after which he resumed drinking fairly soon. Two years later, he again requested substance abuse treatment. This time, in addition to drinking, he also had been involved in intravenous heroin use for 6 months. For his remaining 2 years in the Army, he limited his drinking to beer in barrooms, took no hard drugs, and occasionally used marijuana.

Upon return to civilian life, his drinking escalated. After an embarrassing incident while drunk, he entered an inpatient treatment program, joined Alcoholics Anonymous (AA), and remained substance free for 2 years. During this sober period he met and married his wife and got a stable job as a surveyor technician in a large company. Over the next 9 years, he was mostly abstinent, drinking only for a few weeks on 3 occasions, generally to relieve intense states of anxiety, each of which was followed by a brief treatment center admission.

About 18 months prior to the present hospital admission, Jack began occasional use of morphine obtained from a co-worker. A few months later Jack's employer of 7 years had large-scale layoffs due to an economic downturn. He returned to drinking at first only occasionally and then to bouts of heavy drinking lasting for many days. He also increased frequency of morphine use. Financial stress and marital conflict increased as he continued without steady employment. When Jack lost a temporary job due to drinking about the same time as the bank began foreclosure proceedings on his home, Jack's wife insisted that he leave. After the separation Jack quickly progressed to daily heavy drinking and regular morphine use.

Assessment. In terms of drinking and drug-taking behavior, the time-line interview showed that he had spent 65% of the days in the previous year drinking a pint to a quart of vodka daily and 35% of these days taking morphine. On the Michigan Alcoholism Screening Test (MAST), he received a score of 49, a very elevated score indicating multiple and serious adverse consequences of substance use. Jack's score of 30 on the Alcohol Dependence Scale, his experience of severe shakes and sweats when trying to stop drinking on his own, and the fact that he had gone to a detox center whenever he stopped drinking in the prior 10 years all indicated a substantial physical dependence on alcohol. He also had become dependent on morphine.

Jack's current and previous behavior warranted multiple diagnoses. Substance use disorders included current alcohol dependence and morphine dependence and lifetime diagnosis for heroin dependence, marijuana abuse, and inhalant abuse. In addition, he suffered from a long-standing generalized anxiety disorder. Both the early family dysfunction and instability and his father's alcoholism probably contributed to the development of Jack's problems. The challenges of late adolescence and young adulthood led to increased anxiety largely dealt with through drinking and drug use. After the Army when he joined AA, got married and had a steady job, he remained mostly abstinent except for brief relapses when he felt extremely anxious. When faced with the emotional, financial, and marital stresses of extended unemployment during a recession, Jack increased his substance use. Once he was separated from his wife and children, his substance use increased even further leading to admission to the treatment center.

Treatment. After a week-long detoxification period, Jack entered a 28-day alcohol and drug treatment program. During this inpatient stay, he renewed his involvement with AA but complained that anxiety made it difficult for him to feel comfortable and get involved in the AA meetings the way he should. To deal with the anxiety disorder, Jack received a prescription from the treatment center's psychiatrist for BuSpar® (generic name buspirone), a relatively new antianxiety medication that has very low potential for psychological or physical addiction.

Jack also was referred to an anxiety management therapy group when discharged from the treatment center. He went to live in a substance-free halfway house upon discharge from the treatment center because his wife was reluctant to take him back at that time.

As of this writing, it has been 9 months since Jack's discharge from the treatment center. He has remained alcohol and drug free. He attends AA three to four times a week and is actively involved. His anxiety is much improved. Jack and his wife are continuing in outpatient couples' therapy, having reconciled 3 months after his hospital discharge. Although still unemployed, he has enrolled in a job retraining program.

COURSE AND PROGNOSIS

The course and prognosis for substance use disorders are somewhat complex. These vary from one substance to another as well as within one type of substance use problem. Further, information drawn from clinical samples seeking treatment often is not applicable to the large numbers of people who do not seek treatment.

Evidence from Epidemiological Studies of the General Population

The picture that emerges from epidemiological studies of the course and progression of alcohol and drug problems is relatively clear. Data from the ECA study already described above will be presented since the information from the ECA study is relatively consistent with other epidemiological studies (e.g., Cahalan, 1970; National Institute on Drug Abuse, 1989).

In general, alcohol and drug problems, when viewed from the perspective of the ECA general population epidemiological study, began by about age 20, and over half the cases who ever experienced the disorder were in remission (i.e., had no problems related to substance use in the past year) at the time of the ECA interview. Substance use disorders had among the highest rates of remission of any of the psychiatric disorders assessed in the ECA study.

When examined in more detail, there were some differences noted between drug and alcohol problems. Drug problems, when compared with alcohol problems, have a consistently more youthful onset, a shorter period of risk, and a shorter duration for cases that enter remission. The first drug problem occurs at a median age of 18 years with the age of risk for onset of most drug problems occurring between age 16 and age 21 with onset being rare after age 25. For those whose drug problems were in remission at the time of the interview, the period of active problems had lasted a mean of 2.7 years. Alcohol problems appear more variable in course and progression than drug problems. Although almost 40% of those who develop alcoholism have their first alcohol-related problems between age 15 and 19, cases of alcoholism continue to develop in the 20s, 30s, and 40s. The age of risk for developing alcoholism extends through the late 30s, at which time 90% of those who develop alcohol-related problems will have done so. Duration of alcoholism for those in the ECA study who were in remission (i.e., had no alcohol-related problems in the last year) was 9 years on average, with three quarters in remission within 11 years.

Robins et al. (1991) remark that the high rates of remission for alcohol and drug disorders in the ECA study differ from results for clinical samples, where relapse rates are traditionally very high. Nonetheless, the ECA data agree with previous follow-up studies in the general population, which also show high rates of remission and high rates of instability in the reporting of current problems between interviews a few years apart (Taylor & Helzer, 1983).

Helzer et al. (1991) comment on these ECA findings noting the differences between alcoholics in treatment samples and in general population studies:

> These results (of high remission rates and short duration of the disorder) are very different from those seen in patients, who frequently come to treatment for the first time only after many years of alcohol problems. Our findings may help to explain why so few persons with alcohol problems in the general population seek care. Many appear to be able to reduce their drinking sufficiently to terminate their difficulties quite early in the course of their disorder. It is those who try and fail that appear for treatment (Helzer et al., 1991, pp. 97–98).

From the vantage point of epidemiological studies of the general population, substance use disorders appear to show considerable change over time with many cases in remission at any given time. This is in marked contrast with substance use treatment experience in which substance use disorders are seen as very difficult to treat, unlikely to have good and enduring remission after treatment, and (in the case of alcoholism) as a progressively deteriorating disease that inevitably gets worse and leads to either death or abstinence (Jellinek, 1960). A number of factors may explain the disparate perspective. As already indicated, the general population studies may contain many more substance abusers with less severe problems than do treatment populations that consist mostly of the more severe cases. General population studies generally are cross-sectional and retrospective (i.e., they interview individuals at one point in time and ask them about their current and former problems). Those with the worst substance abuse outcome—death—are eliminated from consideration. Further, the future course of the disorder in those with active substance use disorders at the time of the interview cannot be determined. Longitudinal studies of treatment samples provide an additional perspective on the course and prognosis of substance use disorders.

Evidence from Longitudinal Studies of Treatment Samples

Prior to the mid-1970s, the course and progression of substance use disorders, especially alcoholism, was thought to be relatively straightforward and simple. Alcoholism was seen as a progressively worsening disease that has a natural progression of symptoms that got increasingly severe over time, ending inevitably in death or disability unless the disease was arrested through lifelong abstinence, generally obtained through regular attendance at Alcoholics Anonymous meetings (Jellinek, 1960).

More recently, the course and progression of alcoholism, among those with problems serious enough to seek treatment, are seen as much more complex than had been thought heretofore. *First*, no one course applies to all or most of the cases seen in treatment centers. Clearly, the belief that all or most alcoholics show a progressive deteriorating course is not supported by recent evidence. Alcoholics are seen as having a variety of outcomes to their disorder. *Second*, although this finding has caused considerable controversy, it also is clear that some alcoholics can drink without experiencing problems, suggesting that total abstinence may not be the only way for all alcoholics to resolve their problems. A well known study that illustrates these two important changes will be described next.

OUTCOMES FOUR YEARS AFTER ALCOHOLISM TREATMENT

Table 7 describes outcomes of over 600 alcoholics 4 years after they were treated at one of eight Alcoholism Treatment Centers (Polich, Armor, & Braiker, 1981). The sample was chosen to be representative of all males admitted to treatment at the eight designated centers. The centers' patient populations were very similar to all patients treated in a U.S. government network of treatment centers at the time of the study. Therefore, the results come from a large, fairly representative sample of alcoholics in U.S. treatment centers.

Before considering Table 7, we must note that 15% of the patients were dead, over half of these from alcohol-related causes, 4 years after treatment. This represents over two and a half times the expected death rate for men with demographic characteristics similar to those in the sample. This subgroup would seem to fit the progressive deteriorating course described by Jellinek and other disease model proponents. The 20% in Group 6 who fairly consistently drank and had drinking-related problems might also be considered to have a continuing if not progressive course after treatment. Those who stayed abstinent the entire 4 years, a small minority at 7%, also could fit the progression through abstinence. Group 3, the 9% who were drinking without problems, provided the greatest challenge to the disease model and the most controversy. Drinking without problems meant the patient did not experience any alcohol-related serious adverse consequences (e.g., health problems, legal problems, work or family problems) or dependence symptoms (e.g., tremors, morning drinking, blackouts). These patients tended to be younger and have fewer signs of physical dependence (i.e., tolerance and withdrawal symptoms) on alcohol when they entered treatment, indicating they had less severe, less chronic problems. Group 4, the 6% who had periods of abstinence and of nonproblem drinking, also would not appear to fit the progressive disease model. The largest group of patients, the 52% in Group 5, consisted of those who alternated between periods of problem drinking and short-term abstinence.

The Polich et al. data provide a different picture of the course of alcoholism from that seen in epidemiological general population studies, where about one-half are in remission. Only 28% of the treatment sample are in remission (Groups, 1 to 4 of Table 8) 4 years after treatment. For the most part, these data do not fit the

TABLE 7.   Outcomes during 4 Years after Alcoholism Treatment

1. Continuously abstinent	7%
2. Long-term abstainers	6%
3. Nonproblem drinkers	9%
4. Either abstainer or nonproblem drinker	6%
5. Alternated between drinking with serious problems and short-term abstinence	52%
6. Consistently drinking with serious problems	20%

Note: This table was constructed from information contained in Polich, Armor, & Braiker (1981, p. 216). The percentages given are for the patients still alive 4 years after treatment.

progressive deteriorating disease concept of alcoholism since the majority do not show such a progressive course and some obtain remission without abstinence.

The picture that emerges from the Polich et al. (1981) data is that the course of alcoholism and paths to remission and recovery vary considerably. Some alcoholics show a progressively deteriorating course in which they continue to drink heavily on a consistent basis and have serious alcohol-related problems, including death. Others improve and enter remission either via long-term abstinence or a return to nonproblem drinking (the latter generally among younger, less severe cases). About half continue to alternate between periods of short-term abstinence and continued problem drinking. Table 8 summarizes important and key points about the course and prognosis of psychoactive substance use disorders.

FAMILIAL AND GENETIC PATTERNS

Familial and genetic patterns of substance use disorders have been studied extensively for alcoholism, and to a lesser extent for drug abuse/dependence. As we shall see, findings regarding familial and genetic patterns for alcoholism vary considerably based on the type of sample studied, gender, and the type and severity of alcoholism.

Alcoholism

FAMILIAL PATTERNS FOR ALCOHOLISM

In a widely cited paper, Cotton (1979) reviewed 39 studies of the familial incidence of alcoholism. Most of the studies reviewed by Cotton focused on samples of alcoholics drawn from inpatient and outpatient psychiatric settings. Cotton concluded that alcoholics were approximately four to five times more likely to have an alcoholic parent than were control groups not seen in psychiatric settings.

TABLE 8. Important and Key Points about the Course and Prognosis of Psychoactive Substance Use Disorders

1. Course and prognosis of substance use disorders differ in studies of the general population, compared to treatment center patients, who have a higher proportion of more severe problems.
2. In the general population, drug problems have a youthful onset from age 16 to 25. Over half enter remission (i.e., at least 1 year without problems) within 3 years of onset of the disorder.
3. In the general population, alcoholism onset occurs by age 20 for 40% of alcoholism problems, but the age of risk extends through the late 30s and early 40s. About half of the cases of alcoholism go into remission within 11 years of their onset.
4. In treatment center patients, alcoholism is no longer seen as having a uniformly progressive deteriorating course that ends in death or is "arrested" by abstinence. This view has been called the unitary disease model.
5. A large-scale study of the course of alcoholism over the 4 years after treatment showed:
   a. Some alcoholics (20 to 35%) do not improve or progressively deteriorate with condtinued heavy drinking and serious alcohol-related problems, including death.
   b. A little more than a quarter have a stable remission either via long-term abstinence or a return to nonproblem drinking.
   c. The remaining cases continue to alternate between periods of short-term abstinence and problem drinking.

In representative community and U.S. national samples, the risk for offspring to experience a problem with alcoholism if their parent was an alcoholic was only 1.4 to 1.7 times greater than for those without parental alcoholism (Russell, 1990). This increased risk is not nearly as great as noted by Cotton (1979) in her review of family patterns of alcoholics from treatment settings. These differences in findings from treatment and community samples are not surprising. Alcoholics who seek treatment are more likely to have severe alcoholism problems and to suffer from concomitant psychopathology (Helzer & Pryzbeck, 1988). Thus, it may be that familial patterns for alcoholism differ as a function of the severity of the alcoholism.

GENETIC STUDIES OF ALCOHOLISM

As already indicated, alcoholism runs in families. Such a familial pattern can be caused by genetic inheritance of a predisposition to alcoholism, shared environmental factors within families (e.g., modeling of expectancies and patterns of use for alcohol), or both. Based on a sizable literature examining genetic factors in alcoholism, most researchers would, no doubt, agree that genetic factors exert *some* influence on risk for alcoholism. Currently, the debate centers on the strength of the genetic influence and on the degree to which the importance of genetic factors varies by gender and type of alcoholism (McGue, Pickens, & Svikis, 1992).

McGue et al. (1992) studied inheritance of alcohol problems among men and women who were further divided into those with an early onset (age 20 or less) or late onset (age 21 or older) of alcohol-related problems. The results were clear and also appeared to be consistent with much current thinking and recent prior results. Using the twin study method, McGue et al. found no evidence for a genetic inheritance among females. Results supporting a genetic inheritance were found among males, and most strongly among males with an early onset of alcohol-related problems. These early onset males also showed greater use of illicit drugs and symptoms of conduct disorder in childhood and adolescence. McGue et al. summarized their findings as follows: "Early onset males with concomitant antisocial behavior manifested a highly heritable form of alcoholism, whereas late-onset male and all female alcoholics manifested another form of alcoholism with low to negligible heritability" (McGue et al., 1992, p. 14).

McGue drew two important conclusions from their results. *First,* the role of genetic factors in development of alcoholism may have been overestimated in recent years since only some forms of alcoholism appear to have a substantial genetic basis. *Second,* their results are consistent with the two subtypes of alcoholism described by Cloninger (1987). Type II alcoholism affects men almost exclusively, has an early onset, is associated with antisocial behavior, and is highly inheritable. Type I alcoholism affects both men and women, has a later onset, is associated with anxiety and rigidity, and appears to be low in heritability.

Drug Abuse and Dependence

Familial and genetic influences on the development of drug abuse/dependence have not been investigated intensively. According to M. T. Tsuang (unpublished manuscript), drug problems appear to run in families (Croughan, 1985). A substantial set of studies on which to base conclusions concerning genetic factors in drug addiction is not available currently, although some important studies are being conducted.

Clearly, further studies are required to elucidate the relative contribution of genetic and environmental factors to the development of drug abuse and dependence.

Table 9 summarizes important and key points about familial and genetic patterns pertaining to psychoactive substance use disorders.

DIAGNOSTIC CONSIDERATIONS

Diagnostic criteria for the substance-related disorders of dependence and abuse based on DSM-IV were described at the start of this chapter. Other diagnostic issues will be considered here. These include substance-related disorders of intoxication and withdrawal, substance-induced disorders, other frequently observed co-existing psychopathology, and identification and treatment of substance use disorders and problems.

Substance-Related Disorders of Intoxication and Withdrawal

DSM-IV lists and describes 18 diagnoses that describe behaviors associated with *states of alcohol or drug intoxication or withdrawal*. Complications of the specific intoxication states, such as traffic accidents and physical injury due to alcohol intoxication or potential for serious violence due to PCP intoxication, are also described in DSM-IV for each of the substances. Although intoxication is frequent in those with substance use disorders, it does not necessarily occur in allcases of the disorder, and intoxication can occur without the person suffering from a substance use disorder. Characteristic withdrawal syndromes that occur after regular heavy use when a person stops or reduces intake of the substance also are described for each substance in DSM-IV. Marked physical signs of withdrawal are

TABLE 9.   Important and Key Points about Familial and Genetic Patterns of Psychoactive Substance Use Disorders

---

1. Children of alcoholics are consistently found to have higher rates of alcoholism than are children whose parents are not alcoholic. However, the extent of increased risk for alcoholism varies considerably.
2. Children of alcoholic parents were four to five times more likely to be alcoholic themselves if their parents had been a patient in a treatment center.
3. In representative national and community samples, the risk of offspring to experience a problem with alcoholism was only 1.4 to 1.7 times greater if the child had an alcoholic parent.
4. A genetic influence on risk for alcoholism generally is accepted. The strength of the genetic influence and possible variation based on gender and subtype of alcoholsim are debated.
5. Recent studies propose that two subtypes of alcoholism vary in degree of genetic risk:
   a. Type I alcoholism—low inheritability, affects both men and women, later onset, associated with anxiety and rigidity.
   b. Type II alcoholism—highly inheritable, affects men almost exclusively, early onset, associated with antisocial behavior.
6. Drug problems appear to run in families also, but there is rather limited data to support this conclusion. Genetic factors in drug addiction have not been investigated to any significant extent.

---

common with alcohol, opiods, sedatives, hypnotics, and anxiolytics. Such physical signs are less obvious with amphetamines, cocaine, nicotine, and cannabis, but intense subjective emotional symptoms can occur upon withdrawal from heavy use of these substances. No significant withdrawal is seen even after repeated use of hallucinogens, and PCP withdrawal has not been documented in humans.

Substance-Induced Disorders

Eight *substance-induced disorders*, described in DSM-IV, are behavioral disorders that can be associated with the chronic heavy use of the various psychoactive substances. These include delirium, dementia, amnestic disorder, psychotic disorder, mood disorder, anxiety disorder, sex dysfunction, and sleep disorder. Such mental symptoms that occur as a result of chronic, heavy substance use are diagnosed under the substance that has induced the symptoms (e.g., alcohol hallucinosis, cocaine delusional disorder).

Other Coexisting Psychopathology

Persons with substance use disorders often experience additional types of psychopathology. These additional types of psychopathology generally are described as "coexisting," "co-occurring," or "co-morbid" disorders. We have already seen that two or more types of substance use disorder frequently co-occur. For example, approximately half of those with a drug abuse/dependence problem also experience a problem with alcoholism.

Nearly half (47%) of alcoholics in the ECA study received another diagnosis with additional disorders being more common among female than male alcoholics. While 44% of male alcoholics had a second diagnosis, 65% of females did, no doubt in part because alcoholism is so much less frequent and therefore more deviant in women than men (Helzer et al., 1991, p. 99). In the ECA community study, the most common additional diagnoses for both men and women with alcoholism were antisocial personality, mania, drug abuse/dependence, and schizophrenia. Among alcoholics hospitalized for treatment, antisocial personality disorder and depression are the most frequent co-occurring disorders (Hesselbrock, Meyer, & Keener, 1985). Helzer et al. (1991) argue that treatment-seeking alcoholics have higher rates of coexisting depression than community samples because the occurrence of depression may motivate alcoholics to seek treatment.

Persons with drug abuse/dependence problems are quite likely to have other disorders with 71% overall (75% in men, 65% in women) having at least one additional disorder in the ECA study. The most common additional disorder is alcoholism experienced by nearly half followed by antisocial personality disorder, mania, schizophrenia, and phobic disorder.

When alcohol or drug disorders coexist with other disorders, it often is difficult to know whether or not one disorder caused the other. For example, it is possible that the alcohol or drug use makes already existing problems (e.g., depression, phobic symptoms, antisocial behaviors) worse. Alternatively, the alcohol or drug use may have been made worse by the other disorder when the person drank or used drugs in an effort at self-medication to reduce symptoms of the other disorder (Anthony & Helzer, 1991). At times a "vicious cycle" can occur in which alcohol or drug use leads to other emotional problems, which are temporarily relieved by more alcohol or drug use only to reappear as more serious problems once the temporary escape provided by substance use is over. The case of Frank Johnson described earlier is a good example. This case also illustrates the important clinical point that diagnosis and treatment of coexisting psychopathology require considerable expertise and a degree of patience since some disorders (e.g., depression) coexisting with substance use problems can only be accurately diagnosed after a period of abstinence.

Identification and Treatment of Substance Use Disorders and Problems

Even though substance use disorders are the most common mental or behavioral disorder in the U.S., 85 to 90% of people with substance use disorders never receive treatment for these problems (Robins et al., 1991). Consider also that there are a large number of individuals who do not meet diagnostic criteria for substance use disorder, but nonetheless are heavy substance users who may have problems related to their substance use. These individuals are the heavy problem drinkers noted in Figure 3 and the individuals with mild to moderate alcohol problems noted in Figure 4. Due to their large numbers, these individuals with mild to moderate alcohol problems produce a great burden of costs to themselves and to society for alcohol-related traffic accidents, injuries, lost productivity from work, etc. Still, as we have already discussed, only those with severe problems receive treatment. Finally, even among the more severe cases seen in treatment settings, there is considerable variability in the nature of the substance use symptoms experienced, the type and extent of additional life problems and coexisting psychopathology, the age of onset, course of illness and prognosis for recovery, and in the extent to which genetic and environmental influences are important.

In 1990, the U.S. National Academy of Sciences released a report of a committee on treatment of alcohol problems. Figure 4, taken from the committee's report, conveys the vision of *expanded identification and treatment of alcohol problems* that flowed from the committee's judgments and recommendations. The committee's judgments that efforts to treat alcohol problems in the United States have been too narrowly focused on those people with the most severe problems and that treatment should be matched to a patient's needs even among the more severe cases produced recommendations for a number of significant additions and changes in treatment of alcohol problems.

First, a greatly expanded role for community agencies and settings is proposed. These include health care settings, schools, courts, social welfare agencies, and so forth. This role involves identifying individuals with alcohol problems, providing brief interventions (six or fewer sessions) to reduce or eliminate alcohol consumption of those with mild or moderate alcohol problems, and referring those with substantial or severe problems to the specialized alcoholism treatment sector. The varied professionals in community settings would need considerable additional training to perform these roles.

Second, the specialist treatment of alcohol problems also would be considerably broadened. Specialist treatment refers to public and private inpatient and outpatient centers that specialize in the treatment of alcohol problems. As envisioned, it would begin with a comprehensive assessment by which the person would be matched to the most appropriate type of intervention (e.g., inpatient or residential vs. outpatient). Follow-up data would be gathered after treatment to determine outcomes, and feedback of outcome information would be used to improve the matching guidelines used in assessment and treatment assignment. Although all of the components of the recommended treatment system have been the subject of considerable research and scholarly effort, currently:

> most treatment programs do not offer more than a single treatment option . . . neither do most offer . . . comprehensive assessment . . . With only a single treatment option, matching can not be carried out . . . few treatment programs engage in comprehensive outcome monitoring, and without monitoring, there can be no feedback. (Institute of Medicine, 1990, pp. 334–335)

Third, an explicit goal of all treatment would be to eliminate problems due to alcohol consumption, suggesting that the goal for drinking behavior also might be matched to the type and severity of the person's alcohol problem. Thus, reduced

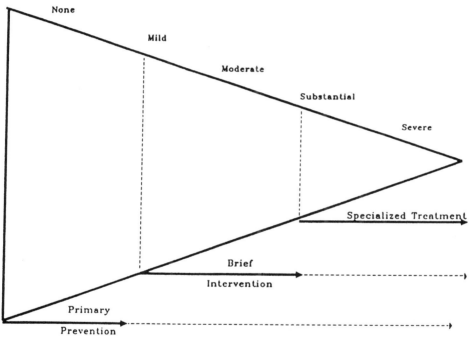

FIGURE 4. A spectrum of responses to alcohol problems. The triangle represents the population of the United States, with the spectrum of alcohol problems experienced by the population shown along the upper side. Responses to the problems are shown along the lower side (based on Skinner, 1988). In general, specialized treatment is indicated for persons with substantial or severe alcohol problems; brief intervention is indicated for persons with mild or moderate alcohol problems; and primary prevention is indicated for persons who have not had alcohol problems but are at risk of developing them. The dotted lines extending the arrows suggest that both primary prevention and brief intervention may have effects beyond their principle target populations. The prevalence of categories of alcohol problems in the population is represented by the area of the triangle occupied; most people have no alcohol problems, many people have a few alcohol problems, and some people have many alcohol problems. *Source*: Alcohol problems and a proposal for their treatment. From Institute of Medicine (1990). *Broadening the base of treatment for alcohol problems*. Washington, DC: National Academy of Science Press. Reprinted with permission.

drinking rather than abstinence might be sufficient to eliminate problems, particularly among persons with mild to moderate alcohol problems.

Finally, the report recommends that a few pilot programs be established to test the feasibility of expanded and comprehensive treatment systems. The committee concludes that, although methods of financing would have to be developed, the social costs saved by appropriate intervention would likely offset the financial costs of a broadened national commitment to treatment of alcohol problems.

The widespread nature of substance use disorders and their associated societal costs have moved those concerned with the treatment of these problems beyond the diagnostic issues of abnormal psychology into the public health arena, where screening and identification of problems replaces diagnosis of disorders. Clearly, this is the thrust of the Institute of Medicine report on alcohol problems just discussed above. No similar report exists for drug abuse problems. Efforts beyond treatment in the drug abuse area have focused on prevention of illicit drug use among school age youth and young adults. Given the decline in frequent use of illicit drugs by U.S. youth (HHS, 1992), these prevention efforts, along with more negative societal attitudes about drug use, have been at least partially successful. Suburban youth have shown the greatest reductions in drug use, which remains a significant problem among inner city youth.

Table 10 summarizes important and key points about diagnostic considerations pertaining to psychoactive substance use disorders.

SUMMARY

Psychoactive substances can be used to affect moods, thinking, and behavior. When serious negative behavioral effects occur from the use of such substances,

TABLE 10. Important and Key Points about Diagnostic Considerations for Psychoactive Substance Use Disorders

1. Disorders associated with substance use include:
   a. States of alcohol or drug intoxication or withdrawal.
   b. Substance-induced disorders (e.g., dementia, psychotic disorders) associated with chronic heavy substance use.
2. Persons with substance use disorders often experience additional types of psychopathology. Antisocial personality, depression, mania, schizophrenia, and phobic disorders are the most common additional coexisting psychopathology.
3. Most (85 to 90%) of those with substance use disorders never receive treatment. Active disorders and heavy substance use that does not meet diagnostic criteria produce substantial costs to society for traffic accidents, injuries and lost productivity related to substance use.
4. A government panel urged *expanded identification and treatment of alcohol problems* in which:
   a. Community settings (health clinics, courts, etc.) would:
      —identify individuals with alcohol problems
      —provide brief intervention (six or fewer sessions) for those with mild or moderate alcohol problems
      —refer more severe problems to specialized alcoholism treatment centers
   b. Alcoholism treatment centers would:
      —conduct a comprehensive assessment
      —match person to appropriate type of intervention
      —gather follow-up data to measure outcome and to improve success of treatment matching process

these serious psychological problems are called *substance-related disorders*. Essential features of the disorder are a maladaptive pattern of substance use leading to clinically significant impairment or distress.

Substance use disorders are the most common psychiatric disorder in the U.S. A recent study found lifetime prevalence of 17%, and noted that in the past year, 4.5 to 7% of the U.S. population (8 to 12% of men and 1 to 2% of women) experienced a substance use disorder.

Course and prognosis for substance use disorders differ in studies of the general population, compared to treatment center patients who have a higher proportion of more severe problems. In the general population, drug problems have a youthful onset from age 16 to 25, and over half enter remission within 3 years of onset of the disorder. In the general population, alcoholism onset occurs by age 20 for 40% of problems, but the age of risk extends through the late 30s and early 40s, and about half go into remission within 11 years of their onset. In treatment center patients, the course of treatment varies. Some alcoholics (20 to 35%) do not improve, or progressively deteriorate, a little more than a quarter have a stable remission, while the remaining cases continue to alternate between periods of short-term abstinence and problem drinking.

Children of alcoholics are consistently found to have higher rates of alcoholism than are children whose parents are not alcoholic. However, the extent of increased risk for alcoholism varies considerably. Children of treatment center alcoholics were 4 to 5 times more likely to be alcoholic themselves, whereas in representative population samples the risk was 1.4 to 1.7 times greater if the child had an alcoholic parent. A genetic influence on risk for alcoholism generally is accepted. The strength of the genetic influence and possible variations based on gender and subtype of alcoholism are debated.

Substance-related disorders include states of alcohol or drug intoxication or withdrawal. Substance-induced disorders (e.g., dementia, mood disorders) may be associated with chronic heavy substance use. Persons with substance use disorders often have additional psychopathology, of which antisocial personality, depression, mania, schizophrenia, and phobic disorders are most common. Most (85 to 90%) persons with substance use disorders never receive treatment. Recent U.S. government reports have recommended expanded identification and treatment of substance use problems.

ACKNOWLEDGMENTS. Preparation of this chapter was supported by grant R01-AA08637 from the National Institute on Alcohol Abuse and Alcoholism, by a grant from the Smithers Foundation, and by the Department of Veterans Affairs.

REFERENCES

American Psychiatric Association (1980). *Diagnostic and statistical manual of mental disorders*, 3rd Edition. Washington, DC: Author.

American Psychiatric Association. (1987). *Diagnostic and statistical manual of mental disorders*, 3rd Edition, Revised. Washington, DC: Author.

American Psychiatric Association (1993). *DSM-IV draft criteria*. Washington, DC: Author.

Anthony, J. C., & Helzer, J. E. (1991). Syndromes of drug abuse and dependence. In L. N. Robins & D. A. Regier (Eds.), *Psychiatric disorders in America: The Epidemiologic Catchment Area study* (pp. 116–154). New York: The Free Press.

Cahalan, D. (1970). *Problem drinkers: A national survey*. San Francisco: Jossey-Bass.

Cloninger, C. R. (1987). Neurogenetic adaptive mechanisms in alcoholism. *Science, 236,* 410–416.

Cotton, N. S. (1979). The familial incidence of alcoholism. *Journal of Studies on Alcohol, 40,* 89–116.

Croughan, J. L. (1985). The contributions of family studies to understanding drug abuse. In L. N. Robins (Ed.), *Studying drug abuse.* New Brunswick, NJ: Rutgers University Press.

Helzer, J. E., & Pryzbeck, T. R. (1988). The co-occurrence of alcoholism with other psychiatric disorders in the general population and its impact on treatment. *Journal of Studies on Alcohol, 49,* 219–224.

Helzer, J. E., Burnham, A., & McEvoy, L. T. (1991). Alcohol abuse and dependence. In L.N. Robins & D. A. Regier (Eds.), *Psychiatric disorders in America: The Epidemiologic Catchment Area study* (pp. 81–115). New York: Free Press.

Hesselbrock, M. N., Meyer, R. E., & Keener, J. J. (1985). Psychopathology in hospitalized alcoholics. *Archives of General Psychiatry, 42,* 1050–1055.

Hester, R. K., & Miller, W. R. (Eds.) (1989). *Handbook of alcoholism treatment approaches: Effective alternatives.* New York: Pergamon Press.

Institute of Medicine (1990). *Broadening the base of treatment for alcohol problems.* Washington, DC: National Academy of Science Press.

Jellinek, E. M. (1960). *The disease concept of alcoholism.* Highland Park, NJ: Hillhouse Press.

McGue, M., Pickens, R. W., & Svikis, D. S. (1992). Sex and age effects on the inheritance of alcohol problems: A twin study. *Journal of Abnormal Psychology, 101,* 3–17.

National Institute on Drug Abuse (NIDA). (1989). *National household survey on drug abuse: 1988 population estimates.* (DHHS Publication no. ADM 89–1636). Rockville MD: Author.

Polich, J. M., Armor, D. J., & Braiker, H. B. (1981). *The course of alcoholism: Four years after treatment.* New York: Wiley.

Robins, L. N., Locke, B. A., & Regier, D. A. (1991). An overview of psychiatric disorders in America. In L. N. Robins & D. A. Regier (Eds.), *Psychiatric disorders in America: The Epidemiologic Catchment Area study* (pp. 328–386). New York: Free Press.

Robins, L. N., & Regier, D. A. (Eds.). (1991). *Psychiatric disorders in America: The Epidemiologic Catchment Area study.* New York: Free Press.

Russell, M. (1990). Prevalence of alcoholism among children of alcoholics. In M. Windle & J. S. Searles (Eds.), *Children of alcoholics: Critical perspectives* (pp. 9–38). New York: Guilford Press.

Skinner, H. A. (1988). *Executive summary: Spectrum of drinkers and intervention responses.* Prepared for the Institute of Medicine Committee for the Study of Treatment and Rehabilitation Services for Alcoholism and Alcohol Abuse. Unpublished manuscript available from the author at Addiction Research Foundation, Toronto.

Taylor, J. R., & Helzer, J. E. (1983). The natural history of alcoholism. In B. Kissin & H. Begleiter (Eds.), *The biology of alcoholism* (Vol. 6) (pp. 17–65). New York: Plenum Press.

U.S. Department of Health and Human Services. (1992). National Household Survey on Drug Abuse. *ADAMHA News.* January–February, 18–19.

18

Sexual Disorders

Judith V. Becker and Meg S. Kaplan

Introduction

Human sexuality is an integral part of life, and concerns about sexuality may affect an individual throughout the stages of life. Psychologists in clinical practice frequently encounter clients or patients with sexual disorders, and consequently, it is important that such practitioners understand aspects of sexual development and functioning. Many men and women experience a sexual problem at some stage in the life cycle. Some are very open about their problem and may seek help from family, friends, or professionals, while others are ashamed or embarrassed and "suffer in silence."

There are two categories of sexual problems: paraphilias (sexual deviations) and sexual dysfunctions. Paraphilias are characterized by repetitive or preferred sexual fantasies involving nonhuman objects (e.g., sexual attraction to particular articles of clothing) or nonconsenting partners (children and adults who do not or cannot consent). Sexual dysfunctions are characterized by a disruption of the sexual response cycle. Both groups of sexual problems are described in this chapter.

Sexual Dysfunctions

Description of the Disorder

Human sexual functioning consists of the complex interaction of the vascular, nervous, and endocrine systems, which interact to produce sexual desire, arousal,

Judith V. Becker • Department of Psychiatry, University of Arizona College of Medicine, Tucson, Arizona 85724.   Meg S. Kaplan • New York State Psychiatric Institute, College of Physicians and Surgeons, Columbia University, New York, New York 10032.

Advanced Abnormal Psychology, edited by Vincent B. Van Hasselt and Michel Hersen. Plenum Press, New York, 1994.

and orgasm. A number of models of the sexual response cycle have been proposed. A frequently cited model is that of Masters and Johnson (1966). They describe a four-stage model. The four stages are excitement, plateau, orgasm, and resolution. Excitement is characterized by the onset of sexual feelings. During this stage, blood pressure and heart rate increase; males experience erection and in females, vaginal lubrication occurs. The second stage, plateau, is characterized by a more advanced stage of arousal. The third stage, orgasm, is a reflex brought about by vasocongestion and myotonia. For men, semen is ejaculated from the penis and for women, reflex rhythmic contractions of the circumvaginal muscles occur. The final stage is termed the resolution stage, in which specific physiologic responses return to a resting state.

A sexual dysfunction is diagnosed when there are disruptions in any of the stages. A dysfunction might be primary: that is, the person has always had difficulty; or secondary: the person was functioning at one time but has lost the ability to function. A dysfunction may also be present in all sexual situations or may be situational and specific to a particular partner or situation. For example, a woman may be orgasmic with one sexual partner but not with another. Finally, the dysfunction might be related to psychological factors or might be organic in origin, or a combination of both.

It is important for the reader to know there is not universal agreement on the sexual response cycle. Recently, Tiefer (1991) criticized the model of the human sexual response cycle described above, stating that it is flawed from a scientific, clinical, and feminist point of view. She feels the human sexual response cycle is neither objective nor universal and states, "It imposes a false biological uniformity on sexuality which does not support the human uses and meanings of sexual potential" (p. 20).

The *Diagnostic and Statistical Manual of Mental Disorders*, Third Edition, Revised (DSM-III-R) (American Psychiatric Association, 1987) lists the following sexual dysfunctions.

Hypoactive sexual desire disorder. Another term for this disorder is inhibited sexual desire. It is characterized by the persistent inhibition of sexual desire. Usually, a patient who presents with this problem reports an absence of sexual fantasies and a lack of desire or interest to engage in sexual activities. In diagnosing this dysfunction, the clinician must take into account factors that may affect sexual functioning, such as age and the context of the person's life. Some patients indicate that they are distressed by inhibited sexual desire, while others may come into therapy because their sexual partner is concerned that they are not as interested in sex as they once were. In some cases, a patient might be experiencing another form of sexual dysfunction, such as male or female sexual arousal disorder, and has developed hypoactive sexual desire disorder because sex is no longer as pleasurable to them as it had been in the past.

Sexual aversion disorder. This disorder is characterized by a persistent aversion to and avoidance of genital sexual contact with a sexual partner.

Female sexual arousal disorder. Characterized by recurrent partial or complete failure to attain or maintain the lubrication–swelling response of the sexual excitement stage of human sexual response. Patients also report a lack of a subjective sense of sexual pleasure during sexual activity.

Male erectile disorder. This disorder is analogous to the female sexual arousal disorder, in that the male experiences partial or complete failure in attaining or maintaining an erection until the completion of sexual activity. There is also a recurrent lack of a subjective sense of sexual excitement and pleasure during sexual activity.

Inhibited female orgasm. This dysfunction is characterized by a persistent or recurrent pattern in which a woman does not experience an orgasm subsequent to adequate sexual stimulation and excitement, or experiences a delayed orgasm following such stimulation and excitement. Orgasmic dysfunctions may be primary, secondary, or situational. The DSM-III-R notes: "Some females are able to experience orgasm during non-coital clitoral stimulation, but are unable to experience it during coitus in the absence of manual clitoral stimulation. In most of these females, this represents a normal variation of the female sexual response and does not justify the diagnosis of inhibited female orgasm." (Also termed Female Orgasmic Disorder in DSM-IV.)

Inhibited male orgasm. This dysfunction is characterized by a persistent or recurrent delay in or absence of orgasm in a male following normal sexual excitement phase during sexual activity. (Also termed Male Orgasmic Disorder in DSM-IV.)

Premature ejaculation (rapid ejaculation). This dysfunction is characterized by persistent or recurrent absence of voluntary control over ejaculation in that the male ejaculates with minimal sexual stimulation or before, upon, or shortly after penetration and before he wishes to.

Dyspareunia. This dysfunction is characterized by recurrent or persistent genital pain in either a male or female during the course or following sexual intercourse.

Vaginismus. This dysfunction is characterized by involuntary spasm of the musculature of the outer third of the vagina so that penetration is not possible.

The DSM-III-R also denotes a category entitled "Sexual dysfunction not otherwise specified." This category covers dysfunctions that do not meet criteria for the above-stated sexual dysfunctions. Examples would include genital pain during masturbation, no erotic sensation during orgasm, or the female analog of premature ejaculation.

In DSM-IV, two new categories of sexual dysfunctions have been included. These are (1) sexual dysfunction due to a general medical condition in which a sexual dysfunction is present, but there is a medical condition which is etiologically related to the sexual dysfunction; and (2) substance-induced sexual dysfunction, which is characterized by sexual dysfunction whose symptoms developed during or within a month of significant substance intoxication or withdrawal.

Also, in DSM-IV, the Gender Identity Disorders of childhood, adolescence, and adulthood have been included with the Sexual Disorders.

Epidemiology

Although the exact prevalence of sexual dysfunctions is unknown, a significant percentage of men and women in our society experience sexual problems at some time in their lives. Nathan (1986) reviewed 22 general population sex surveys to estimate the prevalence for the various sexual dysfunctions, and found that between 5% and 30% of women experience inhibited female orgasm, 5% of males experience inhibited male orgasm, 35% of males experience premature ejaculation, and between 10% and 20% of males experience male erectile dysfunction. Depending on the particular survey conducted, between 1% and 35% of women experience hypoactive sexual desire dysfunction, with 1 to 15% of males experiencing that dysfunction.

Clinical Picture

The following are case examples of actual patients seen by the first author in her sex therapy practice. Identifying information has been changed to protect the confidentiality of the patients.

M.L. is a 22-year-old graduate student who sought treatment for an erectile dysfunction. During the initial interview, he stated he was "impotent" and was beginning to withdraw from all forms of social contact because of his "impotence." A detailed sex history revealed that M.L. had his first experience of intercourse when he was age 17 and since that time had engaged in sexual relations with four female partners. He reported never having had any difficulty with sexual desire, arousal, or orgasm until an incident that occurred 1 month prior to his coming in for a consultation. He indicated that he had attended a party where he met a woman and asked if he could accompany her home. She agreed and when they reached her residence, she invited him in. He initiated sexual interaction and found that he was unable to attain an erection. He reported that he had consumed a significant amount of alcohol during the course of the party—much more than he usually consumed. M.L. stated that alcohol had never interfered with his erectile responding in the past. He also reported that he found this woman to be particularly attractive and wanted to "make a good impression on her" and be the "best lover she ever had." He reported that she was understanding of his not being able to get an erection, but he felt embarrassed and worried that something was wrong with him. Even though he liked this woman and wanted to see her again, he refrained from dating her because of what he defined as his "failure." M.L. stated that he was able to attain an erection when he masturbated and he continued to have erections upon awakening in the morning. However, he reported that a large part of his day was consumed with thoughts about his "sexual inadequacy." He found that he was beginning to view himself in other areas as a "loser" and did not feel he could date until he was "fixed."

M.L. presented as a case of secondary erectile dysfunction. Treatment is discussed in the following section.

The second case involved a female college student who had been the victim of a sexual assault, which had occurred approximately 1 year previous to the evaluation.

B.L. attended a fraternity party with some friends. When she was ready to leave the party, her friends were not; she subsequently accepted an offer of a ride home from one of the men at the party. She had seen this man at other parties and had spoken with him on several occasions. She had never been out with him socially. Instead of driving her to her dorm, he drove her to a deserted part of town and proceeded to rape her. Throughout the rape, he told her "This is what you want, isn't it?" She was finally able to get out of the car and was subsequently taken to the hospital where she reported the sexual assault. Prior to the sexual assault, she had had a relationship for a period of 1 year in which she experienced sexual desire, arousal, and orgasm. Along with the trauma of having been sexually assaulted, she was also concerned about whether or not she may have contracted HIV or a sexually transmitted disease. It was approximately 1 year before she felt comfortable dating. She met a man to whom she felt attracted and after several months of dating, they became sexually intimate. However, B.L. found that whenever he touched her, she would have flashbacks of her sexual assault and was unable to become aroused. She reported that her sexual partner was very gentle and understanding; however, she was concerned that he might terminate the relationship if she could not enjoy sexual interactions with him.

B.L. meets diagnostic criteria for secondary female sexual arousal dysfunction. Treatment for this dysfunction is discussed in the following section.

Diagnostic Considerations

In general, when a patient presents with a sexual dysfunction, it is important for the patient to be evaluated by either a gynecologist or urologist to rule out any organic basis for the sexual dysfunction. Sexual dysfunctions can be organic in nature, psychological in nature, or a combination of both. Because there are numerous medical conditions that can interfere with sexual responsiveness and functioning, it is important to rule them out. Some of those medical conditions include diabetes mellitus, cardiovascular disease, cancer, end-stage renal disease, and multiple sclerosis, to name a few. Schover and Jensen (1988) present a comprehensive review and approach to sexuality in chronic illness.

Various drugs as well as medications can interfere with sexual functioning. Those medications include certain antipsychotic drugs, certain antidepressant drugs, and certain antihypertensive medications. Steroids and estrogens can also impact on sexual functioning. The abuse of alcohol, opiates, or cocaine can also impact on sexual functioning. Rosen (1991) presents an extremely comprehensive review and description of the impact of prescription and illegal drugs on sexual functioning. Assessment procedures such as Doppler flow studies and penile blood pressure measurement, as well as arteriography and NPT (nocturnal penile tumescence studies) have been utilized to differentiate psychogenic from organic disorders in the male. NPT involves measuring erection responses during REM (rapid eye movement) sleep stages. If a male obtains and maintains an erection during this sleep stage, the psychological basis for the dysfunction is considered.

Unfortunately, development of physiological assessment techniques for sexual dysfunctions in women has lagged behind those developed for the male. However, a vaginal photoplethysmograph has been utilized to study vaginal blood flow (a concomitant of arousal) in the female.

Because certain psychiatric illnesses such as depression may impact on a person's interest or desire for sex, it is important to rule out any psychiatric illness that may be affecting sexual functioning. Prior to beginning therapy with the patient, a comprehensive evaluation of the patient should be conducted, including medical testing, psychological testing, and an assessment of the patient's current relationship. In general, if a patient is in a relationship, it is important to work with the couple in therapy and to address whatever communication or relationship issues might be impacting on sexual functioning. A sexual dysfunction can develop at any point in a person's life and consequently, it is important that the person seek counseling or therapy for the dysfunction so that the person does not experience any further distress.

Course and Prognosis

Over the past two decades, numerous advances have been made in both the diagnosis and treatment of sexual dysfunctions. The etiology of the sexual dysfunctions may be related to physical or organic factors, they may be caused by unconscious psychic conflicts, or they may be the result of negative sexual experiences, as posited by learning theorists. Inadequate sex information may be instrumental in causing certain dysfunctions. Performance anxiety is a very common cause of both erectile and/or orgasmic dysfunctions. Failure of individuals to communicate to their sexual partners what they want or need sexually can contribute to the development of sexual dysfunctions. Sexual trauma, either during childhood or adulthood, can place an individual at risk for developing a sexual dysfunction. Some individuals grow up in families in which they experienced both guilt and anxiety around issues of sexuality; consequently, when they enter a relationship, they experience difficulty relating to their sexual partner.

The following are psychological treatments that have been used on patients with specific sexual dysfunctions. Annon (1976) provides an overview of a model for treating sexual dysfunctions. This model is labeled the PLISSIT model, where P stands for permission. Some patients, when entering counseling, are either seeking permission to engage or to not engage in certain types of behaviors. Limited information (LI) is useful in helping some individuals resolve their sexual problems. Other individuals are in need of specific suggestions (SS), and these will be delineated below. Finally, some patients are in need of intensive therapy (IT) to deal with their sexual dysfunctions.

The treatment of hypoactive (low) sexual desire dysfunction can represent a challenge to clinicians. Treatment has ranged from the use of pharmacological or hormonal agents to a systemic or interactional approach to cognitive behavioral therapy. Psychodynamic therapy has been utilized to address early childhood fears or traumas that may be impacting on the individual.

Female sexual arousal dysfunction has been treated in a number of ways, including the utilization of anxiety reduction techniques as well as behavioral techniques, such as sensate focus exercises. These exercises involve teaching the individual to initially engage in nongenital, undemanding caressing of the partner. The initial emphasis is on the couple pleasuring one another. The exercises become more genitally focused in nature over therapy sessions.

Male erectile dysfunctions, which are psychological in nature, also have been treated with the use of sensate focus exercises and anxiety reduction techniques. Those disorders that are organic in nature (that is, they are the result of either hormonal deficits, or vascular or neurological insufficiency) have been treated in a variety of ways, including exogenous testosterone administration for those men who have low testosterone levels, the use of papaverine to induce erections, and in some cases, the use of penile prostheses, which are implanted into the penis.

Planning for treatment of inhibited female orgasm may vary depending on whether or not it is primary or secondary; that is, if the woman has never experienced an orgasm through any means of stimulation, teaching the female to masturbate is most effective in treating this dysfunction. Success rates from 80% to

90% have been reported. For a woman who is experiencing a secondary orgasmic disorder, that is, at one point was able to attain orgasm but is now unable to do so, the clinician assesses the nature of the relationship that the woman is now in and in general, couples' therapy is recommended. Again, therapy would focus on graded exposure exercises in treatment. The success rate for women with secondary anorgasmia can range from 10% to 75%.

The treatment of inhibited male orgasm, defined as either absent or delayed ejaculation or orgasm, is similar to that for treating inhibited orgasm in females. Masturbatory exercises as well as sensate focus exercises have been utilized. Systematic desensitization has been of help to those men who are uncomfortable ejaculating in the presence of their partner.

Therapeutic techniques for premature ejaculation have involved helping the patient identify the point of ejaculatory inevitability, teaching the patient the stop-start technique, and also utilizing different positions during intercourse.

Dyspareunia has been treated through the use of systematic desensitization. It is critical in cases of dyspareunia to rule out any organic pathology.

Vaginismus also has been successfully treated through the use of systematic desensitization. As part of this treatment, the woman learns to insert dilators of graduated sizes into her vagina.

Sexual aversion disorder also has been treated via systematic desensitization. Sexual phobias have been successfully treated using tricyclic antidepressants with a combination of sex therapy. For more detailed treatment appropriate to the sexual dysfunctions, the reader is referred to *Principles and Practice of Sex Therapy* (Leiblum & Rosen, 1989).

Regarding the two case studies presented above, in the first case of M.L., it was not necessary for this patient to undergo elaborate physiologic evaluations given that he reported that he was able to obtain and maintain full erections while he was masturbating and given the fact that he also had "morning erections." It appeared that several factors affected his ability to achieve an erection on that one date. Specifically, he had consumed a large amount of alcohol, and he was also experiencing "performance anxiety," that is, he was very nervous about how he would come across in sexual interactions with this woman. What appeared to be maintaining the problem was the fact that he was obsessing about his lack of erectile responding on that occasion and self-labeling himself as being impotent. The intervention involved providing him information and educating him about why he had difficulty in obtaining an erection that evening and also treating his performance anxiety and having him do some cognitive restructuring regarding his self-labeling. These techniques were successful and he was subsequently able to experience successful sexual relations.

Regarding the second case of B.L., it is not at all unusual for women who have been the victims of incest or sexual assault to develop sexual problems as a result of their abuse or assault. This patient was experiencing a posttraumatic stress disorder and consequently was experiencing flashbacks of her assault whenever her present partner attempted to interact with her sexually. Therapy involved treating her for the posttraumatic stress disorder with behavioral techniques as well as having her feel more in control in terms of the sexual relations that occurred between her and her present partner. These techniques were successful in helping her achieve her goal of being able to become aroused and enjoy sexual interactions with her new partner.

Summary

While tremendous progress has been made in the understanding, diagnosis, and treatment of sexual dysfunction, further research is needed in this area. The field holds many research opportunities and challenges for sex researchers and therapists.

PARAPHILIAS: DESCRIPTION OF THE DISORDER

Historically, paraphilias were termed perversions. Paraphiliac disorders are characterized by repetitive or preferred sexual fantasies or acts that involve non-human objects or nonconsenting partners. In order to make the diagnosis of paraphilia, the fantasies must have existed for at least 6 months and the person should have either acted on the fantasies or suffered serious distress because of them. There are numerous categories of paraphilias, including:

Voyeurism. Also called "peeping Tom." This paraphilia involves observing unsuspecting people engaging in dressing or undressing or sexual or sexually related behaviors. Voyeurs are sexually aroused by viewing a person naked or engaged in sexual activity. Some voyeurs masturbate while viewing the unsuspecting person; others may wait to masturbate until they return to the privacy of their own homes.

Exhibitionism. Involves exposing the genitals to an unsuspecting stranger. Exhibitionists may expose their genitals to children, adolescents, or adults, and in some cases may masturbate while exposing their genitals.

Frotteurism. A frotteur is an individual who achieves sexual gratification by rubbing up against a nonconsenting person. The behavior usually occurs in crowded places, such as elevators, buses, or subways.

Telephone scatologia. This paraphilia is more commonly known as obscene phone calls. People who have this paraphilia attain sexual excitement and gratification by stating obscenities or describing sexual activities to an unsuspecting person. It is not uncommon for the individual to masturbate while making the phone calls.

Fetishism. The sexual attraction is to inanimate objects and these often include women's clothing, such as shoes, stockings, or undergarments. Or, a person can be attracted to a specific body part. Usually, the person with a fetish fondles the article to which he or she is attracted to achieve sexual gratification.

Transvestic fetishism. An individual with this paraphilia obtains sexual gratification by dressing in the garments of a person of the opposite sex. In many cases, the person masturbates while cross-dressed.

Pedophilia. The sexual arousal to prepubescent children. Some pedophiles are exclusively attracted to girls or boys while other pedophiles, termed bisexual pedophiles, do not discriminate in their attraction and might sexually molest both male and female children.

Sexual masochism. This paraphilia involves sexual attraction to being bound, humiliated, beaten, or made to suffer in other manners. A sexual masochist might engage in the behavior with or without a partner. In some cases, the individual may request that the partner tie and beat him/her up or relate to him/her in a humiliating and demeaning manner. In other cases, the individual might impose harm and suffering upon himself or herself, for example, by sticking pins or needles through the nipples or genitals.

Sexual sadism. A sexual sadist is an individual who is sexually aroused by inflicting pain or suffering on another person. There can be an escalation in the severity of the maltreatment of the victim over time, and some sadists have been known to severely torture their victims.

Other less common forms of paraphilias include the sexual attraction and contact with a corpse (necrophilia), being sexually excited and aroused by urine (urophilia), sexual arousal and excitement by fecal material (coprophilia), and sexual attraction to enemas (klismaphilia).

Epidemiology

The majority of individuals who experience paraphilias are male in gender. About 50% of people with paraphilias experience the development of the paraphiliac disorder in adolescence. Furthermore, it is not unusual for a person to develop two or more paraphilias. The majority of people may have both a paraphiliac and nonparaphiliac (nonsexually deviant) arousal pattern at the same time. An individual who has a paraphilia is rarely distressed by the paraphilia and when this person presents for an evaluation or treatment, it is usually because the sexual partner or the criminal justice system has recommended or mandated that an evaluation and/or treatment be given. This is particularly true of individuals who are pedophiles or ephebophiles (engage in sexual activity with those of pubertal age). The reason for this is that the individual with a paraphilia, in the majority of cases, finds the fantasies and behavior exciting and rewarding and does not want to give these up.

Historically, it was believed that an individual would have only one type of paraphilia. However, recent studies have indicated that it is not uncommon for individuals to have more than one form of paraphilia. Also, in some cases, there can be an escalation. For example, some exhibitionists go on to molest children or to rape adult women. Some people who engage in cross-dressing might go on to engage in sexually aggressive behavior.

Information on what percentage of males and females have paraphilias in the United States is lacking. These data are difficult to obtain because not all people who have paraphilias are forthcoming in interview situations in discussing their sexual proclivities.

A number of theories have been postulated to explain why some people develop paraphilias. Some of these theories rely on biological factors, while others rely on psychodynamic or learning theories to explain the etiology of paraphilias. What is lacking is a theory that is comprehensive and takes into consideration biological, familial, and learning factors. Hopefully, over the next decade, our knowledge base will be advanced regarding the development of paraphiliac behaviors. Biological theories postulate that temporal lobe diseases or abnormal levels of androgens may contribute to the development of paraphiliac behavior.

Psychodynamic theories have discussed the role that early childhood trauma and/or anxiety during the oedipal developmental phase may play in the development of paraphiliac behavior. Learning theorists hypothesize that sexual behavior is learned and stress the importance of reinforcement through sexual fantasies and masturbation.

It is important that we educate adolescents about the nature of the inappropriateness of paraphiliac behaviors and make counseling and treatment available to them if they are having fantasies that are paraphiliac in nature or are having urges to engage in paraphiliac behavior. In some cases, adolescents and young adults are aware that their fantasies and urges are inappropriate, but are unaware that there are treatments available to help them.

Clinical Picture

The following case study describes an adult male pedophile who was referred to the first author because he had been molesting his daughter for a number of years. A number of details have been altered to protect the confidentiality of the client.

Mr. C is a 40-year-old male who was referred for evaluation and treatment following an attempted suicide after his daughter, age 13, disclosed to her mother that he had been molesting her since she was 10 years of age. Mr. C was arrested following this disclosure and was subsequently jailed for a short period of time and then released on bail. The outcome of the criminal justice proceedings was that he received probation and was mandated to enter a treatment program to deal with his paraphiliac behavior. His daughter was removed from the home for her protection. She went to live with her biological mother. Mr. C and his wife had shared custody of this child prior to his arrest. Mr. C is a highly intelligent man who was employed as an executive by a large corporation.

The following sexual history was obtained.

He did not recall ever having been sexually abused as a child. He reported that his first consensual sexual activity occurred, when he was age 12, with a same-age male peer. His first sexual activity with a female occurred when he was age 18. He also recalls one occasion of dressing in his girlfriend's underwear when he was this age. He married at age 21, and this marriage ended after three years. One female child (the victim of his pedophiliac behavior) was born from that union.

He reported a history of having engaged in consensual sexual activity with both adult males and females. He reported that at the age of 18 he engaged in mutual masturbation with a male college friend and that at the age of 26, he engaged in oral and anal sexual activity with a same-age male peer.

He reported that during his lifetime he had engaged in consensual sexual relationships with approximately eight same-age female peers. He remarried at age 30. No children were born from that marriage. As mentioned previously, he and his first wife shared custody of their female child. In addition to having molested his own daughter for a period of three years, he disclosed during the interview that he had molested at least eight other female children between the ages of 9 and 12. These children were relatives of acquaintances. Apparently, none of these children had ever disclosed to their parents his sexually touching them; consequently, he was never arrested for those behaviors. The sexual activity with these little girls consisted of having them remove their clothes and his fondling of their genitals. He reported that he never penetrated these children nor did he have them touch his genitals. He indicated that he would experience an erection while touching the children and then would go home and masturbate to fantasies of that experience and would ejaculate. This behavior began shortly after he married his second wife.

Mr. C reported that he experienced difficulty with erections and being able to have intercourse with his wife during his second marriage. He reported that he turned sexually to the other children and his daughter because he did not need an erection to be sexual with them. The nature of the sexual activity that he engaged in with his daughter included fondling her genitals and oral-genital sexual contact.

Mr. C also had a history of alcohol dependence and, in all probability, the difficulty he had in his sexual relationships with his wife, was related to his chronic use of alcohol and the damage this abuse had done to either the nervous or vascular system. He also presented with a history of several depressive episodes.

Mr. C reported that while he knew that sexual contact with his daughter and other female minors was against the law, he did not believe this behavior was particularly harmful to the children. He stated that because the children did not resist him and because his daughter "allowed" the behavior to continue for a period of time, he felt she must have enjoyed the sexual contact. He reported that he was aroused by female minors and attracted to adult females.

Diagnostic Considerations

Given that most individuals with paraphilias are "motivated" to receive treatment by either other family members or the criminal justice system, it is rare that the full extent of the paraphiliac interest pattern is disclosed during the initial interview. In some cases, it is not until rapport has been established and the patient feels that he or she can trust the therapist that the full extent of the paraphiliac behaviors will be disclosed. In some cases, patients feel if they reveal other paraphiliac acts they have engaged in, particularly if their victims are children, and because mental health professionals are bound by law to report child sexual abuse, they will be open to arrest and further prosecution for such behavior.

In making the diagnosis of paraphilia, it is important for the clinician to remember that not all forms of inappropriate sexual behavior are the result of a paraphiliac interest pattern. For example, a patient with a psychosis may, as part of his delusional system, engage in sexual activity that he might not ordinarily engage in were it not for the psychoses. On occasions, individuals who are diagnosed as manic may become hypersexual and engage in forms of paraphiliac behavior. Once the mania is treated pharmacologically, the inappropriate behavior may cease. A patient with dementia may engage in inappropriate sexual behavior, for example, masturbating in public, as a result of cognitive impairment. There have also been some reports of individuals who are developmentally disabled who have engaged in inappropriate sexual behavior related to either their cognitive impairment, poor impulse control, or lack of sexual knowledge.

In the evaluation of a person who has engaged in inappropriate sexual behavior, it is imperative to conduct a thorough diagnostic interview to rule out any of the abovementioned disorders. A comprehensive assessment consists of a detailed sexual history that includes onset and course of both paraphiliac and nonparaphiliac, fantasies, urges, and behaviors. It is important that patients be asked about every category of paraphiliac behavior. As mentioned previously, it is not unusual for patients to present with multiple paraphilias. It is also important to assess the patient for the presence of faulty beliefs (cognitive distortions) about his or her sexual behavior. Sexual knowledge is also assessed as well as whether or not the patient is experiencing any sexual dysfunctions. Another element of the assessment involves evaluating the patient's social, interactional, and assertiveness skills. A thorough evaluation of alcohol and drug usage must also be conducted because abuse of alcohol or drugs can interfere with the patient's ability to control his behavior. There are a number of paper-and-pencil tests that are used in conjunction with a structured clinical interview to obtain the abovementioned information.

There are two forms of psychophysiologic assessments that have been utilized in evaluating individuals with paraphilias. Penile plethysmography is one such form of assessment. In the privacy of a laboratory, the patient places a transducer (either a thin metal ring or mercury and rubber strain gauge) around his penis, and the degree of erection response is recorded while the patient is exposed to various sexual stimuli (either audiotapes, slides, or videotapes) that depict paraphiliac and appropriate sexual scenes. This information is then recorded on a physiograph (or computer) and the degree of arousal to deviant sexual scenes is compared to arousal to nonparaphiliac scenes. This form of assessment is helpful diagnostically and to assess the outcome of treatment. Some have argued, however, that arousal obtained in a laboratory does not necessarily correlate with arousal in the real world. A major disadvantage of this form of testing is that some men are able to voluntarily control their arousal in the laboratory. This form of assessment appears to work best with individuals who are motivated to undergo the evaluation.

Another form of assessment used with individuals who have engaged in sexual behaviors that are against the law, such as sexual aggression and the sexual abuse of children, is the use of the polygraph. Some clinicians have used polygraphy as an adjunct to a clinical interview to determine whether or not the patient is being truthful in terms of the information which is provided. This form of assessment, however, is not universally accepted and questions have been raised about the reliability and validity of polygraphy with a sex offender population.

In the Case of Mr. C, he underwent a structured clinical interview in which he provided detailed information regarding his past paraphiliac as well as non-paraphiliac behaviors. He also was administered a series of paper-and-pencil tests in which he self-reported that he was sexually aroused by children as well as by adult females, and indicated that he had beliefs that were supportive of sexual contact with children (cognitive distortions). In the laboratory, although he was not able to obtain a full erection, his assessment did show differential responding in which he showed an equal amount of arousal to adult females and to young females. While he had average social interactional skills, he did have difficulty in being assertive in his place of employment. As noted previously, he also was experiencing a sexual dysfunction in that he was unable to obtain a full erection. A referral was made to a urologist to determine whether there was an organic component to his sexual dysfunction. The urological consultation indicated that the erection problem was both organic and psychological in nature. He was mandated to receive treatment, but regardless of this, Mr. C indicated that he was actually highly motivated to undergo such treatment.

Clinical Course and Prognosis

Various forms of treatment have been defined in the psychological and psychiatric literatures for the treatment of individuals with paraphilias. These treatments can be grouped into biological treatments, psychodynamic therapy, and a variety of behavioral therapies. The biologic treatments have traditionally been used for individuals who have committed sexual offenses. These treatments have focused on surgical castration or chemical castration. Surgical castration has been widely used in Europe with incarcerated sex offenders. In North America, chemical castration has been utilized in the form of antiandrogenic medication. In relation to the role that androgens play in the maintenance of sexual arousal, these treatments have focused on blocking or decreasing the level of circulating androgens. These medications may be given orally or intramuscularly. They do not appear to influence the direction of sexual drive toward appropriate adult partners. Their mechanism of action is to decrease libido or the sexual drive and consequently diminish the individual's pattern of compulsive paraphiliac sexual behavior. In essence, the patient's circulating testosterone level is decreased with a concomitant decrease in sexual drive and fantasies. Side effects experienced by patients can include weight gain and lethargy; therefore, compliance is a problem in some cases. While sexual drive is reduced as long as the patient continues on the medication, once the medication is discontinued, sexual drive returns. Consequently, it is important that the patient receive other forms of therapy that will help redirect their sexual interests.

Psychodynamic therapy has been used in treating people with paraphilias. Thus, by identifying and attempting to resolve early conflicts and trauma, it is believed that the patient's anxiety toward appropriate partners will be reduced, and consequently, the individual will lose interest in paraphiliac fantasies and behaviors. While psychodynamic therapy has been effective with some patients, in general, it does not appear to be the treatment of choice for individuals with paraphilias.

A number of different forms of behavior therapies have been used to treat individuals who have paraphilias. Various aversive conditioning procedures have been used, such as apomorphine (to induce nausea), electric shock, ammonia aversion therapy, and covert sensitization. Covert sensitization involves teaching the patient to pair his or her inappropriate sex fantasies with aversive, anxiety-provoking scenes. Satiation is a technique in which the patient uses paraphiliac (deviant) fantasies in a repetitive manner to the point of satiating himself with deviant stimuli. In essence, they learn to become bored and repulsed by their own sexual fantasies. While a major aim of therapy is to reduce the patient's (paraphiliac) deviant sexual fantasies, urges, and behaviors, it is important that the patient also receives treatment to facilitate their nondeviant arousal as well as to ensure that they have the necessary skills to relate to their peers in a functional and nonviolent manner. It is also important to confront the faulty beliefs that these patients have. Cognitive restructuring is a treatment technique that changes the paraphiliac's inappropriate beliefs concerning sexual behavior. Sex education and sex dysfunction therapy should also be an integral part of treatment.

Once the patient completes the structured form of therapy, it is important to program for the maintenance of therapeutic gains. The majority of treatment programs for individuals who have paraphilias set as a goal learning control of the behavior and decreasing the frequency of paraphiliac fantasies, rather than setting as a goal "cure" of the paraphiliac behavior. Consequently, it is recommended that individuals have available to them maintenance groups to assist them in consolidating the gains they have made in therapy. For a review of treatment outcome studies with sex offenders, the reader is referred to Becker and Hunter (1992).

In the case of Mr. C presented above, he received covert sensitization, satiation therapy, and cognitive restructuring. Marital therapy was also provided because, as can be expected, the disclosure of the sexual abuse and the knowledge that Mr. C had been involved with his daughter, affected his relationship with his wife. Mr. C did quite well in therapy and learned control over his pedophiliac urges as well as a modification of his cognitive distortions. Mr. and Mrs. C worked on issues in their relationship and Mr. C continued to be seen at 1-month intervals for maintenance therapy.

Summary

Clinical research studies have demonstrated that treatment interventions utilizing a multicomponent approach have relatively high success rates in treating individuals who have paraphilias. Not only are such treatments effective in teaching control of the paraphiliac behavior and thereby reducing future victimization, but they are also cost-effective. For every individual who is successfully treated, there are tens if not hundreds of people who might be saved from being victimized. Further clinical research needs to focus on early identification of those individuals at risk for developing paraphilias as well as developing new forms of interventions, because there is no intervention that is effective in 100% of the cases.

REFERENCES

American Psychiatric Association. (1987). *Diagnostic and statistical manual of mental disorders*, 3rd Edition, Revised. Washington, DC: Author.
American Psychiatric Association (1993). *DSM-IV draft critiera*. Washington, DC: Author.
Annon, J. S. (1976). *Behavioral treatment of sexual problems: Brief therapy*. New York: Harper and Row.
Becker, J. V., & Hunter, J. A. (1992). Evaluation of treatment outcome for adult perpetrators of child sexual abuse. *Criminal Justice and Behavior, 19*, 74–92.
Leiblum, S. R, & Rosen, R. C. (1989). *Principles and practice of sex therapy*. New York: Guilford Press.
Masters, W. H., & Johnson, V. E. (1966). *Human sexual response*. Boston: Little Brown & Company.
Nathan, S. G. (1986). The epidemiology of the DSM-III psychosexual dysfunctions. *Journal of Sex and Marital Therapy, 12*, 267–281.
Rosen, R. (1991). Alcohol and drug effects on sexual function: Human experimental and clinical studies. In J. Bancroft (Ed.), *Annual review of sex research*, (Vol. 2, pp. 119–179). Lake Mills, IA: Society for the Scientific Study of Sex.
Schover, L. R., & Jensen, S. B. (1988). *Sexuality in chronic illness: A comprehensive approach*. New York: Guilford Press.
Tiefer, L. (1991). Historical, scientific, clinical and feminist criticisms of "the human sexual response cycle" model. In J. Bancroft (Ed.), *Annual review of sex research*, (Vol. 2, pp. 1–23). Lake Mills, IA: Society for the Scientific Study of Sex.

19

Psychophysiological Disorders

Donald A. Williamson, Susan E. Barker, and Staci Veron-Guidry

Description of the Disorders

Some physical or medical problems can be strongly influenced by psychological factors such as stress, emotion, or personality. These medical problems are generally called *psychosomatic* or *psychophysiological* disorders. It is important to recognize that there is a physiological basis to these disorders and, therefore, problems such as headache or ulcer are not just "all in the patient's head." Headaches and ulcers really do hurt. The term psychophysiological means "interaction of psychological and physiological variables." Consequently, a psychophysiological disorder occurs when psychological and physiological variables interact to produce a pathological state.

Common types of psychophysiological disorders are: migraine headache, tension headache, peptic ulcer, irritable bowel syndrome, insomnia, and essential hypertension. These problems share a common etiological theory, which is often called the diathesis-stress model. The term diathesis refers to a constitutional vulnerability toward overactivity in a particular biological system (e.g., cardiovascular or gastrointestinal systems). The diathesis-stress model postulates that stress, worry, anxiety, etc. interact with the vulnerable system to produce a specific psychophysiological syndrome. For example, essential hypertension has been postulated to result from an inherently overactive cardiovascular system such that stress ultimately results in chronically elevated blood pressure. Research evidence supporting the diathesis-stress model is somewhat mixed and is stronger for some psychophysiological disorders than others.

Donald A. Williamson, Susan E. Barker, and Staci Veron-Guidry • Department of Psychology, Louisiana State University, Baton Rouge, Louisiana 70803-5501.

Advanced Abnormal Psychology, edited by Vincent B. Van Hasselt and Michel Hersen. Plenum Press, New York, 1994.

A complete review of all psychophysiological disorders is beyond the scope of this chapter. Thus, we have selected three types of disorders—headache, essential hypertension, and insomnia—to illustrate current knowledge of the psychophysiological disorders. These disorders were selected because they are common problems, are quite diverse, and are generally accepted as having both psychological and physiological determinants. Since 1980, *Diagnostic and Statistical Manual of Mental Disorders* (DSM-III, DSM-III-R, and DSM-IV) (American Psychiatric Association, 1980, 1987, 1993) has used the category Psychological Factors Affecting Physical Condition as the proper diagnostic category for classifying psychophysiological disorders. In DSM-IV, psychophysiological disorders are defined as any medical conditions which are adversely affected by psychological factors such as stress, behavior, or mood.

Headache

Migraine and muscle-contraction (also called tension) headaches are the most common types of headache (Williamson, 1981). Migraine headache is usually described as a severe, throbbing pain that is located on just one side of the head (i.e., either left or right side). Pain is usually located in the temple forehead, or back of the head. Nausea and vomiting often accompany the headache. Patients with what is called "classic" migraine report warning signs that precede the headache by about 30 minutes. Common warning signs are seeing flashing lights or having blind spots in the visual field. Most migraine patients do not experience warning signs; they are diagnosed as having "common" migraine.

A muscle-contraction headache is described as a dull, constant ache in the forehead, neck/shoulders, or around the entire head. Pain generally occurs on both sides of the head. Warning signs of headache are seldom reported by tension headache patients. Also, they generally do not experience nausea or vomiting with headache.

Migraine headaches are believed to be caused by extreme changes in the flow of blood to the head. Prior to a headache, blood vessels inside the brain constrict; during a headache the vessels outside the skull dilate (Diamond & Dalessio, 1982). A variety of factors can bring on a migraine attack including stress, emotions, alcohol consumption, and smoke. Muscle-contraction headaches are thought to be caused by sustained contraction of facial and neck/shoulder muscles. Stress has been implicated as a potential cause of tension headaches.

Essential Hypertension

Hypertension refers to elevated blood pressure; essential hypertension refers to those cases in which the etiology is unknown. The remaining cases of hypertension are secondary to other medical problems. Blood pressure is defined as the pressure within the cardiovascular system (the heart, arteries, veins, and capillaries) that is generated during the beating and resting phases of the heart (Blanchard, Martin, & Dubbert, 1988). Since the circulatory system is a closed system, any alterations in cardiac output or resistance of the circulatory system have the potential to alter blood pressure.

Diastolic blood pressure is the pressure exerted when the heart is at rest. Systolic blood pressure is the pressure exerted during contractions of the heart muscle. These components interact to produce blood pressure, which is a function of total cardiac output and peripheral vascular resistance (Hollandsworth, 1986).

A diagnosis of mild hypertension is given when diastolic pressure is 90–104 mm Hg and/or systolic pressure is greater than 160 mm Hg. Moderate hypertension refers to a diastolic pressure in the 105–114 range. A diagnosis of severe hypertension is given when diastolic pressure is 115 mm Hg or higher (Joint National Committee on Detection, Evaluation, and Treatment of High Blood Pressure, 1984).

Individuals with hypertension are generally a "normal" group as evidenced by psychological testing. They demonstrate less psychological stress than patients with other stress-related disorders, such as headache or irritable bowel syndrome (Blanchard et al., 1988). However, a thorough psychological evaluation is an important part of the assessment of a hypertensive patient, especially regarding anger, hostility, stress, and anxiety.

Insomnia

Chronic insomnia can be defined as an inability to initiate and maintain adequate restorative sleep. Common sleep disturbances are difficulty falling asleep or remaining asleep, early morning awakening with an inability to return to sleep, or any combination of these three. Whereas almost all individuals experience occasional sleepless nights, chronic insomnia produces impairment that interferes with daily functioning. The complaint of insomnia is often subjective. There is no standard definition of insufficient sleep because the amount of sleep needed by different individuals varies widely. Lacks (1987) suggested the following practical criteria for a definition of chronic insomnia: (1) sleep onset latency (time required to fall asleep) of more than 30 minutes; or (2) more than 30 minutes spent awake during the night; or (3) fewer than 6½ hours of sleep in a night; (4) daytime fatigue accompanied by impairments in mood and performance; (5) symptoms that occur at least three nights per week; (6) symptoms that occur for at least several months. Similarly, the DSM-III-R diagnostic criteria for insomnia disorders (APA, 1987) required a complaint of "difficulty in initiating or maintaining sleep, or of non-restorative sleep" that occurs at least three times a week for a minimum of 1 month, and results in daytime fatigue, irritability, or impaired daytime functioning. In DSM-IV (APA, 1993), chronic insomnia is characterized as Primary Insomnia if it is not caused by some other type of medical, sleep, or psychiatric disorder.

Many different factors can cause a person to have disturbed sleep. Psychophysiological insomnia is viewed as a brief or persistent insomnia that develops as a result of psychological factors, physiological tension, and negative conditioning (i.e., emotional arousal prevents sleep, which leads the individual to try harder to sleep, which produces more arousal and causes further sleeplessness). Psychophysiological insomnia is often diagnosed by excluding other types of sleep disorders, such as insomnia associated with serious psychiatric or medical problems.

EPIDEMIOLOGY

Headache

Headache is a widespread problem, and most adults report headache to be an occasional difficulty (Waters, 1974). Severe headaches affect approximately 20% of adults, and prevalence rates in women are twice as high as those in men (Blanchard & Andrasik, 1985). Muscle-contraction headaches are much more prevalent than migraine headaches (Linet, Stewart, Celentano, Ziegler, & Sprecher, 1989). Headaches occur less frequently in children and adolescents, affecting about 5 to 7% of these individuals. No segment of society is spared from headaches; they are common in all races and socioeconomic groups. Studies of common health complaints in outpatient medical clinics have found headache to be among the most common presenting problems of children and adults (Williamson, 1981).

Hypertension

Hypertension is the most common cardiovascular disease. It is estimated to affect as many as 15% of Americans. Hypertension increases one's risk for stroke and renal damage, and it has been identified as one of the major risk factors for coronary heart disease (Garrison, Kannel, Stokes, & Castelli, 1987).

Sex. Hypertension occurs less frequently in women; however, after age 55, the rates for women surpass those for men (Blanchard, Martin, & Dubbert, 1988).

Race. African Americans tend to have higher levels of blood pressure (38.2%) than Caucasians (28.8%) in the United States (Subcommittee on Definition and Prevalence of the 1984 Joint National Committee, 1985). Overall mortality rates are higher for African Americans in comparison to the Caucasian population.

Body mass and obesity. Significant correlations have been found between blood pressure and body mass, and between hypertension and obesity. In addition, weight loss is associated with decreases in blood pressure (Eliahou et al., 1981).

Type A behavior. Type A individuals are described as hostile, impatient, competitive, and ambitious, while Type B individuals are described as relaxed, easygoing, and unhurried. Hypertension has been found to be more prevalent among Type A subjects than Type B subjects (Review Panel on Coronary-prone Behavior and Coronary Heart Disease, 1981).

Insomnia

Surveys of sleep patterns indicate that insomnia is a widespread problem. Hauri (1982) estimated that each year approximately 10 million Americans will visit their physicians with complaints of sleep difficulties. Extensive epidemiological studies consistently indicate that approximately 30% of their respondents complain of some sleep disturbances in the past year (Bixler, Kales, Soldatos, Kales, & Healey, 1979), and as many as 50% have experienced insomnia at some point in their lives (Bussye & Reynolds, 1990). In a recent study, Mellinger, Balter, and Uhlenhuth (1985) reported from a sample of 3161 adults that 18% complained of serious sleep problems, and another 18% reported mild to moderate difficulties. Complaints of insomnia appear to be more frequent in the elderly (Bixler et al., 1979), in women (Bussye & Reynolds, 1990), and among individuals of lower socioeconomic groups (Kales & Kales, 1984). The estimated prevalence of psychophysiological insomnia among all the insomnia disorders is 15% (Bussye & Reynolds, 1990).

CLINICAL PICTURE

Headache

Migraine and muscle-contraction headache patients are generally referred for nonpharmacological treatment only after drug therapy has been found to be ineffective. The following case description illustrates a migraine headache case that was complicated by emotional factors and was resistant to standard medical treatment.

> Sharon was a 50-year-old woman referred by a neurologist for biofeedback treatment of classic migraine. Sharon was married and had three children, two daughters were in college, and one son was working in another state. She described headaches that occurred about two to three times each week and generally lasted for 8–24 hours. The headaches typically started in the right temple and eventually radiated to the entire right side of her head. She felt nauseated and sometimes vomited during headaches. Pain was severe, pulsating with each heartbeat. She usually felt light-headed or "out of it" just before a headache began. She and her husband agreed that she was a "worrier." She reported many of the symptoms of generalized anxiety disorder (see Chapter 14) and worried about the family finances, the well-being of her children, and her own health. Friends and family were afraid to tell her anything that was potentially upsetting because they did not want to cause a headache. As a result, she was treated "with kid gloves" by her husband. Their communication and marital relationship had suffered in the past few years. She had been treated with a variety of medications with no success. We treated her using skin temperature biofeedback, relaxation, and cognitive behavior therapy for generalized anxiety disorder. Within 6 months she was experiencing less than one headache per month.

Hypertension

Individuals presenting for treatment of hypertension are a heterogeneous group and have usually been diagnosed during a previous medical examination. As mentioned before, systolic blood pressure above 160 mm Hg and/or diastolic blood pressure above 90 mm Hg warrants a diagnosis of hypertension. It is important that clinicians be aware of a phenomenon called "office hypertension," which refers to the fact that some people have elevated blood pressure in a physician's office but not in other settings (Kaplan, 1986).

In a 40-year longitudinal study, it was found that middle-aged hypertensive men, on average, had low annual income. Subjects with hypertension were more psychosocially disadvantaged, had more experiences of job dissatisfaction, and had experienced more stress during the previous 5 years. They also were prone to using alcohol on a daily basis for purposes of relaxation, and were heavier than the nonhypertensive controls (Lindgarde et al., 1987). The following case description illustrates how behavioral factors can contribute to hypertension and heart disease.

> Marjorie was a 63-year-old woman referred by a cardiologist for behavior modification after sustaining a nonfatal myocardial infarction (MI). Marjorie had been widowed for 2 years and had one daughter, who lived nearby. She had been diagnosed as hypertensive at age 47, and there were several behavioral factors that contributed to her cardiovascular problems. Marjorie's diet was high in fat; consequently, she was 60 lbs overweight. She had been a heavy smoker since age 20, and continued smoking even after a myocardial infarction. Marjorie had not been compliant with previous hypertension treatments because she "couldn't feel her high blood pressure," and until recently, hypertension had not affected her daily life. In spite of the recent MI, Marjorie was not motivated to make any drastic changes in her lifestyle. She reported that she might consider quitting smoking "later on," and was somewhat interested in

modifying her diet. Marjorie was referred to a nutritionist for dietary information and meal planning and eventually lost 20 lbs, resulting in modest reductions in blood pressure.

Insomnia

Patients with psychophysiological insomnia best fit the common picture of chronic insomniacs. These patients do not meet diagnostic criteria for a specific medical or psychiatric disorder, but they may present with a few symptoms of each. Individuals who experience this type of insomnia regard themselves as "light" sleepers; they do not typically complain of daytime sleepiness, but report that they are tired and lack energy to function well during the day.

Patients with chronic psychophysiological insomnia often report the occurrence of a stressful life event near the beginning of their sleep difficulty. Psychological characteristics of the insomniac may interact with these life events to produce sleeplessness. Studies have consistently shown that compared with those who have no problem with sleep, insomniacs demonstrate more psychopathology. In particular, they are more likely to label themselves as worriers and to have elevated profiles on tests for psychological problems (Kales & Kales, 1984). Some investigators theorize that these psychological characteristics lead insomniacs to internalize their reactions to life events, causing emotional arousal, which, in turn, promotes sleeplessness (Lacks, 1987).

Conditioning factors often combine with psychological factors to produce psychophysiological insomnia. Specifically, attempts to sleep become associated with internal and external factors that are incompatible with sleep (Bussye & Reynolds, 1990). Internal factors include the fear of sleeplessness and its accompanying performance anxiety and frustration. These factors are thought to produce the "vicious cycle" in which sleeplessness leads to frustration and emotional arousal, which leads to more sleeplessness.

External cues that interfere with sleep include those elements of one's environment that become associated with sleep disturbance. Examples are the presence of bedtime behaviors that are incompatible with sleep, such as lying in bed reading or watching television. When an insomniac experiences anxiety and frustration because of sleeplessness, the bed and bedroom can become strong aversive stimuli as well.

Other external factors that have been implicated in psychophysiological insomnia are "sleep hygiene" variables (e.g., level of noise or light in the bedroom). Changes in the sleep/wake cycle (e.g., because of shiftwork) can also lead to sleeplessness. The following case description illustrates the multiple factors that can influence psychophysiological insomnia.

"Gary" was a 34-year-old, married, white male who presented at a psychology clinic with complaints of insomnia and daytime irritability. He reportedly began to have problems sleeping about 3 months prior to his presentation at the clinic. At about the same time that he began to have sleep difficulties, he was experiencing marital problems and had just received a promotion at work. His wife had since sought legal separation. At the initial evaluation, Gary reported that his sleep-onset latency was about 1–2 hours. About two times per week, he wakened about an hour before his scheduled wake-up time and was unable to return to sleep. Recently, he had begun to put some papers from the office on his bedside table, so that he could stay in bed and work on these if he could not sleep. He described the atmosphere at his office as "tense" and stated that he felt pressured to prove himself in his new position. He reported that his mood was somewhat depressed and irritable, and that he was very angry at his wife for initiating their separation. Gary had been diagnosed the previous year with hypertension, and had been placed on beta-blocker medication to control elevated blood pressure. Interview and psychological testing indicated that he was experiencing other symptoms of depression such as decreased appetite and difficulty concentrating. However, he did not meet DSM-IV diagnostic criteria for a mood disorder. Treatment planning for Gary's insomnia included several targets: (1) instruction in appropriate sleep hygiene, (2) stress-management training, (3) consultation with his physician to facilitate management of his hypertension through diet and exercise instead of medication, and (4) psychotherapy to help him adjust to his recent marital separation. After 4 months of therapy, his sleep was much improved.

COURSE AND PROGNOSIS

Headache

Headaches are more common in adulthood relative to childhood and adolescence. Epidemiological studies have found that the prevalence of headaches increases from about 5% to about 20% over the course of adolescence (Bille, 1981). By age 15, approximately 70% of all adolescents have experienced at least one headache. The general course of headaches is one of a worsening pattern over time (Bakal, 1982), becoming more severe with a greater diversity of symptoms representing tension and migraine headache. Further, disability due to headache also generally worsens over a person's lifespan. With treatment, the prognosis for headache is quite positive. Drug treatments for migraine headache have a success rate of about 50 to 80% (Williamson & Waggoner, 1986). Tension headache can often be relieved by over-the-counter pain medication. Biofeedback, relaxation, and cognitive-behavior therapy have been found to be effective for relieving headache in about 60 to 90% of headache patients (Williamson & Waggoner, 1986).

Hypertension

There is a large body of data that supports the importance of treating even mild hypertension. Without treatment, even high-normal diastolic blood pressure of 85–89 mm HG may lead to the development of essential hypertension (Blanchard et al., 1988). The risk of stroke covaries with elevated blood pressure, and the incidence of cerebrovascular accidents increases as blood pressure increases. Similarly, vulnerability to heart disease is greater with higher levels of blood pressure. Men with blood pressure levels over 150 mm Hg are more than twice as likely to have a myocardial infarction than are men with blood pressure levels less than 120 mm Hg (Steptoe, 1981).

There are several psychological treatment procedures that have been developed for hypertensive patients. These include relaxation training and biofeedback, assertiveness training, time-management skills, cognitive therapy, and general supportive therapy, which have collectively come to be known as stress management.

One of the most common of these techniques is relaxation training. Based on the assumption that an increased overall level of arousal can result in elevated blood pressure, relaxation training utilizes techniques that decrease overall arousal.

As early as the 1930s, researchers have reported decreases in blood pressure that accompany deeply relaxed states. Overall, the results from relaxation training research are equivocal. While some studies have found relaxation training to be superior to supportive and/or medical therapies (e.g., Taylor et al., 1977), others have found that relaxation training is no more effective in reducing blood pressure than supportive therapy (e.g., Irvine & Logan, 1991).

Stress management intervention training and management of Type A behavior have recently been evaluated as treatments for essential hypertension. Both stress management training and Type A management were successful in lowering blood pressure and for modifying Type A behaviors. This recent research suggests that reductions of anger, hostility, and cardiovascular reactivity may have stronger therapeutic effects upon hypertension than simple relaxation therapy.

Insomnia

Insomnia that is related to another medical or psychiatric factor generally follows the course of the related disorder. The course of psychophysiological insomnia is quite variable. It may be relatively transient, or it may be persistent and last for years. From the large body of research on psychological treatment for insomnia, the following conclusions about its course and prognosis can be drawn (Lichstein & Fischer, 1985): (1) insomnia appears to be highly reactive, since there is a high frequency of success among many distinct types of treatment; (2) once treatment gains are attained, they appear to be maintained well; (3) there are contradictory findings as to which form of treatment for insomnia works best; (4) persistent insomnia is unlikely to remit if left untreated.

FAMILIAL AND GENETIC FACTORS

Headache

There is considerable evidence for a hereditary basis for migraine headache, though most controlled investigations of heritability have suggested that migraine is not a purely inherited disorder (Bakal, 1982). It is generally believed that tension headache has no direct genetic basis. More likely, tension headache patients either inherit or adopt the neurotic traits of their parents (Sacks, 1985). There is a growing consensus that parental models of pain-related behavior may be a strong determinant of the expression of pain (Osborne, Hatcher, & Richtsmeier, 1989). Bakal (1982) has postulated that biological, social, and psychological factors interact to determine the symptoms and severity of headache over the course of a person's lifetime.

Hypertension

It has been estimated that 36 to 67% of the variance in blood pressure is due to genetic factors (Steptoe, 1981). Roughly 30 to 40% of hypertensive patients have close relatives who have been diagnosed as hypertensive. Racial and familial differences are linked to hereditary factors, and transmission is believed to be polygenic.

Essential hypertension has been identified as a major health problem for African Americans. Research has shown that there is a greater prevalence of hypertension and greater mortality from hypertension diseases in this population. However, no single mechanism has been identified to account for this racial disparity.

The cardiovascular responses of African American men with and without parental history of hypertension have been compared. Results show that sons of hypertensive parents have higher systolic and diastolic blood pressure than sons of nonhypertensive parents (Johnson, Nazzaro, & Gilbert, 1991).

Results of twin-family studies and adoption studies document the influence of additive genetic influences on blood pressure. Several conclusions can be drawn from the existing research regarding the role of genetic factors in the development of hypertension. *First*, cardiovascular reactivity is moderately heritable. Individuals with a family history of hypertension and coronary heart disease demonstrate exaggerated patterns of cardiovascular reactivity. *Second*, blood pressure lability in the natural environment is also reliable and heritable. *Third*, higher blood pressure levels, increased responsiveness to stressors, and a delayed recovery to baseline have been found in individuals with parental history of cardiovascular disease (Rose, 1986).

Insomnia

Psychophysiological insomnia is not thought to be a product of direct familial or genetic transmission. However, since sleep difficulties can be a symptom of other medical and psychiatric disorders, a tendency toward insomnia could possibly be indirectly genetically transmitted (e.g., as in the case of schizophrenia, which is thought to cause sleeplessness). Insomnia due to "restless legs" can also be indirectly transmitted, since restless leg syndrome is familial in up to one third of cases (Parkes, 1985). Also, Lugaresi and Montagna (1990) reported a few rare cases of fatal familial insomnia, which is a progressive genetic disease that begins with insomnia and progresses to a stuporous state. Death occurs within months of the onset of the disease.

DIAGNOSTIC CONSIDERATIONS

Headache

Migraine and muscle-contraction headache must be differentiated from other forms of head pain. Some patients report both migraine and muscle-contraction headaches. These "mixed" headache cases are often much more difficult to treat effectively (Bakal, 1982). Another common type of head pain is caused by dysfunction of the temporomandibular joint (TMJ), which connects the jaw to the skull. Pain from TMJ dysfunction is usually located near the joint and is usually associated with displacement of the jaw (e.g., popping out of joint easily) (Williamson, Ruggiero, & Davis, 1985). Other common causes of headache are hypertension, brain tumors, and encephalitis. These disorders require medical diagnosis.

Hypertension

Assessment of hypertensive individuals should include a comprehensive history, careful measurement of blood pressure, and psychological testing (Blanchard et al., 1988). A comprehensive medical history should elicit information regarding demographic background, the history of the patient's hypertension and drug therapy, physical activities, obesity, habits such as smoking, alcohol usage, nutrition, and life stressors.

Measurements of blood pressure can be taken in the clinic as well as at home by the patient. Home blood pressure measures may be more representative of the patient's 24-hour ambulatory blood pressure than those taken in the clinic (Kleinert et al., 1984).

There are several psychological tests that are useful for assessing emotional determinants of hypertension. A common psychological test battery includes the State-Trait Anxiety Inventory (Spielberger, Gorsuch, & Lushene, 1970), the State-Trait Anger Scale (Spielberger, 1980), the Buss-Durkee Scale (a measure of hostility) (Buss & Durkee, 1957), the Beck Depression Inventory (Beck et al., 1961), the Jenkins Activity Survey (for Type A behavior) (Jenkins, Zyzanski, & Roseman, 1965), and the Social Readjustment Scale (for life stressors) (Homes & Rahe, 1967).

Insomnia

Insomnia is not usually a specific disorder or diagnostic category in itself, but rather a symptom of a variety of psychiatric and/or medical disorders. Therefore, complaints of sleep disturbance require a thorough, individualized assessment for differential diagnosis. Ideally, assessment should include interviewing the patient and significant others to obtain an accurate picture of his or her sleep problem. Also, evaluation should include a medical examination, all-night sleep recordings through polysomnography (if possible), psychological testing, and daily self-monitoring of sleep and daytime activity.

Many medical conditions, such as thyroid dysfunction, pain, central nervous system disorders, and cardiovascular disorders can cause or contribute to sleep problems (Parkes, 1985). Alcohol and drugs such as nicotine, beta-blockers, and other CNS stimulants (e.g., caffeine) also have been shown to interfere with sleep (Parkes, 1985). Hypnotic drugs, which are frequently prescribed to treat insomnia, can lead to the development of tolerance and disruption of natural sleep patterns. These drugs often lead to insomnia of greater severity than before their administration (Parkes, 1985).

Several psychiatric disorders, such as depression, anxiety disorders, and schizophrenia, can cause sleep disturbances and must be ruled out when diagnosing insomnia. In these cases, sleep disturbances usually appear only in conjunction with the presence of the psychiatric symptoms.

Physiological factors that may inhibit sleep include nocturnal myoclonus ("restless legs") during sleep, and sleep apnea, a respiration disorder in which the person stops breathing for about 10 seconds repeatedly throughout the night.

Summary

Psychophysiological disorders illustrate the interaction between mind and body and how this interaction can sometimes produce painful, distressing, and potentially life-threatening syndromes. Effective medical and psychological treatments have been developed for the psychophysiological disorders. One field of study that has furthered treatment advances for these disorders is called *behavioral medicine*. Health professionals in behavioral medicine come from many training backgrounds, including medicine, psychology, nursing, and social work. A related field, *health psychology* studies psychological influences on health. Both areas of study have grown considerably over the past 15 years. From this research, the general public has become much more health conscious than it was only a few years ago. It is probable that behavioral medicine and health psychology research will be used more and more in establishing public policy for the prevention of disease and improvement of the health of our society. From this process, improved psychological and physical health may become a reality in the twenty-first century.

REFERENCES

American Psychiatric Association (1980). *Diagnostic and statistical manual of mental disorders*, 3rd Edition. Washington, DC: Author.

American Psychiatric Association. (1987). *Diagnostic and statistical manual of mental disorders*, 3rd Edition, Revised. Washington, DC: Author.

American Psychiatric Association (1993). *DSM-IV draft criteria*. Washington, DC: Author.

Bakal, D. A. (1982). *The psychobiology of chronic headache*. New York: Springer.

Beck, A. T., Ward, C. H., Mendelson, M., Mock, J. D., & Erbaugh, J. (1961). An inventory for measuring depression. *Archives of General Psychiatry, 4*, 561–571.

Bille, B. (1981). Migraine in childhood and its prognosis. *Cephalalgia, 1*, 71–75.

Bixler, E. O., Kales, A., Soldatos, C. R., Kales, J. D., & Healey, S. (1979). Prevalence of sleep disorders in the Los Angeles metropolitan area. *American Journal of Psychiatry, 136*, 1257–1262.

Blanchard, E. B., & Andrasik, F. (1985). *Management of chronic headaches: A psychological approach*. Elmsford, NY: Pergamon Press.

Blanchard, E. B., Martin, J. E., & Dubbert, P. M. (1988). *Non- drug treatments for essential hypertension*. Elmsford, NY: Pergamon Press.

Buss, A. H., & Durkee, A. (1957). An inventory for assessing different kinds of hostility. *Journal of Consulting Psychology, 21*, 243–248.

Bussye, D. J., & Reynolds, C. F. (1990). Insomnia. In M. J. Thorpy (Ed.), *Handbook of sleep disorders* (pp. 373–434). New York: Marcel Dekker, Inc.

Diamond, S., & Dalessio, D. J. (1982). *The practicing physician's approach to headache* (3rd Ed.). Baltimore: Williams & Wilkins.

Eliahou, H. E., Ianina, A., Gaon, T., Shochat, J., & Modan, M. (1981). Body weight reduction necessary to attain normotension in the overweight hypertensive patient. *International Journal of Obesity, 5* (Suppl. I), 157–163.

Garrison, R. J., Kannel, W. B., Stokes, J., & Castelli, W. P. (1987). Incidence and precursors of hypertension in young adults: The Framington Offspring Study. *Preventive Medicine, 16*, 235–251.

Hauri, P. (1982). *The sleep disorders*. Kalamazoo, MI: Upjohn.

Hollandsworth, J. G., Jr. (1986). *Physiology and behavior therapy*. New York: Plenum Press.

Holmes, T. H., & Rahe, R. H. (1967). The social readjustment rating scale. *Journal of Psychosomatic Research, 11*, 213–218.

Irvine, M. J., & Logan, A. G. (1991). Relaxation behavior therapy as sole treatment for mild hypertension. *Psychosomatic Medicine, 53*, 587–597.

Jenkins, C. D., Zyzanski, S. J., & Rosenman, R. H. (1965). *Jenkins Activity Survey*. New York: Psychological Corporation.

Johnson, E. H., Nazzaro, P., & Gilbert, D. C. (1991). Cardiovascular reactivity to stress in black male offspring of hypertensive parents. *Psychosomatic Medicine, 53*, 420–532.

Joint National Committee on Detection, Evaluation, and Treatment of High Blood Pressure. (1984). *The 1984 report of the Joint National Committee on Detection, Evaluation, and Treatment of High Blood Pressure* (U.S. Department of Health and Human Services, NIH Publication No. 84-1088). Washington, DC: U.S. Government Printing Office.

Kales, A., & Kales, J. (1984). *Evaluation and treatment of insomnia*. New York: Oxford University Press.

Kaplan, N. M. (1986). *Clinical hypertension* (4th Ed.). Baltimore: Williams & Wilkins.

Kleinert, H. D., Harshfield, G. A., Pickering, T. G., Devereaux, R. B., Sullivan, P. A., Marion, R. M., Malloy, W. K., & Laragh, J. H. (1984). What is the value of home blood pressure measurement in patients with mild hypertension? *Hypertension, 6* 574–578.

Lacks, P. (1987). *Behavioral treatment for persistent insomnia.* New York: Pergamon Press.

Lichstein, K. L., & Fischer, S. M. (1985). Insomnia. In M. Hersen & A. S. Bellack (Eds.), *Handbook of clinical behavior therapy with adults.* New York: Plenum Press

Lindgarde, F., Furu, M., & Ljung, B. O. (1987). A longitudinal study on the significance of environmental and individual factors associated with the development of essential hypertension. *Journal of Epidemiology and Community Health, 41,* 220–226.

Linet, M. S., Stewart, W. F., Celentano, D. D., Zielger, D., & Sprecher, M. (1989). An epidemiologic study of headache among adolescents and young adults. *Journal of the American Medical Association, 261,* 2211–2216.

Lugaresi, E., & Montagna, P. (1990). Fatal familial insomnia. In M. J. Thorpy (Ed.), *Handbook of sleep disorders* (pp. 479–489). New York: Marcel Dekker, Inc.

Mellinger, G. D., Balter, M. B., & Uhlenhuth, E. H. (1985). Insomnia and its treatment: Prevalence and correlates. *Archives of General Psychiatry, 42,* 225–232.

Osborne, R. B., Hatcher, J. W., & Richtsmeier, A. J. (1989). The role of social modeling in unexplained pediatric pain. *Journal of Pediatric Psychology, 14,* 43–61.

Parkes, J. D. (1985). *Sleep and its disorders.* London: W. B. Saunders Company.

Review Panel on Coronary-prone Behavior and Coronary Heart Disease. (1981). Coronary-prone behavior and coronary heart disease: A critical review. *Circulation, 63,* 1199–1215.

Rose, R. J. (1986). Familial influences on cardiovascular reactivity to stress. In K. A. Matthews, S. M. Weiss, T. Detre, T. M. Dembroski, B. Falkner, S. B. Manuck, & R. B. Williams, Jr. (Eds.), *Handbook of stress, reactivity, and cardiovascular disease.* New York: John Wiley & Sons.

Sacks, O. (1985). *Migraine.* Berkeley, CA: University of California Press.

Spielberger, C. D. (1980). *Preliminary manual for the State-Trait Anger Scale (STAS).* Tampa, FL: Center for Research in Community Psychology, University of South Florida.

Spielberger, C. D., Gorsuch, R. L., & Lushene, R. E. (1970). *STAI manual for State-Trait Anxiety Inventory.* Palo Alto, CA: Consulting Psychologists Press.

Steptoe, A. (1981). *Psychological factors in cardiovascular disorders.* London: Academic Press.

Subcommittee on Definition and Prevalence of the 1984 Joint National Committee. (1985). Hypertension prevalence and the status of awareness, treatment, and control in the United States. *Hypertension, 7,* 457–468.

Taylor, C. B., Farquhar, J. W., Nelson, E., & Agras, W. S. (1977). Relaxation therapy and high blood pressure. *Archives of General Psychiatry, 34,* 339–343.

Waters, W. E. (1974). *Epidemiology of migraine.* Berkshire, United Kingdom: Boehringer Ingelheim.

Williamson, D. A. (1981). Behavioral treatment of migraine and muscle-contraction headaches: Outcome and theoretical explanations. In M. Hersen, R. M. Eisler, & P. M. Miller (Eds.), *Progress in behavior modification* (Vol. 11). New York: Academic Press.

Williamson, D. A., Ruggiero, L., & Davis, C. J. (1985). Headache. In M. Hersen & A. S. Bellack (Eds.), *Handbook of clinical behavior therapy with adults.* New York: Plenum Press.

Williamson, D. A., & Waggoner, C. D. (1986). Psychophysiological disorders. In M. Hersen (Ed.), *Pharmacological and behavioral treatment* (pp. 312–341). New York: John Wiley & Sons.

20

Organic Mental Disorders

Gerald Goldstein

Description of the Disorders

The organic mental disorders are not a single entity, but rather, constitute a collection of syndromes that have in common the fact that they are caused by some presumed or established impairment of brain function. They are basically brain disorders or diseases produced by pathological agents that may impair any organ of the body. Thus, the major known bases for the organic mental disorders are such processes as trauma, infection, cancer, compromise of cardiovascular or cardiopulmonary function, toxicity produced by metabolic or exogenous agents, nutritional deficiencies, degenerative processes of only partially understood or unknown causation, and genetic and developmental deviations. Some of these disorders are at least partially reversible, some are stable once acquired, and some are slowly or rapidly progressive. Inclusion of all of these disorders under a single heading has been controversial in medicine, but the intent of doing so was to systematically characterize the abnormalities of behavior these disorders produce. Thus, to be an organic mental disorder or syndrome, the illness must in some way be directly related to abnormal behavior. In that these disorders are all also neurological diseases, the disciplines of neurology, neurosurgery, and other neurosciences share an interest in patients with such disorders. Thus, the assessment, treatment, and management of organic disorders is typically interdisciplinary in nature.

Psychologists and psychiatrists have been interested in brain-damaged or -diseased patients essentially since the establishment of these disciplines. This interest has covered the lifespan, ranging from mental retardation and less common developmental disorders of brain function that are present from birth, through trauma that typically occurs during late childhood and young adulthood,

---

Gerald Goldstein • Highland Drive VA Hospital, Pittsburgh, Pennsylvania 15206.

Advanced Abnormal Psychology, edited by Vincent B. Van Hasselt and Michel Hersen. Plenum Press, New York, 1994.

into the systemic and environmentally acquired illnesses of middle age, to the degenerative diseases of the elderly. There have been extensive studies of the consequences of disorders of known cause, such as brain trauma, as well as extensive investigation to find the etiology of brain diseases of unknown cause, such as multiple sclerosis. The discipline that is mainly concerned with behavioral consequences of brain damage, and with the relationship between brain function and behavior in general, is called neuropsychology. Neuropsychology cuts across several professions, and while most of the people engaged in it are psychologists, there are many neurologists and psychiatrists whose work may be viewed as primarily neuropsychological in nature. These individuals are sometimes called behavioral neurologists or neuropsychiatrists.

The organic mental disorders are typically characterized as syndromes, and those syndromes generally concern cognitive processes. While brain dysfunction may alter essentially any aspect of behavior, the most pronounced and apparent changes are generally in some aspect of cognitive function. Thus, the description of the behavioral aspects of brain disorders and syndromes almost always contains some reference to impairment of one or more cognitive abilities. In the broadest classification, those syndromes are called mental retardation, delirium, dementia, and amnesia. In mental retardation, intellectual subnormality is present from birth, while in dementia, there must be evidence of a previously higher level of function. In delirium, attention is mainly involved, such that the patient cannot maintain a consistent response to external stimuli, and may show such signs as rambling speech, difficulty in staying awake, and sometimes illusions or hallucinations. Delirium is often a transitory state with a brief course. In dementia, there is significant loss of intellectual function in general, and it typically involves memory, abstract reasoning, problem solving ability, and other complex cognitive functions. In amnesia, memory is substantially compromised, with relative preservation of other cognitive functions. In cases in which the most prominent symptoms are not in the area of cognitive function, one may use other appropriate syndromal diagnoses, including organic delusional, anxiety, mood, personality, and personality-explosive type syndromes.

The significance of cognitive function as a core consideration in these disorders has been further emphasized in the draft criteria for the forthcoming revised diagnostic criteria for mental disorders to be issued by the American Psychiatric Association (DSM-IV) (1993). These criteria suggest the elimination of the term Organic Mental Disorder entirely, and its replacement by the term Delirium, Dementia, Amnestic and Other Cognitive Disorders. This change has been proposed because of the growing evidence that many of the so-called "nonorganic disorders," notably schizophrenia, have a biological basis. Consistent with this proposed change, the terms organic delusional, anxiety, mood, personality, and personality-explosive type disorders may be eliminated. The recommendation concerning the addition of the diagnosis of organic aggressive syndrome was not implemented. The replacement strategy is to diagnose dementia with predominant features that include delusions, depressed mood, hallucinations, perceptual disturbance, and behavioral disturbance. Another possibility is to diagnose under the new general classification Mental Disorders Due to a General Medical Condition. Within this category, there is the diagnosis of Personality Change Due to a General Medical Condition. This new diagnosis contains a number of types including labile, disinhibited, aggressive, paranoid, other, and combined. A limitation, however, is that this diagnosis may not be used when criteria are met for dementia.

One can also diagnose a psychotic, mood, or anxiety disorder due to a general medical condition, apparently to replace the various noncognitive organic disorders (e.g., organic mood disorder). Brief descriptions of the various syndromes and disorders follow.

MENTAL RETARDATION

Mental retardation is the commonest of a number of developmental disorders in which brain function is compromised at birth. Its etiology is heterogeneous, sometimes resulting from known (e.g., fetal trauma) and sometimes from unknown causes. It is distinguished from the organic mental disorders of adulthood, primarily because cognitive abilities never develop fully, as opposed to the situation in which abilities develop but are later impaired by acquired brain damage. Its severity may vary, but there is typically a course of poor psychosocial, scholastic, and vocational development which is familiar to most clinicians.

DELIRIUM

As indicated, delirium is primarily a disturbance of attention in which the patient cannot maintain contact with the external environment. Sometimes there are illusions and hallucinations, and sometimes rambling and incoherent speech. The sleep/wake cycle is often disturbed, and the patient may have difficulty staying awake. Delirium may occur after a head trauma or seizure, or may be the result of an infection or other systemic illness. The condition typically lasts about a week, and is reversible if the underlying cause is effectively treated or self-limited.

While frank delirium is typically treated in acute medical settings, the psychologist may see it in individuals withdrawing from alcohol (a condition popularly known as *delirium tremens* or DTs), or in elderly individuals with dementia who may acquire a superimposed delirium. This condition has been described as dementia with confusion, and can be described as meeting DSM-III-R (American Psychiatric Association, 1987) criteria for both dementia and delirium. The condition may be produced by intercurrent illness or sometimes by adverse medication effects.

DEMENTIA

Dementia is clearly the most common of the adult organic mental disorders. That is in part an artifact of the broad variety of conditions that the term encompasses, but efforts have been made in recent years to define it more specifically. In its broadest sense, dementia refers to loss of one's previous level of cognitive function as a result of structural brain damage. From this standpoint of course, there are three forms of dementia: progressive, static, and reversible. Dementia may be produced by a wide variety of causes, and the course depends upon the particular etiology. This distinction does not consist of fixed entities because as new treatments develop, some static and possibly some progressive dementias may be reclassified as reversible dementias, or a progressive dementia may become reclassified as a static dementia, if a treatment is developed that arrests the progressive process.

Onset of dementia may take place at any age, and if it occurs in very young children, is readily confused with mental retardation. It is recommended in DSM-

III-R that the diagnosis not be made until age 3 or 4, when the IQ typically stabilizes. Dementia most commonly occurs in children as a result of trauma, malnutrition, or infection. Trauma is the most common cause in adolescents and young adults. Dementias associated with genetic disorders, notably Huntington's disease, may begin during young adulthood. However, most dementias afflict the middle aged and elderly. Dementia associated with alcoholism typically becomes apparent after age 35, while the dementias associated with compromised cardiovascular status typically have their onset during middle age. The most well known dementias are those that arise at the onset of old age. Alzheimer's disease is the most common of these disorders. It is technically called primary degenerative dementia of the Alzheimer type because the original specification of Alzheimer's disease was made on the basis of examination of brain tissue rather than clinical phenomenology. The inexorable deterioration of memory and other intellectual functions produced by Alzheimer's disease is familiar to clinicians who work with elderly individuals.

AMNESIA

Amnesia, or loss of memory abilities, is a part of many of the dementias. However, there are relatively rare occasions when it occurs as an isolated symptom, in which case it is diagnosed as an amnestic syndrome. There are few conditions that give rise to pure amnestic syndromes. They include cardiac arrest, encephalitis, and aneurysms of the anterior communicating artery, but most commonly amnestic disorders are acquired by a combination of excessive use of alcohol accompanied by malnutrition. This disorder (also known as Korsakoff's syndrome or Wernicke-Korsakoff syndrome) leaves the patient with almost total loss of recent memory but with relative intactness of other cognitive abilities. The memory deficit is typically of such severity that it is totally disabling, because the patient is effectively disoriented by it. Thus, patients generally cannot give an appropriate estimate of the time, nor can they accurately identify their location. They may know their identity, but cannot give an accurate account of their life circumstances or recent history.

OTHER ORGANIC MENTAL DISORDERS

In these disorders, cognitive impairment is not the most prominent feature, although dementia or amnesia may be present. When this occurs, the most common changes are seen in personality, mood, and anxiety level. The most common personality changes involve fluctuations in affect, impaired social judgment, apathy, and recurrent, unpredictable outbursts of aggression or rage. When the latter change is most prominent, the diagnosis of organic personality syndrome-explosive type is made. It has been suggested that organic aggression syndrome should become a separate diagnosis. When an episode of depression or mania can be related to a specific organic factor, the condition of organic mood syndrome is diagnosed. The diagnosis of organic anxiety syndrome is suggested when panic attacks or a generalized anxiety state occurs, and that occurrence can be linked to a specific organic factor, such as an endocrine disorder.

As indicated above, this particular terminology is unlikely to appear in DSM-IV, primarily because of the proposed abandonment of the term "organic" syndrome or disorder. However, comparable nomenclature has been developed in the forms of the predominant features of dementia and several of the disorders due to a general medical condition (e.g., Mood Disorder Due to a General Medical Condition).

FOCAL DISORDERS

DSM-III-R does not contain a consideration of so-called focal disorders, or alterations of behavior that are attributable to damage to a specific region of the brain. These disorders are of great interest to neuropsychologists and behavioral neurologists, and their clinical and experimental study make up a great deal of the corpus of clinical neurobehavioral research. The interested reader is referred to clinical neuropsychology or behavioral neurology textbooks such as Heilman and Valenstein (1985), Walsh (1978), Kolb and Wishaw (1980), or Mesulam (1985) for overviews of this field. The assessment and treatment of these disorders are somewhat out of the purview of abnormal psychology and psychiatry, and are now largely accomplished by clinical neuropsychologists, behavioral neurologists, and rehabilitation specialists, notably speech/language pathologists and occupational therapists.

Without going into any detail about the focal disorders, we will simply provide some terminology and descriptions related to the more commonly appearing syndromes. Language is often specifically impaired by brain damage, most commonly by stroke. If an individual loses the ability to speak or to comprehend language as a result of damage to the language dominant hemisphere of the brain (the left hemisphere in most people), the condition is called aphasia. Thus, aphasia occurs frequently following a stroke involving the left cerebral hemisphere. Focal disorders may occur in the various perceptual and motor modalities. In these conditions, the modality itself may remain relatively intact, but the patient is impaired in using it in purposeful behavior. In perception, we call these conditions gnostic disorders, and in movement they are called practic disorders. Thus, the patient with visual agnosia may have intact vision but cannot interpret what is seen. The patient with apraxia can move his or her hand but may have difficulties with performing skilled tasks, such as dressing. Focal disorders also occur in the realms of attention, spatial cognition, memory, and executive or problem-solving behavior. These disorders may become quite complex, and require extensive neurobehavioral investigation to analyze. Ideally, they should not simply be characterized as dementia, since their treatment and management usually require an acquaintance with the specifics of the syndrome.

EPIDEMIOLOGY

The epidemiology of the organic mental disorders varies with the underlying disorders, and so is unlike what is the case for most of the other diagnostic categories in DSM-III-R. Here, we will only sample from those disorders in which epidemiological considerations are of particular interest. There are some exceptionally interesting and well documented findings for multiple sclerosis, in which prevalence is directly related to latitude in which one resides; the farther from the equator the higher the prevalence. Further study of this phenomenon has tended to implicate an environmental rather than an ethnic factor.

The epidemiology of head trauma has been extensively studied, with gender, age, and social class turning out to be important considerations. Head trauma has a higher incidence in males than in females (274 per 100,000 in males and 116 per 100,000 in females in one study) (Levin, Benton, & Grossman, 1982). It is related to age, with risk peaking between ages 15 and 24, and occurs more frequently in individuals from lower social classes. Alcohol is a major risk factor, but marital status, preexisting psychiatric disorder, and previous history of head injury also have been implicated.

The epidemiology of Huntington's disease has also been extensively studied. The disease is transmitted as an autosomal dominant trait, and the marker for the gene has been located on the short arm of chromosome 4. Prevalence estimates vary between 5 and 7 per 100,000. There are no known risk factors for acquiring the disorder, the only consideration being having a parent with the disease. If that is the case, the risk of acquiring the disorder is 50%.

There is great interest in the epidemiology of Alzheimer's disease since the specific cause of the disease remains unknown and prevention of exposure to risk factors remains a possibility. General health status considerations do not appear to constitute risk factors, but some time ago there were beliefs that a transmissible infective agent existed, and that exposure to aluminum might be a risk factor. While an infective agent is apparently responsible in the case of a rare form of dementia called Creutzfeldt-Jakob disease, that does not appear to be the case for Alzheimer's disease. The aluminum hypothesis has largely been discarded because of lack of confirmatory evidence. Recently, episodes of head trauma have been implicated as a possible risk factor for Alzheimer's disease. A reasonably solid genetic association involving chromosome 21 trisomy has been formed between what appears to be an inherited form of Alzheimer's disease and Down's syndrome.

Much of the epidemiology of the organic mental disorders merges with general considerations regarding health status. Cardiovascular risk factors, such as obesity and hypertension, put one at greater than usual risk for stroke. Smoking is apparently a direct or indirect risk factor for several disorders that eventuate in brain dysfunction. The diagnosis of dementia associated with alcoholism is now relatively widely accepted, although it was controversial at one time. Alcohol most clearly, and perhaps several other abused substances, make for significant risk factors. In some cases, the crucial risk factor is provided not by the individual, but by the mother of the individual during pregnancy. Existence of fetal alcohol syndrome is well established, and the evidence for association between birth defects and other forms of substance abuse during pregnancy is increasing. Until recently, risk of brain disease by infection had diminished substantially, but that situation has changed markedly with the appearance of human immunodeficiency virus, or HIV-1 infection, or acquired immunodeficiency syndrome (AIDS) dementia.

In summary, the prevalence and incidence of the organic mental disorders vary substantially, ranging from very rare to common diseases. Number of risk factors also varies, ranging from essentially complete absence to a substantial number of them. The genetic and degenerative diseases, notably Huntington's and Alzheimer's diseases, possess little in the way of risk factors, and there is not much that can be done to prevent their occurrence. On the other hand, such disorders as dementia associated with alcoholism, and perhaps stroke, are preventable by good health maintenance. Indeed, the incidence of major stroke has declined in recent years.

In this section we will concentrate on dementia, since it provides the most common picture clinicians are likely to see. Dementia appears most frequently in the elderly, and it is now thought that the most common form of dementia in the elderly is progressive degenerative dementia of the Alzheimer type (Alzheimer's disease). A recent estimate indicates that there are about a half a million people in this country with Alzheimer's disease. With the continuation of increased longevity, this figure will increase markedly in the future.

Since Alzheimer's disease is a progressive disorder, the clinical presentation changes as time goes by. It is a disease of insidious onset, and its earliest signs may not be recognized, or only recognized retrospectively. Most typically, the first sign is forgetfulness, which then merges into increasingly blatant impairment of memory. It is felt by some investigators that the first indication of the disorder is onset of a depression, followed by progressive loss of memory, but that view has not yet been extensively documented. It has been noted that as the disorder progresses, severity of depression becomes milder, ostensibly because the patient becomes increasingly less capable of assessing his or her status. As the disorder progresses other cognitive functions become impaired, notably abstract reasoning and language abilities. The language deficit may begin with word finding difficulties and develop into impoverished, sometimes incomprehensible speech. Eventually all mental abilities deteriorate to a greater or lesser extent, although basic perceptual and motor skills remain relatively preserved. That is, Alzheimer's disease, unlike other progressive disorders, such as Huntington's disease or multiple sclerosis, does not produce severe difficulties with ambulation or loss of sensory functions. Thus, the representative, middle-stage Alzheimer patient may be ambulatory, but will demonstrate obvious failure to recollect recent events, and may either speak incoherently, or coherently but with limited content. Names of objects and people may be forgotten, and spatial orientation may be significantly impaired. Gradually, names of very familiar people, such as family members, may become increasingly less likely to be recalled, and familiar locations will be forgotten.

The progression of the disorder has functional and psychopathological as well as cognitive aspects. Functionally, there is gradual dilapidation of self-care skills, and while social skills may remain relatively preserved, numerous problems with activities of daily living emerge, increasingly compromising independent living. As time passes, the need for assistance in performing self-care activities increases, and placement in a nursing home is often required during the end-stage of the disorder. Alzheimer's disease patients living with their families become increasingly difficult to manage, and the tragedy of the disorder for family members may become a significant clinical consideration.

With regard to psychopathology, Alzheimer patients may sometimes develop delusions, often characterized by suspiciousness. Agitation may also become problematic, and the patient may occasionally have an angry verbal outburst. Sometimes there is physical aggressiveness, without apparent stimulation. Possible environmental stimuli for these behaviors have been suggested, but it is unclear in any general way that agitation seen in the elderly is either completely endogenous or provoked by perhaps subtle environmental triggers.

It is generally reported that the course of the disorder from appearance of first symptoms until time of death is 5 years. However, with good family and nursing care, patients with Alzheimer's disease often survive longer than that. There is no effective treatment for the disorder itself, but it would appear that adequate health maintenance and support can increase longevity as well as quality of life through the duration of the disorder.

COURSE AND PROGNOSIS

Course and prognosis for the organic mental disorders also vary with the underlying disorder. We will review the basic considerations here by first introducing some stages of acceleration and development. Then we will provide examples of disorders that have courses and prognoses consistent with various acceleration and developmental combinations. The acceleration stages are steady state, slow, moderate, and rapid. The developmental stages are the perinatal period, early childhood, late childhood and adolescence, early adulthood, middle age, and old age. The acceleration stages have to do with the rate of progression of the disorder, while the developmental stages characterize the age of onset of symptoms. By progression we are referring in this particular context to changes in the disease process itself rather than to disability. It is quite possible for a disease process not to progress at all while disability increases dramatically, because of increasing environmental demands. It is therefore really necessary to view progression not only from the standpoint of neuropathology, but also from a disability perspective.

Mental retardation would be a disorder with a course involving onset during the perinatal period and steady-state acceleration. Mental retardation is one of those disorders in which there is little if any progression of neuropathology, but there may be a slowly progressive disability because of increasing environmental demands for cognitive abilities that the individual does not possess. Other developmental disorders, such as specific learning disability, do not have their onsets during the perinatal period but rather during early childhood when academic skills are first expected to be acquired.

In contrast to these disorders, stroke is typically characterized by onset during middle age. The acceleration of the disorder is first extremely rapid and then slows down, gradually reaching steady state. Thus, the stroke patient, at the time of the stroke, becomes seriously ill very rapidly, and this is followed by additional destructive processes in the brain. Assuming a good outcome, a gradual recovery period follows, and there is restoration of the brain to a relatively normal steady state. On the other hand, malignant brain tumors, which also tend to appear during middle age, progress rapidly and do not decelerate unless they are successfully surgically removed.

The progressive dementias generally appear during middle or old age and accelerate slowly or moderately. Huntington's disease generally progresses less rapidly than Alzheimer's disease, and so the Huntington's patient may live a long life with his or her symptoms. Head trauma is a disorder that may occur at any age, but once the acute phase of the disorder is over, the brain typically returns to a steady state. Thus, the head trauma patient, if recovery from the acute condition is satisfactory, may have a normal life expectancy with no dramatic pattern of deterioration following completion of resolution of the acute phase of the disorder. However, the degree of residual disability may vary widely.

Briefly summarizing these considerations from a developmental standpoint, the commonest organic mental disorder associated with the perinatal period is mental retardation and its variants. During early childhood, the specific and pervasive developmental disorders begin to appear. Head trauma typically begins to appear during late childhood and adolescence, and incidence peaks during young adulthood. Systemic illnesses, notably cardiovascular, cardiopulmonary, and neoplastic disease, most commonly impact negatively on brain function during middle age. Dementia associated with alcoholism also begins to appear during early middle age. The progressive degenerative dementias are largely associated with old age. With regard to acceleration, following the time period surrounding the acquisition of the disorder, developmental, vascular, and traumatic disorders tend to be relatively stable. Malignant tumors and certain infectious disorders may be rapidly progressive, and the degenerative disorders progress at a slow to moderate pace.

While the connotation of the term progressive is progressively worse, not all of the organic mental disorders remain stable or get worse. There is recovery of certain disorders as a natural process or with the aid of treatment. In the case of head trauma, there is a rather typical history of initial unconsciousness, lapsing into coma for a varying length of time, awakening, a period of memory loss and incomplete orientation called posttraumatic amnesia, and resolution of the amnesia. Rehabilitation is often initiated at some point in this progression, sometimes beginning while the patient is still in coma. The outcome of this combination of spontaneous recovery and rehabilitation is rarely, if ever, complete return to preinjury status, but often allows for a return to productive living in the community. Recovery from stroke is also common, and many poststroke patients can return to community living. Among the most important prognostic indicators for head trauma are length of time in coma and length of posttraumatic amnesia. General health status is a good predictor for stroke outcome and potential for recurrence. Patients who maintain poor cardiac status, hypertension, inappropriate dietary habits, or substance abuse are poorer candidates for recovery than are poststroke patients who do not have these difficulties. Some patients, particularly those with chronic, severe hypertension, may have multiple strokes, resolving into a condition called multi-infarct dementia.

The efficacy of rehabilitation in and of itself for head trauma and stroke patients remains a controversial area, but there is increasing evidence that rehabilitation may often have beneficial effects over and above spontaneous recovery. With regard to the developmental disorders, enormous efforts have been made in institutional and school settings to provide appropriate educational remediation for developmentally disabled children, often with some success. Effective treatment at the time of onset of acute disorder also has obvious implications for prognosis. Use of appropriate medications and management following trauma or stroke, and the feasibility and availability of neurosurgery are major considerations. Tumors can be removed, aneurysms can be repaired, and increased pressure can be relieved by neurosurgeons. These interventions during the acute phase of a disorder are often mainly directed toward preservation of life, but also have important implications for the outcomes of surviving patients.

FAMILIAL AND GENETIC PATTERNS

The organic mental disorders are based on some diseases of known genetic origin, some diseases in which a genetic or familial component is suspected, and some that are clearly acquired disorders. It is well established that Huntington's disease and certain forms of mental retardation, notably Down's syndrome, are genetic disorders. There appears to be evidence that there is a hereditary form of Alzheimer's disease, although the genetic contribution to Alzheimer's disease in general is not well understood. Whether or not multiple sclerosis has a genetic component remains under investigation, although it is clearly not a hereditary disorder like Huntington's disease.

Of great recent interest is the role of genetics in the acquisition of alcoholism, and subsequently dementia associated with alcoholism or alcohol amnestic disorder. Briefly, evidence suggests that having an alcoholic parent places one at higher than average risk for developing alcoholism. The specific genetic factors are far from understood, but the association in families appears to be present. Whether or not having a family history of alcoholism increases the risk of acquiring dementia associated with alcoholism is not clear, but it has been shown that nonalcoholic sons of alcoholic fathers do more poorly on some cognitive tests than do matched controls. The matter is substantially clearer in the case of alcohol amnestic disorder or Korsakoff's syndrome. A widely cited study by Blass and Gibson (1977) showed that acquisition of Korsakoff's syndrome is dependent upon the existence of a genetic defect in a liver enzyme called transketolase in combination with a thiamine deficiency.

Other genetic and familial factors associated with the organic mental disorders relate largely to the genetics of underlying systemic disorders. Thus, the genetics of cancer might have some bearing on the likelihood of acquiring a brain tumor, while the genetics of the cardiovascular system might have some bearing on the risk for stroke. Disorders such as hypertension and diabetes appear to run in families and have varying incidences in different ethnic groups. Ethnic specificity is sometimes quite precise (but this is rare), as in the case of Tay-Sachs disease, a degenerative disorder of early childhood, that is found almost exclusively in eastern European Jews.

DIAGNOSTIC CONSIDERATIONS

Neuropsychological assessment has become the state-of-the-art method for diagnosing the organic mental disorders. Patients with these disorders are often not amenable to structured diagnostic interviews, nor would an interview be an optimal methodology for determining the presence or absence of the various DSM-III-R criteria for the organic mental disorders. Before describing the various assessment methods, however, something should be said about the purposes of diagnosing the organic mental disorders, because they differ in some respects from those of diagnosing the other mental disorders described in DSM-III-R.

In the case of all disorders, the diagnostic process is concerned with whether or not a patient meets the criteria for a particular disorder or for more than one disorder. In the case of the organic disorders, however, it seems that there may be particular concern with whether or not the patient's condition is treatable and reversible. In view of the dismal prognosis for many of the organic disorders and the aura of pessimism that surrounds them, it seems particularly incumbent upon the diagnostician to consider treatment possibilities. Common examples in the literature are use of shunting to reverse dementia associated with normal-pressure hydrocephalus, and appropriate medical treatment to reverse or reduce dementias associated with various metabolic or endocrinological disorders.

Beyond the issue of treatment and reversibility, the establishment of the presence of an organic mental disorder often does not have the same heuristic value as may be the case for other disorders. For example, establishment of the diagnosis of attention-deficit hyperactivity disorder may immediately suggest a course of effective pharmacological intervention. Establishment of the diagnosis of dementia makes no such suggestion. Generally, one needs a great deal more information to make a reasonable attempt at management and treatment planning. One usually wants to know something about the kinds of deficits present and their severity, and about the presence or absence of potentially compensatory preserved abilities.

The task of gaining this knowledge is generally accomplished by a neuropsychological assessment. If the diagnosis of an organic mental disorder has not been established because of a difficult differential diagnostic problem, neuropsychological assessment may be helpful in answering the diagnostic question. In other words, it can help in determining whether the patient's symptoms are based on the presence of structural brain damage. Recent developments in neuroimaging have allowed diagnosticians to view the brain far more directly than was possible in the past, and so the role of neuropsychological tests has diminished somewhat in regard to answering the presence or absence question. A computed axial tomography (CT) or magnetic resonance imaging (MRI) scan has become a routine part of the diagnostic workup for an organic mental disorder.

In recent years, neuropsychological assessment has become increasingly involved in determining extent of deficit in various cognitive functions and describing patterns of impaired and preserved abilities. There are many neuropsychological tests and many theoretical approaches to neuropsychological assessment. Information concerning these matters will not be provided here, but may be found in the texts cited above. Here, we will provide a general outline of what a comprehensive neuropsychological assessment should contain, regardless of the particular tests used or theoretical approach taken.

General Orientation

A neuropsychological assessment generally consists of the administration of a series of individual tests or a group of tests incorporated into a battery. Typically, the tests are of the performance type with rare use of rating scales or self-report questionnaires. To be characterized as a neuropsychological test, a procedure has to have demonstrated sensitivity to brain dysfunction. In a screening or comprehensive assessment, tests are selected to evaluate a number of functions and abilities. There are also specialized neuropsychological assessments that concentrate on one or a limited number of abilities. Many of the tests commonly used, such as the Wechsler intelligence scales, have been borrowed from the general collection of available tests, but their use in neuropsychology is based primarily on research using these tests with brain-damaged patients. There appears to be a general consensus that the tests included in a comprehensive assessment should tap the areas of abstract reasoning and problem-solving ability, attention, memory, language, visual–spatial skills, and perceptual and motor skills. It is also often useful to obtain academic achievement scores, a general measure of intelligence (IQ), and a global index of severity of impairment.

GERALD
GOLDSTEIN

Reasoning and problem-solving abilities are often significantly impaired in dementia, and such impairment constitutes perhaps the major obstacle to engaging in adaptive behavior. Brain-damaged patients typically have difficulty in organizing varying items of information in such a way that inferences can be drawn in the form of concepts or abstractions. They are described as concrete, meaning that they react to the specific characteristics of environmental events with limited capability of generalizing from experience. Tests of abstraction and problem solving mainly consist of sorting tests in which the subject has the task of organizing varying stimuli according to a concept that has to be learned through exposure to the stimuli. For example, in a procedure called the Wisconsin Card Sorting Test, the subject has to learn that cards containing colored geometric forms can be sorted by form, color, or number of forms on the card.

Attention

While attentional dysfunction is the most prominent symptom of delirium, attentional deficits, albeit of lesser severity, are common in the other organic mental disorders. Brain-damaged patients may be distractible, disinhibited, or unable to maintain concentration. There is a form of attention dysfunction seen only in brain-damaged patients. It is called unilateral neglect and is seen mainly in stroke patients or patients with other forms of unilateral brain damage. The phenomenon is the inability to attend to either the right or the left side of space. Neglect is most apparent in vision, but may occur in the tactile or auditory modalities. Neuropsychologists generally test for neglect as well as for other aspects of attention with such tasks as repeating digits, discriminating between sound patterns, and performing psychomotor tasks that require sustained concentration.

Memory

Some degree of impairment of memory is seen in all of the organic mental disorders, but is most clearly evident in the pure amnesias, or organic amnestic disorders. For purposes of neuropsychological assessment, it is important to distinguish among several forms of memory, because the specific form of memory disorder found is often diagnostic. Thus, tests of short-term and long-term memory are usually administered, as are tests for recall of verbal and nonverbal material. Delayed recall, in which material presented about 20–30 minutes previously must be recalled, is a particularly sensitive neuropsychological measure. The Wechsler Memory Scale or some other short battery of memory tests is often included in a neuropsychological assessment.

Language

Impairment of language is less ubiquitous than is impairment of abstraction and memory in the organic mental disorders, but is commonly seen. It is seen in its most dramatic form in aphasia, and in the impoverished language of the advanced Alzheimer's disease patient. Aspects of language generally evaluated by neuropsychologists are verbal intelligence and basic language functions. Verbal intelligence is generally evaluated with the verbal subtests of the Wechsler intelligence scales (WAIS, WAIS-R, WISC, or WISC-R). Basic language functions are evaluated with one of the many available aphasia tests. As part of a comprehensive evaluation, a full aphasia test is typically not administered, but one of several aphasia screening tests is used. The basic skills usually examined are word finding; repetition of spoken language; comprehension of spoken and written language; ability to read letters, words, and sentences; ability to perform simple calculations; and ability to produce extemporaneous speech. Sometimes the language evaluation also includes the use of educational achievement tests.

Visual–Spatial Skills

Brain-damaged patients may become spatially disoriented, and may have difficulty finding locations without the assistance of verbal cues. More often, however, they have difficulty with forming or analyzing spatial representations such that they become impaired in nonverbal problem solving. They cannot construct objects in two- or three-dimensional space, and may have difficulty in recognition of spatially complex patterns. They often have difficulty copying even relatively simple geometric forms. Those who have used the Bender-Gestalt test may be familiar with the gross distortions patients may produce when attempting to copy simple geometric forms. Neuropsychological assessment makes extensive use of complex perceptual, copying and other drawing, and constructional tasks to assess visual–spatial abilities.

Perceptual and Motor Skills

Patients with organic mental disorders frequently have accompanying significant physical disabilities. On the sensory side they may be completely or partially blind, they may be completely or partially deaf, or they may suffer from significant losses of the senses of touch, smell, or taste. The stroke patient, for example, may have some degree of dementia, aphasia, and paralysis of the right side of the body. Multiple sclerosis sometimes produces progressive blindness. Neuropsychologists may do limited evaluations of basic sensory and motor status, but are typically more concerned with these functions at a skill level. Thus, in the case of vision, the interest would be less in visual acuity than in the capacity to identify objects or recognize faces. The important point here is that these skill-level deficits can exist in the presence of completely normal sensory or motor function. In the case of motor function, the patient may not be paralyzed but may be unable to pantomime or make pretended movements and gestures when asked to do so. Thus, a comprehensive neuropsychological assessment contains tests of a variety of perceptual and motor abilities such as ability to recognize objects by touch, motor speed and dexterity, and ability to identify or analyze simple and more complex visual stimuli, such as overlapping or ambiguous geometric forms.

Academic Achievement and IQ

Academic achievement tests are used for various reasons as components of neuropsychological assessment of children and adults. Some neuropsychological tests require some degree of reading ability, and it is therefore important to know

IV

Child Treatment: Introductory Comments

The growing awareness of etiologic factors in childhood disorders, combined with the burgeoning body of research attesting to their short- and long-term deleterious consequences, has led to a dramatic upsurge in clinical and investigative interest in remediation strategies for youth. Findings attesting to the magnitude and complexity of many childhood disorders have led to an increase in interdisciplinary approaches in this area. In particular, work in the fields of psychiatry, developmental psychology, and special education has had a substantial impact on directions that child treatment has taken in recent years. The chapters in this part of the book reflect the expanded and widened scope of endeavors directed toward the amelioration of childhood disorders.

In Chapter 21, Kevin O'Connor and Elizabeth Wollheim present an overview of psychoanalytically based interventions for children. They provide a variety of strategies under this rubric (e.g., free association, play therapy, transference) and discuss the similarities and differences between child and adult psychoanalytic therapy. The wide range of behavioral interventions is discussed by Mark A. Williams and Alan M. Gross (Chapter 22). These authors examine treatment techniques derived from classical and operant conditioning, observational learning, and cognitive therapy. They also highlight the importance of integrating approaches from other disciplines (e.g., developmental psychology) and emphasize the empirical evaluation of treatment effects. Pharmacological interventions are presented by Mina K. Dulcan (Chapter 23). Here, use of medications to treat psychiatric disorders, emotional problems, and behavioral symptoms in children and adolescents is comprehensively covered. Special considerations (e.g., choice of drug, regulation of dose, monitoring of beneficial and adverse effects) in the utilization of pharmacological approaches are discussed.

21

Psychodynamic Psychotherapy

Kevin John O'Connor and Elizabeth Wollheim

Introduction

The term psychodynamic is used in this chapter to refer to all forms of psychotherapy that derive from classical psychoanalysis as developed by Sigmund Freud (1938). Briefly stated:

> In classical psychoanalysis, a client presents with a *neurotic symptom* that is the result of *internal conflict* operating out of the client's conscious awareness due to the use of *defense mechanisms*. In the therapy sessions the client divulges material related to the areas of conflict, usually in the form of *free associations*. It is the therapist's task to organize this material in a manner consistent with psychoanalytic personality theory, and to offer her understanding of the client's personality dynamics to the client in the form of *interpretations*. Once the client gains *insight*, and then *works through* the material interpreted by the therapist, alleviation of the neurotic symptom occurs. The client is then free to choose to make behavioral changes on the basis of greater self understanding.

As can be seen from this brief summary, psychoanalytical theory and practice tend to be bogged down by a language all its own, which can seem intriguing at its best and undecipherable at its worst. The details of the model presented above, including definitions of the italicized terminology, will be presented in this chapter. The reader should be aware that the definition and use of many psychoanalytic terms vary from one to another psychoanalytic writer. What this chapter attempts to provide is an integrated, consensual view of the range of psychoanalytic and

---

Kevin John O'Connor and Elizabeth Wollheim • California School of Professional Psychology, Fresno, California 93721.

Advanced Abnormal Psychology, edited by Vincent B. Van Hasselt and Michel Hersen. Plenum Press, New York, 1994.

psychodynamic psychotherapies for children. In so doing some liberties have been taken in simplifying the material presented.

While all of the psychodynamic therapies developed for use with adults are derived from classical Freudian analysis, psychodynamic therapies for children generally derive from the child analytic models of either Anna Freud or Melanie Klein. These two fundamental models of child analysis differ with respect to the age at which the child is thought to be a suitable candidate for analysis, the role of the child's play in the analysis, and the way in which interpretations are delivered to the child client. In spite of these differences a general presentation of child psychoanalysis will be used in this chapter to present the range of psychodynamic psychotherapies now available for the treatment of children. Where these differences have had an impact on the development of the field they will be highlighted.

The chapter begins with a discussion of the psychoanalytic theory of personality development and structure that underlies the practice of child psychodynamic psychotherapy. An extensive discussion of the therapy process follows.

Personality Theory

Sigmund Freud's contribution to psychological knowledge and treatment is remarkably comprehensive in that he developed not only the psychoanalytic theory of personality development and functioning, but the treatment model that follows from the theory as well. Important components of his theory include models of: psychosexual development, the structure and topography of personality, and psychopathology. In conceptualizing the relationship between psychoanalytic personality theory and child psychodynamic therapy it is most important to recognize the developmental aspects of the model. Freud conceptualized two parallel lines of development. One line involves the child's progression through five psychosexual stages, and the other consists of the development of a balanced personality structure.

Psychosexual Stages

Psychoanalytic theory proposes that children progress through five psychosexual stages between birth and adolescence (Freud, 1905). Each stage is grounded through the anatomical or bodily focus of the child's instinctual sexual energies. It should be note that Freud used the term sexual rather loosely to include all bodily functions that give an individual pleasure. All such sexual energy was thought to drive individuals toward survival. This drive to survive was labelled *libido* and the underlying sexual energy is referred to as *libidinal* energy. Each stage also includes developmental tasks that must be negotiated in order for development to proceed optimally.

The first stage is called the *oral stage*, which lasts from birth until approximately the age of two. The focus of libidinal energy during this first phase is the mouth, which is biologically adaptive in that it focuses the infant on receiving nourishment. The most significant developmental task of the oral stage is the formation of a secure attachment to a primary caretaker(s). To the extent that this is achieved, trust is also developed, and the stage is set for successful negotiation of the process of separation and individuation from the caretaker as the child transitions out of the oral stage.

From approximately the ages of 2 to 4 years, children are expected to negotiate tasks associated with the *anal stage*, when libidinal energy is focused on the process of elimination. The major tasks of this period include the development of both internal and external control as well as *self-* and *object-constancy*. These last two terms refer to the child's ability to view herself and those around her as separate individuals with stable characteristics that endure over time. If development proceeds as expected, the child emerges from the anal stage with a rudimentary sense of autonomy.

During the *phallic* stage, libidinal energy is concentrated on the penis, its presence in the case of boys and its absence in the case of girls. It is during this time that the *Oedipal conflict* occurs. The Oedipal conflict refers to the period of a child's development when, it is theorized, boys hope to eliminate their fathers and keep their mothers to themselves while girls hope to eliminate their mothers in hopes of obtaining a penis or its substitute, a child, from their fathers. Boys successfully negotiate the Oedipal conflict by defensively identifying with their fathers and relinquishing their mothers as objects of sexual desire. Girls must abandon their fantasy of impregnation by their fathers and identify with their mothers in order to resolve the conflict. It should be noted that the female child's experience of the Oedipal conflict remains one of the most controversial aspects of psychoanalytic theory.

From the resolution of the Oedipal conflict until the onset of adolescence the child is in the *latency stage*. During this long period cognitive and social development are more prominent than psychosexual development. The tasks of this period include the formation of peer relationships, adjustment to major changes in body development and body image, and the development of new cognitive skills and interests.

Finally, at adolescence, the child enters the *genital stage*, where she remains throughout adulthood. During this phase libidinal energy is focused on the genitals. The primary task of the stage is the development of a stable, one-to-one, intimate relationship with another adult.

Personality Structures

Simultaneous to the child's progress through the psychosexual stages just described, Freud (1933) postulated that human behavior can be understood in terms of three psychological configurations or structures that account for all of human experience and behavior.

The first of these, the *id*, is the original structure, present at birth. Driven by biological forces, including libido, the id acts on impulse and operates according to the *pleasure principle*, in that it is solely interested in the gratification of basic needs, irrespective of external constraints. It is the domain of instincts, wishes, needs, and fantasies. Id-dominated thought is referred to as *primary process*. Primary-process thought is magical, grounded in imagery, based on internal rather than external stimulation, and unconcerned with the limitations present in reality.

Next to develop is the *ego*, which compels the id to work within the constraints of reality. The word ego, as originally intended by Freud, means "self," and is a shorthand way of speaking about the entire range of conscious mental functioning.

KEVIN JOHN
O'CONNOR and
ELIZABETH
WOLLHEIM

The ego operates according to the *reality principle*. It is dominated by *secondary process* (goal-directed, logical, reality-oriented) thinking. It is assumed that the ego begins to develop as the child separates from her primary caretaker because it is at this point that external reality begins to have meaning for the child. That is, infants do not concern themselves with reality so long as their id impulses are satisfied. As children separate they recognize that some of the sources of their satisfaction are external to themselves and that they must delay gratification in some circumstances. These realizations are the beginnings of ego functioning.

Last to develop is the *superego*. It is the internal representation of the traditional values and ideals of a society as reflected and imposed by the parents through rewards, punishment, and overt as well as unconscious communication. It is this structure that is colloquially referred to as the "conscience." Sigmund Freud and Anna Freud (1936) hypothesized that the superego forms as the child resolves the Oedipal conflict at approximately the age of five. On the other hand, Melanie Klein (1932) hypothesized that the successful negotiation of separation and individuation, which occurs at about the age of two, results in the child's development of a primitive superego. This superego is the result of the child's virtual absorption of an image of the primary caretaker, including all of the caretaker's rules and expectations, in order to make separations tolerable. In other words, the child's mental representation of the parent serves to console the child *and* to control her behavior in the parent's absence. The relevance of this theoretical debate to the treatment of young children will be discussed in a later section.

Personality Topography

In addition to conceptualizing the human psyche as being structured according to the tripartite model discussed above, Freud (1900, 1915) also developed a *topographical* or depth model. This paradigm divides the mind into the *conscious*, the *preconscious*, and the *unconscious*. The conscious, which includes everything in awareness at any given point in time, accounts for a very small portion of that which is contained in the mind or psyche. It has often been referred to as the "tip of the iceberg." The dominant portion of the psyche is the unconscious, which includes most id and superego elements. Thus, most behavior is driven and/or contained by forces outside of a person's awareness. According to Freudian theory, unconscious thoughts enter consciousness only in veiled or symbolic form. Finally, the preconscious, which is topographically located "between" the conscious and the unconscious, includes thoughts that, although not part of one's continuous awareness, can be easily brought to consciousness.

Normality and Pathology

Optimal functioning is evidenced when the id, ego, and superego interact in a delicate balance (Freud, 1923). The id pushes the child to seek to have basic needs and drives gratified, while the superego strives to direct the child to satisfy the id within the constraints imposed by her parents and society. When a conflict arises between the two structures, the ego mediates and attempts to find a realistic way to gratify the id within the constraints imposed by the superego. When a compromise is not possible in reality the ego uses *defense mechanisms* to circumvent the conflict in a way that allows the child to continue functioning. The term *defense mechanisms* refs to characteristic ways the ego has of distorting reality so as to diffuse a conflict. As the child progresses through her psychosexual stages she learns more complex and adaptive defense mechanisms. The ego of a young child is likely to use the defense of *denial*, where the ego simply refuses to recognize that a conflict or conflict-producing situation exists. For example, a young child may simply act as if her mother has not died even when faced with evidence of the reality of the event. The ego of an older child might respond to the same event with the defense of *projection*, where the child attributes her own pain to someone else, perhaps by talking about how sad her dolls are about mom's death while stating that she is not suffering. When older children use more primitive defenses it is considered diagnostic of serious problems.

Within a psychoanalytic framework psychopathology is generally thought to ensue from one of two underlying phenomena. *Neurotic* pathology is seen as resulting from conflict between the id and superego, which the ego is unable to resolve either in reality or through the use of defense mechanisms (A. Freud, 1926). The child then becomes overwhelmed by anxiety or comes to use defense mechanisms excessively and reflexively, resulting in the development of a neurotic symptom.

When the child begins to experience a neurotic symptom, *regression* or *fixation* becomes a possibility. This refers to the tendency, during times of psychological tension or distress, to revert to developmentally earlier patterns of responding. The particular developmental phase to which the child regresses is determined by the extent to which she successfully negotiated the tasks associated with each of the psychosexual stages. If the child was overly frustrated or gratified at a particular stage, she will continue to proceed through the subsequent stages, but respond to stress in a manner consistent with the stage at which the frustration occurred. If the frustration was so severe or the gratification so overwhelming that further development becomes impossible, then fixation is said to have occurred.

The other form of psychopathology noted in psychoanalytic theory involves the failure of either the ego or the superego to develop, due to environmental or physiologic interference. When the ego fails to develop, autism and/or childhood schizophrenia are among the postulated results (Bettelheim, 1967). The development of only partial or weak ego structures is postulated to result in such disorders as borderline or narcissistic personality (Kernberg, 1975). Finally, if the child fails to develop an adequate superego the child is likely to display antisocial behavior and/ or sociopathy.

CLIENTS

Inclusion Criteria

Neurotic symptoms and related regression is the type of pathology that is thought to be most responsive to psychoanalytic interventions. Anna Freud (1945) believed that children under the age of five, who have not yet resolved the Oedipal conflict or developed a superego, are unable to experience internalized conflict and subsequent neurosis. Therefore, pre-Oedipal children are considered to be unsuitable candidates for psychoanalysis, as are those who suffer from personality level pathology. In addition to the presence of internalized conflict, Neubauer (1978) suggests that children are suitable for analysis if the child has some verbal abilities and the parents are both willing to participate in the child's treatment and able to tolerate therapeutic gains leading to an improvement in the child's development. An additional criterion is the ability to establish a relationship with the therapist, which may preclude the treatment of children younger than three. This is due to the fact that, under normal circumstances, relationship skills begin to develop during the oral stage and become solidified through separation and individuation during the anal stage of development.

Melanie Klein's (1932) contention that children develop a primitive type of superego by the age of two led her to view very young children as capable of experiencing internalized conflict, and thus to be suitable candidates for psychoanalysis. Additionally, dynamic modifications of psychoanalysis, most notably ego psychology and *object relations theory*, allow for the *creation* and *strengthening*, as well as the modification, of personality structures in therapy. This opens up the possibility of treating children with more severe forms of psychopathology, which are thought to have their roots in earlier, that is, pre-Oedipal experience, and may be manifest by apparent insufficient ego or superego development.

Indications for Treatment

With children at different developmental levels, there are likely to be particular symptoms and manifestations of psychopathology, which we will briefly discuss below. Some behaviors or symptoms should be considered pathologic regardless of the age of the child in which they appear. For example, homicidal thinking would be considered pathologic in all children. Alternatively, some behavior or symptoms are only viewed as pathologic when they are not consistent with the child's current developmental level. For example, while extreme fear of strangers is very common and developmentally appropriate in 9-month-old children, it would be considered unhealthy in a 4-year-old. The same principle applies when one looks at the types of ego defense mechanisms used by children of different ages.

CHILDREN UNDER SIX

Children in this age range are most likely to present in therapy as a result of failure to meet developmental milestones. Examples of such departures may include a 2-year-old child who is evidencing extreme separation anxiety, a 3-year-old who is not speaking, or a 5-year-old who is not toilet trained. As opposed to the older child or adult who regresses to earlier ways of functioning in the face of stress, these types of presenting problems represent current fixations.

CHILDREN 6–11

When children enter the school system, parents are likely to bring them for therapy to address what they perceive to be peer-related difficulties. At the lower end of this age range children make the sometimes difficult transition from functioning only within their families to having to function in a large peer group. Because this is a new step in the process of separation and individuation, children who have been able to function previously may begin to manifest symptoms at this time. Depression is also a somewhat common presenting problem among school-age children, and because a complete personality structure should have developed by now, early signs of defects in that structure are sometimes observed.

ADOLESCENTS

Major developmental tasks for adolescents include achievement of independence and responsibility, and the development of their own identity within the context of family and peer group. Parents of adolescents are often concerned that these tasks are not being negotiated adequately, and are particularly worried about their adolescents' peer group identification. Adolescents often enter treatment secondary to these concerns and fears. Most adolescents present with symptoms of either behavioral or affective disturbances, particularly oppositional behavior and depression.

THERAPISTS

The theory of personality, psychopathology, and treatment underlying child analysis is remarkably complex, and a thorough grasp of all of the above is necessary in order to competently and ethically engage in its practice. Therefore, advanced postdoctoral training at an analytic institute is required (O'Connor, 1991). This level of training is not required of all therapists who adhere to one or another of the psychodynamic modifications as these treatment modalities are often less complex and intensive. However, regardless of the therapeutic modality one practices, it is still of great importance to operate from a strong theoretical base.

THEORY OF TREATMENT

Strategy/Cure

Theoretically, the task of psychodynamic work with children consists of two parts and is much the same as work with adults as it was described in the opening paragraph of this chapter. Initially, the neurotic conflict is brought to consciousness by means of interpretation. Once this is accomplished, the work of analysis involves reorganization of the personality structures to allow the conflict to be addressed in reality rather than through the excessive use of defense mechanisms (O'Connor, Lee, & Schaefer, 1983). If this work is successful, the optimal result is behavioral change and a subjective experience of no longer being "stuck."

Since the reorganization of the personality structures that the child spent years developing is viewed as such a labor-intensive task, analytic work has always consisted of high-frequency sessions conducted over a long period of time. The frequency of therapy sessions is one of the things that distinguish analysis from its psychodynamic modifications. Traditionally, both child analysis and adult analysis have, by definition, occurred daily, either five or six times per week. Some analysts, including Anna Freud (Sandler, Kennedy, & Tyson, 1980), maintain that the reasons for modification of this practice are extratherapeutic (e.g., financial or a matter of convenience for parents) rather than in the best interest of the child, and thus are not justifiable. Most psychodynamic therapists do not see their clients more than one or two times per week, which is considered adequate contact to do the work indicated. Similarly, analysts tend to continue their client's therapy for a period of years, whereas many psychodynamic therapists terminate therapy in a matter of months. This difference is largely due to the fact that psychodynamic therapies do not attempt to accomplish the same degree or depth of reorganization that analysis attempts.

Regardless of the frequency and duration of the therapy and whether the treatment is analytic or dynamic, the client's *free association* and *transference* provide the primary sources of material to be interpreted by the therapist.

Free Association and Play

Briefly, free association is a "talking-out" technique that involves the patient articulating everything that enters her mind without allowing her internal censor to screen out thoughts, feelings, or fantasies that her conscious mind considers inappropriate. Although to an outside observer the succession of articulations would likely appear random or even bizarre, the assumption is that there are extremely relevant unconscious connections amongst the sequential thoughts in the free associations. It is the therapist's role to recognize, make sense of, and ultimately interpret the repetitive patterns (O'Connor, 1991).

Not surprisingly, children often have cognitive and emotional difficulty in trying to free-associate. In response to this Melanie Klein (1955) viewed the child's play as the virtual equivalent of free association, and thus directly interpretable. Alternatively, Anna Freud (1926) viewed play primarily as a tool the analyst uses to develop a relationship with her clients. Hence, she saw the function of play as a preparation for the "real," that is, verbal, work of therapy rather than as the substance of treatment itself. Consistent with current practice in the United States, the model presented here tends to take an integrative position on this issue. Play may be used both for relationship building and as a source of symbolic content to be interpreted. Therapeutic play is not recreational, and although sometimes skills are attained, the purpose of therapeutic play is not primarily educational. Finally, play is not conducted for its abreactive value, although in cases of acute traumatic neurosis there is a place for abreaction (O'Connor, 1991).

Because play is such a significant part of therapy with children, the use of toys becomes important. Two important questions to consider are: "Which toys should be made available to the child?" and "How should the toys be used?" A discussion of therapy rooms and the materials used in child therapy provides an excellent opportunity to represent the wide range of approaches legitimately referred to as psychodynamic.

Within the context of traditional analysis, there is a split regarding which toys should be made available to children when they enter treatment, and which ones in subsequent sessions. Anna Freud (Sandler et al., 1980) discusses how, historically, a large number of very realistic-looking miniature toys were made available to all children, the thinking being that children would use them to recreate the issues most pressing in their own lives as well as to express their fantasies. Similarly, in treatment settings that employ a very child-centered, nondirective approach, all materials are available, and very few restrictions, if any, are placed on either what the child may use or the manner in which he uses them (Axline, 1947).

Alternatively, other analysts disagree with the notion of making all toys available to all children, believing instead that a few toys should be chosen for each child. Often the toys selected are those that are most likely to elicit material relevant to the issues being addressed in therapy; "in order to provide the most suitable way for the child to display what he cannot express in words." (Sandler et al., 1980, p. 127.) In addition, the therapist almost always has information about what is occurring in the child's life outside of therapy. If a client is hesitant or resistant to bringing that material to sessions, the therapist might provide toys related to that event. For example, knowing that her client responded strongly to having witnessed a fight between her parents, a therapist might provide obvious "Mommy" and "Daddy" figures for that session. This is very different from Anna Freud's view that the analytic situation itself pulls for enough regression, which should not be encouraged by the use of toys which elicit even greater regression.

Transference/Relationship

The importance of the therapeutic relation or *transference* is two fold. First, a strong relationship serves the function of sustaining the child through the inevitable stress of analysis. Second, the transferential aspects of the relationship, to be defined below, provide a vital source of material to be interpreted. Since she did not believe in the appropriateness of directly interpreting children's play, this was the focus of Anna Freud's (1926) work.

The term transference refers to a central component of the psychoanalytic therapist–client relationship. Sandler et al. (1980) define transference as *"the ways in which the patient's view of and relations with his childhood objects are expressed in his current perceptions, thoughts, fantasies, feelings, attitudes, and behavior in regard to the analyst"* (p. 78). In other words, when the therapeutic relationship evokes feelings for an important person in the client's life, and this client responds to the therapist as he or she would to that person, the client is responding transferentially. By strict definition, anything that is evoked by the "real" relationship between patient and therapist is not transferential. However, in most dynamic therapies today, the term transference is used more loosely to refer to any strong feelings or responses the patient has to her therapist.

Transference is considered by all psychodynamic theorists to be an extremely useful phenomenon primarily because it is usually more beneficial to observe a client's characteristic ways of responding than it is to hear such client tell you about his or her experiences retrospectively and in an inevitably subjective manner. However, even in the case of adult analysis, the determination of what is real and what is transference-based is a difficult one. In working with children, the issue of transference is both more complicated and, not surprisingly, more controversial (O'Connor & Lee, 1991). By definition, as we have discussed, transference responses are related to events and relationships in the patient's past, usually connected to the parents and the psychological environment of the family of origin. When adult clients respond to their therapists in a similar manner to the way they respond to their mothers, it is not difficult to point out and/or interpret the "unreality" of such a response. However, for a child, whose relationship with primary caretakers is immediate and currently developing rather than entrenched in characteristic patterns, it is illogical to talk about the "re-creation" of early, that is, parental, relationships within the analytic setting (O'Connor, 1991). Further, with young children in particular, all relationships with adults are characterized, *in*

KEVIN JOHN
O'CONNOR and
ELIZABETH
WOLLHEIM

reality, by dependency needs and a hierarchical structure. It is unrealistic to expect a child to see the "unreality" of treating the therapist in a parentified manner, particularly when the child's parents have participated in creating a caretaking role for the analyst. In fact, the child client's perception of the therapist as a caretaker or authority figure is accurate.

In working with a child client, a therapist is likely to engage in developmentally appropriate activities that would rarely if ever occur in the context of a therapeutic relationship with an adult. Some of these activities may be maternal in nature and will elicit or provoke both transferential and reality-based responses in the child. That there is a response at all is *not* transferential, but rather based on something very real that the therapist did. Conversely, the idiosyncratic nature of the response may indeed contain transferential elements. For example, it would be unusual for a child to fail to respond to being hugged or touched. However, assuming the touch is relatively neutral and in reality neither seductive nor threatening, it can be assumed that the child who responds by refusing to let go of the embrace, as well as the child who turns away in terror, is responding to something beyond the physical action of the therapist. There is clearly an element of transference in both of these responses.

The possibilities for the manifestation of transference reactions are limitless. However, certain types of responses are encountered with greater frequency than others in children. At various ages children are likely to respond to their therapist as a primary love object, as a parent, as a mirror image of the parent, or as a powerful and magical being. Any and all of these manifestations would provide suitable content for interpretation and therapeutic work.

Countertransference

The counterpoint to the client's transference is the therapist's countertransference. Perhaps no psychoanalytic concept is more controversial or anxiety provoking, particularly for a novice therapist, than the thought that her own intrapsychic issues may be unconsciously interfering with the course of her patients' treatment. The definition of countertransference offered by Chethik (1989) is closely aligned with the above statement, as well as with the traditional psychoanalytic meaning of the term: ". . . special feelings a child may elicit in a therapist that stem from a therapist's unique childhood experiences and his own neurotic tendencies " (p. 23). Generally, there is the assumption that countertransference is a phenomenon to guard against, and that strong feelings elicited by a client signal that something is amiss or inappropriately occurring.

Most psychodynamic therapists—those who work with adults as well as those who work with children—adopt a much broader and more balanced view of countertransference, and of the phenomenon of affective responses to clients in general. In fact, the emotions reported by child therapists need not signal the therapist's "latent neurotic tendencies," but rather be thought of as predictable, natural, and in many cases quite useful in terms of the therapeutic work. Some of the more common feelings that emerge with clients are overattachment, detachment, or anger toward the child, her parents, or others in her environment. Such countertransferential feelings can be useful in that they are, in most cases, reality-based and as such a good indication of the way a particular child is responded to by others in her extratherapeutic life. That is not to say that child as well as adult therapists and analysts do not have to be aware of the ways in which they bring their own individual, particularly childhood, issues into the treatment relationship with their clients. It is the rare adult who does not carry some unresolved feelings about their early life into *all* interpersonal relationships, and it is reasonable to expect therapists to strive to become and remain as conscious of the impact of such feelings on their work as possible.

Interpretation

Interpretation is the most powerful intervention used by psychoanalysts to help their patients bring unconscious conflicts to consciousness (O'Connor, 1991). Although this is the primary function of interpretation for both child and adult clients, interpretation serves an additional, preliminary function in work with children. To the extent that their verbal capacities are limited, much of what children experience and store in memory occurs in the absence of linguistic labels. It is thus difficult if not impossible for memories of these experiences to be retrieved using language (O'Connor, 1991). Interpretation can be a powerful way of providing verbal meaning to children's experiences.

Anna Freud (1928) and Melanie Klein (1955) differed in how they proposed to use interpretation in child analysis. Anna Freud believed that a child's ego structure was too fragile to tolerate deep interpretation. In fact, since the child's experience and conflict were all viewed as relatively recent and available, deep interpretation was seen as unnecessary. Alternatively, Melanie Klein favored the use of primary process interpretation, often directly labeling the child's primitive, sexualized fantasies from the outset of the treatment. This is considered one of the most controversial aspects of Kleinian analysis, as it tends to offend the sensibilities of most parents and even therapists in the United States. Beyond these two views there are various models of interpretation, as well as numerous systems for classifying them (Lewis, 1974; Lowenstein, 1957). The model presented here (O'Connor, 1991) integrates important aspects of various other classification systems.

LEVELS OF INTERPRETATION

The first level of interpretation in this system is called *reflection*. This differs somewhat from Carl Roger's (1951) use of the term. Rogerian reflections are generally simple restatements of the client's verbalizations or behavior. In the present model a reflection includes an emotional component that is added to the observation or paraphrase of the child's words or actions. Reflections serve three purposes. They help the child to label her internal experience, expand her affective vocabulary, and have an educative function in that they teach children that feelings are an integral part of therapy.

The second level is *present-pattern* interpretation, in which current and observable patterns of behavior are identified and labeled. Initially, only the patterns within session are interpreted. Later, when the therapist has gathered sufficient data, patterns of behavior observed across sessions are interpreted. Present pattern interpretations teach the child that her behavior is consistent and meaningful rather than random and arbitrary.

Simple dynamic interpretations move beyond the interpretation of behavior to making the explicit connections between affect and patterns of behavior, thus combining and expanding the two previous levels of interpretation. Simple dynamic interpretations are still limited to the content of the child's sessions.

Generalized dynamic interpretations "identify for children the operation of their personal dynamics across both in- and out-of-session behaviors" (O'Connor, 1991, p. 249). In addition to preparing children for the final level of interpretation, generalized dynamic interpretations assist children in applying the therapy process outside of the sessions.

Genetic interpretations draw connections between the child's current behavior and her personal history, and are the types of interpretations considered most useful by psychoanalysts. These interpretations are generally made after the therapy has been underway for some time and the child has been suitably prepared.

REGULATING THE IMPACT

Just as the therapist should gradually build up to genetic interpretations in order to maximize the child's receptiveness and diminish the possibility that she will become overwhelmed, the impact of interpretations can be modulated in various other ways. First, interpreting *within the play* by focusing on the dolls or figures the child is using can be significantly less disruptive or threatening than directly interpreting the child's behavior or feelings. Second, using *as if* interpretations, which suggest that the client's experience is common to many children, provides distance from the content and allows the child to feel less isolated from others. Finally, the impact can be limited by focusing the interpretations primarily on the content of the therapeutic relationship. In addition to reducing anxiety, this can be helpful in building therapeutic rapport.

Finally, interpretations must be conceived and offered according to the child's developmental level. The cognitive and particularly the linguistic abilities of the child will be the most important determinant of how much interpretive work can be accomplished in session. For children under the age of six, interpretation will need to be concrete and conducted primarily within play. Much of the therapeutic work may have to be done through activity and experience rather than discussion and interpretation. For children between the ages of six and eleven, a balance can be struck between language and action, depending on the particular characteristics and needs of the child. With most adolescents, interpretation will load heavily on language, with a minimal emphasis on play.

Working Through

In psychoanalysis, interpretation is followed by the principal work of treatment, a process known as *working through*. Anna Freud defined this process as the "constant reiteration of the interpretation . . . the elaboration and the extension of the interpretation in different contexts" (Sandler et al., 1980, pp. 182–183). If one thinks about how easily things slip out of the minds of adults, let alone children, it becomes obvious that a single interpretation, while potentially effective and even powerful, is insufficient to create any kind of lasting effect or change. Rather, change occurs as "patient's behavior and mental life gradually take in and integrate new knowledge and patterns of behavior as the process of working through proceeds" (Sandler et al., 1980, p. 182). Working through can be observed when the course of development is reestablished along expected lines.

If the above description of working through sounds elusive and difficult to grasp, it is probably because many practitioners of psychoanalysis have difficulty defining the process, and speak of knowing that working through is in process or has been sufficiently completed in very intuitive terms. However, some psychodynamic modifications view working through as a process of *ego-based problem solving* (O'Connor, 1991), or of finding an affectively satisfactory way of "being in the world." Again, developmental considerations are of paramount importance in structuring the experience for the child client.

The burden of helping the very young child work through her conflicts falls primarily on the therapist, who is often quite involved in working to change the client's real, that is, extratherapeutic, environment. While there may still be some environmental manipulation needed in work with 6- to 11-year-old clients, working through now begins to focus on helping the child to think about her interactions with family and peers. Group psychotherapy may be suggested for the child in this age group as a collateral activity aimed at furthering the working through of peer-related conflicts. With children older than eleven the process of working through resembles adult work, with the goal of fostering as much independent ego-based problem solving as possible.

Collateral Involvement of Parents

In adult treatment, the closer one is to the analytic end of the analytic–dynamic continuum, the greater the emphasis on preventing the contamination of the therapist–client relationship and the less likely it is that the therapist will involve anyone other than the client in the treatment process. In child treatment, such "purity" is neither possible nor desirable. It is not possible because the continuity of the therapy depends on the parents bringing the child to treatment and paying the bills. It is not desirable because successful child therapy necessitates the support of parents, and in most cases that means some involvement.

Anna Freud (Sandler et al., 1980) believed that the age of the child and the pathology of both the child and parent(s) should be considered in deciding upon how to involve parents. Contexts in which parents may be seen by their child's therapist range from a true analytic relationship with the parent as client to one in which the therapist provides didactic parenting skills training. Most psychodynamic therapies fall somewhere in-between these polar extremes, where parents are not themselves considered clients, yet are more actively involved in their child's treatment than didactic training implies. The more traditionally psychoanalytic the treatment, the less likely it is that collateral involvement will extend beyond the child's parents. However, more systemic therapists may involve other significant persons in the child's life, including members of family, and medical, educational, and legal systems in which a particular child may be embedded (O'Connor, 1991).

Confidentiality also affects the decision as to how to involve the parents, as information from both parties is received by the therapist at various points during treatment. It is of vital importance that an explicit agreement be made among therapist, child, and parents *at the outset of treatment* regarding the sharing of such information, and that the boundaries around this issue be clear and protected.

Termination

Given the central importance of the analytic relationship, the question of when to end analysis is obviously of great significance. Theoretically, the answer is quite simple: When there is evidence that the child understands and is better able to mediate the conflicts that brought her to therapy, it is appropriate to consider termination. Such evidence includes recognition by the therapist that the child has returned to an appropriate developmental level, and maintained the concomitant behavioral changes (O'Connor, 1991).

Unfortunately, in practice, the question of when to terminate is much more complex than this simple guideline implies. First, it is not always clear when the treatment goals have been accomplished, largely because treatment goals are often modified during the course of therapy. In addition, there are unfortunate circumstances in which a particular client and a therapist cannot work together, in which case all efforts should be made to smoothly transfer the child to another therapist. Finally, there are often external (i.e., extratherapeutic) circumstances that dictate the timing of termination, such as the therapist or client leaving the area, financial constraints, or parental unwillingness to continue to support treatment.

SUMMARY

This chapter presented an overview of psychoanalytic or psychoanalytically derived psychodynamic interventions with children. Because of the close connection between theory and treatment in the analytic paradigm, a review of the psychoanalytic theory of personality was provided prior to discussing the types of clients best suited to and the mechanisms of treatment. An attempt was made to convey the wide range of perspectives and practice in the field, despite the common heritage of Freudian thought. Additionally, reference was made on numerous occasions to the ways in which child and adult psychoanalytic treatments converge and differ. With regard to child treatment, a developmental frame was emphasized. Given the advances that have been made in psychoanalytic treatment for children and the expansion of the original model into a wide array of psychodynamic interventions in the last half century it is certain these will continue to be a dominant force in child psychotherapy well into the future.

REFERENCES

Axline, V. (1947). *Play therapy*. Cambridge: Houghton Mifflin.

Bettelheim, B. (1967). *The empty fortress: Infantile autism and the birth of the self*. New York: Free Press.

Chethik, M. (1989). *Techniques of child therapy: Psychodynamic strategies*. New York: The Guilford Press.

Freud, A. (1926). *The psychoanalytic treatment of children*. London: Imago Press, 1946.

Freud, A. (1928). *Introduction to the technique of child analysis* (L. P. Clark, Trans.). New York: Nervous and Mental Disease Publishing.

Freud, A. (1936). *Ego and the mechanisms of defense*. New York: International Universities Press.

Freud, A. (1945). Indications for child analysis. *Psychoanalytic Study of the Child, 1,* 127–149.

Freud, A. (1965). *Normality and pathology in childhood: Assessment of development*. New York: International Universities Press.

Freud, S. (1900). *The interpretation of dreams*, Standard Ed. (Vol. 5). London: Hogarth Press, 1957.

Freud, S. (1905). Three essays on the theory of sexuality. In J. Stratchey (Ed.), *The complete works of Sigmund Freud* (Vol. 7). London: Hogarth, 1957.

Freud, S. (1915). *The unconscious*, Standard Ed. (Vol. 14). London: Hogarth Press, 1957.

Freud, S. (1923). The ego and the id. *Collected papers*. London: Hogarth.

Freud, S. (1933). *Collected papers*. London: Hogarth.

Freud, S. (1938). *An outline of psychoanalysis*, Standard Ed. (Vol. 23). London: Hogarth Press, 1961.

Kernberg, O. (1975). *Borderline conditions and pathological narcissism*. New York: Jason Aronson.

Klein, M. (1932). *The psycho-analysis of children*. London: Hogarth.

Klein, M. (1955). The psychoanalytic technique. *American Journal of Orthopsychiatry, 25*, 223–237.

Lewis, M. (1974). Interpretation in child analysis: Developmental considerations. *Journal of the American Academy of Child Psychiatry, 13*, 32–53.

Lowenstein, R. (1957). Some thoughts on interpretation in the theory and practice of psychoanalysis. *The Psychoanalytic Study of the Child, 12*, 127–150.

Neubauer, P. (1978). The opening phase of child analysis. In J. Glenn (Ed.), *Child analysis and therapy* (pp. 263–274). New York: Jason Aronson.

O'Connor, K. (1991). *The play therapy primer: An integration of theories and technique*. New York: John Wiley & Sons.

O'Connor, K., & Lee, A. (1991). Advances in psychoanalytic psychotherapy with children. In M. Hersen, A. Kazdin, & A. S. Bellack (Eds.), *The clinical psychology handbook: Second Edition* (pp. 580–595). New York: Pergamon Press.

O'Connor, K., Lee, A., & Schaefer, C. (1983). Psychoanalytic psychotherapy with children. In M. Hersen, A. Kazdin, & A. S. Bellack (Eds.), *Clinical psychology handbook* (pp. 543–465). Elmsford, New York: Pergamon.

Rogers, C. (1951). *Client-centered therapy*. Boston: Houghton-Mifflin.

Sandler, J., Kennedy, H., & Tyson, R. (1980). *The technique of child analysis: Discussions with Anna Freud*. Cambridge: Harvard University Press.

22

Behavior Therapy

MARK A. WILLIAMS AND ALAN M. GROSS

INTRODUCTION

Behavior therapy with children gained impetus in the 1960s and 1970s, when principles of operant conditioning were effectively applied to the treatment of severe behavior problems in retarded and autistic children. These populations had previously been neglected, in that traditional treatments could not be effectively applied to them. These successes were followed by an expansion and acceleration of published reports demonstrating the effective treatment of numerous problem behaviors (Hersen & Van Hasselt, 1987).

Behavior therapy focuses on behavior–environment relationships. Behavioral assessment involves determining environmental contingencies supporting problem behaviors. The resulting "functional analysis of behavior" is used to design environmental manipulations in order to produce desired behavior change.

Early behavior therapists emphasized an exclusive reliance upon the functional analytic method and thus did not refer to sources of information about children from other disciplines, such as psychiatry and developmental psychology. This separatism was fostered by the difficulties that behavior therapists encountered in gaining acceptance of their treatment approach (Hersen, 1981). The radical rejection of contributions from other disciplines has gradually faded. In recent years, behavior therapists have begun to pursue information from other empirical disciplines. At the same time, behavioral approaches to evaluation and treatment have moved to the status of mainstream practice.

This chapter begins with a brief overview of issues to be considered when treating children, as well as with a look at some of the trends in child behavior

MARK A. WILLIAMS AND ALAN M. GROSS • Department of Psychology, University of Mississippi, University, Mississippi 38677.

Advanced Abnormal Psychology, edited by Vincent B. Van Hasselt and Michel Hersen. Plenum Press, New York, 1994.

therapy. The focus of this chapter is on the review of specific treatment procedures that fall under the umbrella of the "behavior therapies." Theoretical foundations, treatment considerations, and empirical findings about the use of behavioral approaches with children and adolescents are reviewed.

ETHICAL ISSUES IN THE TREATMENT OF CHILDREN

Children are seldom self-referred for treatment. Typically, parents, teachers, or other authority figures (e.g., a judge) identify a behavior they consider to be problematic and refer the child for evaluation and treatment. In many cases, the child is not consulted in the decision-making process about the need for treatment. Such decreased freedom of choice obligates the therapist to be keenly aware of ethical responsibilities.

No simple formula exists for determining the extent to which children should be involved in decisions concerning treatment. In cases of severe disability, such as profound retardation, or where the child is very young, it is relatively easy to conclude that the youngster is not capable of making a significant contribution. However, in the case of older children and adolescents without intellectual deficits, it is more difficult to determine the extent to which they are competent to participate in the treatment decision-making process.

The issue of children's competence to make treatment decisions has been empirically examined. After evaluating normal children's responses to several vignettes concerning psychological and physical problems, Weithorn (1980) concluded that 14-year-olds were comparable to adults in their understanding of treatment issues. Moreover, 9-year-olds were found basically to agree with the treatment decisions reached by the older groups, with the qualification that the responses were judged to be more immature. These findings suggest that often adolescents are competent to be fully involved in treatment decision making. Younger children as well should contribute to the decision-making process to the extent that they are competent.

Child therapists have a commitment both to the child as the identified client and to the parents. At times this dual commitment can elicit challenging questions over the issue of confidentiality. In some cases confidentiality between the therapist and child client may be considered necessary in order to facilitate effective treatment. However, in most states parents have the right by law to access their child's records (Ehrenreich & Melton, 1983). This problem should be anticipated and the therapist should address issues of confidentiality with the children and their parents prior to beginning therapy. An agreement should be reached among all three parties about the extent to which communications between the therapist and the child may be restricted from the parents.

DEFINITION OF CHILD BEHAVIOR THERAPY

The first behavior therapies were derived from principles of operant and classical conditioning. With the growth of behavior therapy numerous new interventions have emerged, many of which are only loosely related to principles of learning. Despite the broadening of the theoretical base represented within behavior therapy, behavioral methods continue to share in common a commitment toward the empirical evaluation of their treatments.

Most behavior therapists concern themselves with the assessment of three modalities of behavior: motor, cognitive, and physiological. It is assumed that problem behaviors across all three modalities are the result of faulty or inadequate learning and not symptomatic of some underlying intrapsychic conflict. Behavior therapists emphasize the role of the environment in the acquisition, maintenance, and modification of behavior. Identifying the functional relationship between environmental factors and problem behaviors is primary in the development of behavioral interventions. Although behavior therapists recognize that information concerning the child's past experiences may be helpful in suggesting possible stimuli that may be maintaining the current problem behavior, the actual focus of treatment is upon current behaviors (Ollendick & Cerny, 1981).

MULTIDISCIPLINARY INFLUENCES ON CHILD BEHAVIOR THERAPY

Developmental Psychology

In recent years, behavioral clinicians have begun incorporating empirical information about development into their clinical assessments and treatments of children. It is recognized that qualitative changes take place as children mature. An understanding of what problem behaviors commonly occur at various ages is necessary to determine whether or not intervention is warranted. For example, normative data on fears have indicated that as children mature, qualitative changes take place with regard to the focus of their fears (e.g., Jersild & Holmes, 1935; Lapouse & Monk, 1959; Ollendick, Matson, & Helsel, 1985; Scarr & Salapatek, 1970). As a result, the presence of fear of separation from one's parents in a 4-year-old is relatively common when compared to the prevalence of this fear in adolescents.

Although usefulness of establishing developmental norms for problem behaviors is recognized, this task is in its early stages of development. Achenbach and his colleagues (Achenbach, 1974; Achenbach & Edelbrock, 1978, 1979, 1981) have made a large contribution to this endeavor. Extensive normative data on children ages 4–16 have been collected using the Child Behavior Checklist (CBCL) (Achenbach & Edelbrock, 1983). The CBCL consists of numerous items addressing common problem behaviors and social competencies that the parent or teacher is asked to complete. Responses are compared to the normative data for a specified age. A profile is then generated that compares the child against the normative sample across a number of dimensions (e.g., depressed, aggressive). The CBCL can be useful as a clinical or research tool. However, limitations in the generalizability of the current data must be considered in each case. For example, the current norms do not include a wide sampling of children representing varied socioeconomic and ethnic groups (Underwood & Gross, 1989).

Recognition of developmental issues is also increasingly reflected in the development of behavioral treatment strategies. For example, knowledge regarding the development of cognitive and attentional processes is used to determine whether or not to expect that a child can benefit from a specific type of intervention. Behavior therapy researchers have begun evaluating the efficacy of specific interventions as a function of the developmental capacities of children at various ages (e.g., Sawin & Parke, 1979; Wurtele, Marrs, & Miller-Perrin, 1987).

Developmentally related changes in behavior problems also have implications for the evaluation of child therapies. When high rates of improvement in problem behaviors occur with development alone, it is difficult to determine to what extent behavior change can be attributed to treatment effects or developmental factors. Also, it has been suggested that over the course of development, symptom progression or substitution may occur. That is, a child's specific problem behaviors may change and become more relevant to his or her current developmental level. This possibility points to the necessity of obtaining long-term follow-up data using multiple indicators of adjustment.

Psychological Testing

During the developing years of child behavior therapy, standardized psychological tests were generally considered to be of little value. Instead, behavioral assessment that emphasized direct observations of behavior was considered to be necessary and sufficient in the evaluation of a child's behavior problems. In recent years, norm-referenced tests of intelligence and achievement as well as neuropsychological evaluations have gained acceptance as potentially providing additional useful information about a child's functioning (Hersen & Last, 1988).

Several articles have appeared arguing for the integration of intellectual and neuropsychological tests with behavioral assessments (e.g., Goldstein, 1979; Horton & Miller, 1985; Nelson, 1980). Intelligence and neuropsychological tests can in some cases be helpful in identifying specific deficits that may need to be the focus of treatment, as well as in serving as dependent measures in the evaluation of treatment effectiveness (Nelson, 1980).

Behavioral Assessment and Psychiatric Diagnosis

DSM-III-R (American Psychiatric Association, 1987) provided a much improved attempt at delineating useful classifications of childhood disorders over previous editions. As a result, child behavior therapists have begun to integrate this diagnostic system into treatment and research (Hersen & Ammerman, 1989). Behavioral assessment strategies continue to be viewed as invaluable for describing the specific characteristics of problem behaviors. However, the emerging view is that the two approaches should be used to complement each other. Hersen and Last (1988) proposed a "two-tiered" approach to assessment in which DSM-III-R provides the broad-based assessment, and behavioral assessment strategies provide the detailed assessment of target behaviors.

Hersen and Van Hasselt (1987) have presented the disadvantages of an exclusive reliance upon behavioral assessment as follows:

> Exclusive reliance on a narrow-band approach represented by sole reliance on behavioral assessment strategies that only focus on the immediate target(s) for intervention may yield an incomplete evaluation. That is, a narrow-band behavioral assessment approach frequently does not consider: (1) the etiology of the disorder, (2) precipitating stresses, (3) specific onset, (4) chronicity and past episodes, (5) severity, and (6) the complicated interrelationship of targets and symptoms that may be subsumed under a particular diagnostic label (e.g., childhood depression) (p. 8).

The use of a common diagnostic system allows for better communication between researchers and comparisons among studies. With recent increased acceptance of the DSM-III-R, numerous studies have emerged which have evaluated the effectiveness of behavior therapies for treating children represented by different diagnostic groups (e.g., conduct disorder, depression). Previous studies that have limited themselves to "idiosyncratic" terms such as "social skills deficits" to describe their treatment population have limited the potential relevance of their findings (Kazdin, 1988).

THERAPIES BASED ON RESPONDENT CONDITIONING

Respondent conditioning (also known as classical or Pavlovian conditioning) is the learning paradigm typically used to explain how physiological and emotional behaviors may be brought under stimulus control (Ollendick & Cerny, 1981). The basic model states that by pairing a neutral stimulus with a stimulus that produces an unlearned response (called the unconditioned stimulus), the neutral stimulus takes on properties that allow it to elicit a response similar to the unlearned response. Principles derived from the study of respondent conditioning have led to the development of effective treatments for many fear and avoidance behaviors.

Systematic Desensitization

Systematic desensitization was developed by Joseph Wolpe in the early 1950s. Since that time it has become one of the most frequently used behavior therapy interventions for the alleviation of anxiety and fears in both children and adults (Morris & Kratochwill, 1991). Systematic desensitization attempts to decrease problematic anxiety and fear by systematically associating the fear eliciting stimuli with physiologically opposing states such as relaxation. The treatment as originally presented consisted of three components: (1) relaxation training, (2) developing an anxiety/fear hierarchy, and (3) performing the systematic desensitization procedure.

The first treatment component involves teaching the child how to relax. Progressive muscle relaxation involves systematically tensing and relaxing different muscle groups while attending to the differences in the sensations of tension and relaxation. Unfortunately, most relaxation training scripts have been written for use with adults. When these are used with children they should be modified to reflect the developmental level of the child (Morris & Kratochwill, 1991). For example, Koeppen (1974) has incorporated fantasy statements for use with young children, such as "pretend you are a furry, lazy cat. You want to stretch. Stretch your arms out in front of you. . ." (Koeppen, 1974, p. 17).

It is generally recommended that relaxation training sessions should not extend beyond 15 to 20 minutes and that no more than three muscle groups be emphasized per session. The child is asked to practice the relaxation procedure several times until the child has demonstrated skill in quickly becoming relaxed (Ollendick & Cerny, 1981).

Assessment of the relaxation response is done primarily by observing the child's behavior during the relaxation exercise. Persistent movements, laughter, tension in the face, and excessive eyelid movement can be signs that the child is having difficulties relaxing (King, Hamilton, & Ollendick, 1988). The therapist may

MARK A.
WILLIAMS and
ALAN M. GROSS

need to model the particular steps in the relaxation process as well as provide some physical assistance in teaching the relaxation exercise (Morris & Kratochwill, 1991).

The fear hierarchy is developed by having the child and/or parents write down the specific situations or objects that produce fear. The feared situations are then arranged on a hierarchy from least to most anxiety producing. The therapist may assist in the development of additional hierarchy scenes such that the hierarchy represents a gradual change in anxiety-provoking situations. Anxiety hierarchies usually include 20 to 25 items (Morris & Kratochwill, 1991).

Once these two components have been completed, the systematic desensitization procedure begins. During the first few minutes of the session, the child performs the relaxation exercise. The therapist then begins asking the child to imagine vividly scenes from the hierarchy. The least anxiety-provoking scenes are presented first. The child is asked to hold the image for only a few seconds (until he experiences slight anxiety) and then instructed to return to a pleasant image while focusing on maintaining the relaxed state. Progression through the hierarchy is determined by the speed at which the child learns to imagine each scene with little to no anxiety. The process of switching back and forth between relaxing and fear arousing images continues throughout desensitization sessions until the child can imagine all of the scenes and remain relaxed (Morris & Kratochwill, 1991).

In recent years, *in vivo* desensitization has increased in popularity and is perhaps preferred to systematic desensitization proper in many cases. This technique involves gradually presenting the feared stimuli in the real environment while the child performs a fear-incompatible response (e.g., relaxation). This approach is more appropriate for children who have poor imagery abilities, or for youngsters who are frightened in the presence of the stimulus but not frightened by the thought of the stimulus (King et al., 1988).

Beyond the standard and *in vivo* systematic desensitization procedure, other variations of this treatment have been used. These include replacing relaxation with game playing, story telling, feeding, and physical contact. The imaginal component has also been replaced with such things as pictures and toys that represent the feared object (Barrios & O'Dell, 1989).

As an illustration of the clinical application of systematic desensitization, Van Hasselt, Hersen, Bellack, Rosenblum, and Lamparski (1979) provide an interesting case report on the treatment of an 11-year-old boy named Peter, who had multiple phobias. The assessment identified three primary fears: blood, test-taking, and heights. Peter's fear of blood resulted in dizziness and nausea while he was observing bloody wounds as part of health and safety films at school. This led to his removal from health courses. Peter's fear of heights and his test anxiety also produced observable difficulties.

Motor, cognitive, and physiological measures of the phobias were obtained throughout treatment. A multiple baseline design across behaviors was used to evaluate the impact of treatment. After this baseline evaluation, Peter was taught relaxation strategies. Hierarchies were constructed for each fear. Systematic desensitization was conducted for four to six sessions for each phobia. Fear of heights was treated first followed by the blood phobia and test-taking phobia.

The results demonstrated substantial improvements on the motor (e.g., approach behaviors) and cognitive measures for all three phobias. Decreases in physiological indicators of fear (e.g., heart rate) were less substantial. Treatment gains were maintained at a 6-month follow-up. Peter had returned to his health class and was able to ride tall amusement park rides (e.g., a ferris wheel); his teacher reported less observable signs of test anxiety.

Systematic desensitization procedures have been demonstrated to be effective in the treatment of fears and anxieties among children (see Barrios & O'Dell, 1989). However, the standard approach to systematic desensitization fares less well with children under the age of nine. This is likely due to the fact that younger children find it more difficult to maintain a relaxed state for extended periods of time, they tend to display difficulty focusing attention toward imagined situations, and they may have less motivation for treatment than older children (Morris & Kratochwill, 1991).

Flooding

Flooding procedures differ from systematic desensitization in that in flooding, the child experiences prolonged exposure (imaginally or directly) to the most intense aspects of the feared situation early in treatment (Barrios & O'Dell, 1989). The length of exposure is determined by the child's responses. It is usually recommended that escape from the feared situation be prevented and that exposure continue until the fear response decreases and the child is able to remain calm. Flooding is based upon the principle of extinction. That is, exposure to the feared stimulus (conditioned stimulus) in the absence of the unconditioned stimulus will result in decreased ability of the feared stimulus to elicit a fear response (conditioned response).

Four variations of the flooding paradigm have been presented in the treatment literature. "Imaginal flooding" involves the creation of a fear hierarchy like that developed as part of the systematic desensitization procedure. However, in imaginal flooding the child is asked to begin the process by imagining an anxiety-producing scene that had been ranked about midway down the hierarchy. The child is asked to continue imagining the anxiety-producing scenes until little to no fear remains. "In vivo flooding" involves having the child face the feared object or situation, without escape, until the fear response diminishes. "Implosion" is similar to imaginal flooding except that in implosion the child is asked to imagine an exaggerated version of the feared object or situation. The child is asked to continue until he or she is no longer bothered by it. Finally, in "reinforced practice" the child is rewarded for staying in the presence of a feared stimulus for exceedingly longer periods of time (Barrios & O'Dell, 1989).

Kolko (1984) provides an example of the use of in vivo flooding in the treatment of a 16-year-old female with panic attacks and agoraphobia. The youngster began experiencing panic attacks, and worries centered around physical harm and death, following the sudden death of her grandfather. As these worsened she severely restricted her activities, became very uncomfortable when left alone, and required the company of others when leaving her home.

Behavioral assessment identified 10 phobic situations. These included: walking outside in the dark, sitting alone in the basement, walking through a cemetery, watching a scary movie, and viewing a dead body. The youth was instructed to expose herself to the phobic situations over a period of 3 weeks. She was encouraged to stay in the phobic situations for extended periods of time. In order to insure that she was exposed to the aversive cognitive aspects as well (e.g., thoughts of death), she was instructed to intentionally exaggerate these cognitions during the exposure episodes. The youth monitored her anxiety during each exposure trial and her mother monitored her exposure sessions unobtrusively. The procedure led to rapid decreases in anxiety and avoidance behaviors. At the 3- and 9-month follow-up, she continued to be capable of performing all 10 phobic tasks without difficulty, and she reported reductions in general levels of anxiety.

Few experimental studies have been completed evaluating the effectiveness of these procedures for reducing fears and anxieties in children. Case studies have demonstrated effective outcomes and have generally shown good maintenance of treatment effects (see Barrios & O'Dell, 1989). The relative deficit in experimental studies of treatments involving prolonged exposures (i.e., relative to the wealth of studies on systematic desensitization) is partly due to the poor acceptability of these treatments among therapists, parents, and children (e.g., King & Gullone, 1990). Most child behavior therapists prefer to use these procedures only if less aversive interventions are determined to be ineffective or undesirable.

Flooding procedures may be a preferred first treatment when relatively rapid extinction of fear is critical. For example, a child with a strong fear of needles who requires a blood test for an important medical evaluation is in a situation in which the potential swifter effects of flooding may make this the treatment of choice. Ethical considerations about the use of flooding with children is more complicated than with adults. Whereas adults can chose to escape an aversive situation elicited by the flooding procedure, children have less freedom to do so.

THERAPIES BASED ON OPERANT CONDITIONING

The classical conditioning model has been useful in demonstrating how "involuntary" behaviors such as physiological or emotional reactions can be learned and unlearned. However, the majority of human responding is not a reflexive reaction to environmental stimuli. Most behavior appears to be goal directed. B. F. Skinner called these behaviors *operants*. Operants are behaviors that are altered (with regard to future occurrences) by the consequences they produce. Therapies based upon operant procedures form the foundation of child behavior therapy. The basic operant procedure involves identifying the environmental factors that support target behaviors. Intervention involves systematically arranging the antecedents and consequences of these behaviors in an attempt to alter their probability of occurrence.

Positive Reinforcement

A wealth of research on the use of positive reinforcement has been conducted. Reports demonstrating the effective use of positive reinforcement across numerous target behaviors and settings have pushed reinforcement therapies into the status of being almost a necessary, if not sufficient, therapeutic approach for changing behavior in children (Masters, Burish, Hollon, & Rimm, 1987).

Positive reinforcement involves the delivery of a reinforcer, following the performance of a desired behavior. Reinforcers are identified empirically by observing changes in the target behaviors when the delivery of a stimulus is made contingent upon the performance of the response. If the delivery of a stimulus following a behavior results in an increase in the future occurrence of that behavior, then by definition the stimulus is a reinforcer.

Several variations of positive reinforcement have been described in the literature. However, there are three basic methods commonly used (Matson & Coe, 1991). The first approach involves providing the child with a primary (e.g., food) or social (e.g., praise) reinforcer immediately following the performance of a target response. Secondly, token reinforcers that can be traded for desired objects or privileges are commonly used to increase appropriate behavior. Finally, "differential reinforcement" of behaviors incompatible with undesirable behaviors may be used to decrease the occurrence of undesirable behaviors.

Sometimes the child does not possess a desired behavior in his or her behavioral repertoire. In this case, a reinforcement procedure called "shaping" is appropriate. Shaping is a process in which components of the desired response are systematically taught. Reinforcement is provided to the child, following the performance of a response that approximates the desired goal behavior. Systematically, the performance criteria required to obtain the reinforcer are altered until eventually the child performs the target behavior accurately and consistently. Despite the fact that shaping procedures have been used frequently, there is little research to guide behavior therapists about the optimal speed at which to progress through a shaping procedure. Most researchers have recommended that an 80 to 100% reinforcement-to-attempts ratio be met prior to changing the performance criteria (Ollendick & Cerny, 1981).

Mizes (1985) provides an interesting case example of the use of positive reinforcement to treat a conversion disorder in a 13-year-old girl named Jane. Jane was bedridden due to reported low-back pain and an inability to bend at the waist. Jane's difficulties began 5 months prior to treatment, when she underwent a painful lumbar puncture diagnostic procedure. Examinations by numerous physicians found no evidence of organic pathology that could explain the symptoms. Psychological treatments had been attempted without success by several mental health professionals prior to the behavioral intervention.

Treatment was evaluated using a multiple baseline design across behaviors. Target behaviors included stomach contractions during biofeedback sessions, raising her legs, and mobility behaviors (e.g., back-bending exercises, sitting correctly in a chair). Treatment consisted of providing Jane with visiting time with her parents (social reinforcement) contingent upon meeting performance criteria for the target behaviors. Stomach contractions were the first target behaviors placed under the reinforcement contingencies. Across treatment sessions, performance criteria were gradually increased. As treatment continued, leg-raising and mobility behaviors were systematically incorporated into the reinforcement program.

The contingent use of parental visits resulted in steady improvements in target behaviors. Two weeks after discharge from the hospital, parent reports indicated that Jane was doing well. Unfortunately, at 4 weeks posttreatment Jane developed a respiratory infection and was hospitalized. She again began complaining about back pains. The 1-year follow-up indicated that Jane had entered a behaviorally based pain clinic and had successfully responded to treatment.

Research has revealed that the immediacy of reinforcer delivery, magnitude of the reinforcer, and the schedule of reinforcement are factors that influence the effectiveness of positive reinforcement. Small reinforcers that can be delivered frequently and immediately following the target response are more effective in controlling behavior than large, delayed reinforcers. Also, when reinforcement contingencies are first established, the therapist should attempt to provide the reinforcer after each occurrence of the target response (continuous reinforcement). After the target behavior has been substantially increased, the therapist will generally begin providing the reinforcer intermittently.

Punishment

Whereas positive reinforcement is used to increase the occurrence of desirable behaviors, punishment procedures are used to decrease undesirable behaviors. Punishment procedures involve the delivery or removal of specific stimuli contingent upon the occurrence of undesirable behaviors. Punishers can include a variety of stimuli ranging from what would generally be considered nonaversive to extremely aversive.

The decision to use punishment procedures should be made only after reinforcement procedures have been considered and it has been determined that more aversive procedures are the appropriate treatment choice. Some therapists have recommended that a hierarchy of interventions be followed in which the therapist first attempts to reduce problem behaviors by using nonaversive and minimally restrictive procedures. After evaluating the effectiveness of these procedures, the therapist decides whether or not aversive procedures may be required. This approach to therapeutic decision making seems appropriate when dealing with behaviors that are considered problematic yet not extremely dangerous to the child or to others. In cases in which quick suppression of a threatening behavior is needed, aversive procedures may be the treatment of first choice. This is not to imply that severe behavior problems always require the use of aversive procedures. The point is that the decision-making process regarding how to make changes in a problem behavior should primarily be determined by the information gained from a complete assessment and not by a generic instruction to proceed through a specific treatment hierarchy.

Punishment procedures have been divided into two categories. The first type involves the removal of a rewarding stimulus contingent upon the occurrence of undesirable behavior. Response cost and time out are examples of this type of punishment. The second type involves delivery of an aversive consequence contingent upon the occurrence of the undesirable response. Overcorrection and physical punishment are examples of this type of punishment.

Response cost involves removal of a positive reinforcer following display of an undesirable behavior. Response cost has frequently been used to decrease aggressive and disruptive behavior (Ollendick & Cerny, 1981). However, response cost components are commonly included in treatment packages covering the whole gamut of childhood problems. In order for response cost to be an appropriate intervention, it is necessary that the child have a number of reinforcing possessions or activities that can be contingently removed.

Time out involves making positive reinforcers unavailable to a child for a specified period of time. This is generally achieved by removing the child from a reinforcing environment (e.g., placing the child in another room). In this approach, it is important that the child have very limited opportunities for reinforcement in the time out room.

Overcorrection is a punishment procedure in which the child is made to practice "overly" correct forms of appropriate behaviors contingent upon the occurrence of inappropriate behaviors. "Restitution" and "positive practice" are the two types of overcorrection commonly described. In restitution, the child is made to correct environmental disturbances created by the inappropriate behavior. For example, a child's aggressive outburst may lead to the throwing of a garbage can full of trash all over the playground. The child is then made to pick up the trash he spilled, as well as the rest of the trash on the playground.

In positive practice, the child is made to repeat (several times) behaviors that are incompatible with the inappropriate behavior. For example, a child who hits himself in the face with his fist may be made to repeat alternative arm movements directed away from the face.

Occasionally, physical punishment procedures are used to eliminate or decrease problem behaviors. These punishers have included electric shocks, lemon juice applied in the mouth, water mist to the face, and a visual screen. Ethical considerations require that these procedures be used only when less aversive procedures are ineffective.

Barrett, McGonigle, Ackles, and Burkhart (1987) provide an illustrative case of the use of punishment procedures to suppress high-frequency aerophagia in a 5-year-old, profoundly retarded girl. Aerophagia is typically regarded as a form of stereotypic behavior. It is characterized by the intentional swallowing of air followed by breath holding for several seconds. Assessment of this child indicated that aerophagic responses occurred in excess of 1000 times per day. Radiologic studies indicated the presence of distension in the stomach and upper intestine due to excessive air swallowing. Following collection of baseline levels of aerophagic responses, an alternating treatment design was used to evaluate the effectiveness of several interventions. Differential reinforcement of nonaerophagic behaviors, response cost, and visual screening when evaluated separately did not produce significant suppression of aerophagia. However, a treatment package consisting of an auditory cue, gentle nose occlusion (nose pinch), and visual screening (covering her eyes with experimenter's hand) when used contingent upon the initiation of the aerophagic response was effective in suppressing this behavior to near-zero levels during the laboratory sessions. Treatment effects generalized to the child's classroom and residential facility. Radiologic follow-up studies indicated that the subject's gastrointestinal structure returned to normal.

Although a large number of studies have demonstrated the effectiveness of punishment procedures, negative side effects occasionally occur (Kazdin, 1989). A consideration of these is imperative when evaluating the desirability of such procedures. Responses such as crying, anger, aggressiveness, and avoidance behaviors (e.g., lying, apathy) have been reported (e.g., Becker, 1971; Matson & Ollendick, 1977). Also, individuals (e.g., parents or teachers) who dispense the aversive consequences run the risk of becoming less desirable and nonreinforcing to the child (e.g., Morris & Redd, 1975). By combining positive reinforcement for appropriate behaviors with punishment procedures, the probability of negative side effects can be decreased (e.g., Carey & Bucher, 1986).

Extinction

Another procedure used to reduce the frequency of undesirable behaviors is extinction. Extinction involves intentionally withholding the reinforcers that are believed to be maintaining an undesirable response. Extinction is part of most behavior treatment programs even when not explicitly stated. For example, in a positive reinforcement program, a child is selectively reinforced for desired behaviors, while undesirable responses are ignored.

Several factors have been discussed with regard to the efficacy of extinction procedures. It is important that the reinforcers maintaining the problem behaviors be accurately identified. This is best determined by observing the problem behavior while systematically withholding specific consequences. When reductions or increases in the behavior are observed contingent upon such a manipulation (e.g., teacher's attention), then it is assumed that these consequences are responsible for maintaining the problem behavior. Unfortunately, identifying reinforcers can be difficult. For example, if the problem behavior is maintained on an intermittent schedule of reinforcement, then numerous observations may be required before the maintaining reinforcers can be identified (Kazdin, 1989). Moreover, different reinforcers may maintain the same problem behavior across different settings.

Reinforcers must be consistently withheld in order for extinction to occur. Controlling reinforcers can be difficult, even in a relatively controlled environment. For example, in a classroom, peers may inadvertently provide social reinforcers for a child's problem behaviors. As such, treatment must involve prompting the teacher and students to ignore inappropriate responses.

The schedule of reinforcement on which the problem behavior has been maintained affects the extinction process. Behaviors maintained on a "thin" schedule of intermittent reinforcement are highly resistant to extinction.

Application of extinction procedures frequently results in a relatively brief increase in frequency and/or severity of target response. Such increased responding is referred to as an "extinction burst." With continued withholding of reinforcement, this burst of problem behaviors is expected to subside.

The withholding of reinforcement may produce negative emotional responses, such as crying, frustration, and aggression (e.g., Rekers & Lovaas, 1974). By using positive reinforcement for appropriate behaviors in conjunction with extinction, one can minimize the probability of negative side effects (Kazdin, 1989).

"Spontaneous recovery" refers to a phenomenon in which behaviors eliminated by extinction recur. These behaviors quickly drop out if they are not followed by further reinforcement. However, if reinforcement follows the behaviors, they will become increasingly resistant to extinction.

Mansdorf (1981) provides an interesting case example of the use of extinction combined with positive reinforcement.

> Ann was an 8-year-old girl who was referred for treatment by her pediatrician due to frequent complaints of headaches and stomach aches. Medical examinations failed to find an organic basis for her symptom reports.
> Based on a functional analysis suggesting that Ann's physical complaints were being maintained by her mother's attention, an extinction procedure was initiated. Ann's mother was instructed to ignore Ann's physical complaints. At the same time, Ann's mother was instructed to increase the amount of positive attention she gave Ann for performing appropriate behaviors. With the initiation of these contingencies, rapid decreases in somatic complaints occurred. Behavioral gains were maintained at the 2-year follow-up.

The successful application of extinction has been demonstrated across a wide range of problem behaviors, including complaining, vomiting, excessive speech, and tantrums (Kazdin, 1984). Extinction may be useful in situations in which the problem behavior appears to be maintained by easily identified and controlled reinforcers. The addition of a positive reinforcement component can help to establish more appropriate behaviors and may lessen the potential problematic side effects of extinction. Extinction is not recommended for dangerous behaviors, given the gradual nature of response elimination it produces (Kazdin, 1984).

Contingency Management

Contingency management involves the use of a combination of operant methods, including reinforcement, extinction, and punishment procedures. Target behaviors are identified and treatment mediators (e.g., parents, teachers, peers) are trained in the systematic use of these methods.

Contingency contracting is a contingency management procedure in which the child and the parents indicate the consequences of specific behaviors in a written contract. Contingency contracts have been used for a variety of problem behaviors, including parent–child conflicts, studying problems, and weight control.

Five criteria for developing effective contingency contracts have been suggested (Stuart, 1971). First, the contract should specifically explain what rewards or privileges the child can obtain. Second, the behaviors that are required to obtain the rewards must be made very specific. Vague descriptions of the required behaviors may lead to disagreement between the child and parent about whether or not the child has met the reward criteria. Third, when it is judged necessary to include punishment contingencies, rules indicating what behaviors will be penalized must be very specific. A "bonus clause" should be included to provide a special reward for desired behavior, which continues for an extended period of time. Finally, a contingency contract should include a statement describing the conditions under which reconsideration or termination of the contract can take place.

Token systems are contingency management procedures in which reinforcers are dispensed, contingent upon the performance of specified behaviors. The term "token economy" is usually employed to indicate that a group of individuals are participating in the token system. Token economies have been used effectively within a variety of institutional settings, including psychiatric hospitals, group homes, and workshops (Masters, Burish, Hollon, & Rimm, 1987).

Tokens can take many forms. Such items as poker chips, points on a work-sheet, punched holes in a card, and gold stars can be exchanged for backup reinforcers. Reinforcers are often chosen from a reinforcer menu. Having the option to select from a variety of reinforcers is considered to be a primary advantage of token systems. Also, tokens can be helpful in bridging the time gap between the performance of appropriate behaviors and obtaining reinforcers.

"Teaching-family" group homes for juvenile offenders are an example of a multicomponent contingency management approach. The best known of these programs is Achievement Place (in Lawrence, Kansas), which has served as the prototype for the development of "teaching-family" group homes (Wolf, Braukman, & Ramp, 1987). The program is conducted by "teaching-parents," who have been trained in behavioral management procedures. Approximately six to eight boys or girls (ages 10 to 16) who have been adjudicated for criminal activities are assigned to each home. The children participate in a token economy in which points are earned for meeting a variety of behavioral criteria. Points may also be lost for exhibiting inappropriate behavior. Points are used to obtain rewards and privileges. Vocational training, academic skills, and self-management skills are also taught. Furthermore, the program provides children with an opportunity to experience a close interpersonal relationship with the teaching parents and their peers in the context of a structured environment (Kazdin, 1991).

Kirigin, Braukman, Atwater, and Wolf (1982) evaluated the efficacy of this approach by comparing 12 teaching-family group homes (replications of Achievement Place) with nine comparison group home programs. The findings indicated that during treatment, youths in the "teaching-family" group homes engaged in fewer criminal offenses than those in the comparison programs. Unfortunately, during the posttreatment year these differences were not maintained. This finding is consistent with the other treatment literature on antisocial behaviors and conduct disorders. Generally, little success has been demonstrated in maintaining substantial treatment effects. The current trend in treatment is to combine multiple approaches and to address each of the problematic domains the child presents (e.g., academic problems, peer relations, family relations). For severely antisocial youth, it has been suggested that prolonged treatments lasting for several years may be necessary (Kazdin, 1991).

MODELING

Modeling therapies are derived from principles of observational learning. When a child learns from observing the behavior of others, modeling is said to have occurred. According to Bandura (1977), modeling is one of the primary means by which behavior is acquired and changed.

Bandura emphasizes the distinction between learning and performance. Although behaviors can be learned through observing a model perform the behavior, response consequences that follow the model's behavior, as well as the direct consequences experienced when performing the behavior, will determine the extent to which learned behaviors are actually performed.

Modeling can serve several functions. It can assist a child in acquiring a new behavior. For example, learning a series of finger movements on a typewriter can be acquired from observing a model perform the movements. Modeling procedures are also used to teach more appropriate use of already acquired skills. For example, social skills may be improved by observing a model interact with others across various social interaction scenarios. Much of the early research on modeling was centered around decreasing fear and avoidance behaviors (Masters et al., 1987).

The basic modeling procedure involves exposing the child to a model (live or filmed) who is demonstrating target behaviors. However, numerous procedural variations exist. "Graduated modeling," "guided modeling," and "guided modeling with reinforcement" all have been used to describe the procedure in which the child first views the model perform a behavior and then practices the behavior while receiving feedback from the model. This approach is typically used to teach new skills or improve existing behaviors.

"Participant modeling" and "contact desensitization" are terms that have been used to describe procedures in which the therapist provides physical contact and assistance to the child as the child gradually performs the desired behavior. For example, to treat a child with a dog phobia, the therapist may first allow the child to observe a model petting a dog. This is followed by placing the child's hand on the model's hand and gradually moving the child's hand on to the dog. This procedure is commonly used to reduce fear, anxiety, and avoidance behaviors.

"Covert modeling" is a procedure in which the child is instructed to form an image of a model (himself or a contrived model) performing target behaviors. For example, a shy child can be asked to imagine that she is engaging in conversations with peers. The therapist helps in skill development by instructing the child to imagine performing specific behaviors that are components of adequate social functioning (Masters et al., 1987). Research indicates that covert models should be similar to the child in sex and age and perhaps other physical characteristics (e.g., Kazdin, 1974).

A distinction has been made between mastery models and coping models. Coping models depict a model experiencing difficulties with a specific task. The model exhibits a number of coping behaviors and eventually successfully handles the situation. Mastery models display immediate mastery of the situation. There is some evidence that coping models may be more effective than mastery models (e.g., Kazdin, 1973; Meichenbaum, 1972).

An illustrative case example of the use of modeling procedures to treat social withdrawal has been presented by Ross, Ross, and Evans (1971).

> The child was a 6-year-old boy whose fears and avoidance of social interactions with peers was so pronounced that he was unable to enter kindergarten. At the time of treatment, the child was enrolled in a preschool program. The cause of the child's social withdrawal was unknown. Other than severe social withdrawal, the child appeared normal and scored in the average range on an intelligence test. A 9-week baseline of social interaction behaviors was obtained prior to treatment. In general, the child refused to make verbal or visual contact with his peers and became distressed when presented with pictures of young children.
>
> Treatment was conducted three times per week for 7 weeks at the preschool. During the first 4 sessions, the goal was to have the child practice imitating simple behaviors provided by an adult model. The child's imitations were rewarded with tangible rewards and attention from the model. The next phase of treatment was directed toward teaching social interaction skills and game skills, and eliminating the child's fear of interacting with his peers. To accomplish this, several procedures were used repeatedly and concurrently. Initially the child observed a model interacting with the other children. Gradually, the child was incorporated into the interactions. Pictures, stories, and movies depicting children playing together were also presented to the child for brief periods of time while the model discussed the positive value of interacting with other youngsters. Role-playing procedures depicting appropriate social behaviors were incorporated into treatment. Finally, a nearby park was used to have the child practice interacting with other children (strangers).
>
> At the end of the 7-week treatment program, posttest measures of social interaction and avoidance indicated that the treatment was effective in increasing social interaction behaviors and decreasing avoidance behaviors. Moreover, when compared to a peer group on social interaction measures, no differences in interaction rates were observed. At a 2-month follow-up, the child continued to demonstrate competent social behaviors and appeared to enjoy his interactions with peers.

Modeling procedures have been used in the treatment of a wide range of problems. Skills training programs (e.g., social sills training) have incorporated modeling components and have demonstrated improvements in treatment outcome (e.g., Eisler, Blanchard, Fitts, & Williams, 1978). Numerous controlled group studies have demonstrated the efficacy of modeling procedures in reducing children's fears and phobias (Barrios & O'Dell, 1989). However, these studies have focused on animal fears, fear of medical or dental treatment, and test anxiety. More research is needed to evaluate the treatment of other fears, such as fear of the dark, speech anxiety, fear of heights, and separation anxiety (Morris & Kratochwill, 1991).

COGNITIVE–BEHAVIORAL APPROACHES

Cognitive–behavioral therapy with children began to develop in the late 1960s and early 1970s. Cognitive–behavioral models recognize the influence of environmental factors on behavior. However, these models suggest that cognitions act as mediating factors that are influential in determining the impact of environmental variables upon behavior.

The concept of reciprocal determinism is fundamental to the cognitive–behavioral model. This concept asserts that environmental factors (e.g., stimulus–response relationships) interact reciprocally with personal factors (e.g., cognitions) to produce behavior. Thus, changes in cognitions should result in changes in corresponding behaviors and vice-versa. Cognitive–behavioral interventions attempt to modify directly both factors (Braswell & Kendall, 1988; Craighead, Meyers, & Craighead, 1985).

The cognitive–behavioral view postulates that disturbances in the cognitive processing of environmental events can contribute to the development of internalizing disorders in children. These include disorders such as school phobias, childhood depression, and social anxiety. Cognitive–behavioral interventions for children with these difficulties have focused upon teaching youths to recognize, evaluate, and change distorted cognitions. These interventions are often combined with behavioral interventions. Externalizing disorders, such as impulsivity, hyperactivity, and conduct disorders, are viewed as resulting from deficiencies in the cognitive mediation or verbal control of behavior. Thus, cognitive–behavioral interventions addressing these problems have focused upon increasing the cognitive mediation of behaviors and teaching problem-solving strategies (Braswell & Kendall, 1988).

Self-Instructional Training

Self-instructional training was developed by Donald Meichenbaum (e.g., Meichenbaum & Goodman, 1971). Self-instructional training involves teaching children to use "self-talk" to guide themselves through the performance of an overt behavior or a problem situation.

Much of the treatment research on self-instructional training has been performed on impulsive children (Masters et al., 1987). The training procedures begin with the therapist modeling appropriate behaviors while overtly producing self-instructional statements. The child then imitates this behavior while the therapist verbalizes the self-instructions corresponding to the child's behavior. The youth performs the desired behavior while vocalizing the self-instructional statements that are being whispered by the therapist. This procedure is repeated several times while the prompts are faded, until the child is performing the desired behavior and producing the self-instructions covertly. As can be seen, several procedures, including instructions, modeling, behavioral rehearsal, prompts, feedback, fading, and reinforcement, as well as the actual self-instruction, are involved in this approach (Ollendick & Cerny, 1981).

Meichenbaum and Goodman (1971) first demonstrated use of self-instructional training with second-grade children who had been identified as having problems in self-control. They showed that with just four 30-minute sessions of self-instructional training, they were able to show improved performance on experimental measures of impulsivity. Unfortunately, no changes were evident in the actual classroom behaviors of these children.

Kendall and Braswell (1982) describe a self-instructional training intervention in which coping modeling and a behavioral contingency component were included. The behavioral contingency component involved giving the child 20 tokens at the beginning of each session. Tokens were lost when the child did not perform the self-instructional task correctly. At the end of each session tokens were exchanged for a prize. Treatment resulted in improvements in teacher's ratings of self-control and hyperactivity in the classroom. However, parent ratings of behavior at home did not improve. Also, a 1-year follow-up showed no differences between treated and untreated groups on any of the outcome measures.

While several case studies and controlled studies have demonstrated effectiveness of self-instructional training at decreasing impulsive behavior in some disruptive children, studies examining its effectiveness with children meeting the DSM-III-R criteria for attention-deficit hyperactivity disorder (ADHD) or conduct disorder are scarce. Treatments involving a self-instructional component show promise; however, more research with clinical populations is needed.

Problem-Solving Skills Training

Numerous studies have assessed the relationship between interpersonal cognitive problem-solving skills and behavioral adjustment (e.g., Spivack, Platt, & Shure, 1976). Compared to controls, children with adjustment difficulties supply fewer alternative solutions to interpersonal problems and identify fewer consequences that may follow specific behaviors. These children also exhibit deficiencies in recognizing why others behave the way they do as well as a tendency toward focusing on desired goals, rather than on the steps required to achieve goals (difficulty in "means–ends thinking"). Problem-solving skills training (PSST) is a cognitive–behavioral therapy designed to teach disturbed children the interpersonal problem-solving skills in which they are considered to be deficient.

Training programs have been developed to teach children interpersonal problem-solving skills (Spivack & Shure, 1982). Training scripts, games, and dialogues between the therapist and child are used to expose the children to various interpersonal conflict situations. The children practice generating possible solutions and are given feedback and praise for demonstrating good problem-solving abilities. The focus of training is upon teaching the youngsters how to think and not what to think. PSST research suggests that children who perform well on PSST training tasks tend to show improvements in behavioral adjustment (Spivack, Platt, & Shure, 1976).

Kazdin, Bass, Siegel, and Thomas (1989) compared the effectiveness of PSST with and without *in vivo* practice opportunities with a client-centered relationship-oriented therapy. Children aged 7–13 who had been referred for treatment due to severe antisocial behavior received 25 (50-minute) individual treatment sessions. PSST consisted of instruction in problem-solving skills using pertinent interpersonal examples. Modeling, role-playing, corrective feedback, and social reinforcement were active components of the training. A response-cost component was also included in which subjects lost tokens (which could be exchanged for prizes) for making errors when practicing the problem-solving steps. The second PSST treatment group included an *in vivo* practice component. These subjects were given assignments to practice the problem-solving steps in a variety of real-life situations. The "client-centered relationship therapy" group emphasized providing a warm, empathic, accepting therapeutic environment. Within this context, various problematic interpersonal situations were discussed and the therapist facilitated the child's expression of feelings. Reductions in problem behaviors and increases in prosocial responding at home and at school were demonstrated only for the PSST subjects. These gains were maintained at a 1-year follow-up. Unfortunately, when compared with a normative sample, children who participated in PSST continued to display behavior problems beyond the normal range.

PSST has been demonstrated to be an effective treatment for some clinically referred antisocial youth. Research examining factors that predict success in such treatment packages shows promise. It has been suggested that treatment response may be improved by individualizing PSST such that each child's most problematic domain of functioning is emphasized (e.g., academic functioning, family conflicts). Continued work should result in more refined treatments for children with antisocial behaviors (Kazdin, 1991).

Lewinsohn's Coping with Depression Course

Empirical evaluation of the use of cognitive–behavioral treatments for internalizing disorders (e.g., depression and anxiety) in children is scarce (Braswell & Kendall, 1988). Although articles have appeared calling for the adaptation of cognitive–behavioral procedures for use with children and adolescents, few controlled outcome studies have appeared. A recent report by Lewinsohn, Clarke, Hops, and Andrews (1990) describes a promising cognitive–behavioral treatment for depressed adolescents.

> The subjects consisted of 59 high school students (ages 14–18) who met the DSM-III criteria for major depression or the Research Diagnostic Criteria (RDC) for minor or intermittent depressive disorder. Subjects were randomly assigned to one of three conditions: adolescent only, adolescent and parent, and wait-list. The treatment program, "Coping with Depression Course for Adolescents" (CWD-A), was a modification of a treatment package used previously with adults. Treatment was delivered over fourteen 2-hour sessions spanning a period of 7 weeks. Treatment included relaxation training, encouraging the scheduling of more pleasant events, teaching the youth how to identify and control irrational and negative thoughts, social skills training, communication skills training, and problem-solving skills training. Homework assignments

were de-emphasized (relative to the adult version) and the skills were learned through experiences arranged during the therapy sessions. The parents of those assigned to the "adolescent-and-parent" group met separately from the teenagers for seven 2-hour sessions. Parents were provided with a summary of the specific skills that were being taught to their teenagers. It was hoped that this would facilitate the parental reinforcement of the changes being attempted by their teenagers.

At the end of treatment, approximately one-half of the adolescents receiving treatment continued to meet diagnostic criteria for depression. However, 95% of the wait-list controls were still classified as depressed. Parental involvement was not reliably related to outcome. Follow-up data showed that treated subjects continued to evince a decline in depression over a period of 2 years.

Inclusion of cognitive-based procedures in the treatment of children and adolescents has led to the development of many promising interventions. Although short-term treatment gains have been reported, evidence of treatment generalization and maintenance of behavior change across time is limited. Also, little research has evaluated the question of whether cognitive–behavioral strategies are more effective treatments than more traditional behavioral and nonbehavioral treatments. Much work remains to be done to determine the extent to which cognitive based interventions contribute to the treatment of children.

GENERALIZATION OF TREATMENT EFFECTS

The technology of child behavior therapy has been shown to be effective in treating a variety of problem behaviors in children and adolescents. Recently, the focus of child behavior therapy has been directed toward examining treatment generalization issues. Generalization is concerned with the extent to which treatment gains are evidenced across time, settings, behaviors, and nontreated individuals.

Generalization across time (response maintenance) examines whether treatment gains are maintained after formal treatment is discontinued. Generalization across settings is concerned with the extent to which behavior changes are evident across nontreatment environments. Assessment of changes in behaviors not specifically targeted for treatment is the focus of "response generalization" (generalization across behaviors). Finally, generalization across nontreated individuals (e.g., classmates, siblings, parents) examines whether behavior changes are noted in persons who share the same environment as the treated child.

The four generalization domains (time, setting, behaviors, subjects) can be further broken down into 16 classes (Drabman, Hammer, & Rosenbaum, 1979). A recent review of the child and adolescent behavior therapy literature (1978 through 1989) found that approximately half of the studies presented generalization data (Allen, Tarnowski, Simonian, Elliot, & Drabman, 1991). Generalization across time (response maintenance following treatment cessation) was the most commonly assessed generalization class. However, studies assessing the other classes of generalization were found for 15 of the 16 classes.

Numerous strategies for programming generalization of treatment effects have been offered (Stokes & Baer, 1977; Stokes & Osnes, 1989), and these include the following (Kazdin, 1989):

1. Teach behaviors to the child (perhaps initially with extraneous reinforcers) which, when developed, will come under the control of naturally occurring reinforcers and punishers.
2. Teach family members and peers to use behavioral procedures in the natural environment.
3. Gradually fade the treatment contingencies to eventually resemble the contingencies present in the child's natural environment.
4. Increase the number of discriminative stimuli that exert control over the child's problem behaviors. This may be accomplished by using various therapists and by delivering the treatment under circumstances similar to the posttreatment environment.
5. Teach the child self-control strategies such as self-monitoring, self-evaluation, and self-reinforcement.
6. Use cognitive-based procedures, such as self-instructional training and problem-solving skills training, to increase the cognitive mediation of behaviors.

Strategies designed to maintain treatment gains should be allotted as much importance as strategies designed to establish behavior changes. The "train and hope" (Stokes & Baer, 1977) approach to treatment, in which generalization is not actively programmed, should be abandoned. Behavior therapy has moved beyond the point of demonstrating its ability to produce behavior change. The current challenge is to demonstrate the effective programming of generalized behavior changes.

In some cases, it may be inappropriate to expect generalized behavior changes. This expectation is akin to the notion of a "cure" (Allen et al., 1991). The "chronic disease model" provides an alternative treatment perspective. This model indicates that some behavioral disorders may be chronic conditions (e.g., conduct disorder, ADHD). As with the treatment of chronic medical conditions (e.g., diabetes mellitus), this model indicates that treatment needs to consist of acute interventions as well as long-term monitoring (Kazdin, 1988). Continued work in child psychopathology is needed to determine the utility of this intervention model.

SUMMARY

Currently, child behavior therapy enjoys widespread acceptance. This has been facilitated by incorporation of ideas and methods from other empirical disciplines (e.g., developmental psychology and psychiatry). With its conceptual beginnings springing from principles of classical and operant conditioning, child behavior therapy has expanded to include a collection of therapies derived from varied conceptual models. Cohesiveness within child behavior therapy is maintained by a continued emphasis upon the empirical validation of treatment procedures.

Systematic desensitization and flooding are therapies derived from principles of classical conditioning. They have been effectively applied to the treatment of fear-based disorders. Therapies based upon operant conditioning principles form the core of behavioral interventions. These include positive reinforcement, punishment, and extinction. Such procedures have been used individually. However, many interventions involve the combined use of these procedures. A wealth of research exists that demonstrates the effective use of operant procedures across the entire range of problem behaviors.

Modeling therapies have been developed from principles of observational learning. These techniques have been effectively used in helping children acquire new behaviors, refine existing behaviors, and decrease fear and avoidance responding. Cognitive–behavioral therapies have been developed for the treatment of internalizing and externalizing disorders. Treatments for externalizing disorders (e.g., ADHD, conduct disorder) have included "self-instructional training" and "problem-solving skills training." Treatments for internalizing disorders (e.g., depression, social withdrawal) have focused on changing dysfunctional cognitions that putatively produce depression or anxiety as well as on training children in skills to help them cope with difficulties that can lead to disorders, such as depression.

Demonstrating generalization of treatment effects continues to be a primary empirical challenge for child behavior therapy. This continued emphasis upon empirical evaluation promises an evolving and challenging future for child behavior therapists.

ACKNOWLEDGMENTS.   Preparation of this chapter was supported in part by National Institutes of Health Grant DE08641 to Alan M. Gross.

REFERENCES

Achenbach, T. M. (1974). *Developmental psychopathology*. New York: Ronald Press.
Achenbach, T. M., & Edelbrock, C. S. (1978). The classification of child psychopathology: A review and analysis of empirical effects. *Psychological Bulletin, 85*, 1275–1301.
Achenbach, T. M., & Edelbrock, C. S. (1979). The Child Behavior Profile II. Boys aged 12–16 and girls aged 6–11 and 12–16. *Journal of Consulting and Clinical Psychology, 47*, 223–233.
Achenbach, T. M., & Edelbrock, C. S. (1981). Behavioral problems and competencies reported by parents of normal and disturbed children aged four through sixteen. *Monographs of the society for research in child development, 461*, (No. 188).
Achenbach, T. M., & Edelbrock, C. S. (1983). *Manual for the child behavior checklist and revised child behavior profile*. Burlington, VT: University of Vermont Press.
Allen, J. S., Tarnowski, K. J., Simonian, S. J., Elliott, D., & Drabman, R. S. (1991). The generalization map revisited: Assessment of generalized treatment effects in child and adolescent behavior therapy. *Behavior Therapy, 22*, 393–405.
American Psychiatric Association. (1987). *Diagnostic and statistical manual of mental disorders*, 3rd Edition, Revised. Washington, DC: Author.
Bandura, A. (1977). *Social learning theory*. Englewood Cliffs, NJ: Prentice-Hall.
Barrett, R. P., McGonigle, J. J., Ackles, P. K., & Burkart, J. E. (1987). Behavioral treatment of chronic aerophagia. *American Journal of Mental Deficiency, 91*, 620–625.
Barrios, B. A., & O'Dell, S. L. (1989). Fears and anxieties. In E. J. Mash & R. A. Barkley (Eds.), *Treatment of childhood disorders* (pp. 167–221). New York: Guilford.
Becker, W. C. (1971). *Parents are teachers*. Champaign, IL: Research Press.
Braswell, L., & Kendall, P. C. (1988). Cognitive–behavioral methods with children. In K. S. Dobson (Ed.), *Handbook of cognitive–behavioral therapies* (pp. 167–213). New York: Guilford.
Carey, R. G., & Bucher, B. B. (1986). Positive practice overcorrection: Effects of reinforcing correct performance. *Behavior Modification, 10*, 73–92.
Craighead, W. E., Meyers, A. W., & Craighead, L. W. (1985). A conceptual model for cognitive-behavior therapy with children. *Journal of Abnormal Child Psychology, 13*, 331–342.

Drabman, R. S., Hammer, D., & Rosenbaum, M. S. (1979). Assessing generalization in behavior modification with children: The generalization map. *Behavioral Assessment, 1,* 203–219.

Ehrenreich, N. S., & Melton, G. B. (1983). Ethical and legal issues in the treatment of children. In E. Walker & M. Roberts (Eds.), *Handbook of clinical child psychology* (pp. 1285–1305). New York: Wiley.

Eisler, R. M., Blanchard, E. B., Fitts, H., & Williams, J. G. (1978). Social skill training with and without modeling for schizophrenic and non-psychotic hospitalized psychiatric patients. *Behavior Modification, 2,* 147–172.

Goldstein, G. (1979). Methodological and theoretical issues in neuropsychological assessment. *Journal of Behavioral Assessment, 1,* 23–41.

Hersen, M. (1981). Complex problems require complex solutions. *Behavior Therapy, 12,* 15–29.

Hersen, M., & Ammerman, R. T. (1989). Overview of new developments in child behavior therapy. In M. Hersen (Ed.), *Innovations in child behavior therapy* (pp. 3–31). New York: Springer.

Hersen, M., & Last, C. G. (1988). How the field has moved on. In M. Hersen & C. G. Last (Eds.), *Child behavior therapy casebook* (pp. 1–10). New York: Plenum.

Hersen, M., & Van Hasselt, V. B. (1987). Developments and emerging trends. In M. Hersen & V. B. Van Hasselt (Eds.), *Behavior therapy with children and adolescents. A clinical approach* (pp. 3–28). New York: Wiley.

Horton, A. M., & Miller, W. G. (1985). Neuropsychology and behavior therapy. In M. Hersen, R. M. Eisler, & P. M. Miller (Eds.), *Progress in behavior modification* (Vol. 19, pp. 1–55). New York: Academic Press.

Jersild, A. T., & Holmes, F. B. (Eds.). (1935). *Children's fears* (Child Development Monograph No. 20). Chicago: University of Chicago Press.

Johnson, J. H., Rasbury, W. C., & Siegel, L. J. (1986). *Approaches to child treatment.* New York: Pergamon.

Kazdin, A. E. (1973). The effect of vicarious reinforcement on attentive behavior in the classroom. *Journal of Applied Behavior Analysis, 6,* 71–78.

Kazdin, A. E. (1974). Covert modeling, model similarity and reduction of avoidance behavior. *Behavior Therapy, 5,* 325–340.

Kazdin, A. E. (1984). *Behavior modification in applied settings* (3rd ed.). Homewood, IL: Dorsey.

Kazdin, A. E. (1988). *Child psychotherapy: Developing and identifying effective treatments.* New York: Pergamon.

Kazdin, A. E. (1989). *Behavior modification in applied settings* (4th ed.). Pacific Grove, CA: Brooks/Cole.

Kazdin, A. E. (1991). Aggressive behavior and conduct disorder. In T. R. Kratochwill & R. J. Morris (Eds.), *The practice of child therapy* (2nd ed., pp. 174–221). New York: Pergamon.

Kazdin, A. E., Bass, D., Siegel, T., & Thomas, C. (1989). Cognitive–behavioral therapy and relationship therapy in the treatment of children referred for antisocial behavior. *Journal of Consulting and Clinical Psychology, 57,* 522–535.

Kendall, P. C., & Braswell, L. (1982). Cognitive–behavioral self-control therapy for children: A components analysis. *Journal of Consulting and Clinical Psychology, 50,* 672–689.

King, N. J. & Gullone, E. (1990). Acceptability of fear reduction procedures with children. *Journal of Behavior Therapy and Experimental Psychiatry, 21*(1), 1–8.

King, N. J., Hamilton, D. I., & Ollendick, T. H. (1988). *Children's phobias. A behavioural perspective.* New York: Wiley.

Kirigin, K. A., Braukmann, C. J., Atwater, J. D., & Wolf, M. M. (1982). An evaluation of teaching-family (achievement place) group homes for juvenile offenders. *Journal of Applied Behavior Analysis, 15,* 1–16.

Koeppen, A. S. (1974). Relaxation training for children. *Elementary School Guidance and Counseling, 9,* 14–21.

Kolko, D. J. (1984). Paradoxical instruction in the elimination of avoidance behavior in an agoraphobic girl. *Journal of Behavior Therapy & Experimental Psychiatry, 15,* 51–58.

Lapouse, R., & Monk, M. A. (1959). Fears and worries in a representative sample of children. *American Journal of Orthopsychiatry, 29,* 223–248.

Lewinsohn, P. M., Clarke, G. N., Hops, H., & Andrews, J. (1990). Cognitive-behavioral treatment for depressed adolescents. *Behavior Therapy, 21,* 385–401.

Mansdorf, I. J. (1981). Eliminating somatic complaints in separation anxiety through contingency management. *Journal of Behavior Therapy & Experimental Psychiatry, 12,* 73–75.

Masters, J. C., Burish, T. G., Hollon, S. D., & Rimm, D. C. (1987). *Behavior therapy: Techniques and empirical findings* (3rd ed.). New York: Harcourt Brace Jovanovich.

Matson, J. L., & Coe, D. A. (1991). Mentally retarded children. In T. R. Kratochwill & R. J. Morris (Eds.), *The practice of child therapy* (2nd ed., pp. 298–327). New York: Pergamon.

Matson, J. L., & Ollendick, T. H. (1977). Issues in toilet training normal children. *Behavior Therapy, 8,* 549–553.

Meichenbaum, D. H. (1972). Examination of model characteristics in reducing avoidance behavior. *Journal of Behavior Therapy & Experimental Psychiatry, 3,* 225–227.

Meichenbaum, D., & Goodman, J. (1971). Training impulsive children to talk to themselves: A means of developing self-control. *Journal of Abnormal Psychology, 77,* 115–126.

Mizes, J. S. (1985). The use of contingent reinforcement in the treatment of a conversion disorder: A multiple baseline study. *Journal of Behavior Therapy & Experimental Psychiatry, 16,* 341–345.

Morris, R. J., & Kratochwill, T. R. (1991). Childhood fears and phobias. In T. R. Kratochwill & R. J. Morris (Eds.), *The practice of child therapy* (2nd ed., pp. 76–114). New York: Pergamon.

Morris, E. K., & Redd, W. H. (1975). Children's performance and social preference for positive, negative, and mixed adult-child interactions. *Child Development, 46,* 525–531.

Nelson, R. O. (1980). The use of intelligence tests within behavioral assessment. *Behavioral Assessment, 2,* 417–423.

Ollendick, T. H., & Cerny, J. A. (1981). *Clinical behavior therapy with children.* New York: Plenum.

Ollendick, T. H., Matson, J. L., & Helsel, W. J. (1985). Fears in children and adolescents: Normative data. *Behaviour Research and Therapy, 23,* 465–467.

Rekers, G. A., Lovaas, O. I. (1974). Behavioral treatment of deviant sex role behaviors in a male child. *Journal of Applied Behavior Analysis, 7,* 173–190.

Ross, D. M., Ross, S. A., & Evans, T. A. (1971). The modification of extreme social withdrawal by modeling with guided participation. *Journal of Behavior Therapy & Experimental Psychiatry, 2,* 273–279.

Sawin, D. B., & Parke, R. D. (1979). Development of self-verbalized control of resistance to deviation. *Developmental Psychology, 15,* 120–127.

Scarr, S., & Salapatek, P. (1970). Patterns of fear development during infancy. *Merrill-Palmer Quarterly of Behavior and Development, 16,* 53–90.

Spivack, G., & Shure, M. B. (1982). The cognition of social adjustment: Interpersonal cognitive problem solving thinking. In B. B. Lahey & A. E. Kazdin (Eds.), *Advances in clinical child psychology* (Vol. 5, pp. 323–372). New York: Plenum.

Spivack, G., Platt, J. J., & Shure, M. B. (1976). *The problem-solving approach to adjustment.* San Francisco: Jossey-Bass.

Stokes, T. F., & Baer, D. M. (1977). An implicit technology of generalization. *Journal of Applied Behavior Analysis, 10,* 349–367.

Stokes, T. F., & Osnes, P. G. (1989). An operant pursuit of generalization. *Behavior Therapy, 20,* 337–355.

Stuart, R. B. (1971). Behavioral contracting within the families of delinquents. *Journal of Behavior Therapy & Experimental Psychiatry, 2,* 1–11.

Underwood, S. L., & Gross, A. M. (1989). Developmental factors in child behavioral assessment. In M. Hersen (Ed.), *Innovations in child behavior therapy* (pp. 57–77). New York: Springer.

Van Hasselt, V. B., Hersen, M., Bellack, A. S., Rosenblum, N. D., & Lamparski, D. (1979). Tripartite assessment of the effects of systematic desensitization in a multi-phobic child: An experimental analysis. *Journal of Behavior Therapy & Experimental Psychiatry, 10,* 51–55.

Weithorn, L. A. (1980). Competency to render informed treatment decisions: A comparison of certain minors and adults. *Dissertation Abstracts International, 42,* 3449B–3450B.

Wolf, M. M., Braukman, C. J., & Ramp, K. A. (1987). Serious delinquent behavior as part of a significantly handicapping condition: Cures and supportive environments. *Journal of Applied Behavior Analysis, 20,* 347–359.

Wurtele, S. K., Marrs, S. R., & Miller-Perrin, C. L. (1987). Practice makes perfect? The role of participant modeling in sexual abuse prevention programs. *Journal of Consulting and Clinical Psychology, 55,* 599–602.

23

Pharmacological Intervention

Mina K. Dulcan

INTRODUCTION

This chapter will cover *psychopharmacology* (i.e., the use of *psychoactive* medications or *psychotropic* drugs to treat disorders of emotions and behavior in children and adolescents). Medications are commonly called drugs. It is important to distinguish therapeutic drugs from street drugs, or abused substances. Following a section on general principles, each class or group of medications has its own section, with a description, indications for use, *efficacy* (evidence that the drug works), risks and side effects, and how the drug is generally used. Medications are commonly classified by one of their uses (e.g., antidepressant), a description of their pharmacologic activity (e.g., stimulant or antihistamine), or their chemical structure (e.g., benzodiazepine or lithium). This chapter will not cover doses of medicine. (For more details, see section under Additional Reading.)

Any psychotherapeutic, environmental, or pharmacologic treatment powerful enough to be helpful is also powerful enough to cause negative or side effects. The most common drug side effects will be listed, but not rare or unusual ones. Whenever a new medical or psychological symptom appears in a person taking medication, the index of suspicion should be high that it may represent a side effect, and consultation with a physician should be sought.

Each medication has a *generic*, or chemical, name and one or more trade or brand names. Different brands may not be exactly the same, just as Bounty or Viva paper towels differ from each other and from generic towels. Although generic brands are generally less expensive, their actual potency may vary considerably (the Food and Drug Administration requires equivalent action within 20% of the

MINA K. DULCAN • Department of Child Psychiatry, Children's Memorial Hospital, Division of Child and Adolescent Psychiatry, Northwestern University School of Medicine, Chicago, Illinois 60614.

Advanced Abnormal Psychology, edited by Vincent B. Van Hasselt and Michel Hersen. Plenum Press, New York, 1994.

standard). Substitution may result in new side effects or increased or decreased therapeutic effect, particularly when switching from one generic formulation to another.

The practice of psychopharmacology is both an art and a science, combining knowledge of the basic sciences of medicine and the results of experimental studies to predict therapeutic and side effects (paying close attention to individual characteristics and medication response to tailor the choice of drug, doses, and schedule of administration to each patient and family). Even more difficult is the simultaneous use of more than one drug. Many psychotropic medications interact with each other, and with drugs prescribed for medical conditions or purchased without prescription ("over-the-counter"). Alcohol and abused drugs can be especially dangerous in combination with prescribed medication. Many medications can cause birth defects or withdrawal symptoms in newborn babies, so extreme care must be used when treating sexually active girls who may become pregnant.

Ideally, psychoactive medications are prescribed by child and adolescent psychiatrists, physicians with at least 5 years of postmedical school training in adult, child, and adolescent psychiatry, who often work as a team with one or more other mental health professionals, such as a psychologist, social worker, or psychiatric nurse. Because there is a shortage of child psychiatrists, many pediatricians and family practitioners prescribe psychotropic drugs. Although some of these nonpsychiatric physicians are well informed, others have extremely limited training in psychology and psychopharmacology. In the latter situation, the collaborating mental health professional is often the key to effective treatment.

In many cases, a nonmedical mental health professional will be in the position of deciding whether an evaluation for a trial of medication is indicated, and for making the referral and preparing the patient and family. When there is collaborative treatment (more than one professional, working as a team), the psychologist, social worker, or nurse may be seeing the patient more frequently than the physician does, and can provide valuable assistance in assessing if the drug is working, or if there are side effects.

Questions for the child psychologist to consider regarding the use of psychotropic medication for a particular child include:

1. Who (child, parent, teacher, etc.) will benefit from the medication?
2. What are the target symptoms to be addressed, and have these been sufficiently communicated?
3. Have the target symptoms been defined in ways that can be assessed and monitored, and are procedures in place to monitor them?
4. Have the parent(s) and child been fully informed regarding the possible risks and benefits of the medication, as well as about alternative treatments?
5. Are there financial constraints on obtaining (or medically monitoring) the medication?
6. Is there potential for abuse or misuse of the medication?
7. Is the parent (and is the school) likely to be able to follow the prescribed schedule for medication doses?
8. Have other treatments been conducted or considered, either prior to the use of medication or in conjunction with it?
9. At what intervals will medication response be evaluated, and by whom?

10. What will be the criteria for deciding that the medication response has been sufficient to continue, or that the ratio of positive to negative effects is too low and the medication should be stopped? How long should the medicine be continued in the absence of apparent improvement?

(Adapted from the report of a task force of the Section on Clinical Child Psychology of the American Psychological Association [Barkley, Conners, Barclay, Gadow, Gittelman, Sprague, & Swanson, 1990].)

GENERAL PRINCIPLES OF PSYCHOPHARMACOLOGY IN CHILDREN AND ADOLESCENTS

The Use of Medications in Youth

The life tasks of children and adolescents are physical, cognitive, social, and emotional growth and development. Both medications and untreated psychiatric disorders have the potential to interact with the developmental process in ways that do not occur in adults. No adverse effects on brain development of the use of psychotropic drugs in children have been proven, but the risks of prenatal exposure have been clearly documented. Specific medications may affect physical growth. Interference with attention or alertness may impair learning of academic and social skills. Young patients are more at risk than adults for *behavioral toxicity*: the worsening of preexisting problems or the development of new behavioral or emotional symptoms.

Parents and, to the extent appropriate for developmental status and disorder, the patient, should be fully informed of the potential risks and benefits of each type of treatment, as well as of the risk from no treatment. Laws vary from state to state about the age at which a young person may consent to treatment, rather than assenting to the parent's decision. Some parents or teachers are overly eager to request medication to control a child or adolescent's behavior. It is the role of the mental health professional to advocate for the best interests of the young person, while working to educate parents and teachers.

Assessment

The first step is to conduct an evaluation. Although the majority of the information is gathered by interviewing the patient and family, key additional data are obtained from the pediatrician and the teacher. Specialized medical or psychological tests may be required for a full understanding of the problems. Of particular relevance to pharmacologic treatment is a detailed description of the symptoms, including frequency and severity, and any previous drug treatment, specifying each medication with its schedule, doses, duration of treatment, and therapeutic and adverse effects. Family psychiatric history and family members' response to drug treatment may provide important clues to diagnosis and choice of medication. Past or current medical disorders or drugs prescribed to treat them can cause emotional or behavioral problems, or complicate the use of psychotropic medication. It is important to understand the attitudes of the patient, family, and teacher toward the use of medication. Extreme skepticism and resistance, as well as magical expectations for cure, are common.

Treatment Planning

The initial treatment plan is based on psychiatric diagnosis, target symptoms, and the strengths and weaknesses of the patient, the family, the school, and the community. *Indications* are the reasons for using a selected treatment. They may be syndromes, such as attention-deficit hyperactivity disorder (ADHD) or major depression, or symptoms such as excessive activity, inability to pay attention, aggressive behavior, or hallucinations. In each case, the target symptoms for improvement must be delineated. Based on the scientific literature, as well as clinical experience, some symptoms respond best to medication, others to psychotherapy or special education, and still others to a combination of interventions. This chapter focuses on biological treatment, but should be read with the understanding that for most children and adolescents the best treatment is an integrated multimodality approach.

In the past, clinicians have erred in both directions: on the one hand depriving a patient of a possibly helpful medication, due to lack of knowledge or to prejudice against drugs, or on the other hand using a medication that was not effective or that caused unwarranted side effects, or when psychotherapy, behavior modification, or a change in environment would have been more beneficial. Some people avoid medication because of concerns that the child will be labeled as "crazy." In fact, the child's symptoms would far more likely be stigmatizing among peers and teachers than would taking a helpful medication.

The *Physician's Desk Reference* (PDR), now commonly available to the lay public, is a poor source of information about indications or doses for children and adolescents. It merely reports the U.S. Food and Drug Administration (FDA) guidelines regulating advertising by drug companies, but not the clinical practice of physicians. Because FDA drug trials are expensive to conduct, and children and adolescents do not represent a lucrative market, companies rarely test new medications in young people. This often results in overly conservative doses or lack of "approval" for well-accepted uses. For older drugs, the PDR may recommend indications that are no longer considered appropriate or doses that are too high.

Measurement of Outcome

All medication use should be viewed as a trial to assess whether sufficient benefits are obtained in the presence of minimal or acceptable side effects. Some side effects are inconvenient or uncomfortable; others may have serious consequences. There is a constant balance between the impairment and suffering that would result from the untreated disorder, the benefits of the medication, and the severity of side effects. Target symptoms are specified, and baseline emotional, behavioral, and physical data are gathered, with regular monitoring throughout treatment. Effects can be assessed by interview, observation, standard rating scales, and/or specific medical or cognitive tests. Patient, parent, and teacher are all important data sources. It is essential to ask and look actively for both therapeutic and adverse effects, since many young patients will not report them spontaneously, and adults may not know what to observe.

Obtaining accurate *compliance* with a prescribed regimen is more difficult than for adults. Not only the child, but also parents and frequently school personnel and child care workers must understand, remember, and be willing to cooperate. Factors such as lack of perceived need for treatment, failure to understand how the medicine works, bias against medication, carelessness, lack of money, misunderstanding of instructions, or complex schedules of drug administration can result in missed doses, and therefore reduced effectiveness. Because of the need for regular administration and the danger of many medications in accidental or purposeful overdose, the pill bottle should be supervised by an adult, who takes responsibility for giving the medication as prescribed. Some children will pretend to take their medicine but will hold the pills under the tongue or in the cheek and later throw them out or hide them. Even closer supervision is required in these cases.

STIMULANTS

Description

This category of drugs (see Table 1) is the most studied and most often used in pediatric psychopharmacology. In 1987, nearly 6% of elementary school children in Baltimore County received stimulant treatment for hyperactivity (Safer & Krager, 1988). Contrary to popular belief, stimulants do not have a "paradoxical effect" in children with attention-deficit hyperactivity disorder (ADHD). Hyperactive boys, normal boys, normal adults, and adults with ADHD have similar cognitive and behavioral responses to comparable doses of stimulants, except that children report feeling "funny," while adults report euphoria (Donnelly & Rapoport, 1985).

Indications and Efficacy

The most well established indication is the syndrome of hyperactivity, impulsivity, and inattention currently known as *ADHD*. (Studies conducted before 1987 use the older terms ADD or hyperactivity.) A recent study of boys diagnosed with ADD with hyperactivity demonstrated that 96% responded with reduced behavioral symptoms to methylphenidate and/or dextroamphetamine (Elia, Borcherding, Rapoport, & Keysor, 1991). Although the majority of stimulant research has been conducted with boys, girls appear to be equally responsive.

Before the age of five, stimulant efficacy is less than for older children. Contrary to prevalent myths, stimulants retain their efficacy in adolescents with

TABLE 1.   Stimulant Medications

Brand name	Generic name
Ritalin	methylphenidate
Ritalin Sustained-Release	methylphenidate
Dexedrine	dextroamphetamine
Dexedrine Spansule	dextroamphetamine
Cylert	magnesium pemoline

symptoms of ADHD (Klorman, Brumaghim, Fitzpatrick, & Borgstedt, 1990). There is preliminary evidence that some children who are inattentive and distractible but not hyperactive or impulsive respond positively to stimulants.

When *conduct disorder* or *oppositional defiant disorder* coexists with ADHD, stimulant medication may reduce defiance, negativism, impulsivity, and aggression. In children and adolescents with *mental retardation, fragile X syndrome, autism,* or *organic brain damage*, stimulants may improve target symptoms of inattention, impulsivity, and overactivity, and improve response to behavior modification and special education, although the core social and cognitive deficits remain.

Stimulant effects on individual target symptoms are highly variable from child to child, and even in a single patient. A given dose may produce improvement in some areas, and no change or worsening in others. Positive effects commonly seen with stimulant treatment are listed in Table 2. Stimulants have no effect on learning disabilities in the absence of an attention deficit.

The onset of clinical effect for both methylphenidate and dextroamphetamine is within an hour after each dose. A single dose is effective for 3 to 4 hours. The onset of full action of pemoline is later and the duration longer than the other stimulants.

Stimulants have not been demonstrated to have long-term therapeutic effects, but all existing studies have serious methodological problems (e.g., inappropriate control groups; discontinuing the drug too soon; using doses that are too high, too low, or poorly timed; not measuring compliance; not taking individual variation in response into account; and using inappropriate outcome instruments) (Pelham, 1983). There has been no study of children with ADHD but without conduct disorder randomly assigned to long-term medication versus placebo and/or other treatment.

Although research studies have had difficulty demonstrating that psychological interventions add to the efficacy of stimulant treatment, for many children medication alone is insufficient treatment. Even children who respond positively continue to have deficits. Specific learning disabilities and gaps in academic

TABLE 2.   Therapeutic Effects of Stimulant Medication

Motor
  Decrease inappropriate physical activity
  Decrease excessive vocalization, noise and disruption in the classroom
  Improve handwriting

Social
  Reduce off-task behavior
  Improve compliance to adult requests
  Reduce verbal and physical aggression
  Improve peer interactions

Cognitive
  Improve sustained attention
  Improve short-term memory
  Reduce distractibility
  Reduce impulsivity
  Enhance use of existing cognitive strategies
  Increase academic productivity and accuracy

knowledge and skills require educational remediation. Social skills deficits and family pathology may need specific treatment. Parent education and training in techniques of behavior management are generally useful.

Risks and Side Effects

Even in youngsters who have a positive behavioral response to stimulant medication, side effects may limit the dosage or even require changing to a different medication. Most side effects are similar for all stimulants (see Table 3). An individual patient, however, may have side effects from one of the stimulants but not another.

Possible *emanative effects* (indirect and inadvertent cognitive and social consequences) of medication, such as reduced self-esteem and self-efficacy; attribution by child, parents, and teachers of both success and failure to external causes (rather than to the child's effort); stigmatization by peers; and dependence by parents and teachers on medication rather than making needed changes in the environment (Whalen & Henker, 1991) can be avoided by careful education of the child and adults.

Certain groups of children appear to have a higher rate of side effects; among these are: those under the age of five (more prone to sadness, irritability, "clingi-

TABLE 3. Side Effects of Stimulant Medications

Common immediate side effects often related to dose and to initial adjustment to medication
  Decreased appetite
  Weight loss
  Irritability
  Abdominal pain
  Headaches
  Emotional oversensitivity, easy crying

Less common side effects
  Insomnia
  Sadness
  Decreased social interest
  Impaired cognitive test performance (especially at very high doses)
  Less than expected weight gain
  Rebound overactivity and irritability (as dose wears off)
  Nervous habits (e.g., picking at skin)

Rare but potentially serious side effects
  Motor tics
  Tourette's disorder
  Depression
  Growth retardation
  Rapid pulse
  High blood pressure
  Psychosis with hallucinations
  Stereotyped activities or compulsions

Side effects reported with pemoline only
  Writhing motor movements
  Night terrors
  Lip licking or biting
  Liver damage (very rare)

ness," insomnia, and anorexia), those with co-morbid anxiety disorders (Tannock, 1991), and those who are mentally retarded (more likely to develop motor tics or social withdrawal) (Handen, Feldman, Gosling, Breaux, & McAuliffe, 1991). These patients should not necessarily be denied a medication trial, but indications should be stronger, alternative treatments tried more vigorously, doses should be lower, and surveillance for side effects more rigorous.

In the late 1980s, Ritalin® received a great deal of negative media attention, promoted by the Citizens' Commission for Human Rights, a group affiliated with the Church of Scientology (see Baren, 1989). News stories and law suits alleged a variety of unproven ill effects attributed to the use of Ritalin®. Complications of the disorder itself or consequences of misdiagnosis or inadequate monitoring and therapy were blamed on the medication. As a result, many parents became unnecessarily anxious regarding the use of Ritalin®. The use of Ritalin® decreased, often with negative consequences for child adjustment (Safer, 1991). The truth is that there is no evidence that stimulant therapy promotes addiction, drug abuse, or delinquency.

A cautionary note: the combination of methylphenidate and imipramine may produce confusion, emotional lability, marked aggression, and severe agitation (Grob & Coyle, 1986).

Principles of Use

The decision to medicate is based on inattention, impulsivity, and hyperactivity not due to another treatable cause, which is persistent, sufficiently severe to cause functional impairment at school, and usually also at home and with peers. For safety, parents must be willing to monitor medication and to attend appointments. Other interventions should be considered first, unless severe impulsivity and noncompliance create an emergency situation. It is difficult to predict drug responsiveness among a group of hyperactive children. Neither behavioral signs, inattention, neurological examination, nor EEG predict stimulant responsivity. In addition, there are no empirical data that are helpful in indicating which stimulant drug or formulation is best for a particular child. A significant number of those who respond poorly to one stimulant medication have a positive response to another.

Multiple outcome measures are essential, using more than one source and setting. Baseline data from the school on behavior and academic performance are obtained prior to initiating stimulant medication. The physician should work closely with parents on dose adjustments and obtain frequent reports from teachers and annual academic testing. The CAP (Child Attention Problems) rating scale (see Appendix 1) is useful in gathering weekly data from teachers (Barkley, DuPaul, & McMurray, 1990).

The use of the longer-acting formulations (sustained release methylphenidate, dextroamphetamine spansule, or pemoline) has been advocated in order to avoid a midday dose at school. However, for many ADHD children, the long-acting forms are less effective than an equivalent dose of the standard preparation after breakfast and lunch. There is often a delay in onset of action, and more variability from day to day (Pelham, Sturges, Hoza, Schmidt, Bijlsma, Milich, & Moorer, 1987). Some individual children respond better to a long-acting formulation than to standard Ritalin® (Pelham, Greenslade, Vodde-Hamilton, Murphy, Greenstein, Gnagy, Guthrie, Hoover, & Dahl, 1990). Unpredictably high doses may result if a child chews a time-release pill instead of swallowing it. The longer-acting preparations may be useful if it is impossible or detrimental to give medicine during the school day, if the child suffers from severe medication rebound, or if the standard formulation lasts less than 3½ to 4 hours.

Stimulant medication should be initiated with a low dose and titrated weekly according to response and side effects. Anorexia can be minimized by giving stimulants after meals. Starting with only a morning dose may be useful in assessing drug effect, by comparing morning and afternoon school performance. Pulse and blood pressure are taken initially and at times of dosage change. Weight is followed during initial titration, and weight and height are measured two to three times a year. Observation and inquiry for tics should be made at baseline and at every visit.

The dosage schedule (e.g., whether medication should be given after school, on weekends, and during school vacations) is individually determined by the nature and severity of the target symptoms being treated. Some children may require only morning and noon doses, on school days only, with perhaps a smaller dose after school to assist with homework completion. Children with more prominent behavioral symptoms outside of the school setting, with peers and family, may require three doses a day, 7 days a week. If possible, the young person may have an annual drug-free trial of at least 2 weeks, or even the whole summer. As symptoms improve, each youngster may have a trial off medication during the school year (preferably not at the beginning of the year) to assess whether the medication is still needed. Periodic reevaluation of the need for a dose increase or decrease will optimize effect.

Tolerance (decreased effect of a constant dose of drug) has occasionally been reported, but compliance is often irregular, and should be considered when medication "becomes" ineffective. Children should generally not be responsible for self-administering medication, since these youngsters are impulsive and forgetful, and many dislike the idea of taking medication even when they can verbalize its positive effects. They may try to avoid, "forget," or outright refuse medication. Decreased drug effect may also be due to an increase in the patient's weight, a reaction to a stressful change at home or school, or autoinduction of hepatic metabolism that may require a 10 to 20% dose increase after several months of treatment.

TRICYCLIC ANTIDEPRESSANTS

Description

This is the most commonly used class of antidepressants. Examples are in Table 4. These drugs were developed to treat depression, but have also been used for patients with a variety of other problems. The following information applies

TABLE 4. Tricyclic Antidepressants

Brand name	Generic name
Tofranil	imipramine
Norpramin or Pertofrane	desipramine
Elavil or Endep	amitriptyline
Pamelor	nortriptyline
Anafranil	clomipramine

only to tricyclic antidepressants. Other classes of antidepressants are covered briefly in the next section.

MINA K.
DULCAN

Indications and Efficacy

The usefulness of medication in the treatment of *depression* in youth, compared to that in adults, has been much more difficult to demonstrate. Children are more likely to respond than adolescents, although the high placebo response rate in all but the most ill children complicates assessment of efficacy. For this reason, psychotherapy is generally tried first, with antidepressants being reserved for the most severe cases and for those who do not respond to therapy.

Although an early study demonstrated that imipramine was useful in the treatment of *separation anxiety* and *school phobia*, a recent report has questioned antidepressant efficacy in this disorder (Klein, Koplewicz, & Kanner, 1992). In any case, family therapy, work with school personnel, and behavior therapy should be used before medication is tried for this disorder.

Imipramine, desipramine, and nortriptyline have been found to be equally effective in the treatment of *nocturnal enuresis* (bedwetting). The mechanism of action remains unclear, but it is not by altering sleep stages, by treating depression, or via peripheral anticholinergic activity. In 80% of patients, within 1 to 7 days, tricyclics substantially reduce frequency of bed wetting, but total dryness is achieved in less than 25% (Fritz & Rockney, 1991). Wetting returns when the drug is discontinued, but the success rate may be higher if the drug is tapered gradually. Behavioral treatments, which avoid drug side effects and show better maintenance of improvement, are the first choice. Imipramine may be useful on a short-term basis or for special occasions (e.g., overnight camp).

Tricyclic antidepressants are used occasionally for severe *night terrors* or *somnambulism* (sleepwalking).

Tricyclics are second-choice drugs for children and adolescents with ADHD who do not respond to stimulants, who develop significant depression or motor tics while being treated with stimulants, who have severe rebound symptoms, or who are at risk for Tourette's disorder or substance abuse. Tricyclics have a longer duration of action than methylphenidate, so a dose during the school day is not needed and rebound is less of a problem. Drawbacks include serious potential cardiac side effects, especially in prepubertal children, and the danger of accidental or intentional overdose. Imipramine has been used for ADHD, but desipramine is preferred because it has fewer side effects and better maintenance of therapeutic effects over time (Biederman, Baldessarini, Wright, Knee, & Harmatz, 1989). Desipramine may reduce symptoms of hyperactivity, impulsivity, and inattention in youth with *Tourette's disorder*.

Clomipramine, but not the other tricyclics, is useful in the treatment of *obsessive–compulsive disorder* in children and adolescents (Deveaugh-Geiss, Moroz, Biederman, Cantwell, Fontaine, Greist, Reichler, Katz, & Landau, 1992). Some cases of *trichotillomania* (an irresistible impulse to pull out one's own hair) in adults have responded to clomipramine (Swedo, Leonard, Rapoport, Lenane, Goldberger, & Cheslow, 1989). One small controlled study has demonstrated clomipramine to be helpful in reducing obsessive–compulsive, autistic, and anger-related symptoms in young persons with *autism* (Gordon, Rapoport, Hamburger, State, & Mannheim, 1992).

Although there are side effects common to all tricyclics (see Table 5), each drug within this group has a different side effect profile. All tricyclics predictably slow the conduction of electrical signals in the heart. This is not usually dangerous if monitored, and in the absence of preexisting conduction abnormalities. At moderate to high doses, children and adolescents may develop a rapid pulse, elevated blood pressure, or, rarely, a change in heart rhythm. There has recently been a great deal of media attention to a few cases of children who died suddenly while taking desipramine. It is not clear whether there was a causal relationship between the medication and death, and most experts believe that desipramine is a safe drug, when used with appropriate monitoring and caution (Riddle, Nelson, Kleinman, Rasmusson, Leckman, King, & Cohen, 1991; Schroeder, Mullin, Elliott, Steiner, Nichols, Gordon, & Paulos, 1989).

In the treatment of depression, as the child improves, transient apparent worsening of sadness and crying are sometimes seen in those who previously had been relatively silent. On the other hand, cognitive toxicity may be mistaken for a worsening of the original depression (Preskorn, Weller, Hughes, & Weller, 1988). In children with tics, tricyclics may either improve or worsen motor symptoms.

Sudden withdrawal of moderate or higher doses results in a flulike gastro-intestinal syndrome with nausea, cramps, vomiting, headaches, and muscle pains. Behavioral manifestations may include social withdrawal, hyperactivity, depression, agitation, and insomnia. Tricyclics should therefore be tapered over a 1- to 2-week period rather than being abruptly discontinued. The short half life of tricyclics in prepubertal children may produce daily withdrawal symptoms if medication is given only once a day. These symptoms may also indicate that poor compliance is resulting in missed doses (Puig-Antich, Ryan, & Rabinovich, 1985).

TABLE 5. Side Effects of Tricyclic Antidepressants

Gastrointestinal	*Behavioral*
Abdominal pain	Nightmares
Nausea or indigestion	Agitation
Appetite decrease (may lead to weight loss)	Irritability or anger
Constipation	Psychosis
Weight gain	Mania
Cardiovascular	*Miscellaneous*
Dizziness or fainting	Blurred vision
Rapid pulse	Headache
High blood pressure	Dry mouth (may lead to
	increased dental cavities)
Neurologic	Difficulty urinating
Insomnia	Skin rash
Sedation	Worsening of asthma
Confusion	
Stuttering	
Seizures	

Principles of Use

Due to the potential lethality of an accidental or intentional overdose, parents must be reminded to supervise closely the administration of a tricyclic and to keep the pills in a safe place.

Due to differences between children and adults in fat-to-muscle ratio and in liver size relative to body weight, prepubertal children are likely to need a higher weight-corrected dose of imipramine than adults, and are prone to rapid dramatic swings in blood levels from toxic to ineffective. Tricyclics should be given to children in three divided doses to produce more stable levels (Puig-Antich et al., 1985), but may be given once or twice daily in adolescents.

Before the use of a tricyclic antidepressant, routine evaluation is done, which covers weight, pulse, blood pressure, and presence of involuntary motor movements. EEG (electroencephalogram) and baseline laboratory screening may be indicated. Except in the treatment of enuresis, where very low doses are used, an initial electrocardiogram (ECG) is essential to establish a baseline and to detect a preexisting defect in heart rhythm, which could result in fatality. The ECG, pulse, and blood pressure should be repeated at intervals as the dosage increases (at least 48 hours after an increase), and monitored periodically thereafter. Extremely high pulse rate or blood pressure, or ECG changes greater than a set limit, may require a decrease in dose. Use of blood levels is controversial and is not generally needed, except in patients who fail to respond to usual doses (possibly low levels) or in those who have severe side effects at usual doses (possibly very high levels). Nortriptyline may have fewer side effects and may be more precisely titrated by blood level. It may be given twice a day in children.

Prior to starting imipramine for enuresis, a baseline measure of wet and dry nights should be obtained, with daily charting used to monitor progress. Much lower doses are needed than for the treatment of depression, and medication is given at bedtime only. Tolerance to medication may develop, requiring an increased dose. Tricyclics lose their effect entirely in some children. If medication is used for a long time, there should be a drug-free trial at least every 6 months, since enuresis has a high spontaneous recovery rate.

OTHER ANTIDEPRESSANT DRUGS

Monoamine Oxidase Inhibitors

Monoamine oxidase (MAO) inhibitors are a class of antidepressants completely different from the tricyclics. The most commonly used are phenelzine (Nardil) and tranylcypromine (Parnate). In adults they are used to treat *depression* that does not respond to other drugs, especially in manic–depressive patients, or in those with greatly increased sleep and appetite. MAO inhibitors may be more effective than the tricyclics in the treatment of depression in adolescents.

Suicidal or impulsive outpatients should not be given MAO inhibitors because of the risk of severe (life-threatening) high blood pressure when a MAO inhibitor is combined with certain foods, medications, or abused drugs. Even for relatively responsible adolescents, repeated dietary instruction and review are necessary.

Fluoxetine (Prozac) is a new antidepressant medication with a very different mechanism of action from the older drugs. It has received a great deal of attention, as it has been tried in a variety of patients who have not responded to previous treatment. It is available in capsules and in liquid form (for greater dose flexibility and ease of administration). Although there is a moderate amount of research and clinical experience in using this drug to treat adults, work with children and adolescents is just beginning. More than most medications, fluoxetine has significant interactions with other drugs, and combinations must be approached with great caution.

Although preliminary data suggest that fluoxetine may be useful for children and adolescents in the treatment of *obsessive–compulsive disorder*, obsessive and compulsive symptoms in *Tourette's disorder* (Riddle, Hardin, King, Scahill, & Woolston, 1990), or *depression*, much more experience must be gathered before these uses can be viewed as anything other than experimental.

In general, fluoxetine appears to have fewer and less serious side effects than older antidepressants, but adverse effects do occur and may limit the dose or require discontinuation of the medication. The side effects are different from the tricyclics and the MAO inhibitors, so a patient who cannot tolerate one of those may be able to take fluoxetine. Of particular importance in the treatment of depressed patients is fluoxetine's safety when taken in overdose, compared to the tricyclics and MAO inhibitors. The more common side effects are listed in Table 6. As with all new medications, a number of rare side effects are being identified.

Fluoxetine has recently been the focus of a great deal of media attention, promoted by the Citizens Commission on Human Rights, affiliated with the Church of Scientology. There have been accusations that the drug causes suicidal and violent behavior. Whatever treatment they receive, depressed patients (as well as those with other psychiatric disorders) are at risk for suicide and must be carefully monitored. There is no evidence that fluoxetine has caused dangerous behavior, but in rare, very complex cases it appears to have stimulated thoughts about harming self or others.

Bupropion

Bupropion (Welbutrin) is one of the newest antidepressants, and is chemically different from the others. There are few empirical data regarding its use in children and adolescents, but there are suggestions of modest efficacy in the treatment of

TABLE 6.   Side Effects of Fluoxetine (Prozac)

Nausea or indigestion	Headaches
Vomiting	Tremor (shaking)
Weight loss or gain	Agitation or excitement
Anxiety or nervousness	Akathisia (restlessness)
Insomnia	Overactivity and rapid speech
Nightmares	Hypomania or mania
Excessive sweating	

ADHD (Casat, Pleasants, Schroeder, & Parler, 1989). The most serious potential side effect is increased susceptibility to seizures (convulsions). Other side effects include rash, nausea and vomiting, increased or decreased appetite, weight loss or gain, constipation, dry mouth, dizziness, tremor, insomnia, and rapid pulse.

LITHIUM

Description

Lithium is a naturally occurring salt that is available in several different forms, including lithium carbonate tablets or capsules, controlled-release capsules (Eskalith CR) and lithium citrate syrup.

Indications and Efficacy

Lithium may be considered in the acute or maintenance treatment of children and adolescents with *bipolar affective disorder* (Puig-Antich et al., 1985). Lithium may be efficacious for *children of bipolar parents* who have *behavior disorders* without an apparent mood disorder, or for children and adolescents who have *behavior disorders accompanied by mood swings*. It may be useful as a supplementary drug in a minority of *depressed* adolescents who have not responded to tricyclic antidepressants.

In young people with severe *aggression*, especially with impulsivity and explosive affect, lithium is equal or superior to haloperidol in reducing aggression, hostility, and tantrums with fewer side effects (Campbell, Small, Green, Jennings, Perry, Bennett, & Anderson, 1984). Lithium may also be useful in mentally retarded youth with severe aggression directed toward themselves or others (Campbell, Green, & Deutsch, 1985).

Risks and Side Effects

Side effects (see Table 7) are generally similar to those seen in adults. Risk of side effects increases with decreasing age, and autistic children develop more adverse effects than children with conduct disorder (Campbell, Silva, Kafantaris, Locascio, Gonzalez, Lee, & Lynch, 1991).

Because of its potential to cause birth defects, lithium should not be prescribed for sexually active girls without assurance of a reliable method of birth control. Lithium effects on blood glucose are controversial, but reactive hypoglycemia is possible.

As in adults, toxicity is closely related to serum levels, and the therapeutic margin is narrow. Adequate salt and fluid intake is necessary to prevent levels rising into the toxic range. The child and family should be instructed in the importance of preventing dehydration from heat or exercise, and in the need to stop the lithium and contact the physician if the patient develops an illness with fever, vomiting, diarrhea, and/or decreased fluid intake. Erratic consumption of large amounts of salty snack foods may cause fluctuations in lithium levels (Herskowitz, 1987).

Lithium should not be prescribed unless the family is willing and able to comply with administering regular multiple daily doses and obtaining lithium blood levels. In addition to the usual medical history and physical exam, laboratory tests of blood count, and of liver, thyroid, and kidney function, as well as ECG, should be done prior to starting lithium. An EEG may be indicated. Height, weight, and thyroid and kidney functions should be monitored at least every 3 to 4 months. It is important to be alert to possible clinical signs of low thyroid function (e.g., dry skin, sluggishness, feeling cold) that could be mistaken for fatigue or depression.

Lithium levels (drawn 12 hours after the last dose) are obtained once or twice weekly during initial dose adjustment (allowing 4 days to reach steady state) and monthly thereafter. Therapeutic levels are generally similar to those of adults. Three or four doses per day are usually required. Lithium should be taken with food to minimize stomach irritation. Since most children and adolescents have more efficient kidney function than adults, they may require higher lithium doses for body weight (and sometimes higher apparent blood levels) than adults (Puig-Antich et al., 1985; Weller, Weller, & Fristad, 1986). The use of controlled-release lithium (Eskalith CR) is often advisable, especially in younger children. Twice-daily administration is sufficient and more steady blood levels are attained.

Following lithium treatment of an acute manic episode, medication should be discontinued after 3–6 months, and the patient observed for possible relapse. Many patients will require 1 to 2 years of lithium treatment.

TABLE 7.   Lithium Side Effects

Common side effects	*The following are signs that the lithium level may be too high. Call the doctor immediately, and do not give lithium for at least 24 hours.*
Weight gain	
Stomachache	
Diarrhea	Vomiting or diarrhea more than once
Nausea	Severe trembling
Vomiting	Weakness
Weight loss	Lack of coordination
Increased thirst (polydipsia)	Extreme sleepiness or tiredness
Increased frequency of urination	Confusion
(polyuria): may lead to enuresis	Severe dizziness
Hand tremor	Trouble speaking, slurred speech
Tiredness, weakness	
Headache	*The following are serious toxic effects. SEE THE*
Dizziness	*DOCTOR OR GO TO AN EMERGENCY ROOM*
	IMMEDIATELY.
Occasional side effects	Irregular heartbeat
Low thyroid function, or goiter (enlarged	Fainting
thyroid)	Staggering
Acne	Blurred vision
Skin rashes	Ringing or buzzing sound in the ears
Hair loss	No urination
Metallic taste in the mouth	Muscle twitches
Irritability	High fever
	Convulsions
	Unconsciousness

MINA K.
DULCAN

Description

This group of very powerful medications, including several different chemical classes, are also called antipsychotic drugs. They are listed in Table 8 in order of increasing potency per milligram of drug.

Indications and Efficacy

The most common use is in the treatment of *schizophrenia*, although in general, younger schizophrenics are less responsive to pharmacotherapy than adults, and continue to have substantial impairment, even if the more florid symptoms such as hallucinations, anxiety, tension, and agitation abate with neuroleptics (Campbell et al., 1985). These medications can decrease hallucinations, delusions, and thought disorder. There has been little study, however, of the use of these drugs to treat other psychoses in adolescents (e.g., psychotic depression, mania).

Clozapine (Clozaril) is a newly developed antipsychotic drug that has demonstrated efficacy in adult schizophrenic patients unresponsive to other neuroleptics, and that minimizes motor side effects and the risk of tardive dyskinesia. It has been tried with a few adolescents (Birmaher, Baker, Kapur, Quintana, & Ganguli, 1992), but at present is used only as a last resort because it has the potentially lethal side effect of agranulocytosis (absence of white blood cells). It must be monitored with weekly blood tests.

In certain hyper- or normoactive *autistic* children, very low doses of haloperidol may decrease hyperactivity, aggressiveness, temper tantrums, withdrawal, and stereotypies and, in combination with a structured behavioral/educational program, enhance certain types of learning. Hypoactive autistic children do not generally respond well to haloperidol (Campbell et al., 1985).

Haloperidol in low doses is initially effective for up to 80% of patients with *Tourette's disorder*, but discontinuation may lead to severe withdrawal exacerbation of symptoms for up to several months. Other neuroleptic agents may also be effective, but efficacy is often difficult to evaluate due to the natural waxing and

TABLE 8. Neuroleptics or Major Tranquilizers

Brand name	Generic name
Thorazine	chlorpromazine
Mellaril	thioridazine
Clozaril	clozapine
Serentil	mesoridazine
Loxitane	loxapine
Moban	molindone
Trilafon	perphenazine
Stelazine	trifluoperazine
Navane	thiothixene
Prolixin or Permitil	fluphenazine
Haldol	haloperidol
Orap	pimozide

waning of symptoms. Pimozide may be useful for patients who do not respond well to either haloperidol or clonidine.

Studies of hospitalized children with severe solitary *aggressive conduct disorder* unresponsive to other interventions have found several neuroleptics effective, compared with placebo in reducing aggression, hostility, negativism, and explosiveness. Chlorpromazine, however, leads to unacceptable sedation at relatively low doses.

Very low doses of chlorpromazine can be used to decrease aggression and explosiveness in children and adolescents with *bipolar mood disorders* and *borderline personality disorder*. In the past, some advocated the use of thioridazine or other major tranquilizers in the treatment of hyperactivity, but this has been discredited due to risk of tardive dyskinesia. Neuroleptics are not indicated for insomnia, simple anxiety, or nonspecific behavioral problems.

Risks and Side Effects

The rate of various side effects varies among the drugs in this category. Table 8 lists them in order of decreasing risk of sedation and "anticholinergic" side effects, and increasing tendency to cause muscular side effects ("extrapyramidal").

Side effects are listed in Table 9. Acute dystonia may be treated with diphen-

TABLE 9. Neuroleptic Side Effects

Common "nuisance" side effects
  Dry mouth
  Sleepiness or tiredness
  Constipation
  Abdominal pain
  Mild trouble urinating
  Blurred vision
  Dizziness (especially when getting up in the morning)
  Weight gain
  Increased risk of sunburn

Occasional side effects (may be especially distressing to adolescents)
  Decreased sexual interest or ability
  Changes in menstrual periods
  Increase in breast size (boys and girls)

Serious side effects
  Muscular symptoms (common): "extrapyramidal"
    Akathisia: restlessness or inability to sit still
    Acute dystonia: stiffness of tongue, jaw, neck, back, or legs
    Tongue or throat spasm
    Parkinsonian rigidity: shaking of hands and fingers
    Drooling
    Decreased movement
    Decreased facial expression
  Tardive dyskinesia
  Inability to pass urine
  Overheating (hyperthermia)
  Neuroleptic malignant syndrome
  Seizures

hydramine (Benadryl) or benztropine mesylate (Cogentin) orally or as a shot. Adolescent boys seem to be especially vulnerable to acute dystonic reactions. Chronic extrapyramidal side effects such as muscle stiffness can be treated in adolescents with diphenhydramine or benztropine three or four times a day. In children, however, reduction of neuroleptic dose is preferable to the use of antiparkinsonian agents (Campbell et al., 1985). Akathisia is extremely uncomfortable, and may result in increased symptoms of psychosis, agitation, or aggression. It may be mistakenly interpreted as agitation due to worsening of the underlying disorder, and incorrectly treated with an increase in neuroleptic. Akathisia may be treated by reducing the neuroleptic dose or by adding biperidine (Akineton), propranolol (Inderal), clonidine (Catapres), lorazepam (Ativan), or clonazepam (Klonopin).

Tardive (delayed) or *withdrawal dyskinesias* are involuntary movements of parts of the body, most commonly the mouth and tongue. The movements may be jerky and ticlike, or fine, wormlike movements of the tongue, or chewing motions. In children and adolescents, most are transient, but they may be permanent. They are seen in 8 to 51% of neuroleptic-treated children and adolescents (Campbell et al., 1985) after as brief a period of treatment as 5 months (Herskowitz, 1987). Especially in children with autistic disorder or Tourette's disorder, it may be difficult to distinguish medication-induced movements from those characteristic of the disorder itself. Before being placed on a neuroleptic, and periodically thereafter, each patient should be examined for abnormal movements, using a scale such as the AIMS (Abnormal Involuntary Movement Scale) (Munetz & Benjamin, 1988). Parents and patients (if they are able) should receive regular explanations of the risk of movement disorders.

Neuroleptic malignant syndrome, a potentially fatal side effect, is manifested by very high temperature, muscle rigidity, autonomic hyperactivity (unstable blood pressure, rapid irregular heartbeat, sweating), and mental confusion.

Abnormal laboratory findings seem to be less often reported in children than in adults, but the clinician should be alert to the possibility, especially of blood disorders and liver dysfunction. If yellowing of eyes or skin (jaundice) or an acute illness with fever occurs, medication should be withheld and complete blood count and liver function should be measured.

Of particular concern is behavioral toxicity, manifested as worsening of preexisting symptoms or development of new symptoms, such as hyper- or hypoactivity, irritability, apathy, social withdrawal, stereotypies, tics, or hallucinations (Campbell et al., 1985). Low potency antipsychotic drugs (such as chlorpromazine and thioridazine) can produce cognitive dulling and sedation interfering with ability to benefit from school. Children and adolescents are more vulnerable to this sedation than adults.

Thioridazine is associated with damage to the retina of the eye (at high doses) and retrograde ejaculation (particularly disturbing to adolescent boys).

Side effects are a significant problem in the long-term use of haloperidol for Tourette's disorder. In addition to the side effects noted in Table 9, frequent complaints include: lethargy, feeling like a "zombie," personality changes, and intellectual dulling (Towbin, Riddle, Leckman, Bruun, & Cohen, 1988). Sadness, anxiety, "clinginess," and school avoidance also have been reported (Mikkelsen, Detlor, & Cohen, 1981).

Some side effects of pimozide are similar to those of haloperidol but seem to be less severe. On the other hand, pimozide causes ECG changes in up to 25% of patients, although these appear to be less significant than originally thought.

Principles of Use

Prior to initiating medication, a complete physical examination, including evaluation of involuntary motor movements, should be done. At baseline and at regular intervals blood count and liver function tests are needed.

In almost all cases, neuroleptics can be given once or twice a day, rather than more frequently. An initial trial of about 4 weeks is often needed to assess efficacy (barring serious side effects requiring immediate discontinuation). If the drug appears to be helpful, it should be continued for at least several months. At 3- to 6-month intervals, the drug should be discontinued to observe for withdrawal dyskinesias (involuntary motor movements) and to determine if the drug continues to be necessary. Some children may have physical withdrawal symptoms (stomach pains, nausea, vomiting, insomnia, tremors) or behavioral rebound for up to 8 weeks after the medication is stopped (Campbell et al., 1985).

Tourette's disorder is chronic and not usually an emergency. Careful monitoring for several months prior to starting medication is possible, and is especially useful in mild cases because of the natural waxing and waning of symptoms. During this period, a baseline of symptoms is established, and psychological and educational interventions can be implemented. Prior to starting pimozide, an ECG should be obtained, in addition to the tests listed for all drugs in this section.

In a crisis caused by acute psychosis or severe agitation, small doses of chlorpromazine, haloperidol, or droperidol can be given orally or by intramuscular injection every 2 hours until symptoms are controlled or side effects appear. Patients must be monitored closely, watching particularly for low blood pressure or acute muscle stiffness or spasm.

MINOR TRANQUILIZERS, SEDATIVES, AND HYPNOTICS

Description

Three different chemical groups that are used to treat children and adolescents fall into this category (see Table 10): benzodiazepines, antihistamines, and buspirone (a new drug that is chemically different from all others available).

Indications and Efficacy

Diazepam and lorezapam have been used in the short-term treatment of children with severe anticipatory *anxiety*. Alprazolam may reduce anxiety prior to procedures in children with cancer (Pfefferbaum, Overall, Boren, Frankel, Sullivan, & Johnson, 1987). Anecdotal experience that alprazolam may be helpful in children with avoidant and overanxious disorders has not been systematically confirmed (Simeon, Ferguson, Knott, Roberts, Gauthier, Dubois, & Wiggins, 1992). Diazepam may be used for sleep disorders, such as severe *night terrors*, persistent

TABLE 10. Antianxiety Medications

Benzodiazepines (sedatives or tranquilizers)	
Usually used to reduce anxiety, panic, or night terrors	
Brand name	*Generic name*
Valium	diazepam
Ativan	lorazepam
Xanax	alprazolam
Librium	chlordiazepoxide
Klonopin	clonazepam
Usually used for sleep	
Brand name	*Generic name*
Dalmane	flurazepam
Halcion	triazolam
Antihistamines	
Brand name	*Generic name*
Benadryl	diphenhydramine
Atarax or Vistaril	hydroxyzine
BuSpar (buspirone)	

true *insomnia* (as distinguished from separation anxiety or oppositional resistance to bedtime), or *somnambulism* (sleepwalking). Clonazepam, a benzodiazepine typically used to treat epilepsy, may reduce *akathisia* secondary to neuroleptic treatment; it has also been used to treat *panic* (Biederman, 1987).

Antihistamines (diphenhydramine or hydroxyzine) are most commonly used to treat allergies. Psychiatric indications include *agitation* and severe *insomnia* that has not responded to psychological interventions. Medication to induce sleep should be used only for a short time, to interrupt maladaptive sleep habits, or to manage a brief crisis. Diphenhydramine may also be used to treat acute *dystonic reactions* (muscle spasm) resulting from antipsychotic drugs.

Very little is known about the use of buspirone in children and adolescents, but anecdotal data suggest that it may be useful in reducing *aggression* that is related to anxiety in patients with *mental retardation* or *autistic disorder* (Realmuto, August, & Garfinkel, 1989).

Risks and Side Effects

The three classes of medication differ in their side effects (see Table 11). Unlike other antianxiety agents, buspirone rarely causes sedation and it does not interact with alcohol, or lead to physical dependence.

ANTICONVULSANTS

Description

Anticonvulsant drugs are generally used to treat epilepsy (seizures, convulsions). Several of them, including carbamazepine (Tegretol) and valproic acid (Depakene), are also used to treat psychiatric disorders, more commonly in patients who have a history or signs of brain damage.

TABLE 11. Side Effects of Antianxiety Medications

Benzodiazepines

Sedation	Paradoxical reaction (disinhibition)
Emotional dependence on medication	Excitation
Substance abuse and addiction	Irritability
Decreased coordination (ataxia)	Increased anxiety
Confusion	Hallucinations
Emotional lability	Hostility, rage, or aggression
Worsening of psychosis	Insomnia
	Nightmares
	Euphoria
	Memory loss
	Seizures or agitation if drug stopped suddenly

Antihistamines

Sedation	Decreased coordination
Dizziness	Agitation
Dry mouth	Worsening of asthma
Blurred vision	Increased risk of seizures (at high doses)
Nausea, decreased appetite	Motor tics and other involuntary movements
Stomachache	Tardive dyskinesia (when used for long periods)
Constipation	

Buspirone

Dizziness	Insomnia
Anxiety	Excitement
Nausea	Depression
Headache	Confusion
Restlessness	Muscle stiffness

Indications and Efficacy

Patients with severe impulsive *aggression* with emotional lability and irritability who have an abnormal EEG or a strong clinical suggestion of episodic phenomena may deserve a trial of carbamazepine (Evans, Clay, & Gualtieri, 1987). Carbamazepine and valproic acid have also been used to treat *mania* in bipolar patients (primarily adults) who respond poorly to lithium.

Risks and Side Effects

Anticonvulsants can cause birth defects, so great caution must be used to be sure that sexually active girls do not become pregnant. Side effects are listed in Table 12.

Adverse behavioral reactions may be more frequent in children than in adults (Evans et al., 1987). There are multiple interactions between anticonvulsants and psychotropic (and other) drugs.

Principles of Use

Blood counts and liver functions should be measured before starting and at regular intervals thereafter, or if a rash, sore throat, or fever occurs. Drug blood levels must be followed. Carbamazepine deteriorates in humid environments, so pills must be kept in a dry place.

TABLE 12. Anticonvulsant Side Effects

Tegretol (carbamazepine)

Common side effects, especially at first
- Sleepiness
- Dizziness
- Clumsiness or decreased coordination (ataxia)
- Nausea, vomiting
- Blurred or double vision
- Mild decrease in the number of white blood cells
- Hair loss (grows back when the Tegretol is stopped)
- Increased sensitivity to the sun
- Muscle cramps

Behavioral and emotional side effects
- Anxiety
- Agitation
- Impulsive behavior
- Irritability
- Aggression
- Hallucinations (hearing voices or seeing things that aren't there)
- Mania

Serious but very rare side effects
- Decrease in blood cells
- Liver or kidney damage
- Lung irritation
- Worsening of seizures
- Motor or voice tics
- Severe skin rashes

Depakene (valproic acid)
- Nausea
- Vomiting
- Liver damage (rare over age three)
- Decrease in blood cells (rare)

CLONIDINE

Description

Clonidine (brand name Catapres) is a medication developed for the treatment of high blood pressure.

Indications and Efficacy

In children and adolescents with ADHD who can not take stimulants (e.g., because of tics), who develop unacceptable side effects (e.g., depression), or in whom stimulants do not completely control symptoms, clonidine can improve frustration tolerance and compliance and reduce hyperactvity, impulsivity, temper tantrums, and explosive anger, although it does not directly improve attention (Hunt, Capper, & O'Connell, 1990). Clonidine can be used alone or in combination with a stimulant. It appears to be most useful for highly excitable, "hyperaroused" youngsters. Clonidine works extremely gradually, and no effect other than improved ability to fall asleep at bedtime may be noticed for several weeks. The full beneficial effect may not be apparent for 6 months after reaching a therapeutic dose.

Efficacy in reducing tics in *Tourette's disorder* is controversial. Measurement of response is difficult because of significant placebo response and the natural waxing and waning of symptoms in Tourette's. In certain cases, clonidine may be helpful in improving the behavioral symptoms that may be more problematic than the tics. It may be combined with the neuroleptics haloperidol or pimozide.

Pilot data suggest that clonidine may be useful in reducing symptoms of hyperactivity and impulsivity in *autistic* children (Ghaziuddin, Tsai, & Ghaziuddin, 1991).

Risks and Side Effects

Side effects are listed in Table 13.

Principles of Use

Blood pressure and pulse are necessary, and blood count, thyroid studies, and ECG are advisable before starting clonidine. Clonidine is initiated with a low dose at bedtime and increased gradually over several weeks to three or four daily divided doses. The skin patch lasts only 5 days in children, compared to 7 days in adults (Hunt, 1987). Clonidine should be tapered rather than stopped suddenly, to avoid withdrawal symptoms (see Table 13) (Leckman & Ort, 1986).

TABLE 13.   Side Effects of Clonidine

Common side effects
  Sleepiness, especially when inactive or bored (usually the worst in the first 2 to 4 weeks)
  Local redness and itching from the skin patch
  Weight gain
  Temporary worsening of tics in Tourette's disorder (may be due to small or infrequent doses wearing off)

Side effects sometimes seen as dose is increased
  Headache
  Dizziness
  Abdominal pain
  Nausea or vomiting

Side effects reported in adults, rare in children
  Depression
  Irritability
  Low blood pressure or pulse
  Dry mouth
  Constipation
  Sleep disturbance or nightmares
  Fluid retention and swelling
  Nervousness
  Increased blood sugar (mainly in persons with diabetes)
  Sensitivity to light
  Nosebleed

Effects of sudden drug withdrawal
  Very high blood pressure, even if the blood pressure was normal before starting the clonidine
  Temporary worsening of behavioral problems or tics
  Rapid or irregular pulse
  Chest pain
  Nervousness
  Headache
  Stomach cramps, nausea, vomiting
  Trouble sleeping

MINA K.
DULCAN

BETA BLOCKERS

Description

This group of medications has been used for over 20 years for the treatment of high blood pressure, chest pain, and cardiac arrhythmias. Other medical uses include the treatment of migraine headaches and certain types of tremor. Propranolol (Inderal) is the oldest. Newer beta blockers, such as atenolol (Tenormin), pindolol (Visken), and nadolol (Corgard), are longer acting and have fewer effects on the central nervous system.

Indications and Efficacy

The primary mechanism of action appears to be by blocking the peripheral physical sensations (e.g., dizziness, rapid pulse, shaking) associated with anxiety and anger. These drugs may be useful in patients with otherwise uncontrollable *rage reactions* and impulsive *aggression*, especially those with evidence of organic brain damage (Williams, Mehl, Yudofsky, Adams, & Roseman, 1982). They may reduce aggression and increase socialization in persons with *autistic disorder* or *mental retardation*. Largely anecdotal data suggest usefulness in the treatment of *stage fright* or *test anxiety* and *posttraumatic stress disorder*. Propranolol may also be useful in the treatment of *akathisia* (restlessness) caused by neuroleptic treatment.

Risks and Side Effects

Beta blockers are relatively contraindicated in patients with asthma, diabetes, or heart failure. Side effects are listed in Table 14. Propranolol significantly increases blood levels of neuroleptics such as chlorpromazine and thioridazine.

Principles of Use

In children and adolescents, the initial dose is low. The dose may be increased every 3 to 7 days, if the pulse rate is above 50 beats per minute and the blood

---

TABLE 14.   Side Effects of Beta Blockers

Occasional side effects
Tingling, numbness, or pain in the fingers
Tiredness or weakness
Decreased sexual interest or performance
Slow heartbeat
Low blood pressure
Dizziness (especially when standing up fast)

More serious side effects
Wheezing
Sadness or irritability (if more than a few days)
Hallucinations

24

Dynamic Psychotherapy

Morris Eagle and David Wolitzky

Introduction

The terms "dynamic psychotherapy" and "psychodynamic psychotherapy" have been used interchangeably with psychoanalytic psychotherapy or psychoanalytically oriented psychotherapy. It is useful to remember that Freud borrowed the term "psychodynamic" from physics, where "dynamics" refers to the interaction of forces as in thermodynamics or aerodynamics and is intended to convey the idea of an interplay of forces in the mind, particularly conflicting forces.[1] Indeed, Kris (1947), an influential psychoanalytic theorist, defined psychoanalysis as that discipline that views behavior from the point of view of *inner conflict*. Thus, one of the basic questions a traditional psychodynamic psychotherapist would pose to himself or herself in clinical situations would be: with which inner core conflict is this patient struggling? As we shall see, in some recent psychoanalytic developments, such as self-psychology, there appears to be a relative de-emphasis on inner

---

[1]*Psychodynamic* has come to be a broad term that subsumes Freudian treatment approaches as well as theories and intervention methods since Freud's time. It also stresses intrapsychic conflict but does so in the context of basic assumptions concerning human motivation that are at variance with Freud's. We should also point out that while some clinicians (whether Freudian in orientation or not) make a sharp distinction between "psychoanalysis" as a particular form of psychodynamic psychotherapy, others tend to blur the distinction and see it on a continuum with psychoanalytic psychotherapy (or psychoanalytically oriented psychotherapy). Those who stress the distinction emphasize that in psychoanalysis there is a more systematic focus on transference and resistance (concepts we shall define later), a greater reliance on dreams and free associations, and the exploration and interpretation of the patient's past history as well as current realities. These differences are said to be facilitated by the use of the couch and the frequency of sessions (usually three to five sessions per week in psychoanalysis, as opposed to one or two sessions per week in psychoanalytic psychotherapy).

Morris Eagle and David Wolitzky • The Ontario Institute for Studies in Education, Toronto, Ontario M5S 1V6, Canada.

Advanced Abnormal Psychology, edited by Vincent B. Van Hasselt and Michel Hersen. Plenum Press, New York, 1994.

conflicts and corresponding increased emphasis on other factors (such as self-defects and developmental arrests). However, the emphasis of traditional psychodynamic theory has been on inner conflict.

What is the nature of inner conflict? According to traditional psychoanalytic theory, our basic conflicts consist of the opposition between unconscious wishes and the defenses employed against these wishes so that they are blocked from conscious awareness and from being implemented in actions. Based on both clinical experience with early cases and his understanding of Darwinian evolutionary theory, Freud believed that it is primarily sexual wishes and desires that are implicated in conflict and defense.[1]

How did Freud come to emphasize the centrality of unconscious conflict in psychic life and the therapeutic goal of making these conflicts conscious? When Freud first came on the scene, available methods of therapeutic intervention were rest, massage, hydrotherapy, and faradic stimulation (the application of low voltage electrical stimulation to parts of the body that were symptomatic). These methods did not address the causes of the patient's tensions and suffering. Instead, they were aimed at providing symptomatic relief. They were relatively ineffective and rarely produced stable results.

Freud had studied with two famous hypnotists of his era, Charcot and Bernheim. He came away impressed with the power of hypnosis to induce and remove symptoms. He began to use these methods in his own work. At first, he would put the patient in a hypnotic trance and suggest that the symptoms disappear and that the patient have a posthypnotic amnesia for his directive. This approach met with limited success. Freud then experimented with variations of this approach. In one instance, he was called in to treat a woman who had just given birth and was morose, agitated, and unable to nurse (that is, there was no breast milk forthcoming despite her conscious desire to feed her infant). The direct hypnotic suggestions that the milk start flowing had only a temporary effect. Freud then suggested, again with the directive for posthypnotic amnesia for the fact of his suggestion, that when she awoke from the hypnotic trance the patient would become angry at her family and complain that they were giving her insufficient care and attention, demand food, and insist that under the conditions that had existed they could not expect her to feed her baby adequately. She awoke, carried out the suggestions, and very quickly became symptom-free (Freud, 1892–1893).

What was the underlying basis of this patient's difficulties and what was the insight, though not fully articulated at the time, that led Freud to this successful therapeutic maneuver with this patient who apparently was suffering from a postpartum depression? We assume that the patient both did and did not want to feed her infant. That is, she was in a state of psychological conflict. Further, we assume that part of this conflict was unconscious; as far as the patient consciously knew, she wanted to nurse her baby. To consciously wish not to feed and to thereby harm her infant would produce painful feelings of guilt. Freud discerned that she was angry at having to assume the role of the nurturant one, particularly if it meant

---

[1]It should be noted that for Freud, the term "sexual" includes *infantile sexuality*, such as oral and anal wishes and impulses. "Sexual" should be understood in the sense of *sensual*. The term "infantile" means early in development and should have no pejorative connotations. Freud's point was that from an early age certain bodily zones (mouth, anus, genitals) were special sources of bodily pleasure.

that she would not have any of her passive-dependent wishes satisfied. The inability to nurse was implicitly seen as a psychological symptom based on this conflict. Being given permission by an authority figure to express indirectly this side of her feelings apparently was necessary to shift the dynamic balance of the conflict. (Actually, this is an interesting example in that a psychodynamic understanding was used as the basis for a behavioral manipulation, a kind of assertiveness training through hypnotic suggestion.)

Cases such as these formed the basis for Freud's psychodynamic approach and for the key concepts of psychic determinism and unconscious motivation. By psychic determinism, Freud meant to emphasize that mental activity can be shown to have lawful regularities. Unconscious motivation refers to the idea that a great deal of psychological activity goes on outside of awareness, that it is actively kept out of awareness, and that it nonetheless exerts a continuing, powerful impact on conscious experience and behavior.

Although Freud certainly was not the first major thinker to postulate that there are unconscious influences on conscious thought, he was the first to develop a systematized, comprehensive theory of the dynamic unconscious as the underpinning of the development of normal as well as pathological behavior. It is in this sense that repression (the automatic exclusion of conflict-laden ideas from awareness) was regarded as the "cornerstone" of psychoanalysis.

DEFENSE, ANXIETY, AND SYMPTOM FORMATION

At first, Freud used the terms repression and defense as synonymous. Later, repression came to be regarded as only one form of defense. Other common defenses include reaction formation, projection, and denial, to name just a few. Any mental activity or behavior that a person engages in, in an effort to avoid anxiety, may be said to have a defensive function. Thus, an idea that one might think would generate considerable anxiety could be fully in awareness if its emotional significance is not consciously experienced. For instance, in the defense of isolation of affect one might consciously contemplate murderous ideas, cut off from their normal emotional accompaniments. Freud believed that it was the disavowal of unacceptable wishes that was the critical factor which rendered the person vulnerable to a neurosis. Defense required the expenditure of mental (psychic) energy. If the unconscious wishes were sufficiently strong and/or the defenses could not adequately conceal the wishes, the result would be an outbreak of neurotic symptoms.

In Freud's original (so-called topographic) theory, the mind was divided into an unconscious, a preconscious, and a conscious portion. Freud thought that the moral prohibitions directed against sexual wishes were consciously opposing the unconscious wishes. Initially, conflict was conceptualized as opposition between conscious (or preconscious) psychic elements and unconscious ones. By 1923, Freud had realized that moral prohibitions and defenses against instinctual wishes could and often were unconscious and that repression was not the only way of defending against unacceptable wishes. Thus, Freud maintained the centrality of conflict, but came to realize that its essential nature was not the opposition between unconscious and conscious forces.

These are some of the main reasons that Freud developed the tripartite structural theory of id, ego, and superego as reflecting the major sources of conflict in the human mind. Freud also came to recognize aggression as coequal with sex, the two being the major instinctual drives. Finally, Freud realized that conflict was not an abnormal condition, but an inevitable, ubiquitous feature of mental life. Emotional disturbance occurred not because of conflict *per se*, but because of the maladaptive solutions to which it could give rise in the person's effort to avoid the outbreak of serious anxiety.

In its final form, Freud's theory of anxiety focused on key so-called danger situations that could lead to traumatic anxiety in which the person feels totally helpless, overwhelmed, and unable to satisfy his or her essential needs. These danger situations, in order of their appearance in the course of development, are loss of the object, loss of the object's love, castration anxiety, and superego anxiety (guilt). Each of these potential anxieties persists throughout life and signals of the full-blown experience of any of them is an automatic trigger for the initiation of defenses. Hence, this theory is referred to as the signal theory of anxiety. A fuller statement of these concepts can be found in Waelder (1960), Brenner (1982), and Eagle and Wolitzky (1992).

THE GOALS OF AWARENESS AND CONFLICT RESOLUTION

Two basic assumptions in the traditional psychoanalytic theory of pathology and of treatment—ones that have their roots in the prepsychoanalytic thinking of Charcot and Janet—are that the isolation of mental contents from the rest of the personality is pathogenic and that the bringing to consciousness and the assimilation of such material is therapeutic. These basic prepsychoanalytic ideas remained central. Indeed, a good part of the early history of psychoanalytic treatment can be understood as a continuing evolution of conceptions regarding those mental contents that are to be made conscious, and the techniques employed in achieving this goal. For example, in Freud's earliest writings, it was primarily traumatic memories that were to be made conscious and it was originally through hypnosis that this goal was to be achieved.

Freud believed that if we could restore to conscious awareness what was banished from it, we would free the patient of his or her disabling symptoms. Early on, Freud believed that so-called pathogenic or traumatic, unconscious memories were the cause of symptoms. The affect connected to these memories was thought to exist in a "strangulated" state. If the memory could be retrieved into consciousness, the feelings associated with it could be "abreacted" (reexperienced), lose their intensity, and be "associatively reabsorbed" into consciousness (i.e., take their place in the patient's mass of conscious ideas and memories). At first, hypnosis was the way to achieve these ends. However, matters quickly became more complex. Hypnotic "cures" were often short-lived, and some patients were resistant to hypnosis, leading Freud to try related methods. He would let patients talk (have a catharsis) in the context of which he would urge them to recall traumatic events. Sometimes he would use the so-called pressure technique of placing his hand on the patient's forehead and insisting that a forgotten memory would be retrieved. As one can see, these methods, including the use of the supine position, were remnants of the hypnotic procedure and were still based on the idea that the recovery of specific memories would lead to symptom removal.

Eventually, Freud came to the famous "fundamental rule" of free association. The directive now was to speak freely, without inhibition or editing, the thoughts and feelings that came into one's mind. Over time, Freud came to several realizations that increased the complexity of his task: (1) patients experienced not only the pain of ego-alien, discrete symptoms, but also had disturbed patterns of adaptation for which they sought help; the aim of treatment expanded to deal not only with specific symptoms but with the person's total character; (2) accordingly, it was not that a few key repressed memories were the source of all the patient's suffering, but rather the maladaptive patterns of thought, feeling, and behavior that developed over many years; the reduction of the symptoms as well as the amelioration of the maladaptive patterns now came to be approached more indirectly through a more general, open-ended exploration of the patient's personality; (3) whereas Freud originally thought that memories of sexual seduction played a major role in the patient's emotional disturbances, he came to believe that for many patients what he had taken as memories of actual seduction turned out to be *fantasies*.

The abandonment of the "seduction theory" was a decisive turning point in the history of psychoanalysis for it put in the primary position the issue of the patient's "psychic reality" as a major determinant of psychopathology. This should not be taken to mean that what happens to one is unimportant or that seductions and other traumatic events never take place. Rather, it broadens one's focus to include not only the events themselves, but the *personal meanings*, both conscious and unconscious, of the events. The task for treatment is the uncovering of these personal meanings as expressed in the context of the patient's relationship with the therapist. And, treatment should aim for not only the increasing *awareness* of who one is, how and why one got to be that way, and what unacceptable needs and wishes one has been hiding from one's self, but also the increasing ownership, acceptance, and integration of those aspects of one's self. Thus, Freud's epigrammatic statement of the goal of psychoanalysis as "making the unconscious conscious" was later replaced with the idea of "where id was, there shall ego be" (1933).

RESISTANCE

One important factor that complicates or interferes with achieving the goal of awareness and resolution of inner conflict is the operation of defenses in the treatment. Thus, just as outside therapy one generally defends against becoming aware of certain wishes because of the anxiety that such awareness would entail, so in the therapy situation one continues to resist awareness for the same basic reason. There is no reason to expect that such anxiety would disappear simply because one is in treatment. Indeed, under certain circumstances in treatment, anxiety may be intensified. Resistance has therefore been defined as defense operating in the interpersonal context of treatment. The term resistance has had a pejorative connotation since it suggests opposition to the aims of treatment. However, when we recognize that its primary motive is the avoidance of anxiety, then this connotation should be removed. Resistance may take many forms, both blatant and subtle. For example, refusing to talk is an overt opposition to self-exploration, while forgetting one's dreams is a more indirect form of avoidance.

Another basic way to conceptualize resistance is in terms of the patient's reluctance to relinquish infantile wishes (e.g., that one will be loved or nurtured unconditionally and endlessly) and the fantasy that such wishes can be and will be gratified. Although patients consciously want to change and be rid of their neurotic symptoms and distress, they do not necessarily link (except perhaps in a highly intellectual way) their distress to the compulsive pursuit of infantile wishes. And for many patients the prospect of giving up of central infantile wishes and fantasies is experienced at some deep unconscious level as rendering life empty or meaningless. Patients often experience a period of mourning following their recognition of the need to relinquish core infantile fantasies and wishes. Clearly, patients need to feel emotionally convinced that more realistic meanings, pleasures and gratifications are possible in order to be able to yield essentially unattainable gratifications or fantasies—what Eugene O'Neill in *The Iceman Cometh* referred to as people's "pipedreams."

One of the concrete implications of giving heed to the important role of resistance in treatment is the practical rule-of-thumb that identification and analysis of the patient's defenses (including resistances) should precede analysis of wishes and impulses. Unless defenses are dealt with, awareness of wishes and impulses will be essentially intellectualized and/or will be re-subjected to repression and other defenses. In the development of psychoanalysis, the analysis of defense increasingly became an important part of treatment. Also, the concepts of resistance and defense became broadened to include stable and ego syntonic personality characteristics.

TRANSFERENCE

One of the most central concepts in the psychoanalytic theory of treatment is the concept of transference. Indeed, at one point Freud stated that if central to a therapeutic approach were the concepts of transference and resistance, then whatever the approach might be called, it was psychoanalytic in nature. It is interesting that Freud singled out both transference and resistance, for in the psychoanalytic theory of psychotherapy, transference is understood both as a kind of resistance and perhaps as the most important tool for therapeutic change.

In what way is transference a form of resistance? If transference is understood as transferring on to the therapist one's infantile wishes and fantasies and the conflicts and defenses in which they are embedded, then one can see that at an unconscious level the patient hopes that the therapist will gratify his or her infantile wishes. Indeed, from a traditional psychoanalytic perspective, the essence of the transference can be understood as an expression of a persistent fantasy that this time one's basic wishes and needs will be gratified—by the therapist. But as noted earlier, the fantasy that one's infantile wishes will be gratified is precisely a core aspect of resistance. Hence, the conclusion that the transference is a primary expression of resistance.

In what way(s) is the transference an important, indeed indispensable, tool for therapeutic change? Generally speaking, as Freud (1912a) recognized, a positive transference is often a precondition for therapeutic change and for interpretations to "take hold." A more specific function of the transference is that it provides experiences that have a here-and-now emotional immediacy. It is one thing to talk about wishes, conflicts, and reactions to persons from one's distant past; it is another matter to relive in an emotionally vivid way new editions of these past experiences in relation to the therapist, who is immediately present. And, as Freud (1912a) observed, it is difficult to slay a dragon in effigy.

In fact, most analysts would agree that a good part of psychoanalytic psychotherapy consists in analyzing the transference—that is, in making interpretations that help bring the patient's transference reactions to awareness and that help the patient understand these reactions as a mirror of his or her neurotic patterns. In his study of brief psychodynamic psychotherapy, Malan (1963, 1976) found a positive relationship between the tendency of the therapist to make transference interpretations, and the positive therapeutic outcome. Malan describes the ideal transference interpretation as one that facilitates a "triangle of insight," by which he means interpretations that help the patient make insightful connections among patterns of reactions to the therapist, to other important current figures (e.g., wife, husband, lover, boss, friend, etc.) and to parental figures in the patient's past.

According to classical psychoanalytic theory, therapeutic change consists essentially in bringing to awareness, analyzing and "dissolving," or at least reducing, the "transference neurosis," that is, a full-blown version of his or her neurotic pattern, but now in relation to the therapist. Some analysts take the position that nontransference interpretations are virtually a waste of time; however, most therapists believe that nontransference interpretations are of value. Some analysts no longer consider it necessary even for patients in long-term psychoanalysis, to develop a full blown "transference neurosis" in order for treatment to be effective. It is held by many to be even less necessary for patients in psychoanalytically oriented dynamic psychotherapy.

One final set of comments regarding the concept of transference needs to be made. In recent years, the traditional view of transference as a *distortion* (that is, the patient distorts the therapist and reacts to him or her as if he or she were a parental figure) has been severely criticized by Gill (1982). He argues for a relativistic position in which the therapist attempts to understand the patient's perceptions and behaviors not as distortions, but as plausible reactions to cues emitted by the therapist and to aspects of the therapist's real behavior. For Gill, the transference is broadly conceived and seems to be virtually synonymous with the patient's experience of the therapeutic relationship. For many, including the authors of this chapter, Gill's views constitute a welcome corrective to the classic and mistaken position that the analyst is a "blank screen" onto which the patient projects his or her wishes, fantasies, conflicts, defenses, and so on. Some classical analysts failed to recognize that even silence is a communication and that one is constantly emitting cues even when one is assuming a stance of "analytic neutrality" (we will have more to say about the concept of analytic neutrality later in the chapter). Having endorsed Gill's corrective, we still find it useful to regard transference as a selective and biased reading of the present in terms of the past even though that reading is based on current "reality hooks."

COUNTERTRANSFERENCE

The concept of countertransference is complementary to the concept of transference, but the focus is now on the therapist rather than the patient. That is, in its early meaning (Freud, 1910) the countertransference referred to the therapist's reactions to the patient, particularly to the patient's transference, that were strongly influenced by the therapist's unresolved unconscious conflicts, wishes, fantasies, and so on. Thus, it was of primary importance that the therapist attempt to become aware of and attempt to deal with his or her countertransference reactions, lest they seriously interfere with his or her understanding of the patient and the progress of treatment. Indeed, Freud (1910) maintained that the progress of therapy was limited by therapists' unresolved countertransference reactions. If the therapist could not deal with countertransference reactions on his or her own through introspection and self-analysis or consultation with a colleague, for example, then further psychoanalytic treatment for the therapist was in order.

It can be seen that in the above traditional account of countertransference, it is essentially an impediment, an obstacle to treatment, that must be resolved. In more recent years, however, the concept of countertransference has been broadened so that for some it includes virtually every aspect of the therapist's reactions to his or her patient. Note the parallel between the broadening of the concept of countertransference so that it includes the totality of the therapist's reactions to his or her patient, and the earlier noted extension of the meaning of transference so that it includes the totality of the patient's reactions to the therapist.

Instead of viewing countertransference reactions as an unwanted intrusion, the more recent view emphasizes their potential usefulness in treatment, particularly as a possible clue to what the patient might be "pulling for" in the therapist and to subtle features of the patient–therapist interaction. It seems to us that the key words in the above account are "potential" and "possible." That is, the therapist's emotional reactions to the patient are *potentially* useful and represent *possible* clues to what the patient is "pulling for" and to important aspects of the patient–therapist interaction. However, as a therapist one cannot automatically make the assumption—as seems to be the case in some of the recent literature—that one's emotional reactions to the patient are precisely those that the patient is "pulling for" and are *necessarily* clues to what is going on in the patient. The therapist must reflect upon his or her emotional reactions to the patient and attempt to understand their origin and their nature. They are likely to be the complex product of many different sources and factors. For example, there can be many different reasons for feeling angry (or bored or anxious or sexually aroused or pitying or many other feelings) with a patient. One cannot automatically assume that the anger (or boredom or anxiety or sexual arousal or pity) can be accounted for simply on the basis that this emotion is what the patient was unconsciously "pulling for" in the therapist.

FREE ASSOCIATION

As noted earlier, Freud moved from a reliance on hypnosis to the eventual use of free association, which remains as a basic psychoanalytic technique. In classical psychoanalysis the patient lies on the couch, with the analyst sitting behind and out of view, and is expected to follow the "fundamental rule of psychoanalysis" (Freud, 1912a) of saying whatever comes to mind regardless of how trivial, irrational, irrelevant, or embarrassing it may seem. This is the patient's primary task in psychoanalysis. Based on an association model of the mind, Freud believed—as do most, if not all, contemporary analysts—that free association, in contrast to more directed and socially conventional thought, would facilitate the emergence of unconscious material that would at least partly escape defense and censorship. Of course, because defenses and censorship continue to operate during free association (just as they continue to operate during dreams), the material that emerges continues to be disguised and hence requires deciphering and interpretation (a topic we will cover in the next section). Although the "basic rule" is a simple one—merely saying what comes to mind—it is not that easy to follow. The difficulties patients encounter are not unlike the ones people experience when they attempt to practice meditation—habitual modes of thought keep intervening and taking over.

A basic theoretical assumption underlying use of free association is that unconscious ideas and wishes will influence and direct the course and content of the patient's associations. Thus, contiguous ideas, though of very different manifest content, are assumed to possess an underlying thematic connection. For example, a patient begins an early analytic session by saying that she finds it difficult to express her thoughts, but fears that once she begins, she may not be able to stop. Her next thought is to ask the therapist where the ladies room is located. On the face of it, these two ideas have no apparent connection. The therapist, however, may begin to form the tentative hypothesis that the patient is making an unconscious equation between control of thought and speech and control of bowel and bladder functions.

Although free association (in the context of the use of the couch) is the "fundamental rule" in long-term psychoanalysis, its use is modulated and modified in psychodynamic psychotherapy, particularly when the therapy is carried out with the patient sitting up and facing the therapist. In that situation, the patient would normally be encouraged to speak about what is on his or her mind and what is of immediate concern rather than to free associate. Indeed, in many forms of time-limited brief psychodynamic psychotherapy where there is an agreement between patient and therapist that primarily certain focal or core conflicts will be dealt with in the treatment, the therapist may well take a directive role in influencing what will be discussed in the treatment sessions.

INTERPRETATION

As noted above, the patient's free associations (as well as dreams) are subject to defense and disguise, and hence require interpretation to make their meaning clear. Interpretation is the main psychoanalytic tool for achieving the therapeutic goals of "making the unconscious conscious" and facilitating the patient's resolution of his or her underlying conflicts. We noted earlier that in contemporary conceptions of psychoanalytic treatment, analysis of resistance and defense takes up a major part of therapeutic work. This means that many interpretations made in treatment are likely to deal with the patient's defenses and resistances. They will attempt to clarify not only that the patient is resisting, but why, what, and how he or she is resisting.

There is widespread agreement among analysts and psychodynamic therapists that the most effective interpretations are those that are presented tactfully and with proper timing, that is, at a point at which the patient is almost able to reach the same understanding himself or herself. It should be apparent that there are many interventions, other than interpretations, that the therapist makes in the course of treatment. Examples of these are questions, confrontations, clarifications, explanations about the rationale of treatment, and occasional suggestions and advice (though there is general agreement that this last type of intervention should be used quite sparingly, since a basic value that undergirds the entire process is that the patient will benefit from moving in a more autonomous direction). There is also general agreement that interpretations that focus on the transference and its links to the patient's current and past unconscious conflicts, wishes, and fantasies are the most effective interventions. As noted above, Malan (1963, 1976) has presented some evidence that such interpretations, which presumably facilitate a "triangle of insight," are related to positive therapeutic outcome.

As we shall see, in some of the recent psychoanalytic literature, interpretation and insight have been pitted against other therapeutic factors, in particular, the therapeutic relationship. Thus, some have argued that it is the therapeutic relationship rather than interpretation and insight, that is the primary therapeutic agent. It seems to us, however, that it is misleading and not especially fruitful to dichotomize between these two therapeutic factors: they operate together, synergistically, one might say. Thus, the therapeutic impact of an interpretation, including how it is heard and received, is likely to reflect the nature of the patient–therapist relationship; and conversely, an empathic, well-timed, tactful, and insightful interpretation is likely to strengthen the relationship.

Finally, we will comment briefly on the issue of the validity of interpretations. There is a rather large literature, both psychoanalytic and philosophical, on the question of how one validates an interpretation. For example, what kind of evidence would serve to validate (or invalidate) to a patient an interpretation involving the attribution of an unconscious wish? The answers that have been given to this question include the impact of the interpretations of the patient's subsequent associations (e.g., Schmidl, 1955) and the patient's ultimate conscious acknowledgment of the wish attributed to him or to her (Mischel, 1963, 1966). Consider another question: What kind of evidence would validate (or invalidate) an interpretation pertaining to the patient's early experiences? The difficulties inherent in answering this kind of question have led some theorists to argue that in making interpretations and reconstructions of the patient's past, the analyst cannot claim "historical truth," but only "narrative truth"—that is, a plausible and convincing account (Spence, 1982).

Some recent work by Luborsky and his colleagues (e.g., Luborsky & Crits-Christoph, 1990) suggests possible means of determining the validity of at least some interpretations. Luborsky has developed a method by which clinical raters can assess patients' "Core Conflictual Relationship Themes" (CCRTs) from transcription of psychotherapy sessions. Based on the patient's account of relationship episodes, clinical raters can reliably assess the dominant *wishes (W)* expressed, the *experienced and expressed reactions from others (RO)* and consequent *reactions from the self (RS)*. Luborsky and his colleagues find that patients are characterized by a limited number of stable CCRTs. Of particular relevance in the present context: For a given patient one can operationally evaluate the accuracy of a therapist's interpretations by determining their degree of agreement with independently assessed ratings of the patient's predominant CCRTs. Luborsky reports that accuracy of interpretation defined in the manner described above, is positively correlated with positive therapeutic outcome. As far as we know, this is the first systematic demonstration that accuracy of interpretation is related to positive therapeutic outcome.

The therapist's ability to offer an "accurate," well-timed interpretation reflecting optimal tact is facilitated by his or her awareness and proper management of countertransference reactions and by a capacity for empathy. By empathy we mean that the therapist is able to experience a partial, transient identification with the patient in which there is a cognitive/affective "knowing" of the patient's inner world of experience. In this sense, empathy is a process of data gathering and forms the basis for whatever interpretation the therapist ultimately offers. In some theories, which we shall refer to later, empathy is not only seen as essential to understanding, but the act of empathic communication of one's understanding is regarded as a vital therapeutic factor in itself.

ANALYTIC NEUTRALITY AND ABSTINENCE

Most analysts agree that the therapist should assume a neutral role in the treatment. How neutrality is defined, however, is of great importance. Freud (1912b) recommended that the analyst remain an "opaque" or "blank screen" on to which the patient would project his or her wishes, conflicts, fantasies, and so on. According to this view, the "blank screen" role of the therapist would ensure that the patient's projections were "pure," uncontaminated by real characteristics of the therapist. A similar rationale was provided for the "principle of abstinence" (i.e., the withholding of transference gratification). It was assumed that frustration of transference wishes would most efficaciously stimulate the patient's wishes, conflicts, and fantasies and center them on the person of the analyst.

As discussed earlier, the idea that the therapist could remain a "blank screen" is really not a very tenable one. We are always emitting cues to others, whether we intend to or not. Furthermore, this unrealistic conception of analytic neutrality led to its caricatured implementation and enactment. That is, many analysts mistakenly equated neutrality with coldness, aloofness, stodginess, and excessive and unresponsive silence.

Given the untenability of the "blank screen" idea, what remains of the concept of analytic neutrality? It seems clear to us that a very useful and defensible aspect of analytic neutrality refers to the therapist's not taking sides in the patient's inner conflicts and instead attempting to remain equidistant between the two sides of the conflict. If the conflict is truly an intrapsychic one, the therapist's advocacy or alignment with one or another side will not be very useful in achieving the goal of an inner resolution. A clinical anecdote will illustrate this point.

Some years ago one of us was supervising a beginning therapist who presented a case in which an undergraduate female student from a very traditional immigrant family had been considering moving to her own apartment. The patient's father was outraged at this possibility and communicated his opposition in no uncertain terms. The patient was very upset by the situation she found herself in and came to treatment (at a university clinic) for help. As the case was reported, it became apparent that the therapist, a young graduate student herself, identified with the patient and sided with the latter's desire to acquire her own apartment. Indeed, she largely conceived of her therapeutic role as one in which she would support the patient's move toward "autonomy." The supervisor noted that what was being represented solely as a conflict between the patient and her father might well also include and mask an inner conflict (e.g., between the desire to move on the one hand and anxieties regarding separation and independence on the other) in which one side of the conflict (separation anxiety) was externalized and represented by father's opposition and hence, need not be confronted and experienced. The supervisor also cautioned that the therapist's role in supporting the patient's desire to move could also contribute to a shutting out and denial of conflicted feelings about moving. As it turned out, under the impact of the patient's mother's peacemaking and mediating efforts, the father relented somewhat in his opposition and took a "do what you want" attitude. He was now ready to negotiate about such matters as how frequently the patient would return home for meals, etc. At this point, with external opposition softened, the patient's own conflictual and ambivalent feelings about moving away from home fully surfaced. But because the therapist had taken the role of supporter of "autonomy," the patient found it difficult to work on her conflictual feelings and instead left treatment.

THE THERAPEUTIC OR THE HELPING ALLIANCE

Although some analysts (e.g., Brenner, 1979) have not found it useful to distinguish between the transference and the therapeutic alliance, most have found the distinction useful. The concept of therapeutic alliance is generally intended to emphasize the importance of establishing and maintaining a safe, therapeutic atmosphere in which the therapist's compassion, humanness, and respect for the patient is evident (Greenson, 1965) and in which the patient feels that he or she is supported by the therapist as they are cooperatively engaged in pursuing a common goal. Some analysts (e.g., Zetzel, 1966) believe that the therapeutic alliance not only constitutes a precondition for fostering the analytic process, but also is therapeutic in its own right—for example, by facilitating a "new ego identification" (Zetzel, 1966, p. 92) with the analyst and thereby permitting ego motivation and growth.

Some very promising systematic empirical work has been carried out in this area by Luborsky and his colleagues (e.g., Luborsky, 1976; Luborsky, Crits-Christoph, Alexander, Margolis, & Cohen, 1983; Morgan, Luborsky, Crits-Christoph, Curtis, & Solomon, 1982). Luborsky (1984) has used the term "helping alliance" to refer to the "degree to which the patient experiences the relationship with the therapist as helpful or potentially helpful in achieving the patient's goals in psychotherapy" (p. 79). He and his colleagues have been able to operationally define this construct. They found that one could obtain reliable judgments of the helping alliance, that scores on this measure were reasonably consistent from earlier, and later stages of treatment, and that early indications of a positive helping alliance predicted therapeutic improvement.

SOME RECENT CONCEPTIONS OF DYNAMIC PSYCHOTHERAPY

Although many of the concepts we have discussed—transference, counter-transference, resistance, interpretation—play a central role in all "schools" of dynamic psychotherapy, in the above account we have presented mainly a traditional or broadly Freudian view. The history of psychoanalysis has always been marked by dissent and pluralism. Thus, a complete discussion of psychoanalytic theories of treatment would include not only the work of Freud and of ego psychologists, but also the approaches of neo-Freudians, the work of Melanie Klein, the British school of object relations theorists, and the work of Kohut (e.g., 1984). Obviously, in a brief, introductory chapter we cannot cover all these approaches. (Those who want to read further in these areas can refer to Eagle, 1984; Eagle & Wolitzky, 1992; Greenberg and Mitchell, 1983.) What we will do is present some ideas and conceptualizations of psychotherapy that have been especially influential during the past three decades, particularly on the North American scene. These ideas and conceptualizations have been mainly derived from the work of Kohut (1971, 1977, 1984) and other self psychologists, from the writings of Fairbairn (1952) and Winnicott (1958, 1965) on object relations theory, and from the work of Weiss, Sampson, and their colleagues (1986) on control-mastery theory. Although these theoretical approaches differ in important ways on many issues, there are some central features that are common to all of them.

The Therapeutic Relationship

In many contemporary psychoanalytic approaches to psychotherapy there is a reduced emphasis on the therapeutic role of insight and an increased emphasis on the patient–therapist relationship as a *direct* therapeutic agent. Although the importance of the patient–therapist relationship is recognized in traditional psychoanalytic theory, it has largely an *indirect* role. That is, the therapeutic relationship serves a precondition for treatment and makes it possible for insight and analysis of the transference to operate. By contrast, in some contemporary views, the relationship itself is directly therapeutic. The factors and processes that are invoked to account for the supposed therapeutic efficacy of the relationship include identification with the therapist and a resumption of arrested development facilitated by the experience of a benevolent, understanding, and constructive relationship. This relationship partially compensates for what was traumatically missing in early development. Thus, Fairbairn (1952) maintains that in successful psychotherapy, an earlier "bad" object situation is replaced by a "good" object situation. In ordinary language, this means that earlier experiences of deprivation, frustration, neglect, rejection, and nonunderstanding are replaced by understanding and acceptance.

In a similar vein, Kohut (1977, 1984) directly and explicitly conceptualizes the therapeutic process in terms of resumption of developmental growth. In particular, Kohut believes that the patient's self-defects are engendered by early traumatic failures on the part of parents and that the patient enters treatment with a basic drive to repair these self-defects and to complete the development of the self. What makes the achievement of these goals possible is a therapeutic relationship in which early experiences of traumatic empathic failures are replaced by experiences of the therapist's empathic understanding and by "optimal failures." That is, even when the therapist fails to fully understand the patient (and one's understanding of another can never be perfect), his or her failure is not of traumatic proportions. It is "optimal" in the sense that it can be assimilated by the patient and can strengthen his or her ability to cope and to benefit from "good enough" understanding.

One way of contrasting the traditional Freudian view of psychotherapy with that of self psychology is to note that whereas from the perspective of the former, it is the *patient's* insight and understanding that are held to be therapeutic, in the latter view it is the *therapist's* understanding and the communication of such understanding to the patient that are held to be therapeutic. Another way to put this is to say that in the traditional view, *understanding* (one's wishes, conflicts, etc.) is therapeutic, whereas in the self psychology view, *being understood* is therapeutic.

The degree to which the contemporary psychoanalytic conceptions of treatment are similar to the formulations of Rogers (e.g., 1951) should be noted, particularly since these similarities often go unobserved and unacknowledged. According to Rogers, the experience of a relationship in which the other is nonjudgmentally caring, empathic, genuine, and accepting will in itself *automatically* facilitate innate actualizing tendencies and hence bring about change and growth. As a therapist, one does not need to do anything else, such as provide interpretations and insight. One should note that for Rogers the growth that is brought about in successful therapy is not so much a resumption of early arrested development, but rather an expression of a life-long actualizing tendency that needs proper interpersonal conditions in order to find expression.

In the contemporary "control-mastery" theory of Weiss, Sampson, and their colleagues (1986), the therapeutic relationship also plays a critical role, but with a somewhat different emphasis than that given by object relations theory or self psychology. According to Weiss and Sampson, *"unconscious pathogenic beliefs"* acquired in childhood interactions with parental figures are responsible for much neurotic distress and suffering. According to them, patients come to treatment, not to gratify infantile wishes—as is claimed in traditional Freudian theory—but to be rid of their pathogenic beliefs. Furthermore, they are assumed to have an *unconscious plan* as to how to go about achieving this goal. In general, patients attempt to find conditions in which it is safe to bring forth repressed material, to attempt to master the associated conflicts, anxieties, and traumas, and to attempt to disconfirm their pathogenic beliefs. In order to determine whether *conditions of safety* are present in the treatment (i.e., patients need to determine whether or not the therapist will react to them in the same way as parental figures did), patients unconsciously present *tests* to the therapist. If tests are *passed*, the patient is more likely, among other things, to bring forth repressed material, to experience less anxiety, and to show evidence of greater depth of experiencing. These patient responses are *not* associated with *test failures*. Much of the clinical richness of Weiss and Sampson's work is expressed in the accounts of what constitutes test-passing and test-failing for each patient. From a research and methodological point of view, one of the important contributions of Weiss and Sampson's work is the demonstration that one can obtain reliable ratings and measures of such factors as a patient's unconscious plan, whether a therapeutic intervention constitutes test-passing or test-failing, and the behavioral consequences of test-passing and test-failing.

At this point, we should elaborate on and provide some concrete examples of what Weiss and Sampson mean by pathogenic beliefs and what constitutes test-passing and test-failing. The essence of pathogenic beliefs is that, based on early interactions and implicit parental communications, developmentally normal goals, such as striving toward separation-individuation, are experienced as endangering oneself and others, and as threatening vital ties to parents, and hence are fraught with anxiety and guilt. These pathogenic beliefs can be understood as having an implicit if–then form such that *if* I pursue such and such a goal (e.g., to separate and become more independent), *then* I will be punished or I will endanger a vital relationship or I will be hurting someone important to me.

One person might have the pathogenic belief that "*if I pursue the goal of leading an independent life, it can only be at the expense of my parent(s),*" thus engendering intense guilt. Another person may suffer from the pathogenic belief that "*if I pursue my ambition and desire to be successful, I will be severely punished for surpassing my parent(s),*" thus resulting in the experience of "survivor guilt" (Modell, 1983) and the inhibition of ambitious striving.

As to what kind of therapist interventions and behaviors constitute test-passing and test-failing, one can state as a general rule-of-thumb that interventions that tend to *disconfirm* the patient's pathogenic beliefs represent test-passing, whereas those that tend to *confirm* the patient's pathogenic beliefs are experienced as *retraumatizations* and constitute test-failing. Let us provide a simple clinical example taken from a recent paper by Weiss (1990). "A woman who feared she would hurt her parents and her male therapist by becoming independent might experiment with independent behavior in her sessions by disagreeing with the therapist's opinions and then unconsciously monitoring him to see if he feels hurt" (pp. 107–108). Obviously, the therapist's tolerance and acceptance of disagreement would constitute test-passing, while his or her anger, or attempts to direct or control the patient would constitute test-failing.

It will be noted that implicit in Weiss and Sampson's concept of psychotherapy is the idea that test-passing and consequent positive therapeutic changes can occur without interpretations and without explicit insight. And indeed, they have empirically demonstrated that therapeutic changes do occur without interpretation. One can understand these changes largely as a product of the "corrective emotional experiences" (Alexander & French, 1946) provided by the therapeutic relationship. Many contemporary approaches, including those of Rogers and of the object relations theorists, Kohut's self psychology, and the control mastery theory of Weiss and Sampson, all of which view the patient–therapist relationship as the primary therapeutic agent, can be understood as different ways of formulating the primary importance of "corrective emotional experiences" in leading to positive therapeutic outcome.

Another common feature shared by the therapeutic approaches we have been considering is the assumption of a basic drive toward health. This is especially clear and explicit in Rogers' (1951) concept of an inborn and universal actualizing tendency. However, it is also expressed in (1) Kohut's (1977, 1984) idea that patients strive to complete developmental growth and will do so under appropriate therapeutic conditions; (2) Winnicott's (1965) idea that a "facilitating environment" (which includes the therapeutic situation) will automatically facilitate maturational growth; and (3) Weiss and Sampson's (1986) claim that patients are motivated to be rid of their unconscious pathogenic beliefs and have an unconscious plan as to how to accomplish that goal.

All theories of treatment accept the idea that empathy on the part of the therapist is a desirable, and even indispensable, aspect of therapy and of the therapeutic relationship. However, for some approaches (e.g., Freudian; cognitive-behavioral), empathy, like patient–therapist rapport, is a *precondition* for the operation of the presumable active therapeutic ingredients (e.g., interpretation and insight; capturing automatic thoughts and relinquishing irrational beliefs). By contrast, for other approaches (e.g., client-centered), empathy is itself an important active therapeutic agent. Indeed, in self psychology it is the most critical curative agent.

ALTERED CONCEPTION OF TRANSFERENCE

Common to all the more contemporary psychoanalytic approaches to psychotherapy we have been discussing is a revised understanding of the nature of transference. As discussed earlier, according to traditional theory, an essential aspect of the transference is the patient's push for the therapist to gratify his or her infantile wishes. Common to the more contemporary views we have been discussing is the rejection of this assumption and its replacement by the basic idea that patients come to treatment with the hope, not that their infantile wishes will be fulfilled, but that they will have a *new* set of experiences radically different from the traumatic, pathology-generating experiences of the past. Thus, in Weiss and Sampson's control-mastery theory, patients hope to have their pathogenic beliefs disconfirmed by the therapist's interventions and responses. In Kohut's self psychology, patients hope to receive the empathic mirroring necessary for the resumption of developmental growth, and in object relations theory, patients hope to experience the therapist as a "good object," in contrast to the traumatic "bad objects" of the past.

In this new conception of transference, therapeutic change is as likely to come about through such "silent" and implicit processes as disconfirmation of pathogenic beliefs, empathic understanding, and transference–countertransference enactments as through explicit interpretation and insight. Of course, ideally, these implicit and explicit factors will operate together in a congruent fashion.

SOME SELECTED RESEARCH ON DYNAMIC PSYCHOTHERAPY

We think it is appropriate to end this chapter by describing some recent research involving dynamic psychotherapy.

Weiss, Sampson, and Their Colleagues

Many of the formulations of Weiss and Sampson's (1986) control-mastery theory that we have discussed are buttressed by systematic empirical research. Using detailed process notes and transcripts of tape-recorded psychoanalytic sessions in a single case design, they have shown that independent judges can reliably agree regarding the nature of the patient's unconscious plan, which contents have been warded off, when the patient has presented a test to the analyst, and whether the analyst has passed or failed the test. They have also shown that test-passing is reliably followed by the patient becoming less anxious, more relaxed, more flexible and spontaneous, bolder in tackling issues in treatment, and friendlier toward others. Finally, in the course of treatment, the patient showed a steady decline in the number of statements in which she complained that she felt compelled to do something she did not consciously want to do or felt unable to do something she consciously wanted to do. (It should be noted that the issue of feeling driven rather than feeling a sense of control was a central complaint of the patient.) Silberschatz, Fretter, and Curtis (1986) reported that for two cases showing, respectively, very good and moderately good outcome, 89% and 80%, respectively, of the therapists' interventions were independently rated as "proplan" (that is, furthering the patient's unconscious plan), while 2% and 0%, respectively, of the interventions were "antiplan." Contrastingly, in a case showing poor outcome, 50% of the therapist's interventions were rated as "proplan," 6% as "antiplan," and 44% as "ambiguous." In a more recent paper, Silberschatz, Curtis, and Nathans (1989) found that when the therapist was rated low on test-passing, the result was poor outcome "as defined by conventional therapeutic outcome measures" (p. 44) and conversely, when the therapist was rated high on test-passing, the result was good outcome.

Luborsky and His Colleagues

Luborsky has pursued systematic investigation of the process of psychodynamic psychotherapy. Much of his work during the last number of years has been summarized in a recent book (Luborsky and his colleagues, 1988), which presents many complex findings that are difficult to summarize simply and succinctly. As noted earlier, according to Luborsky, patients' relationship episodes narrated in treatment can be reliably broken down into the wish or need the patient expresses (W), the response from the other (RO), and the subsequent reaction of the self (RS). Further, one can reliably find for each patient predominant or core conflictual relationship themes (CCRT). According to Luborsky et al., one finds the following pattern in successful treatment from early to late treatment sessions:

1. Relative stability in the main wish or need expressed.
2. A decrease in the percentage of negative responses from the other.
3. A decrease in the percentage of negative responses from the self.
4. An increase in the percentage of positive responses from the other.
5. An increase in the percentage of positive responses from the self.

As one can see from the above, it appears that even in successful treatment, the main wish or need expressed by the patient tends not to change. What does change is the experienced reaction of the other to one's expressed need or wish and one's own subsequent reaction to the response of the other. That the experienced response of the other changes in the course of treatment provides a clue as to what factors bring about change. The treatment factor that Luborsky most emphasizes as a critical one in effecting change is the patient's experience of a helping alliance or relationship. This general factor includes a "Type 1" helping alliance, which refers to the patient's experience of the therapist as helpful and supportive and a "Type 2" helping alliance, the predominant characteristic of which is the patient's experience of working together with the therapist in a joint effort and struggle.

One can link the importance of the helping alliance to the above noted CCRT changes in experienced responses from others and from the self. According to traditional psychoanalytic theory, the neurotic individual's wishes are linked to conflict and anxiety and set off "expected or remembered helplessness" (Freud, 1926). If the patient has been able to express these wishes in the therapy situation and experience the therapist's responses as helpful and supportive, then he or she will come to modify his or her experience and expectation of a negative response from the other and the consequent negative response from the self. According to Luborsky et al., these changes indicate that the patient has developed an increased sense of mastery and a decreased sense of helplessness in dealing with his or her core relationship problems. The patient is now better able to express his or her wishes and needs (as well as thoughts and feelings) with reduced anxiety and a greater sense of mastery, as shown in his or her experience and expectation of a positive response from the other (and from the self). (Note that from the perspective of Weiss and Sampson's [1986] control-mastery theory this whole sequence can be understood in terms of the therapist's test-passing and disconfirmation of the patient's pathogenic beliefs.)

Strupp and His Colleagues

We come, finally, in our brief sampling of psychotherapy research, to the work of Strupp and his colleagues. Like Luborsky, Strupp has been a pioneer in psychotherapy research. Also like Luborsky, Strupp's work has been too variegated to be subject to a brief summary. However, we can provide a sampling and some highlights.

Strupp understands psychotherapy as, above all, a human relationship and as a process of learning (and unlearning) in the context of that relationship (Strupp, 1986). Along with others, then, for Strupp psychotherapy is more a kind of *education* than a form of treatment. (Interestingly enough, Freud referred to psychoanalysis as "after-education"—that is, so to speak, as a second round of post-childhood socialization and education). In accord with that conception of psychotherapy, much of the research and writing of Strupp and his colleagues has focused on aspects of the *interaction* between patient and therapist in the therapeutic relationship. Thus, like Luborsky, Strupp and his colleagues have stressed the importance of the *therapeutic alliance* between patient and therapist. For example, they have developed a 44-item Vanderbilt University Therapeutic Alliance Scale, which clinical judges can reliably use to rate taped psychotherapy sessions for degree of therapeutic alliance (Hartley & Strupp, 1983).

Employing the Vanderbilt scale, Strupp and his colleagues found that although overall therapeutic alliance scores did not predict therapeutic outcome, there was a strong suggestion that with positive outcome patients the therapeutic alliance was highest during the first quarter of sessions, in contrast to poor outcome patients whose therapeutic alliance scores *fell* by the end of the first quarter of sessions (Hartley & Strupp, 1983). This pattern, suggesting the importance of the *early* therapeutic alliance for outcome, has also been reported by Luborsky (1976). In general, Hartley and Strupp (1983) conclude that the therapeutic alliance may be a necessary but not sufficient condition for determining therapy outcome. They concur with Morgan et al.'s (1982) observation that whereas a poor therapeutic alliance almost always predicted a poor outcome, good outcome occurred in cases both with many as well as with few signs of a therapeutic alliance.

In another study on the interaction between patient and therapist, Henry, Schacht, and Strupp (1986) found that positive and total *complementarity* between patient and therapist (complementarity refers to "a given interaction sequence in which the communication of one participant is thought to 'pull for' a complementary communication from the other" [Strupp et al., 1988, p. 693]) was related to good therapeutic outcome, while *multiple communications* "which simultaneously communicate more than one interpersonal message (e.g., acceptance and rejection) . . . were almost exclusively associated with therapies having poor outcome" (Strupp et al., 1988, p. 693).

Henry, Schacht, and Strupp (1986) found that in poor outcome, therapists' communications tended to be more hostile and negative. However, what is quite fascinating is that the therapists' own self-rated introject "at worst" was significantly related to the number of hostile statements made to the patient. And, quite consistent with this finding, Christensen, Lane, and Strupp (1987) found that the degree of hostility in the therapists' reports of past relationships with their parents was predictive of similarly poor interpersonal process in the therapy interaction.

There is much else one can discuss regarding the work of Strupp and his colleagues—for example, the relation between psychotherapy research and practice (e.g., Strupp, 1989); psychotherapy research and practice and public policy (e.g., Strupp, 1986); a manual for short-term psychodynamic psychotherapy (Strupp & Binder, 1984); and the nature of training in psychodynamic psychotherapy (e.g., Strupp et al., 1988). However, we trust that the foregoing has provided some idea of the range and importance of the contributions of Strupp and his colleagues. And we also trust that the sampling of psychotherapy research that we have presented will provide the reader with an idea of the range and vitality of research, theory, and practice in psychodynamic psychotherapy.

SUMMARY

In concluding this chapter, we should like to underline what we hope has been implicit in our exposition; namely, that currently we do not have a single, agreed upon, comprehensive theory of psychoanalytic psychotherapy which, by the way, would have to include a specification of which particular variants of the approaches outlined above are most suited for particular kinds of patients. It is a healthy sign that there are active discussions and debates concerning the modes of therapeutic action of psychoanalytic psychotherapies and the beginnings of systematic research that will refine our understanding of the therapeutic process, its successes, and its failures.

REFERENCES

Alexander, F., & French, T. M. (1946). *Psychoanalytic therapy: Principles and applications*. New York: Ronald Press.
Brenner, C. (1979). Working alliance, therapeutic alliance and transference. *Journal of the American Psychoanalytic Association, 27* (Suppl.), 137–157.
Brenner, C. (1982). *The mind in conflict*. New York: International Universities Press.
Christensen, J. C., Lane, T. W., & Strupp, H. H. (1987). *Pre-therapy interpersonal relations and introject as reflected in the therapeutic process*. Paper presented at the meeting of the Society for Psychotherapy Research (SPR), Ulm, West Germany.
Eagle, M. (1984). *Recent developments in psychoanalysis: A critical evaluation*. Cambridge, MA: Harvard University Press.
Eagle, M., & Wolitzky, D. L. (1992). Psychoanalytic theories of psychotherapy. In D. K. Freedheim (Ed.), *History of psychotherapy: A century of change* (pp. 109–158). Washington, DC: American Psychological Association.

Fairbairn, W. R. D. (1952). *Psychoanalytic studies of the personality*. London: Tavistock Publications & Routledge & Kegan Paul.

Freud, S. (1982–1893). A case of successful treatment by hypnotism. *Standard Edition* (Vol. 2, pp. 115–128). London: Hogarth Press, 1966.

Freud, S. (1910). The future prospects of psychoanalytic therapy. *Standard Edition* (Vol. 11, pp. 139–151). London: Hogarth Press.

Freud, S. (1912a). The dynamics of transference. *Standard Edition* (Vol. 12, pp. 97–108). London: Hogarth Press, 1958.

Freud, S. (1912b). Recommendations to physicians practising psychoanalysis. *Standard Edition* (Vol. 12, pp. 109–120). London: Hogarth Press, 1958.

Freud, S. (1914). On the history of the psychoanalytic movement. *Standard Edition* Vol. 14, pp. 7–66). London: Hogarth Press, 1957.

Freud, S. (1923). The ego and the id. *Standard Edition* (Vol. 19, pp. 3–59). London: Hogarth Press, 1961.

Freud, S. (1926). Inhibitions, symptoms, and anxiety. *Standard Edition* (Vol. 10, pp. 87–174). London: Hogarth Press, 1959.

Freud, S. (1933). The dissection of the psychical personality. *Standard Edition* (Vol. 17, pp. 57–81). London: Hogarth Press, 1964.

Gill, M. M. (1982). *Analysis of transference*. New York: International Universities Press.

Greenberg, J. R., & Mitchell, S. A. (1983). *Object relations in psychoanalytic theory*. Cambridge, MA: Harvard University Press.

Greenson, R. R. (1965). The working alliance and the transference neurosis. *Psychoanalytic Quarterly, 34*, 155–181.

Hartley, D., & Strupp, H. (1983). The therapeutic alliance: Its relationship to outcome in brief psychotherapy. In J. Masling (Ed.), *Empirical studies of psychoanalytic theory* (Vol. I, pp. 1–27. Hillsdale, NJ: Laurence Erlbaum.

Henry, W. P., Schacht, T. E., & Strupp, H. H. (1986). Structural analysis of social behavior: Application to a study of interpersonal process in differential psychotherapeutic outcome. *Journal of Consulting and Clinical Psychology, 54*, 27–31.

Kohut, H. (1971). *The analysis of the self*. New York: International Universities Press.

Kohut, H. (1977). *The restoration of the self*. New York: International Universities Press.

Kohut, H. (1984). *How does analysis cure?* Chicago: University of Chicago Press.

Kris, E. (1947). The nature of psychoanalytic propositions and their validation. In S. Hook & M. R. Korwitz (Eds.), *Freedom and experience: Essays presented to Horace Kalle* (pp. 239–259). New York: Cornell University Press.

Luborsky, L. (1976). Helping alliances in psychotherapy: The groundwork for a study of their relationship to its outcome. In J. Claghorn (Ed.), *Successful psychotherapy* (pp. 92–116). New York: Brunner/Mazel.

Luborsky, L. (1984). *Principles of psychoanalytic psychotherapy: A manual for supportive–expressive treatment*. New York: Basic Books.

Luborsky, L., & Crist-Christoph, P. (1990). *Understanding transference: The CCRT method*. New York: Basic Books.

Luborsky, L., Crits-Christoph, P., Alexander, L., Margolis, M., & Cohen, M. (1983). Two helping alliance methods for predicting outcomes of psychotherapy: A counting signs versus a global rating method. *Journal of Nervous and Mental Disease, 17*, 480–492.

Luborsky, L., Crits-Christoph, P., Mintz, J., & Auerbach, A. (1988). *Who will benefit from psychotherapy?: Predicting therapeutic outcome*. New York: Basic Books.

Malan, D. (1963). *A study of brief psychotherapy*. New York: Plenum Press.

Malan, D. (1976). *The frontier of brief psychotherapy*. New York: Plenum Press.

Mischel, T. (1963). Psychology and explanations of human behavior. *Philosophy and Phenomenological Research, 23*, 578–594.

Mischel, T. (1966). Pragmatic aspects of explanation. *Philosophy of Science, 33*, 40–60.

Modell, A. (1983). Self preservation and the preservation of the self: An overview of the more recent knowledge of the narcissistic personality. Paper given at Symposium on "Narcissism, masochism, and the sense of guilt in relation to the therapeutic process," Letterman General Hospital, San Francisco, California, May 14–15, 1983.

Morgan, R., Luborsky, L., Crits-Christoph, P., Curtis, H., & Solomon, J. (1982). Predicting the outcomes of psychotherapy by the Penn Helping Alliance rating method. *Archives of General Psychiatry, 39*, 397–402.

Rogers, C. R. (1951). *Client-centered therapy*. Boston: Houghton-Mifflin.

Schmidl, F. (1955). The problem of scientific validation in psychoanalytic interpretation. *International Journal of Psychoanalysis, 36*, 105–113.

Silberschatz, G., Fretter, P. B., & Curtis, J. T. (1986). How do interpretations influence the process of psychotherapy? *Journal of Consulting and Clinical Psychology, 54*(5), 646–652.

Silberschatz, G., Curtis, J. T., & Nathans, S. (1989). Using the patient's plan to assess progress in psychotherapy. *Psychotherapy, 26*(1), 40–46.

Spence, D. P. (1982). *Narrative truth and historical truth*. New York: W. W. Norton.

Strupp, H. H. (1986). Research, practice, and public policy (How to avoid dead ends). *American Psychologist, 41*(2), 120–130.

Strupp, H. H. (1989). Can the practitioner learn from the researcher? *American Psychologist, 44*(4), 717–724.

Strupp, H. H., & Binder, J. L. (1984). *Psychotherapy in a new key: A guide to time-limited dynamic psychotherapy*. New York: Basic Books.

Strupp, H. H., Butler, S. F., & Rosser, C. L. (1988). Training in psychodynamic therapy. *Journal of Consulting and Clinical Psychology, 56*(5), 689–695.

Waelder, R. (1960). *Basic theory of psychoanalysis*. New York: International Universities Press.

Weiss, J. (1990). Unconscious mental functioning. *Scientific American, 262*(3), 103–109.

Weiss, J., Sampson, H., & the Mount Zion Psychotherapy Research Group. (1986). *The psychoanalytic process: Theory, clinical observation and empirical research*. New York: Guilford Press.

Winnicott, D. W. (1958). *Collected papers: Through paediatrics to psychoanalysis*. London: Tavistock Publications Ltd.

Winnicott, D. W. (1965). *The maturational processes and the facilitating environment*. London: The Hogarth Press and the Institute of Psycho-Analysis, 1987.

Zetzel, E. (1966). The analytic situation. In R. E. Litman (Ed.), *Psychoanalysis in the Americans* (pp. 86–106). New York: International Universities Press.

25

Behavior Therapy

Kevin T. Larkin and Jennifer L. Edens

Introduction

Although the term behavior therapy was not employed until the early 1950s, behavioral interventions have been in use for centuries. For example, holding a fearful child's hand when approaching the ocean for the first time, withholding a teenager's allowance for failing to make his or her curfew, and providing salary incentives for exceptional work productivity all represent tactics aimed at altering one's behavior. Centuries of anecdotal evidence have indicated the efficacy of behavioral strategies of this type. As behaviorism became more influential in psychology throughout the twentieth century, it was not surprising that specific behavioral therapeutic applications were formulated to deal with the most severe psychosocial problems seen: that is, those seen in persons manifesting psychiatric disorders.

Despite the uniformity among behavior therapists commonly perceived by the public, not all behavior therapists are alike, and these differences are reflected in the numerous terms that have been employed to describe this general therapeutic approach (e.g., behavior modification, applied behavior analysis, cognitive–behavior therapy). Despite these various terminologies employed to describe one's approach, therapists who have a behavioral orientation hold in common the importance placed upon the scientific method (both in laboratory and clinical settings). They adhere to the belief that current problems are caused and maintained by maladaptive learning experiences, and they deny unconscious or psychodynamic factors in explaining behavioral problems. Traditionally, behavior therapists approach each problem through what is termed a functional behavior

Kevin T. Larkin and Jennifer L. Edens • Department of Psychology, West Virginia University, Morgantown, West Virginia 26506.

Advanced Abnormal Psychology, edited by Vincent B. Van Hasselt and Michel Hersen. Plenum Press, New York, 1994.

analysis, in which the physiological, cognitive, and behavioral facets of a current problem are identified with respect to the context in which it typically occurs. To elucidate such a functional analysis, consider the following case.

> Stan is a 21-year-old college student who exhibits extreme nervousness in dating, classroom, and other social situations. In such situations, he manifests physiological responses of facial flushing, rapid heartbeat, increased rate of breathing, "butterflies in the stomach," and palmar sweating. Also, he commonly believes that others perceive him as socially inept and can detect his degree of nervousness in social settings. Needless to say, he engages in very few social encounters, dates infrequently, and spends most of his free time playing videogames on his home computer. When coerced by his peers, Stan will occasionally go on an outing but rarely does so without drinking a few beers "to calm down." Often, even alcohol fails to reduce his anxiety, and so Stan leaves social functions early and returns to his room alone.

A functional behavioral analysis of Stan's problem is depicted in Figure 1. When confronted with a social situation, Stan responds by becoming physiologically aroused and thinking others will notice his degree of nervousness. He becomes preoccupied with the perceived level of aversiveness of his anxiety, which perpetuates the problem in a cyclic fashion. The more arousal he experiences, the more he is concerned about others detecting his nervousness; the more he worries about his perceived social ineptness, the more physiologically aroused he becomes. Sensing that he cannot tolerate this anxiety much longer, Stan resorts to two coping behaviors that have been shown to reduce tension in the past: drinking alcohol and/or escaping from the situation. A sense of relief and anxiety reduction accompany his return to his room. The removal or reduction of anxious symptoms that occurs following these escape behaviors serves to reinforce such behavioral patterns, thereby maintaining the problem and making it more likely to occur in the future. Therefore, in contrast to other therapeutic perspectives, the primary focus of the functional analysis is on defining the factors that are currently maintaining it.

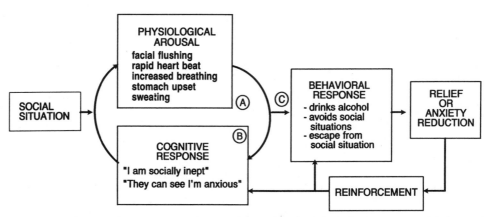

FIGURE 1. A functional behavioral analysis outlining the physiological, cognitive, and behavioral components of social anxiety and consequent negative reinforcement that occurs through anxiety reduction. Interventions employing anxiety reduction strategies occur at point A, cognitive restructuring strategies occur at point B, and operant strategies occur at point C.

Based upon a functional behavioral analysis of the sort described, behavioral treatment plans focus upon a relearning process to change the sequence of events illustrated. Most behaviorally oriented clinicians would have little trouble conceptualizing this case as outlined in Figure 1; however, the specific intervention employed with Stan may differ from clinician to clinician, depending upon where he or she desires to interrupt this pattern of events. Three different approaches can be considered: (1) anxiety reduction techniques aimed at decreasing the phenomenological experience of anxiety (point A), (2) cognitive restructuring techniques aimed at altering specific thoughts that are instrumental in maintaining the problem (point B), or (3) operant extinction techniques aimed at removing the reinforcing properties of the escape and avoidance behaviors (point C). Each of these avenues for intervention will be explored with respect to background information, outcome data pertaining to a number of psychological disorders, and a description of how such a strategy would be employed in treating Stan's problems with social anxiety.

ANXIETY REDUCTION STRATEGIES

Anxiety reduction strategies, including relaxation and meditation, have been used for centuries; however, it has been only recently that such techniques were exposed to experimental scrutiny. It was mainly the work of Joseph Wolpe (1958, 1990) that was instrumental in the scientific exploration and demonstration of the utility of anxiety reduction strategies. Wolpe's procedure aimed at reducing anxiety, termed systematic desensitization, involves three steps: (1) relaxation training during which patients are taught to achieve an ultimate relaxed state; (2) the construction of an anxiety hierarchy, which is a list of anxiety-eliciting situations ranging from situations with low levels of anxiety to events that create extreme anxiety; and (3) the desensitization procedure itself, during which scenes from the hierarchy are imagined during deep relaxation. With time, patients are able to imagine their most feared scenes without anxiety. Wolpe explained the success of systematic desensitization through a physiological process known as reciprocal inhibition. To put it simply, this principle states that a person cannot exhibit the physiological state accompanying relaxation and anxiety simultaneously because each state inhibits the expression of the other. Accordingly, the state of relaxation inhibits the experience of anxiety and serves as the basis for how systematic desensitization works. Others have disagreed with Wolpe, suggesting that systematic desensitization works because of extinction following imaginal or actual (i.e., *in vivo*) exposure to the feared stimulus (Marks, 1976), or that it works because it provides the patient with a highly credible procedure and positive expectancy for improvement (Wilkins, 1971).

Employing an anxiety reduction strategy, such as systematic desensitization, in treating Stan's problem with social anxiety would begin with comprehensive training in relaxation procedures (e.g., progressive muscle relaxation). This is followed by the construction of an anxiety hierarchy composed of scenes that elicit various amounts of social anxiety (see Table 1). Once Stan demonstrates competency in achieving a relaxed state, he would be instructed to relax himself during presentation of progressively more anxiety-evoking images from the hierarchy. Typically within eight to twelve sessions, Stan would be able to imagine the most

TABLE 1. Stan's Hierarchy of Socially Anxious Situations

Step	Scene	SUDS[a]
1	Playing videogames alone in room and roommate walks in	11
2	Playing videogames in Student Union with no other students in the arcade	26
3	Playing videogames in Student Union with roommate	33
4	Playing videogames in Student Union with small crowd	42
5	Going to a quiet party with roommate after two beers	55
6	Going to a quiet party alone after two beers	70
7	Going to a large party with roommate after two beers	75
8	Going to a large party alone after two beers	80
9	Going to a quiet party with roommate with no alcohol	95
10	Going to a quiet party alone with no alcohol	98
11	Going to a large party with roommate with no alcohol	100
12	Going to a large party alone with no alcohol	100

[a]SUDS refers to subjective units of distress, a 0–100 scale measuring anticipated anxiety/distress assoicated with engaging in that particular item (adapted from Wolpe, 1990).

stressful scene on the hierarchy without experiencing anxiety. Successful imaginal presentations without anxiety are often followed by instructions to actually practice engaging in that particular task during intervening weeks of therapy (*in vivo* desensitization).

Anxiety Disorders

As one might expect, there is substantial literature demonstrating the efficacy of systematic or *in vivo* desensitization with a large number of problems, most notably anxiety disorders. In particular, regarding the treatment of phobic disorders, including social and simple phobias, these approaches constitute treatments of choice. Numerous empirical investigations attest to the efficacy of these approaches, their comparatively low cost, and the enduring nature of behavior change observed at follow-up. Desensitization procedures have also demonstrated efficacy for treating the behavioral avoidance exhibited among agoraphobic patients. Furthermore, based upon the principles outlined by Wolpe, several airlines have developed programs to overcome fear of flying, and dental clinics have employed comparable programs to deal with dental anxiety and phobia.

Sexual Dysfunction

Sexual dysfunctions, including impotence, anorgasmia (inability to achieve orgasm), dyspareunia (painful intercourse), and inhibited sexual desire, are commonly thought to be anxiety-mediated phenomena. Following determination that such problems are not organic in nature, a treatment very similar to systematic desensitization can be employed. Masters and Johnson (1970) were instrumental in formalizing an anxiety reduction strategy termed "sensate focus therapy" to deal with problems of sexual arousal. Similar to the desensitization procedures already described, sensate focus involves gradual exposure to progressively more sexually intimate exercises, often preceded by training in anxiety reduction strategies. For example, early exercises involve backrubbing, handholding, and kissing; more moderate exercises involve total body caressing; and advanced exercises involve genital stimulation and intercourse. Although the number of controlled investigations of sensate focus therapy is far inferior to those supporting systematic desensitization, there is considerable case report evidence to support its continued use.

Psychophysiological Disorders

Since the discovery that certain physical disorders (e.g., essential hypertension, ulcer) reflect a person's inability to tolerate or cope with the amount of stress in his or her environment, a large number of stress management programs have arisen. Central to most programs of this type is an emphasis upon developing better strategies for relaxation. These programs include: progressive muscle relaxation, autogenic training, yoga, transcendental meditation, stretch relaxation, self-hypnosis, guided imagery, clinically standardized meditation, breathing retraining, and biofeedback-assisted relaxation. Although the definitive study to compare and contrast the efficacy of these procedures has yet to be carried out, it is safe to assume that there exists considerable overlap among strategies. Almost all require a state of sustained attention in a quiet, comfortable therapy room, the therapist's use of soothing vocal characteristics, and an emphasis upon home practice to learn the technique.

Perhaps the strongest evidence for the use of relaxation training for treating psychophysiological disorders exists in the behavioral treatments for headache. Time-limited courses in relaxation or biofeedback training have shown remarkable success at alleviating pain from either migraine or muscle-tension headaches (Blanchard & Andrasik, 1982). Similar stress management procedures have also demonstrated success at blood pressure reduction among essential hypertensive patients, increased blood flow to the periphery among patients with Raynaud's disease, and improved gastrointestinal motility among patients diagnosed with irritable bowel syndrome.

COGNITIVE–BEHAVIORAL STRATEGIES

In the 1970s, behaviorally trained clinicians were often criticized for ignoring what were perceived as being important mental events relevant to understanding a patient's presenting symptom picture. Although the validity of these assertions can be immediately called into question upon examining the importance cognitive activity plays in the functional behavioral analysis described earlier, these criticisms served to polarize the field: a state that has continued into the 1990s. While some behavior therapists acknowledge the central role of anxiety reduction strategies that evolved from the conditioning models of behavioral pathology (Wolpe, 1989), others have elevated the importance of cognitive or mental events in explaining the etiology of maladaptive behavioral problems (Beck, 1976; Meichenbaum, 1977). This latter group of practitioners, who often are referred to as cognitive–behavioral therapists, have focused on developing new strategies aimed at altering directly the cognitive component of the prevailing problem.

Returning to our socially anxious friend, Stan, a therapist employing a cognitive approach would begin by outlining the maladaptive nature of his prevailing thoughts in response to social situations. Because thought processes are often well learned and may appear to occur automatically, the first phase of treatment would involve training to recognize thoughts of a maladaptive nature. For example, Stan's beliefs, that he is socially inept and that other people can detect his degree of nervousness, are not facilitating optimal functioning in social settings. Indeed, these beliefs would be labeled as maladaptive. Furthermore, these thoughts may be totally false and have no basis in reality! Stan may exhibit satisfactory social skills and his degree of anxiety may go largely unnoticed. After common negative thinking patterns have been identified, treatment would proceed with the second phase of cognitive restructuring, or replacing maladaptive thoughts with more productive beliefs. This can be attained through the active challenging or disputing of the maladaptive belief system as advocated by Ellis (1977), or by rehearsing positive self-statements to use during social situations, as advocated by Meichenbaum (1977). In Stan's case, he would be able to diffuse his negative thinking patterns by asking the question: "Where is the evidence that others can detect my degree of anxiousness?" Because evidence to support this maladaptive thought was lacking, he might conclude that his beliefs were in error. Anxiety reduction and a decreased tendency to engage in escape or avoidance behaviors would follow.

Anxiety Disorders

Complementing the anxiety reduction strategies described above, a number of cognitive–behavioral approaches have been employed with anxiety disorder patients. To parallel the systematic desensitization procedure, Goldfried, Decanteceo, and Weinberg (1974) developed a procedure known as systematic rational restructuring, which involved training in cognitive restructuring skills rather than in relaxation skills and then employing them in the progressively more difficult situations outlined on a patient's hierarchy. Extrapolating from promising results observed with these early cognitive interventions, Heimberg and Barlow (1988) developed a cognitive behavioral group therapy where socially anxious participants practice interactions within the context of the treatment group. These approaches have been demonstrated to be quite effective for dealing with a variety of problems pertaining to social anxiety, including speech anxiety, social phobia, and deficits in assertive behavior.

Perhaps the most intriguing use of cognitive–behavioral strategies with anxiety disorders involves a therapeutic program aimed at treating panic disorder (Barlow & Craske, 1989). As part of this program, participants are taught to identify and question the validity of their catastrophic thinking patterns that occur in response to the physiological burst of activity observed during a panic attack. Recent reports have revealed superior treatment outcome, with the majority of treatment completers remaining panic-free at a 2-year follow-up.

Depression

Although advances in cognitive–behavioral strategies have been made with a number of patient populations, there is no more compelling evidence for the efficacy of these procedures than findings from clinical trials of the cognitive treatment of depression. Stemming from the belief that people depress themselves by engaging in a variety of negative thinking patterns and perceptual styles in response to environmental events, Aaron Beck (1976) developed and formalized this therapeutic approach. Treatment of depression, according to Beck, involves identification and challenging of common maladaptive thoughts and their deeper cognitive roots (i.e., a belief system referred to as a cognitive schema). Through a collaborative relationship with the therapist, the patient learns to consider alternative thought processes that may be just as valid as the depressing thoughts. For example, upon failing a test a student might think that this poor performance is the result of his or her stupidity or ignorance, which leads to a depressive state. Accordingly, the failure itself does not result in depression, but rather it is the belief that, "I failed the test because I am stupid" that results in depressive affect. Alternative conceptualizations discovered through the therapeutic process may include failing the test because it was an extremely difficult test or because the student did not study hard enough. In both cases, if evidence exists for the alternative, the level of depressive mood can be attenuated. Empirical efforts aimed at examining the efficacy of this approach have provided clear evidence that cognitive therapy for depression results in reduced negative affect. Further, the magnitude of mood change parallels the effects of commonly accepted therapy with antidepressant medication or electroconvulsive therapy.

Personality Disorders

The clinical challenges of treating individuals with personality disorders is legend, and until recently, a lack of behavioral treatment conceptualizations existed for these patients. Yet, the frequency with which individuals who manifest maladaptive, temporally stable clusters of behaviors indicative of a personality disorder present in clinical settings demands treatment consideration. Behavioral and cognitive–behavioral interventions can be efficacious, although behavior therapists must spend more time focusing upon collaboration with the patient in developing clear, shared goals as well as fostering positive characteristics of the therapist–patient relationship. In addition, patient noncompliance and slow therapeutic progression typically accompany working with patients with personality disorders.

Despite these difficulties, recent attempts have been made by behaviorally oriented clinicians to evaluate the efficacy of behavioral and cognitive–behavioral treatments with personality-disordered individuals. Depending upon individual presentation, a number of cognitive–behavioral techniques may be useful with this subset of patients (Beck, 1990). Labeling of cognitive distortions, disputing of maladaptive beliefs, decatastrophizing, and application of assertion and problem-solving skills may all be useful with such individuals. In addition, more traditional behavioral strategies may also be integral, such as role playing to facilitate skill development, relaxation training or behavioral distraction, *in vivo* exposure to problematic settings, and behavioral monitoring and other homework assignments used to ensure practice of new skills.

With respect to treating patients suffering from borderline personality disorder, Linehan (1987) has developed a therapeutic program that combines cognitive modification and restructuring with more traditional techniques such as skills training, contingency management, and exposure to emotionally arousing cues in a structured, 1-year treatment package comprising both individual and group therapy components. Recent outcome research has indicated that, when compared with traditional community therapy, severely dysfunctional female borderline patients treated with Linehan's approach had fewer and less severe parasuicidal episodes, were more likely to remain in therapy, and experienced fewer days in inpatient psychiatric units.

OPERANT STRATEGIES

The hallmark of most behavior therapy techniques lies in the use of some facets of operant conditioning. While factors such as respondent conditioning, observational learning, and cognitions may impact on behavioral presentation, reinforcement and punishment paradigms appear universally present in the acquisition, maintenance, and elimination of behavior. Operant methods may be broadly dichotomized into two categories: those techniques that increase the likelihood of a specific behavior occurring, and those that decrease that likelihood. Common methods used to achieve the former include positive and negative reinforcement and shaping. A preponderance of methods have been developed to achieve the latter, including extinction, punishment, and differential reinforcement techniques.

Positive reinforcement methods of behavior change involve the presentation of a desirable stimulus contingent upon emitting an appropriate behavior. Examples of this include providing a salary incentive to a worker who exceeded her productivity goals or providing a new and desired item of clothing for a spouse who has lost weight. Conversely, negative reinforcement involves response-contingent removal of an unpleasant stimulus, resulting in an individual's escape from an undesirable situation. For example, returning to Stan's social fears, escape behaviors employed by this patient result in the termination of the anxiousness experienced in social settings. Therefore, escape behaviors as well as the preceding social anxiety are negatively reinforced by anxiety reduction.

While it is evident that reinforcement strategies can effectively increase the performance rates for behaviors already present within the individual's repertoire, the same can not be said for the development and maintenance of behaviors not currently within the behavioral repertoire. If a novel or unusual response is the target of therapeutic intervention, then the behavior must be "shaped" by systematic reinforcement of activities that successively approximate the desired behavior. Using this shaping technique, the individual is assessed to derive an activity that can be successfully performed and that, although distinct, is similar to the desired behavior. Emission of this distinct behavior is initially reinforced, with the criterion for reinforcement shifting to closer and closer approximations of the desired behavior throughout treatment. For example, in shaping assertive behavioral responses in an extremely passive-dependent patient, reinforcement may be initially provided for a verbal response of any type. Through successive approximations, the specific content and nonverbal style of presentation can be shaped to arrive at the delivery of an appropriate assertive statement.

The list of operant techniques available to decrease response likelihood is much more extensive than the list for targeting response increases. Of course, this is consistent with a bias toward dealing with pathology rather than attempting to prevent its expression. Punishment represents the most basic technique for response diminishment, and can be broadly defined as the provision of a negative

reinforcement, coping strategies, and stimulus control, also shows promise for effective maintenance of treatment gains.

Organic Mental Disorders and Traumatic Brain Injury

Because the range of difficulties and the level of impairment among individuals suffering from traumatic brain injuries (TBI) and dementing processes are highly variable, the therapeutic techniques most suited to these patients must be individualized, with useful strategies running the gamut of behavioral techniques. This specificity makes well-controlled, comprehensive outcome studies of therapy with this population particularly difficult to evaluate with respect to generalization of effects across patients and over time. A second difficulty with these populations concerns onset of psychopathology, particularly mood disorders, secondary to the onset of their cognitive and functional deficits. Presence of depressive features in such patients may not only inhibit treatment of the deficits, but may also make the patients appear more impaired than they actually are.

Traumatic Brain Injury (TBI)

Individuals who have experienced TBI generally undergo some formal means of cognitive rehabilitation or remediation/retraining, which involves a hierarchical progression through cognitive and behavioral goals to achieve maximum functional benefit. Cognitive rehabilitation programs can be broadly categorized as: (1) those individually tailored to ameliorate specific deficits, and (2) more general, fixed curriculum programs. The former method asserts that discrete training will affect global functioning, while the latter conversely asserts that broad retraining will impact on general and residual deficits (Incagnoli & Newman, 1985).

Because TBI patients tend to show constellations of deficits across several cognitive and psychosocial domains, a variety of cognitive and behavioral targets are recommended. Visual and perceptual deficits may be ameliorated by shaping the patient's visual scanning skills and providing performance feedback and reinforcement. Attentional deficits have been targeted using programs that shape skills in the areas of attention, arousal, and concentration. Computer programs to enhance reaction time, attention, and concentration have also shown modest success.

Memory deficits have traditionally been targeted in TBI patients with the use of memory aids, such as date books, notes posted in conspicuous view, and resettable timers. While remediation of language deficits is not routinely pursued by behavior therapists, Melodic Intonation Therapy (singing information that cannot be verbalized) and nonverbal communication strategies (symbol and sign language) have been used successfully with some aphasic patients (Brown, Gouvier, & Blanchard-Fields, 1990).

Dementing Processes

Treatment of TBI patients involves retraining to reestablish as much premorbid functioning as possible and to provide methods to compensate for lost functioning. By contrast, in patients experiencing progressive dementing processes, treatment is more likely concerned with maintenance of current skills and compensation for lost skills. Appropriate orientation and sustained attention can be targeted by providing orienting information to the patient, as well as environmental symbols, such as color-coding and labeling hallways and doors. Declining memory skills can be targeted using mnemonics to aid encoding, and reinforcement to aid in attention, rehearsal, and maintenance of encoded material. Shaping and reinforcement of memory by progressively increasing intervals between stimulus presentation and retrieval may also be modestly effective.

Several operant strategies have been used effectively to treat general behavioral difficulties among both TBI and dementing patients. Excessive or inappropriate behaviors, such as impulsiveness, restlessness, aggressiveness, and affective lability, can be targeted with patient self-monitoring, modeling, and shaping. Punishment procedures, such as time out, differential reinforcement schedules, and extinction, may also be effective with these behaviors. Behaviors that are absent or occur at a lower than desirable rate, such as social interactions, self-control, and positive mood, can be facilitated with role playing, modeling, shaping, self-monitoring, and reinforcement, as well as with assertiveness and social skills training.

COMBINATION STRATEGIES

Due to the enormous body of literature supporting anxiety reduction, cognitive–behavioral, and operant conditioning strategies, it is not surprising that many behavior therapists have integrated components of all three in implementing what can best be termed combination strategies. For example, Meichenbaum's (1985) Stress Inoculation Training involves training in relaxation *and* cognitive restructuring followed by systematic exposure to stressful situations. Variations of this approach to target problems with anxiety and anger expression have also been implemented successfully. Although these approaches have considerable clinical utility, it is difficult, if not impossible, to determine which treatment component or combination of components is responsible for the observed behavior change. Therefore, investigations of combined strategies lend little information about our understanding of the mechanisms responsible for therapeutic behavior change.

SUMMARY

Behavior therapy has advanced considerably over the past 40 years, growing from early single-subject investigations of conditioning strategies to its present application with virtually every diagnostic presentation. For the most part, outcome findings have been impressive and in some cases (e.g., simple phobia, obsessive–compulsive disorder, posttraumatic stress disorder, sexual dysfunction) behavioral therapeutic applications are the treatments of choice.

Despite the significant growth of the field and demonstrated efficacy, continued empirical work is warranted on many strategies employed by behavior therapists. Perhaps the most important unanswered question pertains to the unknown mechanisms of behavior change and what conditioning or learning principles are responsible for the relearning that occurs during therapy. Even well-studied procedures, such as systematic desensitization, lack consistent definition regarding causal mechanisms of change.

Secondly, behavior therapists are beginning to examine their strategies without solely relying on the diagnostic nomenclature employed in psychiatry. It has long been known that despite great efforts to achieve an effective categorization system for psychiatric disturbances, considerable individual differences exist within these diagnostic groupings. It is often such specific information that is crucial in optimizing successful matching of patient problems with treatment strategies. Efforts in this direction will enable a more comprehensive evaluation of pretreatment characteristics in search of prognostic indicators for satisfactory treatment outcome.

Finally, there has been increased impetus among behavioral scientists to integrate the important contributions of behavior therapy not only with other therapeutic orientations, such as psychodynamic and pharmacologic approaches (Bellack & Hersen, 1990), but also with other realms of psychological science, including social, developmental, and cognitive psychology (Martin, 1991). These efforts can assure that behavior therapy will continue to expand into new and exciting areas and continue to make important contributions to understanding and treating emotional and psychological problems.

REFERENCES

Ayllon, T. (1963). Intensive treatment of psychotic behavior by stimulus satiation and food reinforcement. *Behaviour Research and Therapy, 1,* 53–62.

Barlow, D. H., & Craske, M. G. (1989). *Mastery of your anxiety and panic.* Albany, NY: Center for Stress and Anxiety Disorders.

Beck, A. T. (1976). *Cognitive therapy and the emotional disorders.* New York: International Universities Press.

Beck, A. T. (1990). *Cognitive therapy of personality disorders.* New York: The Guilford Press.

Bellack, A. S., & Hersen, M. (Eds.). (1990). *Handbook of comparative treatments of adult disorders.* New York: Wiley.

Blanchard, E. B., & Andrasik, F. (1982). Psychological assessment and treatment of headache: Recent developments and emerging issues. *Journal of Consulting and Clinical Psychology, 50,* 859–879.

Brown, L., Gouvier, W., & Blanchard-Fields, F. (1990). Cognitive interventions across the life-span. In A. M. Horton Jr. (Ed.), *Neuropsychology across the life-span: Assessment and treatment* (pp. 133–153). New York: Springer Publishing Co.

Ellis, A. (1977). The basic clinical theory of rational-emotive therapy. In A. Ellis & R. Grieger (Eds.), *Handbook of rational-emotive therapy* (pp. 31–45). New York: Springer.

Goldfried, M. R., Decanteceo, E. T., & Weinberg, L. (1974). Systematic rational restructuring as a self-control technique. *Behavior Therapy, 5,* 247–254.

Heimberg, R. G., & Barlow, D. H. (1988). Psychosocial treatments for social phobia. *Psychosomatics, 29,* 27–37.

Incagnoli, T., & Newman, B. (1985). Cognitive and behavioral rehabilitation interventions. *Journal of Clinical Neuropsychology, 7,* 173–182.

Linehan, M. (1987). Dialectical behavior therapy for borderline personality disorder: Theory and method. *Bulletin of the Menninger Clinic, 51,* 261–276.

Marks, I. M. (1976). Current status of behavioral psychotherapy: Theory and practice. *American Journal of Psychiatry, 133,* 253–261.

Marlatt, G. (1978). Craving for alcohol, loss of control, and relapse: A cognitive-behavioral analysis. In P. E. Nathan, G. A. Marlatt, & T. Loberg (Eds.), *Alcoholism: New directions in behavioral research and treatment* (pp. 271–314). New York: Plenum Press.

Marlatt, G. (1987). Research and political realities: What the next twenty years hold for behaviorists in the alcohol field. *Advances in Behaviour Research and Therapy, 9,* 165–171.

Martin, P. R. (Ed.). (1991). *Handbook of behavior therapy and psychological science: An integrative approach.* New York: Pergamon Press.

Masters, W. H., & Johnson, V. E. (1970). *Human sexual inadequacy.* Boston: Little, Brown.

Meichenbaum, D. H. (1977). *Cognitive-behavior modification.* New York: Plenum Press.

Meichenbaum, D. H. (1985). *Stress-inoculation training.* New York: Pergamon Press.

Miller, W. R., & Munoz, R. F. (1976). *How to control your drinking.* Englewood Cliffs, NJ: Prentice-Hall.

Morrison, R. L., & Bellack, A. S. (1985). Social skills training. In A. S. Bellack (Ed.), *Schizophrenia: Treatment, management, and rehabilitation* (pp. 247–279). Orlando, FL: Grune & Stratton.

Nemeroff, C. J., & Karoly, P. (1991). Operant methods. In F. H. Kanfer & A. P. Goldstein (Eds.), *Helping people change: A textbook of methods* (pp. 122–160). New York: Pergamon Press.

Paul, G., & Lentz, R. (1977). *Psychosocial treatment of chronic mental patients: Milieu vs. social learning programs.* Cambridge, MA: Harvard University Press.

Wilkins, W. (1971). Desensitization: Social and cognitive factors underlying the effectiveness of Wolpe's procedure. *Psychological Bulletin, 76,* 310–317.

Wolpe, J. (1958). *Psychotherapy by reciprocal inhibition.* Stanford, CA: Stanford University Press.

Wolpe, J. (1989). The derailment of behavior therapy: A tale of conceptual misdirection. *Journal of Behavior Therapy & Experimental Psychiatry, 20,* 3–15.

Wolpe, J. (1990). *The practice of behavior therapy* (4th Ed.). New York: Pergamon Press.

26

Pharmacologic Interventions

Harold M. Erickson, Jr. and Donald W. Goodwin

A desire to take medicine is, perhaps, the great feature
which distinguishes man from other animals.
—Sir William Osler

Introduction

The dictionary defines a drug as a substance used in medicine to treat disease. This includes a very wide range of substances, including food and water. Milk is prescribed for heartburn, the amino acid tryptophan for insomnia and depression, and garlic for anxiety (garlic is a prescription drug in some countries). Other drugs come from plants (digitalis for heart disease) or have a mineral source (lithium for mania). Others are manmade in the laboratory, including all of the currently prescribed drugs for anxiety, depression, and psychosis.

The oldest drugs in medicine come from plants. They include products of fermentation (alcohol), marijuana from *Cannabis sativa*, cocaine from the cocoa leaf, and products of the poppy plant, such as opium, morphine, and heroin (heroin is a slightly modified form of morphine).

These drugs (with the exception of heroin) have been used by humans for as long as there is a historical record, not only medically but also "recreationally," a new word for fun.

All drugs are dangerous, depending on the amount. Dosage is all-important with every drug. Even strychnine is harmless if the amount is small; water is fatal if the amount is large.

Harold M. Erickson, Jr. and Donald W. Goodwin • Department of Psychiatry, University of Kansas Medical Center, Kansas City, Kansas 66160.

Advanced Abnormal Psychology, edited by Vincent B. Van Hasselt and Michel Hersen. Plenum Press, New York, 1994.

HAROLD M.
ERICKSON, JR.
and DONALD W.
GOODWIN

This chapter describes drugs used for psychosis (usually meaning delusions and hallucinations), depression, insomnia, anxiety, substance abuse, and disorders of memory. All require a prescription in the United States. Each category contains a number of drugs—twenty or more for depression alone. Examples of each class will be described. Commercial names will be used rather than chemical names because commercial names are often better known, even by physicians.

DRUGS FOR ANXIETY

Anxiety should be distinguished from *fear*. Fear signifies the presence of a *known* danger. The strength of fear is more or less proportionate to the degree of danger. In general, fear is a desirable emotion because it leads to useful action. *Anxiety* refers to an emotion that signifies the presence of a danger that cannot be identified, or, if identified, is not sufficiently threatening to justify the intensity of the emotion. Anxious people may *think* that they know what they are afraid of: the garden snake, the crowd in the theater, a rebuke from the boss. But, if they think about it, they realize that the anxiety is disproportionate to the threat. Thus, the real source of the distress is unknown, even if some things seem to bring it on more than others. Unlike fear, anxiety can be viewed as an undesirable emotion. It leads to nothing useful because the true source of the danger is unknown (Goodwin, 1985).

The drugs described in this section generally are for anxiety, as defined above; but they are sometimes given for fear, such as fear of surgery. The American Psychiatric Association (1987) lists a number of anxiety *disorders* (see Chapter 11). These include generalized anxiety disorder, panic disorder, phobic disorders, obsessive–compulsive disorder, and posttraumatic stress disorder.

Of these categories, *generalized anxiety disorder* has been least studied. It is characterized by so-called free-floating anxiety, the popular synonym for which is nervousness. Some people are more nervous than others, presumably because of a mix of genetic and acquired traits. Nowadays it is customary to distinguish "state" from "trait." State refers to a temporary episode of anxiety or depression; trait refers to emotional propensities dating back to childhood and perhaps largely influenced by heredity. Generalized anxiety disorder is often a "trait" disorder.

Panic disorder is a phenomenon in which individuals experience attacks of intense anxiety coupled with rapid heartbeat, trouble with breathing, dizziness, and increased activity by the sympathetic nervous system. The sympathetic nervous system—part of the autonomic nervous system—is generally not subject to volitional control and is activated by circumstances requiring the well-known "flee or fight" response to avoid harm. In anxiety disorders, the source of the harm is unknown or incorrectly identified.

Panic attacks often occur spontaneously and are not connected to any perceived danger. As the term implies, panic attacks are terrifying. People often think they are going to die. Episodes may occur frequently or infrequently.

One response to having a panic attack is to avoid situations where an attack might occur without warning and have frightening consequences, such as embarrassment in public. Some people who have panic attacks stay home to avoid being in places where a panic attack might occur. When panic attacks lead to avoidance of public places the condition is called *agoraphobia* (agora from the Greek for "mar-

and antipsychotic effects is highly desirable (e.g., when dealing with an acutely agitated individual).

Although there are approximately 20 antipsychotic drugs in use, there are no scientific data suggesting that one is more effective than another. However, a given patient may respond very well to one drug and not so well to others.

The phrase "chemical restraints" came into use during the 1960s and refers to the potent calming antiagitation/antiaggression effects of these drugs. In past decades they were used excessively to control behavior in psychiatrically disordered patients and mentally retarded persons. These drugs generally should not be used for behavioral control but must be appropriately prescribed for treatment of mental illness. On rare occasions, after discussing the risk–benefit considerations with a patient and his/her family, they are used in the lowest effective dose and in a time-limited manner.

Thorazine is an example of a low-potency phenothiazine. Prolixin is a high-potency phenothiazine. Haldol may be the most widely used high-potency non-phenothiazine drug, and Moban and Clozaril are examples of lower-potency drugs.

Clozaril is an interesting drug first developed about 30 years ago but set aside because it caused agranulocytosis (decreased white blood cell count). In recent years Clozaril has become recognized as effective in treating patients having schizophrenia who have not responded to other drugs. In addition to suppressing hallucinations and delusions, it may benefit so-called negative symptoms: apathy, ambivalence, social withdrawal (Andreasen et al., 1990). In 1990 Clozaril became available in the United States, to be prescribed only with a protocol designed to detect agranulocytosis early (Baldessarini & Frankenburg, 1991). One of the positive attributes of Clozaril is that it does not produce tardive dyskinesia, a serious late-onset side effect of other antipsychotics discussed later in this chapter.

Certain antipsychotic drugs are approved by the Food and Drug Administration for treating Tourette's disorder. This is characterized by tics involving larger muscles of the upper body and involuntary utterances, often profane in nature. Orap and Haldol are most commonly used.

The mechanisms by which antipsychotic drugs have their clinical effect are only partially understood. They block dopamine (an important neurotransmitter) receptors (Davis et al., 1991) thought to be involved in areas of the brain associated with expression of primitive emotions and drives.

Tardive dyskinesia is one of several serious side effects associated with these drugs. It is characterized by involuntary movements, most typically of the tongue and lips. Such oral/facial muscle activity is unattractive and can be so severe as to interfere with eating. It is more likely to occur in patients who have taken the drugs for many years but can develop in adolescents who have only been treated for several months. It may be irreversible. Patients having concomitant organic brain dysfunction seem to be more at risk. Tardive dyskinesia must be differentiated from other involuntary movements of the neck and/or facial muscles, which, although disconcerting and even frightening, can be quickly remedied with medication.

Neuroleptic (a synonym for antipsychotic drug) malignant syndrome is a life-threatening condition associated with fever, muscle rigidity, and dysfunction of the autonomic nervous system. It constitutes a medical emergency requiring immediate attention (Perlman, 1986).

Impaired liver function and cardiotoxic effects of antipsychotic drugs occur.

HAROLD M.
ERICKSON, JR.
and DONALD W.
GOODWIN

Some patients being treated with high potency drugs develop akathesia, which can best be described as an uncomfortable "inner restlessness." Like the involuntary movements of face and neck described above, it responds very well to anticholinergic agents such as Cogentin. These drugs occasionally produce dryness of the mouth and blurred vision, which usually clear spontaneously while the patient continues on medication.

One phenothiazine (Prolixin) and one nonphenothiazine (Haldol) are available in long-acting injectable form. This allows a patient to visit an outpatient setting once or twice a month for an injection of medication. Such an approach greatly increases the likelihood of maintaining the person outside the hospital. These injections are particularly advantageous for patients who habitually forget to take oral medication and/or who have suspicious thoughts about drugs. Some states provide for court-ordered outpatient treatment so that a patient can decrease the chances of being involuntarily hospitalized by coming to a psychiatrist's office or mental health clinic every 2 to 4 weeks for treatment.

Although it has been traditional to avoid polypharmacy (prescribing more than one drug simultaneously for the same condition), current practice allows for certain combinations of drugs. Patients with schizophrenia may experience symptom reduction when lithium is added to their regimen. Beta-blocking drugs can reduce tension. Tegretol may reduce a patient's tendency to become explosive, and antianxiety agents such as Ativan can ameliorate anxiety in psychotic patients.

Lithium's antimanic effects were discovered in 1950, but it was not approved by the Food and Drug Administration until 1970. The FDA's caution was in part due to illness and some deaths attributed to lithium chloride when it was used as a salt substitute during the war years of the 1940s. Lithium can be toxic to the kidneys and thyroid gland (Yassa et al., 1988).

Lithium is useful in preventing recurrence of mania and to some extent depression. Many patients on lithium report decreasing oscillations of mood so that after several months of treatment they are affectively stable. Although lithium has been the basic drug treatment for mania, it is not always effective. In some cases the addition of antiseizure drugs such as Tegretol and Depakote may improve the patient's condition (Small et al., 1991).

Care must be taken, especially with the low-potency drugs, to see that orthostatic hypotension (drop in blood pressure) does not occur. Elderly persons can sustain fractures from falls caused by light-headedness due to insufficient blood reaching the brain.

Some of the antipsychotic drugs have anticholinergic effects, which (especially in combination with other drugs) may produce a paradoxical anticholinergic psychosis. The problem is more likely to occur if certain antidepressant and/or anticholinergic drugs are used concommitantly. These psychoses can be dramatic with visual, auditory, and tactile hallucinations. Symptoms clear when the offending agents are withdrawn. A cholinergic drug such as Antilirium can be administered to determine if in fact the patient's symptoms are due to anticholinergic phenomena.

SUMMARY

Drugs have been used to treat disease for thousands of years. Over the centuries, knowledge slowly evolved about which plant, mineral, or synthetic substance was effective for a certain disease. Modern psychopharmacology has developed rapidly out of greater understanding of brain microstructure and neurochemistry. Current psychiatric drugs have been evaluated in systematically controlled double-blind studies. Although the results of any one study may be more or less positive, the average effectiveness rate of most drugs is about 70%. This chapter reviews drugs for anxiety, posttraumatic stress disorder, depression, insomnia, substance abuse, organic brain syndromes, and psychosis.

Many drugs have multiple effects on neurochemical systems, and often the psychiatrist's choice is based on the drug's side effect profile. Although several drugs in a category (e.g., antidepressants) may be about equal in efficacy, there are significant variations in individual responses to a particular drug.

Special care must be exercised in prescribing drugs for the elderly, as they tend to require lower doses and are more sensitive to side effects. There is increasing awareness of "drug–drug" problems that arise when these agents interact so as to produce adverse reactions. Millions of people suffer from psychiatric disorders. These drugs have a major effect on their quality of life.

REFERENCES

American Psychiatric Association (1987). *Diagnostic and statistical manual of mental disorders*, 3rd Edition, Revised. Washington, DC: Author.

Andreasen, N. C., Flaum, M., Swayze, II, V. W., Tyrrell, G., & Arndt, S. (1990). Positive and negative symptoms in schizophrenia. *Archives of General Psychiatry, 47*, 615–621.

Baldessarini, R. J., & Frankenburg, F. R. (1991). Review article, drug therapy: Clozapine—A novel antipsychotic agent. *New England Journal of Medicine, 324*, 746–754.

Davis, K. L., Kahn, R. S., Ko, G., & Davidson, M. (1991). Dopamine in schizophrenia: A review and reconceptualization. *American Journal of Psychiatry, 148*, 1474–1486.

Goodwin, D. W. (1985). *Anxiety.* New York: Oxford University Press.

Litten, R. Z., & Allen, J. P. (1991). Pharmacotherapies for alcoholism: Promising agents and clinical issues. *Alcoholism: Clinical and Experimental Research, 15*, 620–633.

Lydiard, R. B., & Ballenger, J. C. (1987). Antidepressants in panic disorder and agoraphobia. *Journal of Affective Disorders, 13*, 153–168.

Medical Letter on Drugs and Therapeutics. (1986). Buspirone: A non-benzodiazepine for anxiety, *28*, 117–118.

Perlman, C. A. (1986). Neuroleptic malignant syndrome: A review of the literature. *Journal of Clinical Psychopharmacology, 6*, 257–273.

Pigott, T. A., Pato, M. T., Bernstein, S. E., Grover, G. N., Hill, J. L., Tolliver, T. J., & Murphy, D. L. (1990). Controlled comparisons of and fluoxetine in the treatment of obsessive–compulsive disorder. Behavioral and biological results. *Archives of General Psychiatry, 47*, 926–932.

Pohl, R., Balon, R., & Yeragani, V. (1988). Autoinduction of hypertensive reactions by tranylcypromine? *Journal of Psychopharmacology, 8*, 225–226.

Quitkin, F. M., McGrath, P. J., Stewart, J. W., Harrison, W., Tricano, E., Wager, S. G, Ocepek-Welikson, K., Nunes, E., Rabkin, J. G., & Klein, D. F. (1990). Atypical depression, panic attacks, and response to Imipramine and Phenelzine. *Archives of General Psychiatry, 47*, 935–941.

Small, J. G., Klapper, M. H., Milstein, V., Kellams, J. J., Miller, M. J., Marhenke, J. D., & Small, I. F. (1991). Carbamazepine compared with lithium in the treatment of mania. *Archives of General Psychiatry, 48*, 915–921.

Yassa, R., Saunders, A., Nastase, C., & Camille, Y. (1988). Lithium-induced thyroid disorders: A prevalence study. *Journal of Clinical Psychiatry, 49*, 14–15.

About the Editors

VINCENT B. VAN HASSELT, Ph.D., is Professor of Psychology and Director of the Interpersonal Violence Program at the Center for Psychological Studies, Nova University, Fort Lauderdale, Florida. Over the past several years, he has conducted programs of clinical research directed toward a wide range of severely disturbed clinical disorders. Some of those include visually impaired and multiply disabled (deaf-blind, blind-mentally retarded) children and youth, dually diagnosed substance-abusing adolescents, and perpetrators and victims of spouse and child maltreatment. He has published numerous journal articles, book chapters, and books on behavioral assessment and intervention with these populations, and is coeditor of *Journal of Family Violence, Journal of Developmental and Physical Disabilities*, and *Journal of Child and Adolescent Substance Abuse*, Dr. Van Hasselt is the recipient of grants from the National Institute of Mental Health, the National Institute on Handicapped Research, the March of Dimes Birth Defects Foundation, the Buhl Foundation, and the Pittsburgh Foundation.

MICHEL HERSEN, Ph.D., is Professor of Psychology and Director of the Nova Community Clinic for Older Adults at the Center for Psychological Studies, Nova University, Fort Lauderdale, Florida. Past President of the Association for Advancement of Behavior Therapy and Diplomate, American Board of Medical Psychotherapists, he is the author and coauthor of numerous papers, book chapters, and books. His current research involves the behavioral assessment and treatment of high-risk populations. Dr. Hersen is coeditor of several journals, including *Behavior Modification, Clinical Psychology Review, Journal of Family Violence, Journal of Developmental and Physical Disabilities*, and *Journal of Anxiety Disorders*, and has been the recipient of federal grants from the National Institute of Mental Health, the U.S. Department of Education, and the National Institute on Disabilities and Rehabilitation Research.

Author Index

Subject Index